Goodheart's Photoguide to Common Skin Disorders

Diagnosis and Management

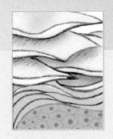

THIRD EDITION

Goodheart's Photoguide to Common Skin Disorders

Diagnosis and Management

Herbert P. Goodheart, M.D.
Assistant Clinical Professor
Department of Dermatology
Mount Sinai School of Medicine
New York, New York

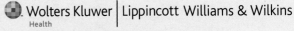
Wolters Kluwer | Lippincott Williams & Wilkins
Health
Philadelphia · Baltimore · New York · London
Buenos Aires · Hong Kong · Sydney · Tokyo

Acquisitions Editor: Sonya Seigafuse
Managing Editor: Kerry Barrett
Developmental Editor: Martha Cushman
Production Editor: Bridgett Dougherty
Senior Manufacturing Manager: Benjamin Rivera
Design Coordinator: Risa Chow
Compositor: Aptara®

© 2009 by LIPPINCOTT WILLIAMS & WILKINS
530 Walnut Street
Philadelphia, PA 19106 USA
LWW.com

Printed in China

Library of Congress Cataloging-in-Publication Data

Goodheart, Herbert P.
    Goodheart's photoguide to common skin disorders : diagnosis and management / Herbert P. Goodheart. — 3rd ed.
        p. ; cm.
    Includes index.
    ISBN-13: 978-0-7817-7143-6
    ISBN-10: 0-7817-7143-9
    1. Skin—Diseases—Handbooks, manuals, etc. 2.
Skin—Diseases—Atlases. I. Title. II. Title: Photoguide to common skin disorders.
    [DNLM: 1. Skin Diseases—diagnosis—Atlases. 2. Skin Diseases—therapy—Atlases. WR 17 G652g 2008]
    RL74.G66 2008
    616.50022'2—dc22

                                                                2008024074

Care has been taken to confirm the accuracy of the information presented and to describe generally accepted practices. However, the authors, editor, and publisher are not responsible for errors or omissions or for any consequences from application of the information in this book and make no warranty, expressed or implied, with respect to the currency, completeness, or accuracy of the contents of the publication. Application of this information in a particular situation remains the professional responsibility of the practitioner.

The authors, editor, and publisher have exerted every effort to ensure that drug selection and dosage set forth in this text are in accordance with current recommendations and practice at the time of publication. However, in view of ongoing research, changes in government regulations, and the constant flow of information relating to drug therapy and drug reactions, the reader is urged to check the package insert for each drug for any change in indications and dosage and for added warnings and precautions. This is particularly important when the recommended agent is a new or infrequently employed drug.

Some drugs and medical devices presented in this publication have Food and Drug Administration (FDA) clearance for limited use in restricted research settings. It is the responsibility of the health care provider to ascertain the FDA status of each drug or device planned for use in their clinical practice.

10 9 8 7 6 5 4 3 2 1

To my family, who have provided immense support and encouragement throughout.

What the mind
does not know,
the eyes cannot see.
ANCIENT PROVERB

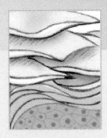

Contents

PART TWO

PART THREE

PART FOUR

The following patient handouts can be found online, on the solution Web site

Acne
Acne: How to Apply Duac Gel, BenzaClin Gel, and Benzamycin Gel
Acne: How to Apply Topical Retinoids
Alopecia Areata
Athlete's Foot (Tinea Pedis)
Atopic Dermatitis
Atypical Nevus (Mole)
Basal Cell Carcinoma
Burow's Solution
Contact Dermatitis
Dry Skin (Xerosis)
Fungal Nails (Onychomycosis)
Genital Warts
Granuloma Annulare
Hair Loss (Androgenic Alopecia)
Hand Eczema
Head Lice
Herpes Simplex
Herpes Zoster (Shingles)
Hives (Urticaria)
Keratosis Pilaris (Rough Bumpy Skin)
Lichen Planus
Lyme Disease

Lyme Disease: Prevention
Malignant Melanoma
Melasma
Molluscum Contagiosum
Pityriasis Rosea
Poison Ivy and Poison Oak (Rhus Dermatitis)
Pseudofolliculitis Barbae (Razor Bumps)
Psoriasis
Rosacea
Scabies
Scalp Psoriasis: Scale Removal
Seborrheic Dermatitis of the Face
Seborrheic Dermatitis of the Scalp and Dandruff
Short-Term Cortisone Therapy
Soak and Smear Instruction Sheet
Solar Keratosis (Actinic Keratosis)
Squamous Cell Carcinoma
Sun Protection Advice
Tinea Capitis
Tinea Cruris (Jock Itch)
Tinea Versicolor
Vitiligo
Warts

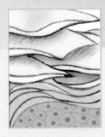

Contributors

Mary Ruth Buchness, M.D.
Associate Professor of Medicine
New York Medical College
Valhalla, New York
Attending Physician
Department of Medicine
St. Vincent's Catholic Medical Center
New York, New York

Herbert P. Goodheart, M.D.
Assistant Clinical Professor
Department of Dermatology
Mount Sinai School of Medicine
New York, New York

Peter G. Burk, M.D.
Clinical Associate Professor of Medicine (Dermatology)
Albert Einstein College of Medicine
Attending Physician
Dermatology Service
Montefiore Medical Center
Bronx, New York

Kenneth Howe, M.D.
Assistant Clinical Professor
Department of Dermatology
Beth Israel Medical Center
New York, New York

Hendrik Uyttendaele, M.D.
Instructor in Clinical Dermatology
Department of Dermatology
Columbia Presbyterian Medical Center
Assistant Attending Physician
New York Presbyterian Hospital
New York, New York

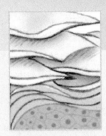

Foreword

As a second-year medical student, I recall studying cardiology one evening when my brother Andrew asked me to look at a rash that developed on his trunk. I did not have a clue as to how to make *any* dermatologic diagnosis. So, after Andrew accused my father of wasting tuition money on my evidently inadequate education, I thought it proper to register for a dermatology elective in my fourth year. I reasoned that, regardless of whatever field I would ultimately choose, I would inevitably be confronted with some cutaneous dilemmas. It was with tremendous fortune that I subsequently trained at the Albert Einstein College of Medicine in the Bronx, New York, under the tutelage of Michael Fisher, M.D., the former head of the illustrious division of dermatology. It was during my training that I befriended the attending physician, Dr. Herb Goodheart. Herb always provided special insights, wisdom, and compassion in the evaluation of even the most rudimentary dermatologic disorders. He is a stellar teacher and dermatologist, who has compiled his years of perspicacity into this guide to dermatology.

As we begin the twenty-first century, the landscape of American medicine and dermatology is changing at an accelerating pace. Even though we can now comprehend many skin disorders at a molecular level and have advanced our therapeutic realm to include laser technology and immunobiology, the cornerstone of all dermatologic endeavors will always be careful clinical observation. As venues of practice shift toward a greater proportion of primary dermatologic care being delivered by nondermatologists, resources for these providers must be accessible, comprehensible, and practical. Dr. Goodheart's guide to dermatology is divided into common disorders, the interrelationship between the skin and systemic diseases, basic and advanced dermatologic procedures, and a very useful appendix that provides patient handout material in both English and Spanish. Importantly, it combines features of an atlas with Herb's pithy perspectives, as though he is standing over your shoulder in the dermatology clinic. Those who use this guide will come to appreciate many of the finer points and opinions that Dr. Goodheart provides and even more so when becoming more facile with the discipline. Use this guide as a primer, an atlas, a consultant, and as a supplement to more in-depth dermatology texts and medical literature. Your dermatologic knowledge base will flourish, your appreciation of the field will blossom, and most importantly, your patients will benefit from your expertise.

Warren R. Heymann, M.D.
Head, Division of Dermatology
UMDNJ—Robert Wood Johnson School of Medicine at Camden
Newark, New Jersey

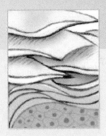

Preface to the Second Edition

In dermatology, the naked eye is our primary tool, and because virtually every skin disorder is visible, the photographic image is an essential teaching aid.

Despite the commonplace occurrence of skin disorders, making a correct dermatologic diagnosis is a customary stumbling block for many health care professionals. It is rather unusual to find a nondermatologist who is comfortable diagnosing or managing most skin problems; in fact, many admit to using the therapeutic approach of "trial and error." Medical schools simply do not emphasize the teaching of dermatology. Skin diseases are generally considered less life threatening and are a lower priority than most of the conditions seen in teaching hospitals. Frequently, this can result in mistreatment, a delay in appropriate treatment, or a referral to a dermatologist.

This book is intended to be an accessible reference for nondermatologists such as family physicians, physician assistants, nurse practitioners, and medical students, who are often on the frontline in treating skin problems. Its focus has been limited intentionally to the diagnosis and management of the most common skin problems encountered in an outpatient setting. Wherever possible, "look-alike" photos are juxtaposed with photos of primary dermatoses to help the reader make the differential diagnosis.

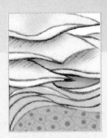

Preface to the Third Edition

Many changes have occurred in the 10 years since the first edition, *A Photoguide of Common Skin Disorders,* was published. This third edition has been expanded and extensively rewritten to reflect these changes. The treatment sections have been updated and offer more therapeutic options that also will serve as a resource for those in dermatology residency training. The photographs, which are fundamental to this text, have been enlarged to achieve greater clarity and detail.

New to this edition is an online Solution site that allows the reader to access the entire contents of the book plus additional material such as patient handouts in English and Spanish. The handouts can be downloaded as PDF files and given to patients to read. They also can serve as an ongoing source of information for health care providers who use this book. Also included online is an image bank that allows the user to download and save the images found on the site as .pdf or .jpg files for teaching and lecturing purposes. International readers should benefit from Appendix A, where Canada and India now appear on the list, allowing the reader to recognize dermatologic agents that often have different brand names in their respective countries.

The addition of Chapter 27, "Special Considerations in the Skin of Pediatric and Elderly Patients," covers many disorders that are not discussed in the preceding chapters. The thumbnail images that appear in this chapter can be viewed in a larger size online.

It is hoped that these changes will make this edition even more useful to those responsible for diagnosing and managing the common problems that account for the vast majority of dermatologic complaints.

Herbert P. Goodheart, M.D.

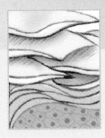

Acknowledgments

I owe a great deal of gratitude to many for making the writing of this third edition a truly satisfying and enjoyable experience. I am immensely pleased with the superb job that my publisher, Lippincott Williams & Wilkins, has done in producing this edition. Beginning with Sonya Seigafuse, who had the foresight and determination to take on the project, I am deeply indebted. Sonya was the catalyst for this book. Martha Cushman, my editor par excellence, practically worked side by side with me in pulling the project together; my heartfelt appreciation goes to her. She has been a terrific partner. Another key player was Kerry Barrett, whose attention to detail and availability to answer a multitude of questions brought this complicated project to completion. Special credit also goes to Brett MacNaughton, who kept track of the illustrations and the multitude of disconnected digital and 35-mm images, and to Risa Clow, whose creative layout and design suggestions always respected the content of the material.

Muchas gracias to Rebeca Barroso, who supplied the Spanish translations of the patient handouts. Many helped with the foreign brand names of drugs, including Danille Luquin (French), Hans J. Kammler (French and German), and Terry Marshall (British)—merci, danke, and thanks. My appreciation also goes to Ashit Mahar and Ben Barankin, who added India and Canada, respectively, to the list of brand names of drugs. Thanks go to Joe Eastern, M.D., my colleague, whose critical judgment and comments concerning the accuracy of the material have been invaluable. I also wish to thank Ross Levy, M.D., my friend, whose advice about wound healing has been a great addition; his hands and surgical skills are featured more than once in this book.

I also would like to express thanks to the people at Aptara, particularly Stephanie Lentz, who helped me finalize the manuscript and whose patience and enthusiasm saved me from many errors. My gratitude also goes to Jenny Ceccotti, General Manager of Aptara, Tom Chronister, who made sure the images were as clear as possible, and Max Leckrone, who assisted with the final editing.

Thanks go to my colleagues at Derm-Chat/Derm-Rx, who kept me up to date on the latest diagnostic and therapeutic issues in dermatology: Art Huntley at UC Davis, who founded and maintains this valuable online resource, as well as "heavy posters" Joe Eastern, Orin Goldblum, Diane Thaler, Ashit Mahwar, Otto Bastos, Bob Rudolph, Sahar Ghannam, Larry Finkel, Bill Danby, Sate Hamza, Noah Scheinfeld, Steve Feldman, Bernie Recht, Barry Ginsberg, Bill Smith, Pierre Jaffe, Omid Zargari, Becky Bushong, Ed Zabawski, Jerry Litt, Skee Smith, Jo Bohanon-Grant, Ben Treen, Norman Winkler, Chuck Fishman, Susan Bushelman, Robin Berger, Maida Burrow, Stu Kittay, Diane Davidson, Chuck Miller, Norm Guzick, Joel Schlessinger, Jane Chew, Mauricio Goihman, Pat Condry, Kevin Smith, Steve Stone, Gail Drayton, Steve Emmet, Linda Spencer, and many others who are too numerous to mention, who have been my "online classmates."

Illustrated Glossary of Basic Skin Lesions

Topical Therapy

LESIONS

Primary Lesions

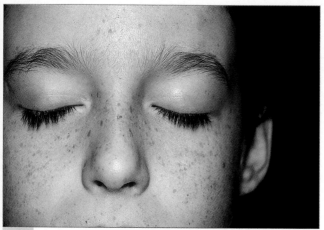

Macule. Freckles (ephelides).

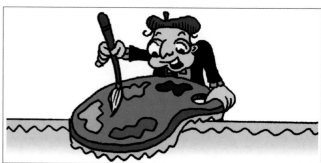

Macules are small, flat, nonpalpable changes in skin color (you cannot feel macules and, if you close your eyes, they "disappear"). They occur in various shapes and sizes.
Examples include tattoos, flat nevi, postinflammatory hyper-pigmentation, postinflammatory hypopigmentation, erythema, purpura, and freckles.

Patches are large macules.

Examples include melasma and vitiligo. There is some confusion regarding patches; some dermatologists refer to a patch as a large macule, whereas others refer to patches as macules with overlying fine scale (e.g., the scaly patches seen in pityriasis rosea and tinea versicolor).

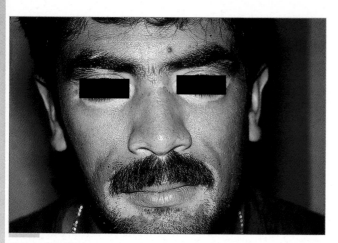

Patch. Vitiligo.

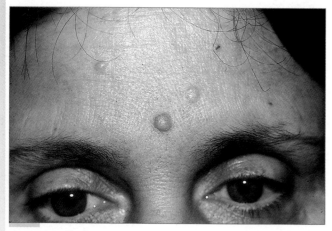

Papule. Multiple nevi

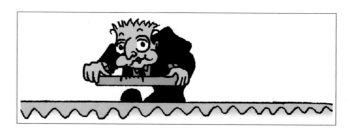

Papules are small, solid lesions that are generally 1 cm or less in diameter.
Examples include, molluscum contagiosum, warts, and palpable nevi (moles).

Note: "Maculopapule" *is a contradiction in terms, and the use of this term should be abandoned (an eruption may be described as being* macular *and* papular, *rather than "maculopapular").*

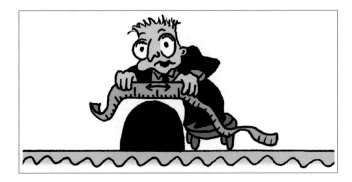

Nodules are firm, solid palpable lesions that are generally 1 cm or more in diameter. They may be seen as elevated lesions or can be palpated without any elevation of the skin.
Examples include erythema nodosum, lipoma, rheumatoid nodules, basal cell carcinoma, and keloid.

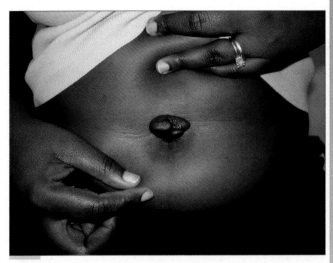

Nodule. Keloid

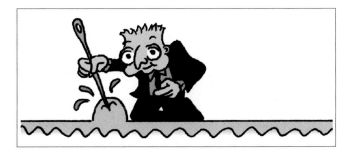

Vesicles (small blisters) are clear, fluid-filled lesions generally 1 cm or less in diameter.
Examples include herpes simplex, acute vesicular tinea pedis, and early chickenpox.

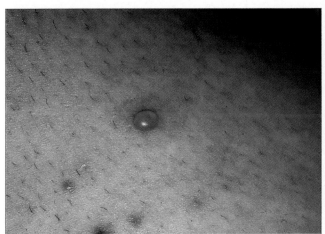

Vesicle. Chickenpox.

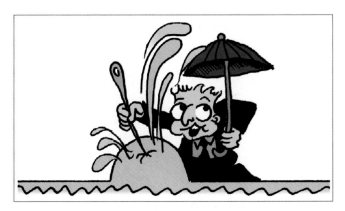

Bullae (large blisters) are clear, fluid-filled lesions generally 1 cm or more in diameter.
Examples include second-degree burns, herpes zoster, and insect bite reactions.

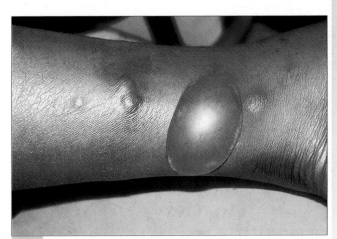

Bulla. Bullous insect bite reaction.

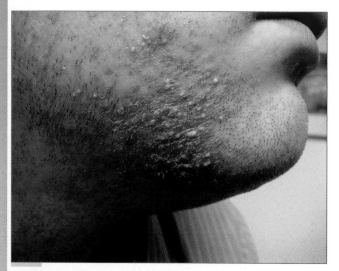

Pustule. Folliculitis barbae.

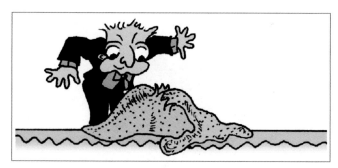

Pustules are superficial lesions that contain purulent, cloudy material.
Examples include evolving chickenpox, folliculitis, and pustular acne.

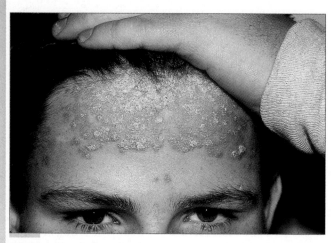

Plaque. Psoriasis vulgaris.

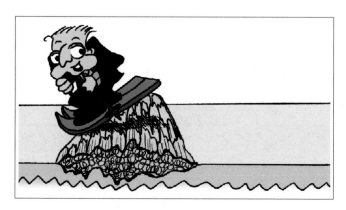

Plaques are solid, elevated, or depressed (*atrophic*) flat-topped, plateaulike lesions that cover a fairly large area; they may arise from papules that coalesce or arise de novo.
Examples include chronic eczematous dermatitis and psoriasis.

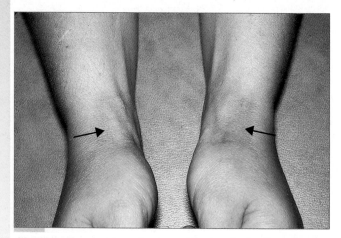

Atrophic plaque. Atrophy caused by intralesional cortisone injections.

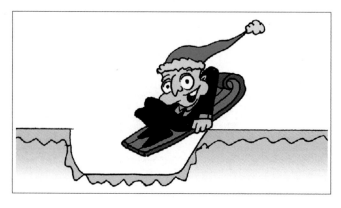

Atrophic plaques *include discoid lupus erythematosus, morphea (localized scleroderma), and steroid atrophy.*

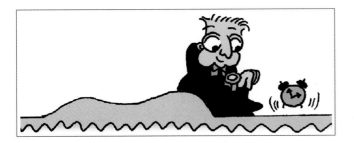

Wheals are raised flesh-colored or erythematous papules or plaques that are transient lesions. They generally last less than 24 hours, during which time they may change shape and size. *Examples include urticaria (hives) and angioedema.*

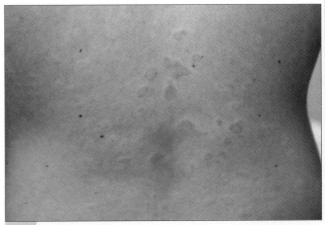

Wheal. Urticaria.

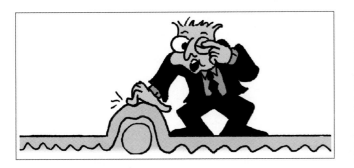

Cysts are walled-off lesions containing fluid or semisolid material. (They feel like an eyeball when you palpate them.) *Examples include pilar and epidermoid cysts.*

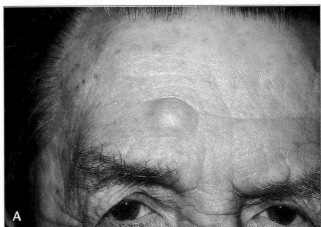

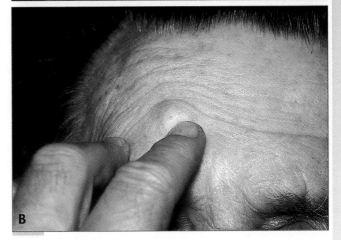

Cyst. Epidermoid cyst.

Secondary (Modified) Lesions

Secondary lesions are those primary lesions that have evolved naturally or have been manipulated by the patient.

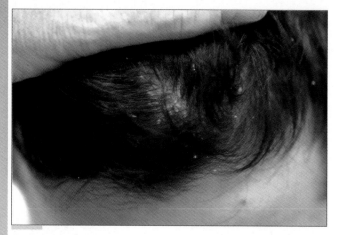

Scale. Dandruff.

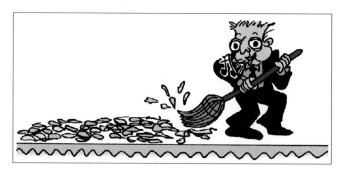

Scales (desquamation) comprise the outer layer of epidermis. The outer epidermis normally desquamates or sheds imperceptibly on a daily basis. In many dermatologic conditions, when this shedding becomes visible, it is abnormal and is called "desquamation" or "scale."
Common examples of conditions that produce scale are psoriasis, ichthyosis, and dandruff.

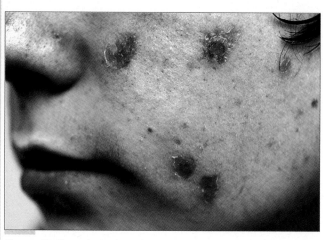

Crust. Bullous impetigo.

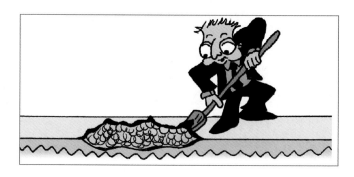

Crusts (scabs) are formed from blood, serum, or other dried exudate. "Honey-colored crusts" (*impetiginization*) are often a sign of superficial bacterial infection.
Examples include excoriated or infected insect bites and evolving bullous lesions of impetigo.

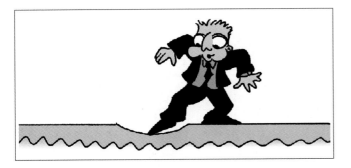

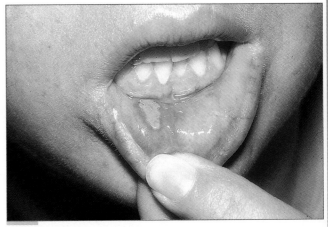

Erosions are shallow losses of tissue involving only the epidermis ("topsoil"). They often result from blisters and pustules and usually heal without scarring.
Examples include the secondary lesions of herpes simplex, herpes zoster, and lesions of aphthous stomatitis.

Erosion. Aphthous stomatitis ("canker sore").

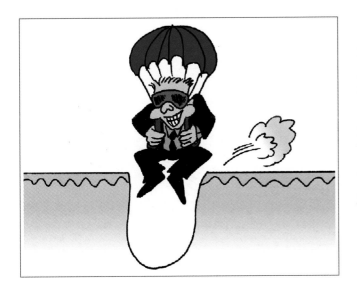

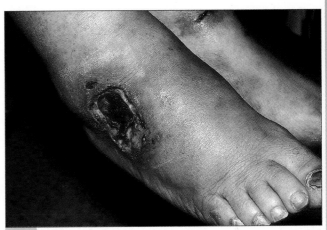

Ulcer. Vasculitis.

Ulcers are defects deeper than erosions. Ulcers involve the dermis or deeper layers and usually heal with scarring.
Examples include pyoderma gangrenosum, venous stasis ulcers, and vasculitis.

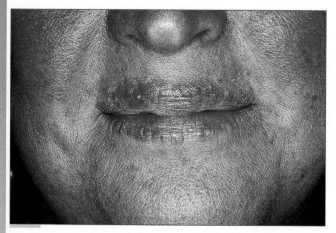

Fissure. Atopic dermatitis of lips (atopic cheilitis).

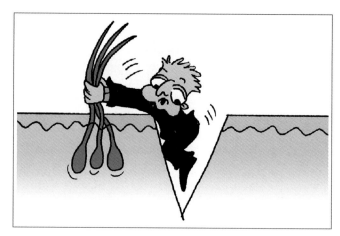

Fissures are linear ulcers or cracks in the skin. They are often painful.
Examples of conditions in which they may be seen include eczematous dermatitis of the fingers, angular stomatitis (perlèche), and eczema of the lips.

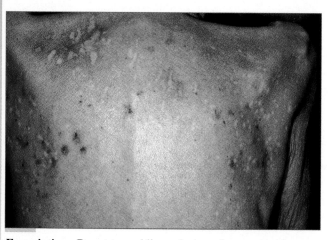

Excoriation. Punctate and linear lesions from scratching.

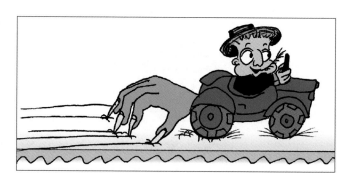

Excoriations are linear or punctate erosions or excavations induced by scratching, picking, or digging.
Examples include insect bites, cat scratches, and self-induced lesions.

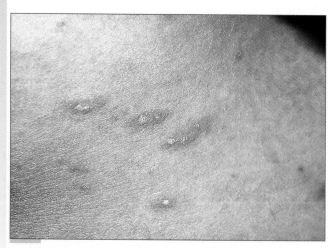

Papulosquamous reaction pattern. Pityriasis rosea.

REACTION PATTERNS, SHAPES, AND CONFIGURATIONS

Diseased skin has a limited number of clinical manifestations. Many skin disorders tend to occur in characteristic shapes, distributions, arrangements, and reaction patterns that often serve as diagnostic clues.

Reaction Patterns

The convention of describing skin disorders in terms of certain reaction patterns is often inexact, and there is a great deal of overlap. However, using these patterns to describe individual skin lesions or eruptions often helps greatly in formulating a differential diagnosis.

Papulosquamous reaction patterns refer to eruptions in which the primary lesions consist of macules, papules, or plaques with scale. Thus, a papulosquamous reaction pattern suggests a diagnosis from a list that includes the following differential diagnoses: psoriasis, tinea corporis, tinea versicolor, lichen planus, parapsoriasis, mycosis fungoides, and pityriasis rosea.

Eczematous reaction patterns are a little more difficult than papulosquamous patterns to describe (see Chapter 2, "Eczema"), because they may have various presentations and, at times, may be impossible to distinguish from papulosquamous patterns.

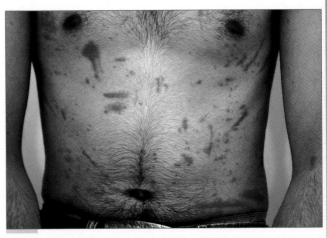

Acute eczematous reaction pattern. Poison ivy.

- **Acute and subacute eczema.** Examples include erythematous "juicy" papules or plaques and/or weeping vesicobullous lesions. A classic example is an acute contact dermatitis such as poison ivy.

- **Chronic eczema.** The hallmark lesion of chronic eczematous dermatitis caused by repeated scratching is known as lichenification, a plaque with an exaggeration of the normal skin markings that looks like the bark of a tree. Typical examples include the lesions seen in long-standing atopic dermatitis and lichen simplex chronicus.

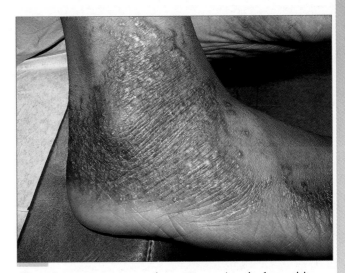

Chronic eczematous reaction pattern. Atopic dermatitis with lichenification.

Vesicobullous reaction patterns consist of fluid-filled blisters. *Examples include second-degree burns, herpes simplex, and herpes zoster infections.*

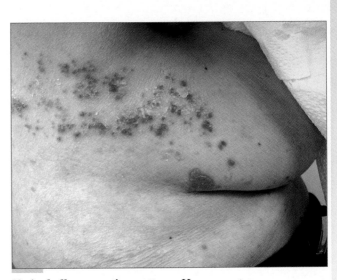

Vesicobullous reaction pattern. Herpes zoster.

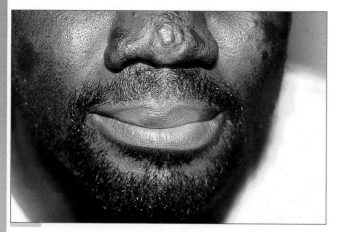

Dermal reaction pattern. Cutaneous sarcoidosis.

Dermal reaction patterns are lesions or eruptions that are confined to the dermis.
Examples include granuloma annulare and cutaneous sarcoidosis.

Subcutaneous reaction patterns are characterized by lesions or eruptions that are confined to the cutis (subcutaneous tissue).
Examples include erythema nodosum and lipomas.

Vascular reaction patterns refer to erythema or edema resulting from changes in the vasculature, such as vasodilatation and vasculitis.
Examples include first-degree burns, viral exanthem, urticaria, erythema multiforme, vasculitis, and drug rashes.

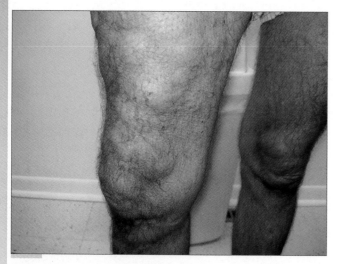

Subcutaneous reaction pattern. Multiple lipomas.

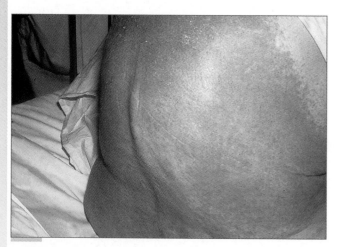

Vascular reaction pattern. Drug rash.

Shape of Lesions

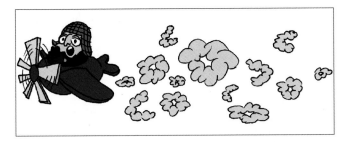

Annular and **arciform** are terms used to describe lesions that are ring-shaped or semiannular.
Examples include urticaria, granuloma annulare, and tinea corporis (ringworm).

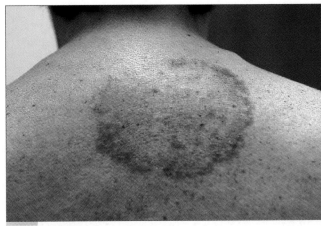

Annular lesion. Tinea corporis.

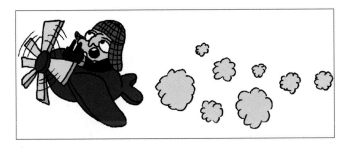

Nummular is a term that describes coin-shaped lesions.
Examples include lesions seen in discoid lupus erythematosus, psoriasis, and nummular eczema.

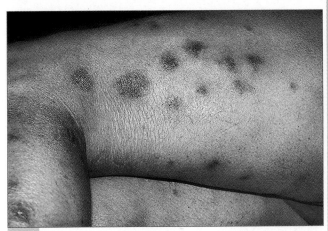

Nummular lesions. Coin-shaped lesions of nummular eczema.

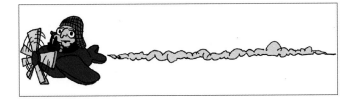

Linear lesions may result from exogenous agents, excoriations, and congenital growths.
Examples include lesions of poison ivy and dermatographism.

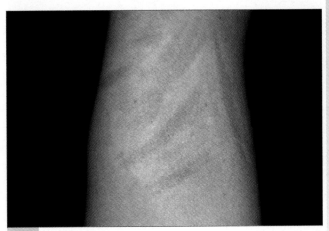

Linear lesion. Dermatographism.

Configuration of Lesions

The arrangement (configuration) of lesions is the interrelationship of multiple lesions.

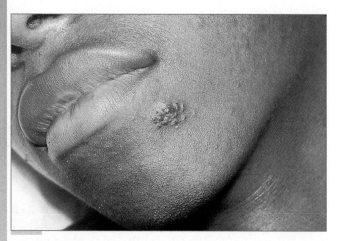

Grouped lesions. Herpes simplex. Grouped vesicles.

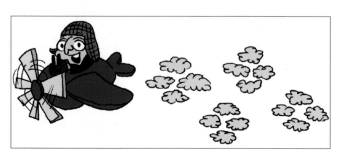

Grouped lesions are noted in herpetiform and zosteriform vesicles or bullae.
Examples are seen in insect bite reactions, herpes zoster, and herpes simplex.

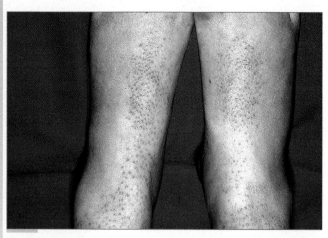

Follicular lesions. Follicular eczema. Note the gridlike pattern of tiny papules.

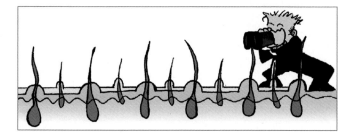

Follicular arrangement of lesions involves hair follicles. Lesions are often papular or pustular, at times with a visible central emerging hair. Lesions are spaced at fairly equal distances in a gridlike pattern.
Examples are seen in keratosis pilaris and folliculitis.

OVERVIEW

Topical therapy, the mainstay in the treatment of many dermatologic conditions, has traditionally been the bailiwick of dermatologists. Thus, it is no surprise that an understanding of the appropriate use and abuse of these agents has been either neglected or misunderstood by other health care professionals. The following is an attempt to provide a practical overview of topical therapy. The primary focus is on the use of topical steroids; other topical agents such as antibiotics and antifungals will be discussed in other sections of the book. (Topical antibiotics used for acne are listed in Chapter 1. Topical antibiotics for other cutaneous infections such as impetigo are described in Chapter 5.)

GENERAL PRINCIPLES

BASICS

- Topical therapy is generally safer than systemic therapy.
- Creams are generally more popular with patients than ointments because they are less greasy and messy; however, they are usually less potent and more drying.
- In addition to their enhanced potency, ointments are more moisturizing than creams, gels, and foams.
- Gels and foams are greaseless; they spread more easily and are very practical for acne and for application to hairy areas of the body. They also dry on contact, leaving a thin, invisible film.
- Solutions tend to be drying but cover large areas more easily than other preparations.
- Lotions are moisturizing to some extent; however, those that contain propylene glycol may have drying effects. They are also easy to apply and can be used on any skin type.
- Although foams may be somewhat drying, they are easy to spread, particularly on hairy areas such as the scalp as well as on the chests and backs of hirsute males. However, foams are expensive. Emollient (nonalcohol-based) foams have recently become available.
- Patients' choice should be taken into account because compliance is often related to patients' personal preference for a vehicle.
- The amount of a topical preparation applied does not affect its penetration or potency. The thicker the application, the greater the wastage—only the thin layer that is in intimate contact with the skin is absorbed; the remainder is rubbed off. More is not always better!
- Once- or twice-daily applications are usually sufficient for most preparations (sunscreens and some moisturizers are generally applied more frequently).

Vehicles

- The active drug is combined with a vehicle, or base. The vehicles vary in their ability to "deliver" to the target site in the skin.
- The rate of penetration and of absorption of a topical preparation into the skin depends on how occlusive its vehicle is (discussion to follow) and on how readily the vehicle releases the active chemical.
- The vehicle should be cosmetically acceptable and nonsensitizing.

Wet Dressings

- There is some validity to the old adage: "If it's dry, wet it; if it's wet, dry it."
- Wet dressings help dry wounds, and they aid in the débridement of wounds by removing debris (e.g., serum, crusts). They also have a nonspecific antifungal and antibacterial effect, especially when chemicals such as aluminum sulfate, silver nitrate, acetic acid (vinegar is dilute acetic acid), and potassium permanganate are added.
  - For example, the application of **Burow's solution** (aluminum sulfate and calcium acetate) helps dry out lesions that are weeping and oozing (e.g., poison ivy, tinea pedis, herpes simplex, herpes zoster) or impetiginized (e.g., impetigo, infected stasis ulcers). It is available without a prescription.
  - However, white vinegar in water, or even, plain unsterilized tap water may serve as less expensive, readily available—although probably less effective—alternatives, if Burow's solution cannot be obtained.

 SEE PATIENT HANDOUT, "Burow's Solution" ON THE SOLUTION SITE

TOPICAL STEROIDS

See TABLES I.1 and I.2

MECHANISM OF ACTION

Topical steroids have two basic mechanisms of action: anti-inflammatory and antimitotic.

- Anti-inflammatory properties are of particular importance when they are used to treat eczematous and other primarily inflammatory conditions.
- Antimitotic properties of topical steroids help to reduce the buildup of scale, as in the treatment of psoriasis, a condition that is both inflammatory and hyperproliferative (rapid cell division).

GENERAL CONSIDERATIONS

- Topical steroids are used to treat most inflammatory dermatoses. They are the cornerstone of therapy in dermatology, and, when used properly, they are quite safe.
- The unwanted effects of topical steroids are directly related to their potencies.
- When possible, the lowest-potency steroid should be used for the shortest possible time. Conversely, one should avoid

using a preparation that is not potent enough to treat a particular condition.

- For severe dermatoses, a very potent steroid may be used to initiate therapy, and a less potent preparation may be used afterward for maintenance ("downward titration").
- **Occlusion,** which involves placing medications under occlusive dressings produces increased hydration of the stratum corneum. Hydration increases penetration, which, in turn, increases efficacy and potency.
- **Tachyphylaxis** (tolerance) occurs when the medication loses its efficacy with continued use. It is most often seen in the treatment of psoriasis and other chronic conditions when very strong topical steroids are used continuously for prolonged periods.
- To help minimize tachyphylaxis, a high-potency preparation is applied until a dermatosis clears ("strong, but not long"), and a lower-potency topical steroid is prescribed for intermittent flares should they occur.

Potencies

- Fluorinated topical steroids are generally more potent than other topical steroids. For example, triamcinolone acetonide, which contains a fluoride ion, is 100 times more potent than nonfluorinated hydrocortisone.
- When treating children and elderly patients, clinicians should take extra measures to avoid the use of potent fluorinated compounds, when possible.
- Even without an added fluoride ion, certain molecular structural changes can increase potency in corticosteroids. For example, hydrocortisone valerate, which contains no fluoride ion, is almost as potent as triamcinolone acetonide.
- Only nonfluorinated, mild topical steroids should be applied to the face and, ideally, only for short periods of time, to avoid atrophy and steroid-induced rosacea. (However, this rule can be broken. For example, for the treatment of severe acute contact dermatitis of the face, a superpotent topical steroid used briefly may be preferable to a mild, ineffective topical steroid or a systemic steroid.)
- Thin eyelid skin requires the least potent preparations for the shortest periods of time. The intertriginous (skin touching skin) areas similarly respond to lower potencies because the apposition of skin surfaces acts like an occlusive dressing. The axillae and inguinal creases are particularly prone to higher absorption and resultant steroid atrophy (see FIG I.3).
- Every potency class has a generic preparation that is generally more economical than the trade-name preparation; however, there is some concern about the bioequivalence between trade and generic formulations.

Delivery (Percutaneous Penetration)

Topical steroids and other topical preparations are ineffective unless they are absorbed into the skin. Percutaneous penetration varies among individual patients, and it can be manipulated by hydrating the skin, occlusive dressings, changing the drug, the vehicle, the length of exposure, or the anatomic surface area to which the drug is applied. It also depends on

whether the skin is inflamed and therefore less of a barrier to penetration (e.g., eczematous skin).

- The barrier to cutaneous penetration resides in the stratum corneum. The thicker the stratum corneum—as on the palms, soles, elbows, and knees—the more difficult it is for the topical agent to penetrate the skin. The ability to penetrate varies by anatomic site as follows:

Mucous membranes ➤ Scrotum ➤ Eyelids ➤ Face ➤ Torso ➤ Extremities ➤ Palms and soles

- Because the stratum corneum serves as a "reservoir"—a storehouse of medication—it continues to release the topical steroid into the skin after application. Consequently, once-daily application is often sufficient to manage many inflammatory dermatoses. The following are methods of decreasing the epidermal barrier to penetration:
  - **Soaking.** Soaking an affected area in water before the application of a topical agent allows water to hydrate the stratum corneum and thus allows the topical steroid to penetrate more deeply into inflammatory foci. The wrinkling

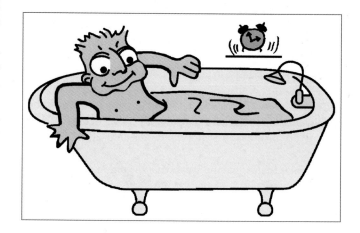

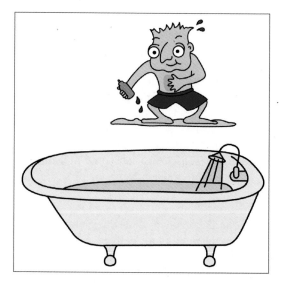

that develops after a hand or foot is immersed in water for a prolonged period results from the skin's increasing its surface area to accommodate the water it absorbs (FIG. I.1).

- **Smearing.** After soaking, the application ("smearing") of a topical steroid (particularly an ointment-based preparation) to wet skin traps the absorbed water, which cannot easily evaporate through the greasy, occlusive barrier.

- **Occlusion.** A "nonbreathing" polyethylene wrap such as Saran Wrap or Handi-Wrap, held in place by tape, a bandage, a sock, or an elastic bandage, can provide occlusion to an area where topical steroids have been applied (FIG. I.2). The wrap may be left on while the patient sleeps or worn for several hours while the patient is awake. Specific areas may be occluded as follows:
  - A plastic shower cap can be used when the scalp is treated with a topical steroid.
  - Cordran tape, which is impregnated with the steroid flurandrenolide, is helpful for occlusive therapy when relatively small areas are treated. However, it is expensive and can be uncomfortable when it is removed from hairy areas.
  - Rubber or vinyl gloves or finger cots may be used for the hands and fingers.
  - Small plastic bags (e.g., Baggies) may be used for the feet.
  - Occlusive garments ("sauna suits") can be worn when extensive areas are involved.

 SEE PATIENT HANDOUT, "Soak and Smear Instruction Sheet" ON THE SOLUTION SITE

A Cream, an Ointment, a Gel, or a Lotion?

- Creams are often preferred by patients for aesthetic reasons. However, their water content makes them more drying than ointments (oil-in-water preparations).
- Generally, ointments are more potent than are creams or lotions, but their inherent greasiness often makes them cosmetically unacceptable. Ointments are helpful for dry skin conditions because of their occlusive properties. They are also more lubricating and tend to be less irritating and less sensitizing.
- Lotions, gels, aerosols, foams, and solutions are useful on hairy areas.
- They are easier than other preparations to apply to large areas but may cause stinging and/or drying.

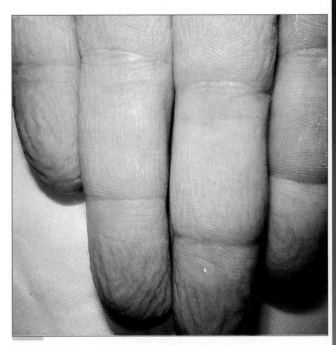

I.1   *Hydration.* These fingers have been immersed in water for a prolonged period to increase the penetration of a topical drug. The corrugated appearance is the result of water absorption.

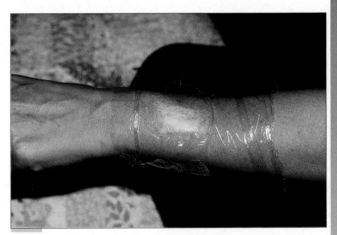

I.2   *Occlusion.* A topical steroid cream has been applied, and a "nonbreathing" polyethylene wrap is used to cover it.

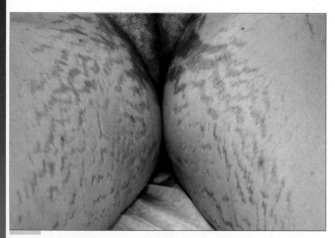

I.3 *Skin atrophy.* Inguinal striae. Linear atrophic scars may develop after repeated use of a potent topical steroid, particularly in an intertriginous (naturally occluded) area.

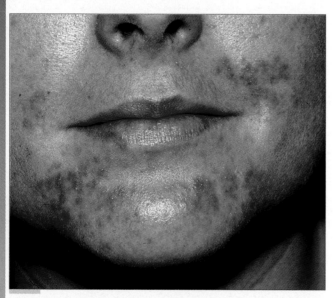

I.4 *Perioral dermatitis resembling rosacea.* This reaction was caused by long-term use of a potent fluorinated topical steroid.

Potential Side Effects

Possible adverse reactions to topical steroids are as follows:

- **Skin atrophy.** Epidermal atrophy is a local reaction demonstrated by shiny, thinned skin and telangiectasias. It generally reverses when topical drugs are discontinued. Striae (linear atrophic scars) may occur after repeated use of a potent topical steroid in one area. These permanent scars are seen most often in intertriginous areas, such as the axillae and groin, where the skin is generally thin, moist, and naturally occluded (FIG. I.3).
- **Acneform eruptions** of the face (FIG. I.4). Lesions resembling acne vulgaris, rosacea, and perioral dermatitis may result from the regular use of topical fluorinated steroids on the face. These eruptions manifest as persistent erythema, papules, pustules, and telangiectasia. The condition often flares once the steroid is withdrawn ("rebound rosacea").
- **Tinea incognito,** a superficial fungal infection. This condition may be misdiagnosed because its clinical signs may be obscured by the use of topical steroids, which reduce inflammation and itching without killing the fungus.

Less common side effects include:

- **Hypersensitivity reactions.** Allergic contact dermatitis to the steroid molecule may occur and may easily be overlooked. The hypersensitivity can be evoked by the steroid, the vehicle, or both, and it is often not suspected clinically. A clue to its presence is a lack of the expected anti-inflammatory effect of the topical steroid.
- **Purpura.** This condition may be noted after prolonged topical steroid use, particularly in elderly patients.
- **Other local effects.** These include hypopigmentation, excess facial hair growth, and delayed wound healing.
- **Systemic effects,** which may result from extensive use of and occlusion with potent topical steroids. Fortunately, these events rarely occur; in fact, hypothalamic-pituitary-adrenal axis suppression is quickly reversible and is unlikely to cause the same side effects as systemic steroid use. Infants, particularly those born prematurely, are more likely to have a greater risk of systemic side effects because of their increased body surface compared to body mass as well as their less efficient cutaneous permeability barriers.

TOPICAL IMMUNOMODULATORS (CALCINEURIN INHIBITORS)*

These topical nonsteroidals inhibit the activity of T-lymphocytes, which produce the cascade of cytokines that increase inflammation and thus have the potential to be "topical steroid-sparing agents." They are approved only for the treatment of eczema and are best used in areas of high risk where skin thinning (atrophy) tends to occur—the face, eyelids, groin, and axillae, as well as the upper chest. Both Protopic and Elidel have been used as effective "off-label" treatments for the management of other dermatoses such as seborrheic dermatitis, oral lichen planus, inverse psoriasis, discoid lupus erythematosus, as well as various other dermatoses.

- **Protopic ointment** in a 0.1% concentration has been approved for treatment in adults. A lower 0.03% concentration is designated for treatment in children.
- **Elidel cream** (pimecrolimus) is available in a 1% formulation.

*The long-term safety of these two agents has been brought into question and has resulted in a "black box" warning by the Food and Drug Administration. Animal studies using high doses of these drugs have suggested an increased rate of malignancy; however, the risk of malignancy in humans has not been established. Currently, these drugs are indicated for short-term or intermittent treatment of atopic dermatitis and are considered as second-line therapy when conventional therapies are inadvisable, ineffective, or not tolerated.

TABLE I.1 TOPICAL STEROIDS ("THE SHORT LIST")[a]

CLASS/POTENCY	GENERIC NAME	BRAND NAMES
Class I: Superpotent	Clobetasol propionate cream/gel/ointment/ foam, lotion 0.05%	Temovate, Olux foam, Clobex lotion, spray, Cormax scalp solution
	Diflorasone diacetate ointment 0.05%	Psorcon
	Halobetasol propionate cream/ointment 0.05%	Ultravate
	Flurandrenolide	Cordran tape (small roll, large roll)
Class II: Very high potency	Desoximetasone cream/ointment 0.25%, gel 0.05%	Topicort
	Fluocinonide cream/ointment/solution/gel 0.05%	Lidex
Class III: High potency	Fluticasone ointment 0.005%	Cutivate
Class IV: Medium-high potency	Triamcinolone acetonide ointment 0.1%	Kenalog
	Hydrocortisone valerate ointment 0.2%	Westcort
Class V: Medium potency	Hydrocortisone valerate cream 0.2%	Westcort
	Triamcinolone acetonide cream 0.1%	Kenalog
	Desonide ointment 0.05%	DesOwen
Class VI: Low potency	Desonide cream 0.05%	DesOwen
Class VII: Very low potency	Hydrocortisone cream/ointment/lotion 0.5%, 1.0%, 2.5%[b]	Hytone, Cortizone 10 and many other brands

[a]Most preparations are available in tubes of 15, 30, or 60 g; lotions and solutions are available in bottles of 20 to 60 mL.
[b]Prescription 2.5% hydrocortisone is hardly more potent than 1% hydrocortisone.
The agents listed should provide more than enough treatment options for the conditions discussed in this book.

TABLE I.2 CLASSIFICATION, STRENGTH, AND VEHICLE OF SOME COMMONLY USED TOPICAL CORTICOSTEROIDS ("THE LONG LIST")

GENERIC NAME	BRAND NAME(S)
Class I: Superpotent	
Betamethasone dipropionate gel/ointment/lotion 0.05%	Diprolene
Clobetasol propionate cream/ointment/gel/lotion/foam 0.05%	Temovate, Olux foam, Clobex lotion, spray, Cormax scalp solution
Diflorasone diacetate ointment/lotion/gel 0.05%	Psorcon
Halobetasol propionate cream/ointment 0.05%	Ultravate
Flurandrenolide	Cordran tape
Fluocinonide cream 0.1%	Vanos
Class II: Very high potency	
Amcinonide ointment 0.1%	Cyclocort
Betamethasone dipropionate ointment 0.05%	Diprosone
Desoximetasone cream/ointment 0.25%/gel 0.05%	Topicort
Diflorasone diacetate cream 0.05%	Psorcon
Betamethasone dipropionate cream 0.05%	Diprolene AF
Fluocinonide cream/ointment/gel 0.05%	Lidex
Halcinonide cream/ointment/solution 0.1%	Halog
Mometasone furoate ointment 0.1%	Elocon

(continued)

TABLE I.2 CLASSIFICATION, STRENGTH, AND VEHICLE OF SOME COMMONLY USED TOPICAL CORTICOSTEROIDS ("THE LONG LIST") *(Continued)*

GENERIC NAME	BRAND NAME
Class III: High potency	
Amcinonide cream/lotion 0.1%	Cyclocort
Betamethasone dipropionate cream/lotion 0.05%	Diprosone
Betamethasone valerate ointment 0.1%	Valisone
Diflorasone diacetate cream 0.05%	Florone, Maxiflor
Fluticasone propionate ointment 0.005%	Cutivate
Triamcinolone acetate ointment 0.1%, cream 0.5%	Aristocort A
Class IV: Medium-high potency	
Betamethasone valerate foam 0.12%	Luxiq Foam
Desoximetasone cream 0.05%	Topicort LP
Fluocinolone acetonide cream 0.2%	Synalar-HP
Fluocinolone acetonide ointment 0.025%	Synalar
Hydrocortisone valerate ointment 0.2%	Westcort
Mometasone furoate cream 0.1%	Elocon
Triamcinolone acetonide ointment 0.1%	Kenalog, Aristocort
Hydrocortisone probutate 0.1%	Pandel
Class V: Medium potency	
Betamethasone valerate cream/lotion 0.1%	Valisone
Desonide ointment 0.05%	DesOwen, Tridesilon
Fluticasone propionate 0.1% cream	Cutivate
Fluocinolone acetonide cream 0.025%	Synalar, Synemol
Flurandrenolide cream 0.05%	Cordran SP
Hydrocortisone butyrate cream/ointment/solution 0.1%	Locoid
Hydrocortisone valerate cream 0.2%	Westcort
Prednicarbate 0.1%	Dermatop-E
Triamcinolone acetonide cream/lotion 0.1%	Kenalog
Triamcinolone acetonide cream 0.025%	Aristocort
Class VI: Low potency	
Alclometasone dipropionate cream/ointment 0.05%	Aclovate
Betamethasone 17-valerate lotion 0.1%	Valisone
Desonide cream/lotion 0.05%	DesOwen
Desonide cream 0.05%	Tridesilon
Fluocinolone acetonide cream/solution 0.01%	Synalar
Fluocinolone acetonide 0.01%	Capex shampoo, Derma-Smoothe
Mometasone furoate cream/ointment 0.1%	Elocon
Class VII: Very low potency	
Hydrocortisone cream/ointment/lotion 0.5%, 1.0%, 2.5%	Hytone, Cortaid, Cortizone-10, Cortizone 5 Creme

PART ONE

Common Skin Conditions: Diagnosis and Management

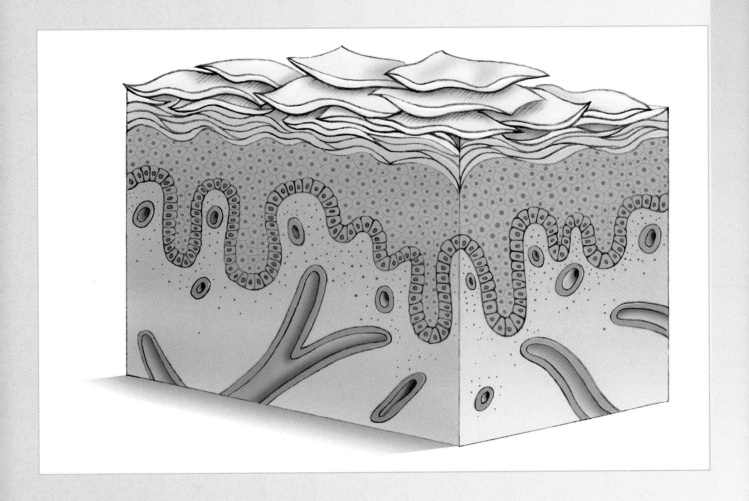

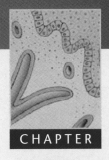

Acne and Related Disorders

OVERVIEW

Acne, the most common skin disorder in the United States, is an embarrassing problem for many teenagers, but it is not limited to that age group. It may develop before puberty in either sex, or it may first be seen in adults, particularly in women.

Acne is a condition that involves the pilosebaceous apparatus of the skin. Acne vulgaris, or common acne (referred to herein as adolescent acne), begins in the teen or preteen years. In general, it becomes less active as adolescence ends but may continue into adulthood.

Acne that initially occurs in adulthood is designated postadolescent acne or adult-onset acne. Despite the clinical similarities and occasional overlapping of adolescent and postadolescent acne, the pathogenesis and treatment of each are somewhat different.

Acnelike disorders, such as neonatal acne, drug-induced acne, rosacea, and other so-called acneiform conditions, are also considered separate entities because of differences in pathogenesis.

That being said, no clear lines separate the various types of acne; much of acne's features overlap and lie along a continuum. However, readers may find the following classifications useful for diagnostic and therapeutic purposes.

> **CLASSIFICATION OF ACNE**

Adolescent Acne (Acne Vulgaris)
- Preteen acne and adolescent acne, which may persist into adulthood

Postadolescent Acne
- Female adult-onset acne, acne excoriée des jeunes filles
- Male adult-onset acne

Acnelike Disorders
- Rosacea
- Perioral dermatitis
- Neonatal acne
- Drug-induced acne
- Endocrinopathic acne
- Physically induced and occupational acne
- Folliculitis (see Chapter 5, "Superficial Bacterial Infections, Folliculitis, and Hidradenitis Suppurativa")
- Hidradenitis suppurativa (see Chapter 5, "Superficial Bacterial Infections, Folliculitis, and Hidradenitis Suppurativa")
- Pseudofolliculitis barbae (see Chapter 10, "Hair and Scalp Disorders Resulting in Hair Loss")
- Acne keloidalis (see Chapter 10, "Hair and Scalp Disorders Resulting in Hair Loss")

Adolescent Acne

BASICS

Teenage acne has a strong tendency to be hereditary and is less likely to be seen in Asians and dark-skinned people. Lesions begin during puberty when androgenic hormones cause abnormal follicular keratinization, which then blocks the sebaceous duct. This blockage results in a microcomedo (the microscopic primary lesion of adolescent acne). The microcomedo enlarges to become the visible comedo: the noninflammatory blackhead or whitehead. Alternatively, the microcomedo may become an inflammatory lesion, such as a papule or pustule.

The development of inflammatory lesions theoretically occurs as follows: Androgenic hormones stimulate sebaceous glands to increase in size and function and thus to produce more sebum. The skin becomes oilier and the microcomedo becomes more hospitable to the anaerobe *Propionibacterium acnes*. Then *P. acnes* produces lipases that digest the lipids into fatty acids, causing a rupture of the microcomedo that incites an inflammatory cell response (ILLUS. 1.1–1.4) will be helpful.

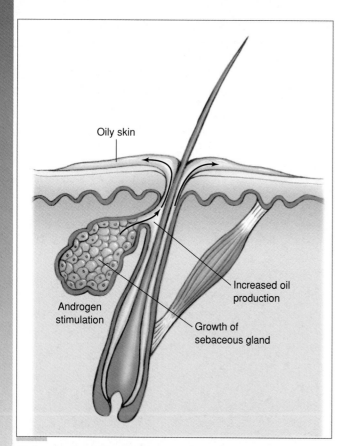

Oily skin

Increased oil production

Androgen stimulation

Growth of sebaceous gland

I1.1 *Androgenic stimulation.* The sebaceous gland over-reacts to androgen stimulation

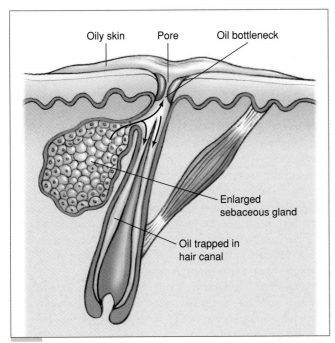

I1.2   *Follicular occlusion*. Pores become clogged and the follicular canal narrows.

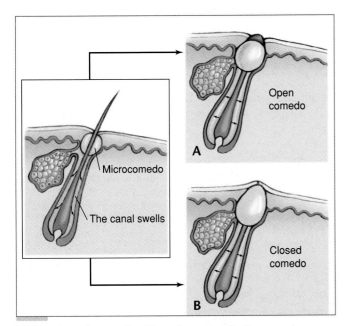

I1.3   *Comedogenesis*. The microcomedo forms and becomes either an open (**A**) or closed comedo (**B**).

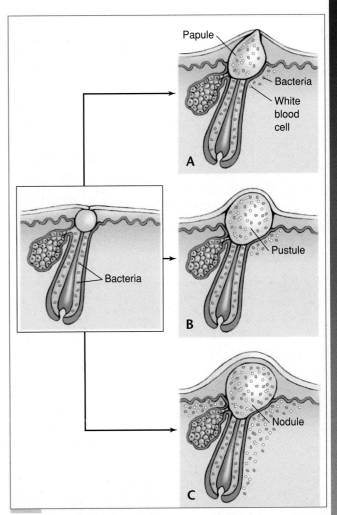

I1.4   *Inflammatory acne*. The microcomedo becomes an inflammatory papule (**A**), pustule (**B**), or nodule (**C**).

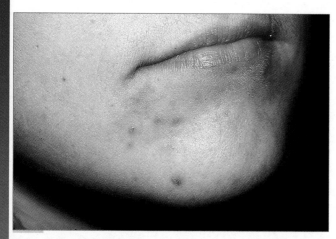

1.1 *Inflammatory acne.* Papules.

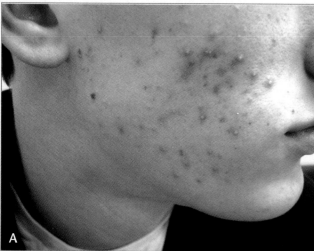

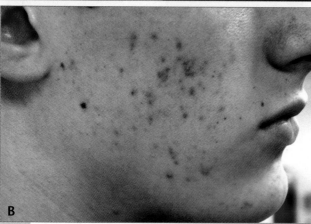

1.2 A and B *Inflammatory acne.* **A:** Papules and pustules. **B:** Macules. The same patient after 6 weeks of treatment. These reddish purple (violaceous) blemishes are frequently evidence of improvement following treatment.

DESCRIPTION OF LESIONS

Acne lesions are designated as inflammatory or noninflammatory (comedonal), or a combination of the two.

Inflammatory Lesions
See FIGURES 1.1–1.3

- **Papules:** Superficial red "pimples" that may have crusted, scabbed surfaces caused by dried pustules or by picking or squeezing.
- **Pustules:** Superficial raised lesions containing purulent material, generally found in the company of papules.
- **Macules:** The remains of formerly palpable inflammatory lesions that are in the process of healing from therapy or spontaneous resolution. They are flat, red or sometimes purple (violaceous) blemishes that slowly heal and may occasionally form a depressed, atrophic scar.
- **"Acne cysts" (nodules):** Large, deep papules or pustules. Acne "cysts" are not really cysts. True cysts are neoplasms that have an epithelial lining. Acne "cysts" do not have an epithelial lining; they are composed of poorly organized conglomerations of inflammatory material.

Noninflammatory (Comedonal) Lesions
A comedo is a collection of sebum and keratin that forms within follicular ostia (pores) (FIG. 1.4).

- **Open comedones (blackheads)** have large ostia that are black as a result of oxidized melanin.
- **Closed comedones (whiteheads)** have small ostia.
- **Follicular prominence.** These blackheadlike, dilated pores are frequently seen on the nose and cheeks in acne patients (FIG. 1.5).

Severity
Acne may be further classified as mild, moderate, or severe.

- **Mild acne** consists of comedones and/or occasional papules and pustules.
- **Moderate acne** is more inflammatory, with relatively superficial papules and/or pustules (papulopustular acne); comedones may also be present. Lesions may heal with scars.
- **Severe acne** ("cystic" or nodular acne, acne conglobata) has a greater degree, depth, and number of inflammatory lesions: papules, pustules, nodules, "cysts," and possibly abscesses. Sinus tracts, significant scarring, and keloid formation may also be evident (FIG. 1.6).

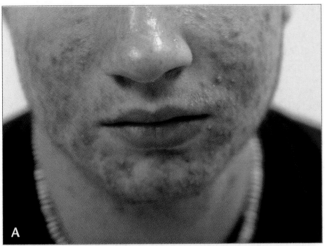

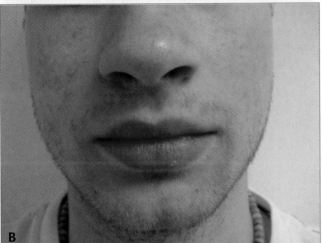

1.3 A and B **A: *Inflammatory acne.*** Nodules. Severe "cystic" acne. **B:** The patient 6 months later after treatment with isotretinoin (Accutane).

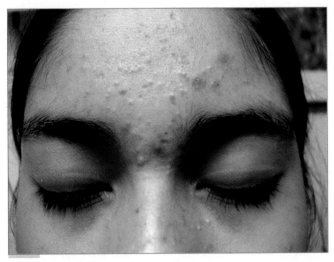

1.4 ***Noninflammatory acne.*** Open and closed comedones, as well as inflammatory lesions are evident.

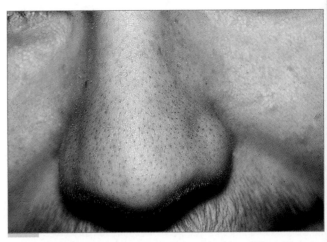

1.5 ***Follicular prominence.*** These blackheadlike, dilated ostia (pores) are frequently seen on the nose and cheeks in acne patients.

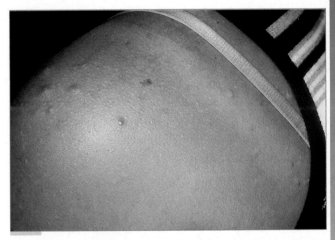

1.6 ***Acne scars.*** Hypertrophic scars are seen on the shoulder of this patient.

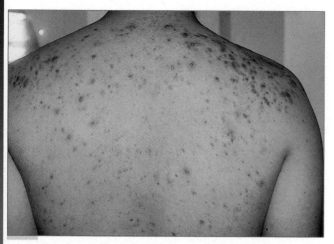

1.7 ***Severe, "cystic" acne.*** This patient's severe acne shows early signs of significant scarring. Involvement of the chest and back predict that this patient will have a poorer prognosis and will be more difficult to treat.

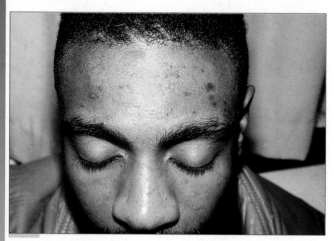

1.8 ***Postinflammatory hyperpigmentation.*** Resolving acne lesions often leave dark macules such as those seen in this African-American patient.

DISTRIBUTION OF LESIONS

- Acne most commonly erupts in areas of maximal sebaceous gland activity: the face, neck, chest, shoulders, back, and upper arms.

CLINICAL MANIFESTATIONS AND SEQUELAE

- The more severe inflammatory lesions of acne are prone to heal with atrophic or pitted ("ice-pick") scars on the face, and hypertrophic scars or keloids on the trunk (FIG. 1.7).
- Postinflammatory hyperpigmentation may occur, particularly in patients with darker skin (FIG. 1.8).
- The negative psychologic effects of acne (e.g., lowered self-esteem) and its impact on limiting employment opportunities and social functioning are among the overriding concerns of individuals who have moderate to severe acne.

DIAGNOSIS

- Adolescent acne is easy for both the patient and practitioner to recognize.
- However, specific underlying causes of acne (e.g., hyperandrogenism) should be considered in certain female patients (see following).

DIFFERENTIAL DIAGNOSIS

Keratosis Pilaris
(See Chapter 2, "Eczema, Atopic Dermatitis.")

- Keratosis pilaris consists of small, follicular, horny spines. The tiny papules may resemble acne when they are inflamed.
- The lesions of keratosis pilaris are most often seen on upper outer arms (FIG. 1.9), back, thighs, and lateral face.

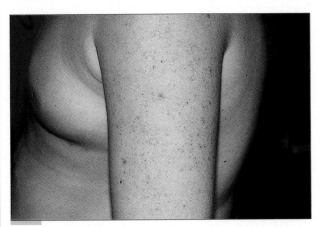

1.9 **Keratosis pilaris.** Acnelike papules located in a typical location.

- In children, the lateral sides of the cheeks are frequently involved. These findings are commonly mistaken for acne (FIG. 1.10).

Folliculitis
See Chapter 5, "Superficial Bacterial Infections, Folliculitis, and Hidradenitis Suppurativa."

Rosacea and Perioral Dermatitis
See the following section for discussion of these conditions.

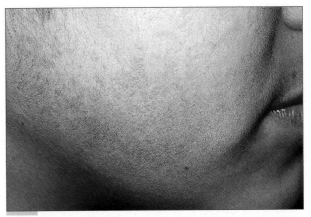

1.10 **Keratosis pilaris.** Often mistaken for acne, these rough-textured acnelike lesions are noted on the lateral face of this child.

 MANAGEMENT

Goals
The three main therapeutic goals are:

- To prevent scarring
- To help improve the patient's appearance
- To make every effort to control acne with topical therapy alone

General Principles
- Treatment of acne should be individualized and frequently involves a trial-and-error approach that begins with those agents that are known to be most effective, least expensive, and have the fewest side effects.
- Acne is a multifactorial disease; therefore, appropriate therapy often involves the use of more than one agent, each of which targets a different pathogenic factor.
- Mild acne can often be managed successfully with over-the-counter (OTC) remedies.
- Oral medications should be tapered as soon as control is achieved.

- A patient should be advised not to squeeze or pick lesions.

Topical Therapies
Notwithstanding the testimonials seen on late-night television infomercials for acne preparations, no "one size fits all" treatment for acne exists. In fact, the active ingredients in these advertised preparations can be obtained less expensively in many OTC products.

Benzoyl Peroxide
See TABLE 1.1.

- In addition to being potent antibacterial agents, benzoyl peroxide preparations improve both inflammatory and noninflammatory lesions (comedones).
- They dry and peel the skin, and they help clear blocked follicles.
- Benzoyl peroxide may be used alone to treat mild acne, but for more severe cases, it should be used in conjunction with topical retinoids, as well as topical or systemic antibiotics.

continued on page 30

Table 1.1 BENZOYL PEROXIDE–CONTAINING PREPARATIONS

OVER-THE-COUNTER PREPARATIONS

Oxy-5, Oxy-10	5%, 10% benzoyl peroxide
Clear by Design	2.5% benzoyl peroxide gel
Clearasil 10%	10% benzoyl peroxide lotion

PRESCRIPTION FORMULATIONS

Desquam-Xerosis	5%, 10% benzoyl peroxide gel (water based)
Desquam-E	2.5%, 5%, 10% benzoyl peroxide gel (water based)
Bevoxyl	4%, 8% benzoyl peroxide gel (water based)
Triaz pads	3%, 6%, 10% benzoyl peroxide gel (water based)

ADVANTAGES	DISADVANTAGES
Available over the counter	Often irritating (causes stinging, redness, and scaling)
No reported bacterial resistance	Contact sensitivity may occasionally occur
Available in many formulations, including cream and liquid (water-based gels less irritating than alcohol-based preparations)	May bleach clothing and bed linen

- Benzoyl peroxide is an ingredient of many brand-name OTC products, such as **Clearasil, Oxy 5,** and **Oxy 10**, as well as less expensive generics. It is available in water- and alcohol-based vehicles, soaps, medicated pads, and washes.
- Lower-strength (e.g., 2.5%) preparations are less irritating and probably as effective as the 5% and 10% concentrations.
- The addition of zinc to benzoyl peroxide in several newer products, such as **Triaz,** may enhance efficacy.
- Benzoyl peroxide is also available in combination with erythromycin (**Benzamycin**) and clindamycin (**Benza-Clin** and **Duac**).

How to Use Benzoyl Peroxide
- Beginning with a lower strength preparation, benzoyl peroxide is applied sparingly once or twice daily, in a thin layer on acne-prone areas.
- Irritation and burning are not uncommon but usually resolve in 2 to 3 weeks.

Topical Retinoids
See TABLE 1.2.
- Topical retinoids are primarily comedolytic (i.e., they treat comedones); they also have potent anti-inflammatory effects.
- In addition, retinoids facilitate the penetration of, and may be used in combination with, other topical antiacne agents such as benzoyl peroxide.
- These agents help "plump up" the skin and make enlarged pores (follicular prominence) less obvious.
- All retinoids may produce sun sensitivity.
- They should not be used during pregnancy or breast-feeding (although no studies have shown them to be harmful to the fetus).

Table 1.2 TOPICAL RETINOIDS

BRAND NAME	GENERIC NAME	ADVANTAGES/ DISADVANTAGES	STRENGTHS	SIZES
Retin-A cream, gel	Tretinoin	Available in various strengths and less expensive generic formulations. Often irritating	Creams: 0.025%, 0.05%, 0.1% Gels: 0.01%, 0.025%	20, 45 g
Retin-A Micro topical gel	Tretinoin	Less irritating than other forms of Retin-A	0.04%, 0.1%	20, 45 g, 50-g pump dispenser
Avita cream, gel	Tretinoin	Less irritating than Retin-A One strength	0.025%	20, 45 g
Differin cream, gel, solution, pledgets	Adapalene	Less irritating than Retin-A; causes less sun sensitivity than Retin-A One strength	0.1%, 0.3%	15, 45 g 30 ml, #60
Tazorac dream, gel	Tazarotene	Possibly more effective and faster acting than Retin-A; two strengths Irritating; expensive	0.05%, 0.1%	30, 100 g

continued on page 31

Table 1.3 TOPICAL ANTIBIOTICS[a]

BRAND NAME	GENERIC NAME	ADVANTAGES/DISADVANTAGES	SIZES
A/T/S solution, gel	Erythromycin 2%	Effective for postadolescent acne, rosacea; irritation is infrequent Often used in conjunction with benzoyl peroxide and/or retinoids	60 ml, 30 g
Akne-Mycin ointment	Erythromycin 2%	Least irritating topical antibiotic; excellent for atopic skin Somewhat messy to apply	25 g
Cleocin T solution, gel, lotion	Clindamycin 1%	Effective for postadolescent acne, rosacea Lotion is less irritating than solution and gel	30, 60 ml
Evoclin foam	Clindamycin 1%	Easy to apply to large and hairy areas	50, 100 g
Theramycin Z	Erythromycin 2%/ zinc acetate	Contains zinc	50, 100 g 60 ml
Ziana	Clindamycin 1.2%/ tretinoin 0.25% gel	New combination drug	30, 60 g

[a]Bacterial resistance is possible with all of these agents.

How To Use Topical Retinoids
- Topical retinoids are applied once daily, usually at bedtime.
- Beginning with lower-strength preparations, such as **tretinoin** 0.025%, **adapalene** cream 0.1%, or **tazarotene** cream 0.05%, they are applied sparingly in a thin layer over the acne-prone areas. In time, higher concentrations can be applied.
- Patients who exhibit sensitivity may use it every other day, or less frequently, until they develop a tolerance to it.
- The area of application should first be washed and thoroughly dried.
- Side effects may include erythema, dryness, and peeling. These usually resolve after 3 weeks.
- Use of a sunscreen should be advised, because tretinoin and adapalene may cause photosensitivity in some patients.

Topical Antibiotics
See TABLE 1.3.

- Preparations that contain the topical antibiotics clindamycin and erythromycin are active against *P. acnes*.

- In addition to their antibacterial action, these drugs have an anti-inflammatory action that helps clear inflammatory acne lesions (papules and pustules).
- Topical clindamycin and erythromycin are considered equally effective.
- Drug resistance has been reported with these antibiotics.

How To Use Topical Antibiotics
- These agents are applied once or twice daily, in a thin layer across the acne-prone areas.
- Irritation and burning are uncommon and may be avoided by using an ointment-based erythromycin such as **Akne-Mycin** or clindamycin (**Cleocin**) in a lotion preparation.
- Topical antibiotics are available in a variety of vehicles, including creams, lotions, ointments, gels, and solutions.

Combination of Topical Antibiotic and Benzoyl Peroxide
See TABLE 1.4.

- **Benzamycin, BenzaClin,** and **Duac** gels are the most commonly prescribed formulations.

Table 1.4 COMBINATION TOPICAL ANTIBIOTIC AND BENZOYL PEROXIDE AGENTS[a]

BRAND NAME	GENERIC NAME	ADVANTAGES/DISADVANTAGES	SIZES
Benzamycin gel	Erythromycin 3%/benzoyl peroxide 5%	Less expensive than comparable products Refrigeration necessary	23.3, 46.6 g
BenzaClin gel	Clindamycin 1%/benzoyl peroxide 5%	No refrigeration necessary; 50-g pump dispenser	25, 50 g
Duac gel	Clindamycin 1%/benzoyl peroxide 5%	No refrigeration necessary	45 g

[a]No bacterial resistance is reported with these agents.

continued on page 32

MANAGEMENT *Continued*

- The combination of erythromycin and clindamycin with benzoyl peroxide helps prevent bacterial resistance furthermore, there appears to be a synergistic effect (the combination appears to be more effective than either drug used alone) when clindamycin and erythromycin are combined with benzoyl peroxide.

How To Use Combination of Topical Antibiotics and Benzoyl Peroxide
- These agents are applied sparingly once daily to acne-prone areas.
- The same cautions apply as for benzoyl peroxide. Dryness, erythema, and pruritus are the most common side effects.

Alternative Topical Prescription Drugs
- These include azelaic acid (**Azelex** 20%), as well as older preparations that contain sulfur and sodium sulfacetamide such as **Sulfacet-R lotion, Novacet lotion,** and **Klaron lotion.**
- These medications are used as alternatives or adjuncts to retinoids, benzoyl peroxide, and topical clindamycin and erythromycin. They are second-line therapy for acne and are also used in the treatment of rosacea (see following).

Topical Nonprescription Agents
Alpha- and Beta-Hydroxy Acids
- Many OTC products contain ingredients that have been used for acne for many generations without great success.
- However, for children just beginning to develop acne or for patients with very mild acne, gentle topical peeling agents such as **salicylic acid** or **glycolic acid,** or anti-inflammatory agents that contain **resorcinol** or **sulfur,** may be helpful.

Multiingredient and Other Over-the-Counter Products
- Numerous products contain various combinations of resorcinol, aloe, glycolic acid, sulfur, and salicylic acid.
- Herbal remedies that contain aloe and benzoyl peroxide are available.
- Such products are difficult to evaluate clinically.

Retinols
- Although retinols were originally marketed to fight aging skin, they are currently being touted for use in treating acne.
- Their efficacy in acne has not been scientifically tested.

Systemic Therapies
Patients who have moderate to severe acne that is unresponsive to topical treatment alone, or acne that tends to scar, are generally prescribed systemic therapy, in addition to topical therapy. Furthermore, significant acne on the chest and back often requires systemic therapy because truncal acne does not respond to topical therapy as readily as does facial acne.

In comparison with topical therapy, systemic therapy has a more rapid onset of improvement, which may enhance patient compliance. However, whenever systemic drugs are administered, the potential dangers—including side effects, drug allergy/intolerance, drug interactions, and fetal exposure in women who are or may become pregnant—must be carefully considered. A risk-benefit calculation is particularly important whenever treating a benign condition, such as acne.

Systemic agents for acne include the following:

- **Oral antibiotics,** most often tetracycline derivatives, are prescribed.
- The **oral retinoid** 13-*cis*-retinoic acid (Accutane) is reserved for more severe, recalcitrant disease.
- In female patients, **hormonal agents,** such as oral contraceptives, and antiandrogenic drugs, such as spironolactone, may be prescribed in carefully selected situations.

Oral Antibiotics
See TABLE 1.6 at end of chapter
Tetracyclines
The tetracycline derivatives are the mainstay of oral acne therapy. They are the first-line antibiotic drugs of choice in the management of moderate to severe acne. As with the topical antibiotics, tetracycline derivatives inhibit the growth of *P. acnes*, which decreases free fatty acid production and pustule formation. In addition, they have a significant anti-inflammatory action as a result of their inhibition of the chemotactic response of neutrophils.

Side Effects
- The use of any of the tetracyclines during a child's tooth development (before 10 years of age) may cause a permanent discoloration of the teeth.
- There are risks to the teeth and bones of unborn fetuses and nursing children.
- Tetracyclines may temporarily stain the teeth of older patients, particularly those with orthodontic braces. While taking any one of the tetracyclines, a patient should be advised to practice good dental hygiene, including flossing.

These drugs may also cause gastrointestinal irritation, phototoxic reactions, and candidal vulvovaginitis.

- In addition, the tetracyclines have been implicated in the development of benign intracranial hypertension

continued on page 33

(pseudotumor cerebri), particularly when taken concurrently with isotretinoin (**Accutane**).

Tetracyclines: Another Concern

Because patients frequently take tetracyclines on a long-term basis (in some instances for years), there is understandably a concern about their consequences. Studies have indicated that routine laboratory supervision of healthy young people receiving long-term tetracycline therapy is not necessary. However, when treatment extends for more than 1 to 2 years, some dermatologists recommend periodically monitoring via appropriate blood tests. This is particularly important if the patient has a history of liver, kidney, or autoimmune disease.

Plain Tetracycline

- Tetracycline is given in dosages ranging from 250 to 500 mg twice a day.
- The dosage may be tapered as inflammatory lesions diminish (usually after 6 to 8 weeks), but this will vary depending on an individual patient's response.
- Tetracycline is taken on an empty stomach (1 hour before or 2 hours after a meal).
- Esophageal irritation may be avoided by taking the drug with a full glass of water.
- Dairy products such as milk or divalent cations that contain iron, magnesium, zinc, or calcium may interfere with tetracycline's absorption from the stomach. Therefore, the drug should not be taken with these compounds.

Minocycline

- Doses are 50 mg twice a day, 75 mg once or twice a day, or 100 mg once or twice a day.
- Minocycline is more expensive but more effective than plain tetracycline for treating inflammatory acne.
- The drug's excellent absorption allows it to be taken with food.
- It causes few, if any, phototoxic problems.
- Minocycline appears to be less likely to induce candidal vulvovaginitis than plain tetracycline. However, it is more likely to cause such side effects as nausea, vomiting, and, in high doses (those that approach 200 mg/day), dizziness owing to vestibular dysfunction. The dizziness usually diminishes after a few days or when the dosage is lowered.
- Less commonly, long-term treatment may cause a reversible bluish hyperpigmentation of the gums and/or skin.
- In rare cases, minocycline is associated with benign intracranial hypertension, hepatitis, and a lupuslike syndrome that is antinuclear antibody positive. This syndrome, which occurs most often in young women, usually develops late in the course of therapy. The symptoms consist of swollen glands, rash, fever, and joint pains and generally disappear following discontinuation of the drug.

An extended-release formulation of minocycline tablets, **Solodyn**, is available and prescribed in a weight-based dosage of 1 mg/kg daily. The tablets are supplied in 45-, 90-, and 135-mg strengths (see TABLE 1.5). It has been shown to have anti-inflammatory effects without acting on *P acnes*, the bacteria involved in causing acne. This approach is intended to prevent bacterial resistance.

Doxycycline

- Doxycycline is given in doses ranging from 50 mg twice a day, 75 mg once or twice a day, or 100 mg once or twice a day.
- Doxycycline is absorbed well and may be taken with food.
- Its main disadvantage is its phototoxic potential—the highest of the tetracyclines. Patients should be advised regarding sun protection.
- Vestibular dysfunction, hyperpigmentation, and the lupuslike syndrome associated with minocycline have not been reported.
- Benign intracranial hypertension may occur.

Second-Line Oral Antibiotics

Erythromycin

- Erythromycin derivatives may be useful as second-line alternative when a tetracycline fails or is not tolerated, or when the patient is younger than 10 years of age or pregnant.
- Erythromycin is generally less effective than tetracycline.
- Gastrointestinal upset is common. An enterically coated erythromycin product such as **E-Mycin** is less likely to cause gastrointestinal symptoms.
- Multiple drug interactions may occur (e.g., erythromycin may elevate digoxin, theophylline, and cyclosporine levels). Reports of *P acnes* resistance to erythromycin, which may be the cause of some treatment failures, are also increasing.
- As with the tetracyclines, candidal vulvovaginitis may occur.

Amoxicillin

- This penicillin derivative is another safer alternative to a tetracycline that can be used during pregnancy.

continued on page 34

Azithromycin (Zithromax)

- The use of azithromycin in a 4- or 5-day pulse therapy regimen has recently gained some interest. Pulse (also called intermittent) therapy refers to taking the drug for several days per week or for 1 week per month, discontinuing it, and then starting it again. For example, the drug could be taken for just 1 week prior to premenstrual flares. Pulsing routines have been suggested to reduce the cost of this expensive drug.
- Azithromycin has no serious side effects; however, as with all of the antibiotics, buildup of bacterial resistance is a concern.

Clindamycin

- Clindamycin is a very effective antibiotic; however, its resistance pattern is similar to that of erythromycin.
- Clindamycin also has the potential serious side effect of pseudomembranous colitis.

Cephalosporins

The new-generation cephalosporin antibiotics appear to have good efficacy against acne. Again, bacterial resistance is a concern.

Trimethoprim-Sulfamethoxazole

- Oral sulfonamides such as trimethoprim-sulfamethoxazole (TMZ) are very effective as antiacne agents. They are reserved for unusually stubborn cases of severe acne that do not respond to any of the other antibiotics listed here. They are sometimes used in situations in which oral isotretinoin (Accutane) is not indicated.
- TMZ has been associated with severe side effects and may precipitate severe allergic reactions.
- The development of resistance is also an issue.

Hormonal Treatment

Oral contraceptives or systemic antiandrogens (such as **spironolactone**) are used in women in whom hormonal treatment may be an effective alternative or adjuvant to antibiotics and oral retinoids. Hormonal treatment is an option when conventional topical and systemic therapies are ineffective or when an endocrine abnormality is discovered. (For a more detailed discussion, see the next section; see also Chapter 11, "Hirsutism.")

Oral Retinoids (Accutane)

Commonly referred to as **Accutane**, **isotretinoin** (13-cis-retinoic acid) is an oral synthetic derivative of vitamin A that promotes long-term remissions in severe acne. The efficacy of isotretinoin in patients with previously unresponsive acne is often profound and long lasting. This powerful drug is reserved for patients with severe nodular acne who are unresponsive to conventional therapy.

The original brand names for oral isotretinoin were Accutane in the United States and Roaccutane in rest of the world. In addition to Accutane and Roaccutane, the drug is now sold under several generic brand names in the United States, including **Amnesteem, Claravis, and Sotret**

Isotretinoin treats acne by:

- Dramatically reducing the size and output of sebaceous glands. It limits the amount of sebum and thus the food supply of *P. acnes*.
- Shedding dead skin cells more normally (stabilizes keratinization), the process through which keratinocytes (epidermal cells) produce the protein keratin. Consequently, the keratinocytes are less likely to clog pores (comedogenesis).

Isotretinoin **can cause severe birth defects if taken by a pregnant woman** or a woman who becomes pregnant while taking the drug, even for a short time. Teratogenic birth defects include skull abnormalities, heart defects, deafness, cleft palate, and central nervous system defects. Because the drug remains in the body for a long time, it can cause birth defects for 1 month *after* a woman has stopped taking it. It also carries an increased risk of miscarriage when used during pregnancy or up to 1 month prior to pregnancy.

Dosage

Oral isotretinoin is available as capsules in strengths of 10, 20, 30, and 40 mg. It is generally taken for 20 weeks; in Europe, the drug is given until a total dosage of 120 to 140 mg/kg is reached. Many prescribers require that women use oral contraceptives before starting treatment, during treatment, and for 1 month after isotretinoin treatment is completed.

Side Effects

General

- Isotretinoin's ability to shut down the oil production in the body accounts for some of its less serious side effects, such as cheilitis, conjunctivitis, dry skin, nose-bleeds, dry eyes, increased sensitivity to the sun, and itching. In general, these reactions are well tolerated because the drug is so effective that patients want to continue taking it despite any side effects.
- Less commonly, a patient experiences musculoskeletal and joint pains.
- Some patients have reported thinning hair during treatment. Rarely has this been a persistent or a permanent

continued on page 35

problem—the hair generally grows back when treatment is discontinued.

- Allergic reactions, decreased night vision, persistent headaches, benign intracranial hypertension, and hearing impairments, are rare findings. Skeletal hyperostosis is limited to those who take a high dosage, one much higher than is used to treat acne, and those undergoing long-term isoretinoin therapy.
- Approximately 25% of patients experience serum triglyceride elevations, and 15% experience decreases in high-density lipoprotein levels.
- Studies performed in men taking isotretinoin showed no significant effects on their sperm and no long-term damage to a man's ability to have healthy children.

Depression and Suicide

- Depression is unfortunately a common problem in the age group that needs isotretinoin most frequently—adolescents. Acne appears most often in patients between 12 and 24 years of age. The onset of depression also commonly occurs at about the same time.
- In the United States, the Food and Drug Administration (FDA) has received reports of depression and suicide in patients who take isotretinoin, and there is concern about a possible link between the drug, psychiatric disorders and suicide.
- Emotional problems in the adolescent population coupled with the stress of having severe acne makes it difficult to determine whether isotretinoin can trigger depression and suicide or whether successful treatment may thwart such problems. Because suicide is a major cause of death in teenagers, particularly in boys, it has been difficult to determine a causal relationship between isotretinoin and these events, and there is a great need for further study.

> **If a patient taking isotretinoin is showing signs of moodiness, depression, or psychosis, the drug should be discontinued!**

The iPLEDGE Program

Isotretinoin's toxicity during pregnancy has long been known, but past efforts to reduce birth defects, including stricter product labeling and a limited pregnancy testing system, failed to resolve the problem. Therefore, in 2005, the FDA established an isotretinoin federal registry program called iPLEDGE. The registry keeps tabs on all isotretinoin prescriptions in the United States. Manufacturers, wholesalers, pharmacists, prescribers, and patients are linked through a centralized computer registry. The registry also connects to the laboratories that perform the required pregnancy testing in this system.

> **Procedures All iPLEDGE Patients Must Follow**
> *Everyone* in the United States who is prescribed the isotretinoin must register with iPLEDGE. After registration, a female patient of child-bearing potential must receive ongoing counseling and pregnancy testing each month while taking the drug. All patients, male or female, are allowed only a 30-day supply of isotretinoin at each office visit. These prescriptions are only valid for seven days after they are prescribed (unless the patient is a man or a woman who is unable to become pregnant).

Other Therapeutic Modalities

Comedo Extraction (Acne Surgery)

- This has been performed less commonly since the topical retinoids have become available.
- Comedones may be removed more easily if the patient is pre-treated with a topical retinoid for 3 to 4 weeks before comedo removal.

Intralesional Corticosteroid Injection

- Intralesional injections of glucocorticosteroids, introduced with a syringe and a 30-guage needle, can reduce the inflammatory response and decrease the size of nodular inflammatory lesions.
- The recommended dose of a triamcinolone acetate suspension is given in a concentration of 2.5 mg/mL to avoid local steroid atrophy. For patients with severe disease and considerable scarring, the concentration can be increased to 5 or 10 mg/mL.
- If too strong a concentration of cortisone is used, atrophy, or depressed scars, may result at the injected sites. These atrophic "dents" usually resolve after several months, but they can be permanent. Similar atrophy may also have been the "normal" healing response of the inflamed lesion if it had not been injected.

Lasers, Lights, and Other Newer Technologies

Because of the concerns over the safety of isotretinoin, hormones, and long-term antibiotic use in the treatment of acne, lasers and other newer technologies will probably play an ever-larger role as future therapies for acne. Laser and light therapies offer a promising, noninvasive treatment alternative. They have shown evidence of

continued on page 36

improving not only inflammatory acne but also acne scarring. Laser and light therapy seem to be most helpful when used in combination with traditional acne medication treatments.

Potential acne treatments currently under consideration include:

- **Photodynamic therapy (PDT):** This involves applying a solution of a photosensitizing agent, aminolevulinic acid (ALA), to the skin. The ALA accumulates in target cells—the sebaceous glands. The skin is then exposed to a high-intensity light source. Light sources used in PDT include visible (nonlaser) or laser light. The *P. acnes* that reside in sebaceous glands produce porphyrins as a by-product of their metabolism. The light activates these porphyrins and thus kills the bacterial cells.
- **Intense pulsed light (IPL):** These devices are similar to lasers, but they use a wider range of wavelengths as opposed to only a single beam of light. These wavelengths can be customized to reach the specific targets such as blood vessels and sebaceous glands.
- **Pulsed dye laser (PDL):** Results for acne have so far been inconsistent. This laser is "tuned" to a specific wavelength of light. It produces a bright light that is absorbed by blood vessels. This laser is also being used to improve the appearance of acne scars and is effective in removing the enlarged blood vessels associated with rosacea.
- **Pulsed light and heat energy (LHE) therapy:** This treatment combines pulses of light and heat, which may target both *P. acnes* and sebaceous glands.
- **Diode laser:** This laser uses infrared frequencies that are longer, invisible wavelengths. It appears to be effective not only on acne but on the acne scars as well.

Office-Based Chemical Peels
- Chemical peels have become popular as antiaging facial rejuvenation procedures; however, they are sometimes used to treat acne as well. In this procedure, a chemical acid solution is applied to the skin, causing the skin to peel off so that new skin can regenerate.
- Chemical peels are probably not effective for the treatment of inflammatory lesions of acne. They seem to work best in the elimination of comedonal acne.
- Deeper peels, with stronger concentrations of acids, are sometimes used to treat acne scars.
- The two most commonly used chemicals for peels are the alpha-hydroxy acids and the beta-hydroxy acids.

POINTS TO REMEMBER

- The patient should be informed that a significant therapeutic response may require 6 to 8 weeks.
- Every effort should be made to try tapering oral medications as soon as acne is controlled.
- If there is evidence of scarring, acne should be treated more aggressively (even mild acne can heal with significant scarring).
- The two Hs—**h**ormones and **h**eredity—underlie teenage acne (one or both parents probably had acne), and not the proverbial poor **d**iet and **d**irty face (the two Ds). A minority of dermatologists believe that there is a connection between certain dairy products and acne.
- In the treatment of females of childbearing potential, isotretinoin should be used only for patients with severe, disfiguring, cystic acne.

HELPFUL HINTS

- Compliance is often a problem for teenagers, who are notoriously poor at dealing with delayed gratification, so it is quite important to clearly explain the treatment regimen, make it simple, and give written instructions. The teenager—or more likely the parent—should be advised to call the health care provider with any questions or concerns.
- Because topical retinoids may *appear* to make acne worse, BenzaClin, Duac, or Benzamycin gel may be used first with inflammatory lesions. Such lesions are usually the first to respond, and thus their quick disappearance can be helpful in obtaining compliance in teenagers.
- For those patients who experience irritation and excessive dryness, topical retinoids may be applied for 2 to 3 minutes and then washed off. This short-contact treatment appears to work quite well and helps avoid irritation. The time of application can be gradually increased as tolerated.
- **"Rollercoasting"** (i.e., titrating or fine-tuning the dosage of oral antibiotics such as tetracycline, minocycline, and doxycycline) may help minimize potential side effects such as vertigo and the total dosage of the medication. For example, a dosage schedule can begin as 50-mg minocycline capsules—two in the morning and one in the afternoon. This method may also lessen the total dosage, and help lower the cost of the medication. (In addition, because the highest recommended dosage is 200 mg per day, this dosage allows for a possible increase of an additional 50 mg per day after the patient's next follow-up visit. However, if the acne shows marked improvement, the dosage can be lowered—to perhaps, 50 mg twice a day.)
- For patients who experience premenstrual flares of acne, increasing the dosage 5 to 7 days before the next menstrual period and then lowering the dosage afterward can help reduce the amount of drug used.

SEE PATIENT HANDOUTS, "Acne: How to Apply Topical Retinoids" AND "Acne: How to Apply: Duac Gel, BenzaClin Gel, Benzamycin Gel" ON THE SOLUTION SITE

➤ FURTHER ACNE FACTS

- In most people, acne tends to improve temporarily during the summer months. Exposure to the sun in small doses diminishes acne, and tanning promotes a blending of skin tones.
- Fall and winter acne flareups are quite common and are often influenced by mood swings.
- Some women may note improvement of acne during pregnancy or while taking birth control pills. Others may note a worsening of acne or no change at all.
- Moderate to severe involvement of the chest and back predict that the patient will have a poorer prognosis and will be more difficult to treat. Severe, unremitting, scarring acne is more prevalent among men.
- Because acne is a visible disease, acne patients may suffer from impaired self-image, depression, anxiety, employment insecurities, social withdrawal, self-destructive behaviors, and even suicidal ideation.
- Acne, hirsutism, and irregular periods may be associated with hyperandrogenism and/or polycystic ovaries.
- Some drugs, including systemic steroids, lithium, epilepsy agents, and antituberculosis medicines, can cause or exacerbate acne.
- Stress seems to worsen acne. College students at examination time, teenagers about to go to the prom, or someone going for a first job interview often provide testimony to this phenomenon. The question is: are these individuals simply more aware of the appearance of their skin at these critical times, or is the acne actually worse at these times because of stress? It is proposed that the release of excess amounts of glucocorticoids and a resulting increase in sebaceous gland activity account for this worsening of acne.
- In darkly pigmented people, the severity of inflammation may be equivalent to that in fairer-skinned people, but it may not be as apparent. Consequently, African-American patients are often as concerned about the acne-related pigmentary changes as they are about the acne itself.

Postadolescent Acne (Adult-Onset Acne)

BASICS

Dermatologists regularly hear the lament "acne, at my age!" expressed by women in whom acne suddenly appears or in whom acne has not resolved by 20 years of age. Adult-onset acne is overwhelmingly a condition of women. In fact, women often develop acne in their 20s and early 30s, sometimes for the first time in their lives. Although frustrating for those women who were spared acne during adolescence, adult-onset acne is often even more upsetting for those who had teenage acne and "grew out of it" only to discover the return of pimples when they reach 32 years of age. Some women continue to have acne into their 40s and 50s. In some cases, teenage acne that persists into adulthood is complicated by the appearance of adult-onset acne.

The prevalence of female adult acne has increased significantly in the past several generations. Proposed hypotheses to explain this apparent increase include:

- The entry of women into the workforce and its attendant stresses
- The use of low-estrogen containing oral contraceptives
- The proliferation of food additives and the injection of hormones and antibiotics into livestock
- The increased use of cosmetics

There is little question that acne is influenced by hormones. For example, many women report premenstrual or (less commonly) midcycle flares of inflammatory acne. Pregnancy, oral contraceptives, and hormonal supplementation also appear to affect a woman's complexion and cause fluctuations in acne.

"Acne cosmetica" is the traditional name for acne that is supposedly caused by cosmetics. Indeed, some reactions to cosmetics can sometimes look like inflammatory acne; however, such "acne" is often the result of an irritating skin reaction.

Acne with an onset in adult males has traditionally been an unusual finding; however, it has been seen increasingly in men and some women who participate in athletic activities. The reason for the recent increased prevalence of this type of acne is unknown. Causes are speculated to be one or all of the following: sweating, mechanical friction, anabolic steroids, and creatine-containing dietary body-building supplements.

DESCRIPTION OF LESIONS

Unless preexisting adolescent acne is a concurrent problem:

- Postadolescent acne is relatively free of comedones and consists of evanescent, inflammatory red papules and/or pustules.
- The lesions more closely resemble those seen in rosacea or perioral dermatitis.
- In general, lesions tend to be few in number.

DISTRIBUTION OF LESIONS

- In women, lesions occur on the face, most often in the peri-oral area, along the jawline, or on the chin—the lower part of the face. Also, the hairline, neck, and upper trunk may also be affected. The acne in this location is probably caused by an increase in the response of hair follicles to male hormones (androgen receptor sensitivity) (FIG. 1.11).
- In men who develop adult-onset acne, lesions tend to be limited to the trunk.

CLINICAL MANIFESTATIONS

- Lesions tend to appear and reappear like clockwork according to a woman's fluctuating levels of circulating hormones. They are more likely to recur premenstrually or at ovulation. They last for several days; sometimes they persist for a month or longer. In some women, lesions occur without any pattern.
- No such fluctuation occurs in men.

DIAGNOSIS

- The diagnosis is made clinically.
- However, in female patients whose acne is not responding to treatment, or for those who have other signs of hormonal excess such as male characteristics (e.g., facial hair) or irregular menstrual periods, hormonal tests are indicated. More often than not, these levels are normal, and it appears that these women may have an end-organ hypersensitivity to their endogenous androgens.

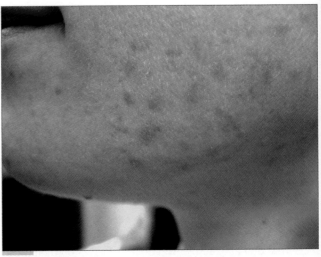

1.11 *Postadolescent acne.* Characteristic location of erythematous acne papules along the jawline in a female adult .

 DIFFERENTIAL DIAGNOSIS

Rosacea and Perioral Dermatitis
See also the following sections.

- These conditions are seen primarily in adults.
- They most often occur on the central third of the face (rosacea) or perioral area (perioral dermatitis).
- In older women, and in some men, rosacea and acne often appear simultaneously, and there are no comedones.

 MANAGEMENT

Topical Treatment
- Skin care should be kept simple and gentle with the use of mild soaps.
- Postadolescent acne in female patients may be treated with many of the same agents used for adolescent acne; however, treating adults who have acne can be more challenging because aging skin is often more sensitive than teenage skin and sometimes cannot tolerate the potentially drying, irritating effects of some topical acne medications.

Systemic Treatment
Oral Antibiotics
For more information on treatment of postadolescent acne with oral antibiotics, see the earlier discussion in TABLE 1.5.

Hormonal Treatment
Indications include:

- Normal serum androgens and intractable acne
- Ovarian or adrenal excess
- An alternative to oral isotretinoin or antibiotics; in women of childbearing potential, oral contraceptives are often taken during a course of oral isotretinoin.
- Relapse after taking a course of oral isotretinoin

Oral Contraceptives
By suppressing gonadotropins, reducing ovarian androgen secretion, and increasing sex hormone–binding globulin levels, oral contraceptives decrease serum testosterone concentrations. Besides suppressing ovulation, the estrogens in birth control pills can help improve acne by blocking the androgenic stimulation of sebaceous glands by acting as androgen receptor blockers.

Oral contraceptives such as **Yasmin** and **YAZ** have, in addition to an estrogen, a progestin, drospirenone, which is a very close chemical relative to spironolactone (see following). Hormonal treatments with oral contraceptives such as **Ortho**

continued on page 40

MANGEMENT *Continued*

Tri-Cyclen, **Ortho-Cyclen**, **Ortho-Cyclen Lo**, **Estrostep**, **Ortho-Cept**, **Alesse**, **Mircette**, and **Desogen** are also relatively low in androgenic activity.

Antibiotics and the "Pill"

A recent study has concluded that the antibiotics used to treat acne probably do not interfere with the efficacy of oral contraceptives. Nevertheless, patients taking oral antibiotics should be advised of this controversy so that they can decide to use an alternative or additional form of birth control.

Oral Antiandrogens

Before oral antiandrogens are prescribed, a hormonal and gynecologic evaluation is appropriate for a small number of acne patients, particularly for women who have treatment-resistant acne, a sudden onset of severe acne, virilizing signs or symptoms, irregular menstrual periods, or hirsutism. Oral antiandrogens (androgen receptor blockers) may also be considered for those women who are reluctant to take oral contraceptives for moral or religious reasons.

Spironolactone (Aldactone) is the antiandrogen used most frequently to treat acne. It has potent antiandrogenic effects and works by decreasing sebum production. Spironolactone is started at a low dosage of 25 to 50 mg per day and may be increased. It may take 3 months for any positive effects to become visible, but results may appear sooner. The dosage may need to be adjusted during the first 6 months of treatment.

The most common side effect of spironolactone is an irregular menstrual cycle; however, if the patient is taking birth control pills, this is less likely to happen. It is recommended that an oral contraceptive be taken concurrently, because there is a risk of feminization of a male fetus if a woman becomes pregnant while taking an antiandrogen. Breast tenderness sometimes occurs.

Flutamide (Eulexin) is another antiandrogen that is sometimes used in unmanageable female adult acne. It has the potential of causing severe liver damage, which greatly limits its use.

Cyproterone is an acetate steroidal androgen receptor blocker. It acts as a competitive inhibitor of testosterone and dehydroepiandrosterone at the level of androgen receptors. A drug with the trade name **Diane-35**, an oral contraceptive that is very effective in the treatment of acne but not available in the United States, contains a combination of cyproterone acetate and ethinyl estradiol.

HELPFUL HINTS

- A minimum of 3 to 6 months of therapy is required to evaluate the efficacy of oral contraceptives and antiandrogen agents in treating adult-onset acne.
- Hormonal birth control methods such as the birth control patch and ring have an unpredictable effect on acne and can actually provoke acne. Depo-Provera, an injectable form of birth control containing synthetic progesterone, can also worsen or trigger acne at times.
- Because it is very common for women to have premenstrual flares of acne, an increased dosage of oral antibiotics can be given 5 to 7 days before her next menstrual period (see earlier discussion of "rollercoasting").

POINT TO REMEMBER

- Every female patient with acne should be questioned about her menstrual history and virilizing symptoms.

BASICS

Rosacea is a common disorder that is frequently mistaken for acne. In fact, as recently as 20 years ago, rosacea was referred to as "acne rosacea." Both conditions look alike, they often respond to the same treatments, and they may coexist.

Rosacea arises later in life than acne, usually when patients are between 30 and 50 years of age. It occurs most commonly in fair-skinned people with an ethnic background from Great Britain (Scotland and Wales), Ireland, Germany, Scandinavia, and certain areas of Eastern Europe. Women are reportedly three times more likely to be affected than men. Rosacea is rare in all dark-skinned people, including Hispanic, African, and African-American populations.

Although the precise cause of rosacea remains a mystery, it is believed that certain environmental factors contribute to its development and progression. Rosacea is not caused by drinking excessive amounts of alcohol—a serious misconception that has been around for ages and should be put to rest! Precipitating factors that may exacerbate rosacea include:

- Sun exposure
- Excessive washing of the face
- Irritating cosmetics

There is no convincing evidence that the following environmental factors have any long-term deleterious effects on rosacea:

- Excess alcohol ingestion
- Emotional stress
- Spicy foods, smoking, or caffeine

Despite their similarities, acne vulgaris and rosacea seem to have quite different pathophysiologies. It has been suggested that the bacterium, *Helicobacter pylori*, which is found in the stomach, may cause or exacerbate rosacea; other investigators have implicated the *Demodex* species of mite that is often found in the hair follicle of patients with rosacea. However, evidence that either organism plays a central role in the pathogenesis of this disorder is lacking. Recent investigations have suggested that an excess of the protein cathelicidin plays a role in the inflammation of rosacea.

DESCRIPTION OF LESIONS

- Rosacea is a facial eruption that consists of acnelike erythematous papules, pustules, and telangiectasias.
- It lacks the comedones ("blackheads" or "whiteheads") that are seen in acne.
- It does not appear to have any relationship to androgenic hormones.
- In general, rosacea does not scar or present with nodules or cysts, unless the patient has concomitant acne.
- When it first appears, rosacea may begin with erythema on the cheeks and forehead that later spreads to the nose and chin. This is referred to as "erythemotelangiectatic rosacea" (formerly known as prerosacea). Often, affected patients describe how they are inclined to flush and blush easily.
- As rosacea progresses, telangiectasias, papules, and sometimes, pustules begin to arise against a background of erythema. The papules and pustules (papulopustular rosacea) tend to come and go in cycles, but the erythema and telangiectasias tend to remain.

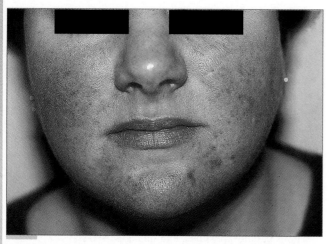

1.12 *Rosacea.* As seen here, rosacea involves inflammatory papules and pustules and telangiectasias that are located on the central third of the face.

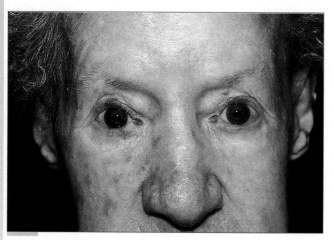

1.13 *Ocular rosacea.* Note the conjunctivitis as well as the typical facial papules of rosacea.

DISTRIBUTION OF LESIONS

- Lesions are most typically seen on the central third of the face-the forehead, nose, cheeks, and chin (the so-called "flush/blush" areas) (FIG. 1.12).
- Lesions tend to be bilaterally symmetric, but they may occur on only one side of the patient's face.

CLINICAL MANIFESTATIONS

- Rosacea is primarily a cosmetic problem; however, burning and flushing can be quite uncomfortable.
- Patients may also have ocular involvement, which results most often in blepharoconjunctivitis. Episcleritis and keratoconjunctivitis sicca are rare complications. Ocular rosacea may precede the skin manifestations in up to 20% of people (FIG. 1.13).

DIAGNOSIS

- Rosacea is diagnosed clinically.
- A biopsy may be necessary in atypical cases.

 DIFFERENTIAL DIAGNOSIS

Rosacea is different from acne vulgaris and adult-onset acne in several ways, although the three conditions are sometimes similar.

Adult Acne
- The microcomedo, the primary lesion of acne, arises in response to hormonal (androgenic) stimulation.
- Lesions are influenced by a woman's menstrual cycle.
- Adult-onset acne tends to occur on the lower part of the face and tends to have a much wider distribution, such as on the chest and back.

Seborrheic Dermatitis
See also Chapter 2, "Eczema."

- The presence of scale and erythema, without acnelike lesions (papules and pustules)
- Appears on the nasolabial area, eyebrows, and scalp

Systemic Lupus Erythematosus
(See Chapter 25, "Cutaneous Manifestations of Systemic Disease")

- "Butterfly" distribution of rash
- Absence of papules and pustules
- Presence of antinuclear antibodies and other manifestations of lupus

continued on page 43

DIFFERENTIAL DIAGNOSIS *Continued*

Sun-Damaged Skin (Dermatoheliosis)

- Rosacea is a condition that is regularly "overdiagnosed" by health care providers; sometimes these patients may simply have "rosy cheeks" (FIG. 1.14). In many instances, rosacea can be difficult to distinguish from weathered, sun-damaged skin that is seen in many fair-skinned farmers, gardeners, sailors, or in people who have worked or spent long periods of their lives outdoors.
- Such long-term sun exposure can also lead to persistent red faces and telangiectasias and can resemble rosacea.

"Flusher/Blushers"

- In a "flusher/blusher" redness occurs in different places than where it is commonly seen in rosacea. Symptoms tend to appear on the sides of the cheeks, the front and side of the neck, and the ears, rather than the central area of the face.

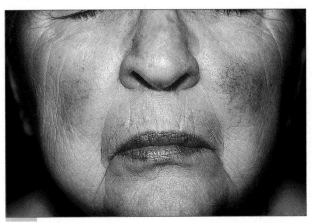

1.14 *Facial erythema.* Frequently misdiagnosed as rosacea, this woman has "rosy cheeks" and telangiectasias.

 MANAGEMENT

Patients should be advised to avoid significant environmental triggers and to apply a sunscreen prior to sun exposure.

Topical Therapy

Some of the topical medications used to treat acne are also very effective for rosacea; however, some precautions must be taken, because many people with rosacea have very sensitive skin. Consequently, standard acne medications such as topical retinoids and benzoyl peroxide can be drying and/or irritating, may sensitize the skin to the sun (retinoids), and can even exacerbate rosacea. If possible, long-term control of rosacea should be attempted with topical therapy alone, and oral antibiotics should be reserved for initial control and for breakthrough flares.

The preparations described in this section can be used in combination with oral antibiotics as well as the other topical medications. It may take 6 to 8 weeks before significant improvement is noted.

Metronidazoles

- The "metros" are the most frequently prescribed first-line topical therapy for rosacea.
- **Noritate** (metronidazole) 1% cream, and **MetroGel** 1% gel are applied once daily on rosacea-prone areas.

Azelaic Acid

- **Azelex** cream and **Finacea** gel are 15% azelaic acid preparations. (**Skinoren** is available in Europe.) They are considered to be as effective as metronidazole in the treatment of rosacea.
- Application is twice a day.

Sodium Sulfacetamide and Sulfur

- Medications containing sodium sulfacetamide and sulfur are also effective for rosacea. **Klaron** and **Sulfacet-R** are preparations containing sodium sulfacetamide 10% and sulfur 5%. Brand names include **Klaron, Plexion, Rosula, Rosac, Rosanil, Novacet,** and **Ovace.** They are available as lotions, creams, and washes.
- Some of these products contain a humectant and can be used in patients with rosacea who have dry, sensitive skin. Others have color tinting to help hide the redness of rosacea. These agents are generally applied twice a day to clean dry skin. When used in combination, they also appear to enhance the effectiveness of the other topical agents (azelaic acid and metronidazole) that are detailed in this section.

Systemic Therapy

See TABLE 1.6 at the end of this chapter

Oral Antibiotics

- The same systemic oral antibiotics used to treat acne also can be used to treat the papules and pustules of rosacea. Most cases can be treated and controlled with topical agents alone; however, if topical treatment is ineffective, an oral antibiotic is generally prescribed.

continued on page 44

Table 1.5 TOPICAL AGENTS FOR ROSACEA AND PERIOROFICIAL DERMATITIS

BRAND NAME	GENERIC NAME	ADVANTAGES/DISADVANTAGES	SIZES
Noritate cream	Metronidazole 1%	Minimal irritation Once-daily application	30 g
MetroGel,	Metronidazole 1%	Once-daily application	60 g
MetroCream	Metronidazole 0.75%	Twice-daily application	45 g
Azelex, Finevin, Skinoren creams	Azelaic acid 15%, 20%	May lighten skin; irritation is common	30, 50 g
Finacea gel	Azelaic acid 15%	May lighten skin; irritation is common	30 g
Rosac cream	Sodium sulfacetamide 10%/sulfur 5%	Contains broad-spectrum sunscreen	45 g
Sulfacet-R lotion	Sodium sulfacetamide 10%	Tinted preparation may be a good camouflage in fair-skinned acne patients	25 g

- **Tetracycline** and tetracycline derivatives, such as **minocycline** and **doxycycline,** are the first-line oral drugs of choice in the management of moderate to severe rosacea. The mechanism of action of these drugs is more likely anti-inflammatory than antibiotic, because no microorganisms have been definitively identified as a cause of rosacea or its variants.
- In comparison with topical therapy, systemic therapy has a more rapid onset of action. With oral antibiotics, improvement of rosacea is usually noticeable in a week or two. The papules and pustules begin to flatten and disappear, and new ones stop appearing. The antibiotic is then tapered when this improvement persists (usually after 3 to 4 weeks).

Dosage
- Tetracycline is given in dosages ranging from 250 to 500 mg, taken twice daily.
- It is tapered when the inflammation has improved (usually after 2 to 3 weeks).

- If tetracycline is ineffective, minocycline (50 to 100 mg bid), doxycycline (50 to 100 mg twice a day), or erythromycin (250 mg twice to four times daily) may be tried. **Oracea,** an anti-inflammatory low-dose (subantimicrobial) doxycycline, is available as a 40-mg capsule that contains 30-mg immediate-release and 10-mg delayed-release beads. It is taken once daily.

Alternative Antibiotics
Azithromycin, clarithromycin, or **amoxicillin** are used as second-line alternatives when a tetracycline fails or is not tolerated.

Other Treatment Options
Electrocautery
- Electrocautery with a small needle is used to destroy small telangiectasias.

Pulse Dye Lasers and Intense Pulsed Light
- These light treatments are used to destroy larger telangiectatic vessels.

HELPFUL HINTS

- Initial treatment with oral antibiotics typically delivers a rapid therapeutic response and helps confirm the diagnosis of rosacea.
- It should be recognized that the "flat" telangiectasias and flushing erythema tend to persist and respond minimally, if at all, to antibiotic therapy.
- Men who have difficulty shaving around the papules of rosacea should try using an electric razor rather than a blade to reduce abrasion.
- The patient should be instructed to avoid irritating cosmetics, astringents, and exfoliating agents. Instead, water-based moisturizers and cosmetics and makeups or moisturizers with a sunscreen already added are recommended.
- Sunscreens that contain zinc oxide or titanium dioxide-the barrier sunscreens-should be used, especially if other sunscreens irritate or worsen rosacea.
- Cosmetic foundations can be applied to cover erythematous areas. Green-tinted foundations can hide the red. Other nonprescription products that may be used to cover up the redness are **Dermablend** and **Covermark**. They can be matched to a patient's normal skin color. These products can be found at makeup counters in some department stores.

 POINTS TO REMEMBER

- Rosacea is a chronic condition with no known cure.
- Acne and rosacea share similar clinical manifestations and overlapping management strategies, yet each has a distinctive course and prognosis; consequently, an attempt at making a specific diagnosis should be made.
- If possible, long-term control of rosacea should be attempted with topical therapy alone, with oral antibiotics used only for breakthrough flares.

➤ TRIGGERS OF ROSACEA

Common factors include:
- **Sun exposure**
- **Excess alcohol ingestion.** Drinking habits have nothing to do with *causing* rosacea; however, it is accepted that the blushing and flushing of rosacea may flare up in the short term when some people drink alcohol—especially red wine. However, it is questionable that the drinking of alcoholic beverages causes a long-term worsening of the condition.

There is no convincing evidence that the following factors have any long-term harmful effects on rosacea. However, they can increase the redness of the face temporarily.

- **Spicy foods, smoking, and caffeine**
- **Cooking over a hot stove or oven**
- **Emotional stress**
- **Physical exertion**

Rosacea Variants

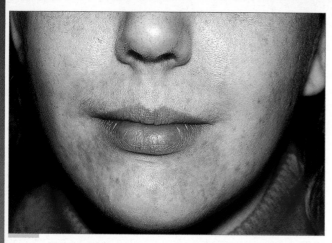

1.15 *Perioral dermatitis.* Multiple, small, acneiform papules can be seen on this young woman. Note the characteristic sparing around the lips.

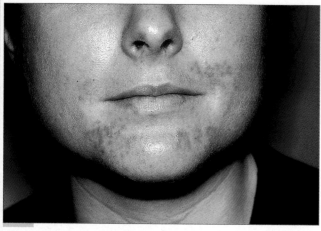

1.16 *Topical steroid-induced rosacea.* This woman has been applying a potent topical steroid every day to her face for eight months.

PERIORAL DERMATITIS

This condition, which is also known as "periorificial dermatitis," perioral dermatitis is a rosacea-like eruption seen primarily in young women and uncommonly in young boys and girls. It is usually found around the mouth, but it may be noted around the eyes and nose (which explains the more inclusive term, "periorificial") (FIG. 1.15). As with rosacea, the etiology is unknown. Potent topical steroids and fluoridated toothpaste have occasionally been implicated, but there is no consistent evidence.

Features that distinguish perioral dermatitis from rosacea include the following:

- Perioral dermatitis appears in women between 15 and 40 years of age.
- It manifests in small, erythematous papules or pustules without telangiectasia.
- It characteristically circles the mouth and spares the vermilion border of the lips.
- Occasionally, there is superimposed scaling.
- Usually it does not recur after successful treatment.

TOPICAL STEROID–INDUCED "ROSACEA"

Rosacea induced by topical steroids is often clinically indistinguishable from ordinary rosacea, but a history of long-term, indiscriminate misuse of potent topical steroids on the face helps confirm the diagnosis. It is sometimes referred to as "steroid use/abuse/misuse/dermatitis" (FIG. 1.16).

- The topical steroids are often prescribed for other skin conditions and then overused by the unsuspecting person, who continues to apply them.
- The condition typically worsens when the topical steroids are discontinued (an occurrence known as "rebound rosacea").
- In an unfortunate cycle, the steroid is sometimes reapplied to diminish the erythema, which only worsens the condition.
- This condition is treated by stopping the offending topical steroid and by taking a tetracycline derivative for a few weeks or more to get over the "hump" of the rebound.

RHINOPHYMA

Rhinophyma can be an unsightly manifestation of rosacea. This condition usually occurs in men over 40. It consists of knobby nasal papules that tend to become larger and swollen over time (FIGS. 1.17 and 1.18). It is quite uncommon and is rarely seen in women.

The usual treatments described in this chapter for rosacea are not effective for rhinophyma. Recontouring procedures with a scalpel or a carbon dioxide laser have been used successfully to remove ("sculpt") the excess nose tissue, resulting in a more normal shape and appearance. This may also be accomplished by electrocautery and dermabrasion.

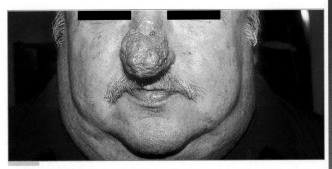

1.17 *Rhinophyma.* This man's enlarged nose is caused by marked sebaceous hyperplasia.

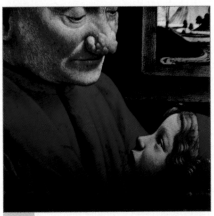

1.18 *Rhinophyma.* Ghirlandaio's portrait of an old man with his grandson (showing a tender human relationship, despite the appearance of his nose).

Acne: Other Types

SYSTEMIC DRUG-INDUCED (OR DRUG-EXACERBATED) ACNE

Several drugs are known to provoke acneiform reactions.

- Oral corticosteroids and adrenocorticotropic hormone produce acnelike lesions that are usually more monomorphic and symmetric in distribution than those seen in adolescent and postadolescent acne. Lesions are located primarily on the trunk. The precise mechanism is uncertain.
- Lithium may exacerbate acne.
- Androgens. including anabolic steroids and gonadotrophins, may precipitate acne, especially in athletes who take such drugs.
- Antiepileptic drugs, especially phenytoin, have been held responsible for causing or exacerbating acne; however, modern anticonvulsants do not appear to have acne as a potential side effect.
- Patients taking isoniazid, especially those who slowly inactivate the drug, appear to be prone to develop acne.
- The management of drug-induced or drug-exacerbated acne includes the following choices: discontinuation of the causative drug, decreasing the dosage, or substituting the drug with another agent. Treatment of acne is described earlier in this chapter.

NEONATAL ACNE

- This self-limiting form of acne is seen mainly in male infants; it occurs from the stimulation of maternal androgens.
- Because it is self-limiting, it requires no treatment. (See Chapter 27, "Special Considerations in the Skin of Pediatric and Elderly Patients.")

ACNE EXCORIÉE DES JEUNES FILLES

This type of acne is routinely picked at by the patient, who almost invariably is female (FIG. 1.19).

- Many of these patients deny that they manipulate their skin, but it is rather obvious because there are no primary lesions present; all have crusts.
- Some of these patients may benefit from selective serotonin receptor inhibitors and psychotherapy.

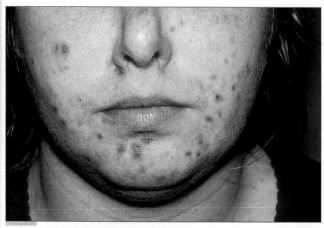

1.19 *Acne excoriée des jeunes filles.* This type of acne has obviously been picked at by the patient.

ENDOCRINOPATHIC ACNE

- The presence of acne, coupled with other signs or symptoms, may indicate an endocrinopathy.
- Hormonal disorders that can produce excessive androgens, as well as those that can manifest with elevated cortisol levels can be responsible for producing or aggravating pre-existing acne (see Chapter 11, "Hirsutism").

AGENT ORANGE AND DIOXINS (CHLORACNE)

- Agent Orange, an herbicide, was used during the war in Vietnam. This herbicide contains dioxins (halogenated aromatic hydrocarbons), a group of chemicals known to increase the likelihood of cancer. Some veterans reported a variety of health problems and concerns attributed to exposure to this agent. The first disease associated with dioxins was the extreme skin disease chloracne, which causes acnelike pustules on the body that can and do last for several years and result in significant scarring.
- The chloracne develops a few months after swallowing, inhaling or touching the dioxin. Most cases are caused by occupational exposure, but chloracne can also develop after accidental environmental poisoning.

HIDRADENITIS SUPPURATIVA (ACNE INVERSA)

(See Chapter 5, "Superficial Bacterial Infections, Folliculitis, and Hidradenitis Suppurativa.")

- This is an acnelike condition.

Table 1.6 SYSTEMIC ANTIBIOTICS FOR ACNE, ROSACEA, AND RELATED DISORDERS

BRAND NAME	GENERIC NAME	DELIVERY	COMMON STARTING DOSE
Tetracycline Generic	Tetracycline	Capsules	250 or 500 mg twice a day
Doxycycline Generic	Doxycycline	Capsules, tablets, liquid	50, 75, 100 mg twice a day
Adoxa	Doxycycline hyclate	Tablets	75 or 100 mg twice a day
Oracea	Doxycycline (subantimicrobial)	Capsules	40 mg per day
Minocycline Generic	Minocycline		50, 75, or 100 mg twice a day
Solodyn	Minocycline	Tablets	1 mg/kg per day
		Extended-release tablets	45, 90, 135 mg once daily
Minocin	Minocycline	Capsules, oral suspension	50 or 100 mg twice a day
Dynacin	Minocycline	Capsules, tablets	50 or 100 mg twice a day

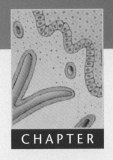

Eczema

OVERVIEW

Despite being the most common inflammatory skin condition, eczema is the most confusing skin ailment for both patients and their nondermatologic health care providers. Eczema is very difficult to define. United States Supreme Court Justice Potter Stewart once said that he could not define pornography, but he knew it when he saw it. Such is the case with eczema, a condition that is best understood through repeated viewing.

The word *eczema* was coined by the Ancient Greeks to mean "a boiling out or over." Conceivably, Greeks viewed certain rashes as boiling out or erupting from under the skin. As a case in point, the acute eczematous eruption of poison ivy often manifests with a fiery red color and a linear, blistered appearance, suggesting an acute boiling, bubbling, second-degree burn.

Terminologic confusion may also arise if the word *dermatitis*—a more generalized, often vague designation that refers to all cutaneous conditions with inflammation—is used synonymously with eczema or is coupled with it. In general, it is acceptable to use *eczema* and *dermatitis* interchangeably. *Eczematous dermatitis*, therefore, is somewhat redundant, although some might argue that the term is more inclusive than either word alone. The diversity of clinical images presented in this chapter is indicative of the protean clinical appearance of eczema.

Histopathology

On a microscopic level, an eczematous epidermis contains intercellular and intracellular fluid that appears in a sponge-like formation (spongiosis).Vasodilatation of the dermis also occurs. These abnormalities result in the clinical manifestations of acute eczema: edema, erythema, vesicles, and bullae (e.g., from poison ivy).

Later, the epidermis thickens (acanthosis) and retains nuclei (parakeratosis), and an abundant cellular infiltrate develops in the dermis. These changes account for the scale and lichenification (see following) of chronic eczema (e.g., chronic lichenified atopic dermatitis).

Acute, Subacute, and Chronic Eczema

In reference to eczema, the designators *acute, subacute,* and *chronic* are somewhat arbitrary because they describe parts of a dynamic spectrum. A patient can present with lesions in any or all of the phases.

The following clinical presentations of eczema or associated conditions are discussed in this chapter:

➤ ATOPIC DERMATITIS (ATOPIC ECZEMA)

➤ CONTACT DERMATITIS AND DIAPER DERMATITIS

➤ CHRONIC HAND ECZEMA AND DYSHIDROTIC ECZEMA

➤ NUMMULAR ECZEMA

➤ LICHEN SIMPLEX CHRONICUS

➤ PRURIGO NODULARIS

➤ ASTEATOTIC ECZEMA

➤ NEUROTIC EXCORIATIONS

➤ NONSPECIFIC ECZEMATOUS DERMATITIS

➤ SEBORRHEIC DERMATITIS

➤ STASIS DERMATITIS

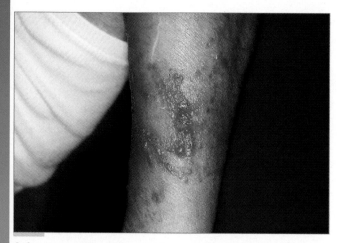

2.1 *Acute allergic eczematous eruption of poison ivy.* The red color and linear blistered appearance suggest an acute "boiling," bubbling, second-degree burn.

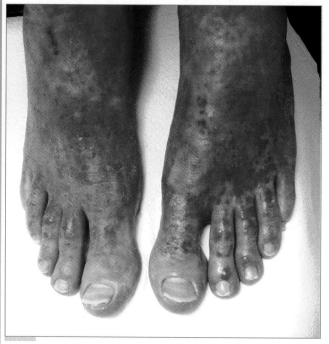

2.2 *Subacute eczema.* The crusts, scales, and erythema of subacute eczema are less intense than those seen in acute eczema.

Acute eczema is manifested by itchy erythematous patches, plaques, or papules that may become "juicy" and develop into vesicobullous lesions (FIG. 2.1). Alternatively, acute eczema may originate and continue as a less florid, non-vesicular, erythematous eruption.

Subacute eczema is an intermediate stage between acute and chronic eczema. The term has little clinical value. It is best simply to be aware that acute oozing lesions dry into crusts (scabs; FIG. 2.2), and they can later develop scales that overlie an erythematous base. Subacute eczema may become chronic, resolve spontaneously, or resolve with treatment.

Chronic eczema is also known as *chronic eczematous dermatitis.* Its hallmark is lichenification—plaque with an exaggeration or hypertrophy of the normal skin markings. Lichenification resembles the bark on a tree trunk; or, as implied, the skin appears lichenlike. (FIG. 2.3). In addition, scale and hemorrhagic crusts can result from scratched or drying vesicles. Older lesions may exhibit postinflammatory pigment alterations (PIPA), i.e., hyperpigmentation and/or hypopigmentation (FIG. 2.4).

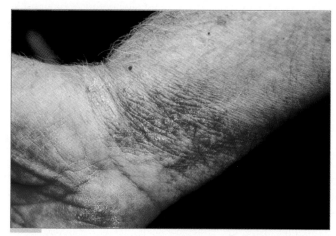

2.3 *Chronic eczematous dermatitis.* This patient shows lichenification, an exaggeration of skin markings, which was caused by repeated scratching.

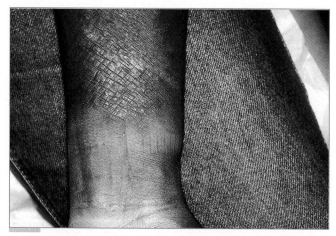

2.4 *Chronic eczematous dermatitis.* This lesion shows no evidence of active inflammation. Lichenification and postinflammatory hyperpigmentation are apparent.

Atopic Dermatitis (Atopic Eczema)

See also Chapter 27, "Special Considerations in the Skin of Pediatric and Elderly Patients."

BASICS

- Atopic dermatitis, also known as atopic eczema or endogenous eczema, is the most commonly seen type of eczema (FIGS. 2.5–2.9). It is a chronic, inflammatory, itchy skin condition with an unpredictable course of flares and remissions that affects an estimated 5% to 10% of the United States population. Atopic dermatitis is the most frequently seen skin condition among patients of Asian descent.
- By definition, atopic dermatitis occurs in association with a personal or family history of hay fever, asthma, allergic rhinitis, sinusitis, or atopic dermatitis itself. A probing history taking is often necessary to uncover symptoms of atopy. For example, patients should be asked whether they or their family members are allergic to pollen, dust, house dust mites, ragweed, dogs, or cats. Inquiries should be made about chronic recurrent symptoms that suggest atopy, such as nasal pruritus and rhinitis, rhinorrhea, paroxysmal sneezing, or itchy or irritated eyes. A personal or family history of allergies to multiple medications is also important. Furthermore, secondary relatives (aunts, uncles, cousins, and grandparents) may have an atopic predisposition.
- Most cases begin in childhood (often in infancy); however, atopic dermatitis may start at *any* age. The disease frequently remits spontaneously—reportedly in 40% to 50% of children—but it may return in adolescence or adulthood and possibly persist for a lifetime. Traditionally, patients and their families were advised that children "will grow out of eczema"; however, this optimistic prognosis is not always realized.

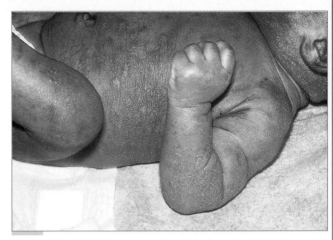

2.6 *Atopic dermatitis.* Lesions are widespread in this infant.

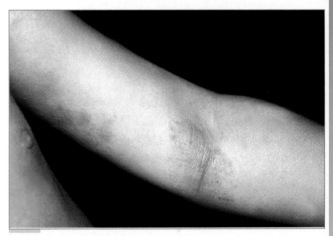

2.7 *Atopic dermatitis.* Antecubital involvement in a 2-year-old child.

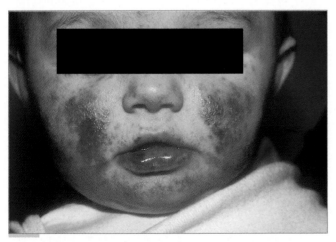

2.5 *Atopic dermatitis.* The cheeks are a typical location in an infant.

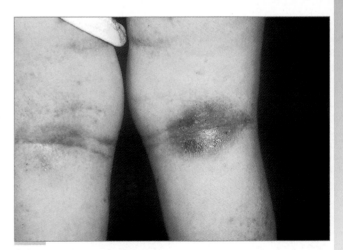

2.8 *Atopic dermatitis.* Popliteal involvement is apparent in this toddler.

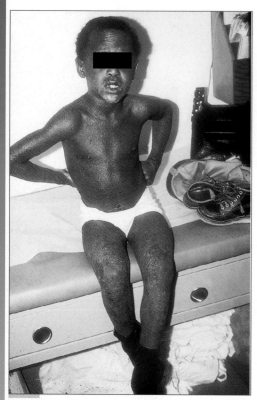

2.9 *Atopic dermatitis, generalized.* Note the marked postinflammatory hyperpigmentation in this African-American child.

- Children with asthma—an increasing population in the inner cities of the United States—appear to have a higher prevalence of atopic dermatitis than do other children; atopic dermatitis often manifests in asthmatic children in a more extensive and chronic form. African-Americans and Asians, particularly those living in an urban setting, tend to develop atopic dermatitis at an earlier age. Severe eczema in childhood portends a worse prognosis in adulthood.
- Atopic dermatitis can present with a wide spectrum of severity. Some patients may have only a mild, recurrent, localized, itchy rash on "dry" or "sensitive" skin; others may experience a more severe, extensive eruption that can be accompanied by unremitting pruritus, sleepless nights, secondary cutaneous bacterial or viral infections, embarrassing alligatorlike lichenification, and, rarely, an exfoliative erythroderma. Many patients with atopic dermatitis have multiple accompanying atopic ailments, as mentioned earlier.
- In addition to the physical discomfort of atopic dermatitis, patients may suffer from embarrassment about the appearance of lesions. Psychosocial problems, such as poor self-image, anger, and frustration, may lead to depression and social isolation.

Pathogenesis

- Atopic dermatitis is an inherited type I (immunoglobulin E–mediated) hypersensitivity disorder of the skin. In comparison with normal skin, atopic skin tends to be more prone to irritation, dryness, barrier abnormalities, and infection; it is also more likely to be negatively influenced by emotional stress.
- The intense itching of atopic dermatitis is presumed to be produced by the release of vasoactive substances from sensitized mast cells and basophils in the dermis. **The itching may be initiated by external agents such as woolen or synthetic fabrics; certain foods; alcohol; and overexposure to dry, cold weather or to very hot, humid conditions that predispose to sweating.** Less commonly, pruritus has been reported to be triggered by house dust mites. There is considerable debate about whether atopic dermatitis is primarily an allergen-induced disease or, rather, an inflammatory skin disorder found in association with respiratory allergy or other atopic symptoms. Individuals find that an allergic condition is permanent, whereas they often outgrow atopic dermatitis; this supports the latter explanation.
- Even though atopic dermatitis frequently remits spontaneously, patients, their families, and their health care providers—in particular, pediatricians and allergists—often relentlessly search for external sources that patients can avoid or eliminate from their environments. Avoidance of milk products and food preservatives and extreme dietary restrictions are not only very difficult to maintain on an ongoing basis, but they may also incite developmental problems in growing children; furthermore, they rarely, if ever, offer a cure.

DESCRIPTION OF LESIONS

- Although the character and distribution of the skin eruption tend to vary according to the patient's age, the different phases of atopic dermatitis are not always clearly distinct.
- Any or all manifestations of atopic dermatitis may exist in a single patient.

Infantile Phase

- In patients aged 2 months to 2 years, the face (particularly the cheeks; see FIG. 2.5) scalp, chest, neck, and extensor extremities are most often involved. The eruption may become generalized (see FIG. 2.6). In many cases, atopic dermatitis first manifests with severe "cradle cap" or severe recalcitrant intertriginous (groin, neck, axillae) rashes.
- As the patient approaches age 2, the flexor creases become involved. Lesions consist of scaly, red, and, occasionally, oozing plaques that tend to be symmetric (see FIGS. 2.7 and 2.8).

Childhood Phase

- Lesions seen in children aged 2 through 12 years tend to become lichenified because of repeated rubbing and scratching.
- Lichenification occurs more commonly in Asian and African-American patients than in Caucasian patients (see FIG. 2.9).
- The hallmark of atopic dermatitis is pruritus; children who have atopic dermatitis are typically very "busy" and cannot often sit quietly because of the pruritus.

Distribution of Lesions

- Lesions tend to occur symmetrically, with a characteristic distribution in the flexural folds: the antecubital and popliteal fossae and the neck, wrists, and ankles.
- Lesions may also occur on the eyelids, lips, scalp, and behind the ears.

Adolescent and Adult Phase

In adolescents and adults, lichenified plaques are generally prominent and tend to blend into surrounding normal skin. Postinflammatory hyperpigmentary and hypopigmentary changes may be seen (FIG. 2.10). Alternatively, lesions may consist of small, itchy, erythematous papules (e.g., follicular eczema; FIG. 2.11) or vesicles on the hands (e.g., dyshidrotic eczema; see below).

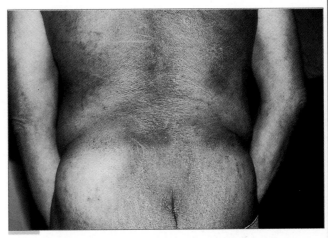

2.10 *Atopic dermatitis.* In this adult, the lichenified plaques tend to blend into the surrounding normal skin. Postinflammatory hyperpigmentation is seen here.

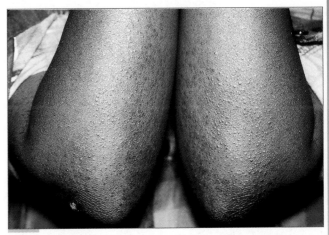

2.11 *Atopic dermatitis, follicular eczema.* Atopic dermatitis of the hair follicles. Note the gridlike pattern of follicular papules. This is a common presentation in African-American patients.

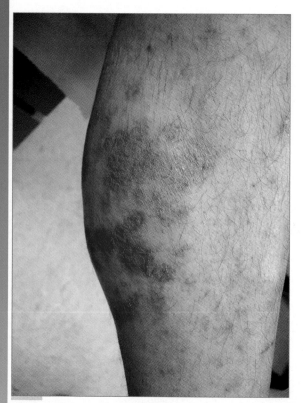

2.12 **_Atopic dermatitis._** Lesions in this patient resemble both nummular and asteatotic eczema (see FIGS. 2.40 and 2.52).

Distribution of Lesions

The distribution of lesions may be similar to that seen in childhood (i.e., in the flexural folds). However, lesions may also appear in extensor locations: the dorsa of the hands, wrists, shins (FIG. 2.12), ankles, and feet, and the nape of the neck (FIG. 2.13). On the other hand, lesions may be limited to the lips (atopic cheilitis; FIG. 2.14); eyelids; vulvar or scrotal areas (FIGS. 2.15 and 2.16, respectively); or hands (as in chronic hand eczema or dyshidrotic eczema; see below), which may be the only features of atopic dermatitis in some adults. Nail dystrophy occurs when the proximal nail fold and the underlying nail matrix (root) are involved (FIG. 2.17).

OTHER CLINICAL ASPECTS

Additional associated features and findings that are clues to the diagnosis of atopic dermatitis include the following:

- Persistent xerosis, or dry, "sensitive" skin.
- Dennie–Morgan lines. These comprise a characteristic double fold that extends from the inner to the outer canthus of the lower eyelid (FIG. 2.18).
- "Allergic shiners." This term refers to a darkened, violaceous, or tan coloring in the periorbital areas. Along with Dennie–Morgan lines, this dark coloring may be an instant clue to the diagnosis of atopic dermatitis (FIG. 2.19).
- Hyperlinear palmar creases (FIG. 2.20).

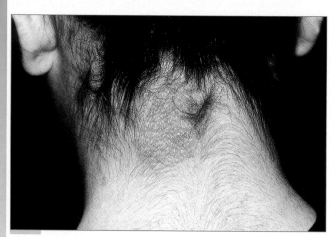

2.13 **_Atopic dermatitis, lichen simplex chronicus._** The nape of the neck is a common site of involvement.

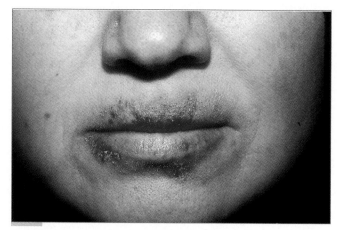

2.14 **_Atopic cheilitis (atopic dermatitis of the lips)._** Note the lichenification and the ill-defined outline of the vermilion border of the upper lip.

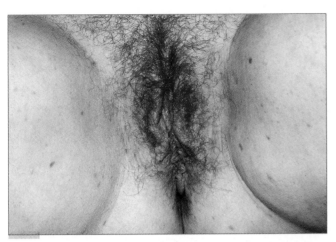

2.15 *Atopic dermatitis limited to the vulvar and inguinal areas.* This eruption was initially diagnosed and treated as a fungal infection by the patient's health care provider.

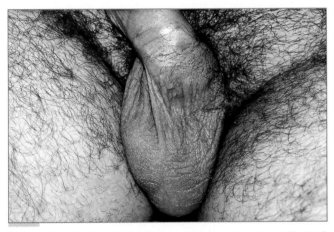

2.16 *Atopic dermatitis (lichen simplex chronicus) limited to the scrotum.* This patient was also initially thought to have tinea cruris. Note the lichenification.

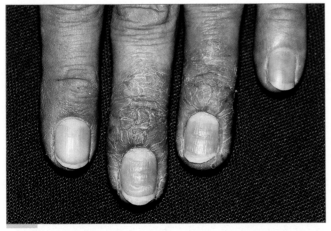

2.17 *Atopic dermatitis.* This patient's middle fingernails show dystrophic changes, transverse ridging, and cuticle loss solely on those fingers where eczema is present in the proximal nail folds.

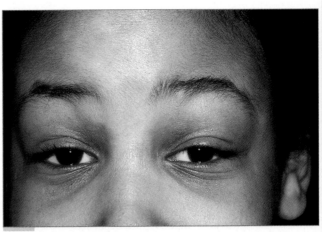

2.18 *Atopic dermatitis, periorbital.* Note lichenification and the characteristic double fold (Dennie-Morgan line) that extends from the inner to the outer canthus of the lower eyelid and the "allergic shiners," the darkening color of the periorbital areas.

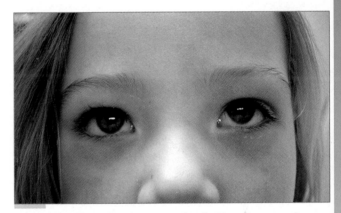

2.19 *Atopic dermatitis, periorbital.* The presence of "allergic shiners"—a darkened or violaceous hue, as in this child—is a clue to the diagnosis of atopic dermatitis.

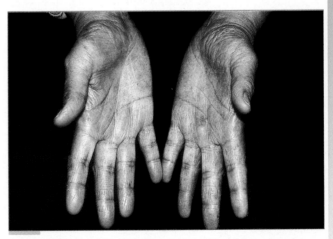

2.20 *Atopic dermatitis.* Hyperlinearity of the palms is evident here.

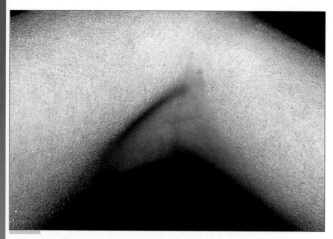

2.21 Ichthyosis vulgaris. Lesions resemble fish scales. Note the characteristic sparing of the popliteal creases.

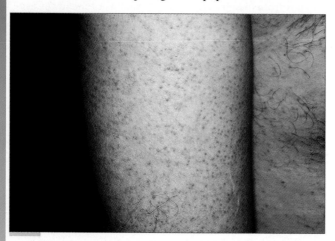

2.22 Keratosis pilaris. This teenager has tiny, rough-textured, red, follicular papules on his lateral upper arms.

Other associated dermatoses include the following:

- Ichthyosis vulgaris. This condition is frequently associated with atopy. Lesions, which are most apparent on the shins, resemble fine fish scales. Characteristically, the flexor creases are spared in this condition (FIG. 2.21).
- Keratosis pilaris. These tiny, horny, rough-textured, whitish or red, follicular papules or pustules occur most often during adolescence. Most commonly, keratosis pilaris is noted on the deltoid and posterolateral upper arms, the upper back and thighs, and the malar area of the face. It is frequently confused with acne (FIG. 2.22).

CLINICAL MANIFESTATIONS AND POSSIBLE COMPLICATIONS

- Pruritus may interfere with sleep. Itching is increased by repeated scratching and rubbing, which leads to lichenification, oozing, and secondary bacterial infection (impetiginization, or "honey-crusted skin").
- Secondary infection with *Staphylococcus aureus* may trigger relapses of atopic dermatitis.
- Secondary infections with herpes simplex virus may result in eczema herpeticum (Kaposi's varicelliform eruption), which is more commonly seen in childhood.

DIAGNOSIS

- Diagnosis of atopic dermatitis depends on excluding conditions such as fungal infections, seborrheic dermatitis, psoriasis, scabies, contact dermatitis, ichthyosis, and cutaneous T-cell lymphoma.

DDx DIFFERENTIAL DIAGNOSIS

- The diagnosis of atopic dermatitis is generally not difficult, especially in patients with an atopic history in whom the following causes of eczema or eczemalike eruptions have been excluded.

Contact Dermatitis
(See later in this chapter).

- Determine whether the patient was exposed to a substance that could cause contact dermatitis. The location of the lesions may suggest an external cause.

Scabies
(See Chapter 20, "Bites, Stings, and Infestations.")

- A history of exposure is important in diagnosing scabies.
- Symptoms are present in other household members.
- Characteristic distribution (e.g., in the webs between the fingers and on the flexor wrists) can mimic that of eczema.

- A positive scabies scraping is diagnostic of scabies.

Psoriasis
See Chapter 3, "Psoriasis."

- Lesions generally appear on extensor locations—the elbows, knees, and other large joints—rather than on flexor creases.
- Patients may have a positive family history of psoriasis.
- Usually, psoriasis is less pruritic than eczema.
- Psoriatic lesions tend to be clearly demarcated from normal surrounding skin, and the scale of psoriasis tends to be thicker and micaceous in appearance. However, psoriasis may at times be clinically indistinguishable from atopic dermatitis.

Tinea Pedis, Corporis, Manuum, and Capitis
(See Chapter 7, "Superficial Fungal Infections.")

- A positive potassium hydroxide (KOH) test or fungal culture result indicates these conditions.

MANAGEMENT

Topical Steroid Therapy

See also "Introduction: Topical Therapy."

General Principles

- The application of an appropriately chosen topical steroid usually results in prompt improvement in most patients with atopic dermatitis.
- Topical steroids should be used only as short-term therapy, if possible, and only to treat active disease (i.e., with itching and erythema).
- Topical steroids should not be used for prevention of future lesions or for cosmetic concerns, such as postinflammatory hyperpigmentation.
- "Stronger" is often preferable to "longer" in the use of topical steroids, because long-term application is more often associated with side effects.
- Without question, the use of a superpotent topical steroid is preferable to the administration of a systemic steroid, with its potential side effects.
- When the condition is under control, the frequency of application and the potency of the topical steroids are reduced ("downward titration"), or the agents are discontinued.

Face and Body Folds

- For the face and intertriginous regions (the axillae and inguinal creases are areas that are "naturally" occluded), treatment should be initiated with a low-potency (class 7) cream or ointment, such as over-the-counter (OTC) **hydrocortisone 0.5% or 1%.**
- In more severe cases of atopic dermatitis, initial therapy may be with a more potent steroid, followed by a less potent preparation for maintenance. For example, a higher-potency (class 5) agent, such as **hydrocortisone valerate 0.2% cream,** could be used for 2 or 3 days, followed by a lower-potency (class 6) agent, such as **desonide 0.05%** or OTC **hydrocortisone 0.5% to 1%,** which is then used for maintenance as needed.

Body

- For nonintertriginous areas of the body, treatment can be initiated with a mid-strength (class 4) cream or ointment, such as **triamcinolone acetonide 0.1%,** or a mid-strength (class 3) agent, such as **fluocinonide 0.05%.** Even a superpotent (class 1) agent, such as **clobetasol 0.05%,** may be used for limited periods (no more than 2 weeks) until control is achieved. Then therapy may be switched to a lower-potency (class 5) agent, such as **hydrocortisone valerate 0.2%. Fluticasone 0.05%** cream **(Cutivate)** is another lower-potency agent that has been shown to be effective as maintenance therapy when it is used twice weekly.

- Ointments are helpful for dry skin. Because of their occlusive properties, they are more lubricating than other formulations. They also tend to be less irritating and less sensitizing. Their popularity increases in colder, drier weather. For patients with widespread skin involvement, a **1-lb jar of triamcinolone acetonide cream** or **ointment** 0.1% is quite economical.

Infection

- If necessary, topical steroids can be given concurrently with systemic antibiotics. This combination is sometimes helpful if evidence of coexisting staphylococcal or streptococcal infection ("impetiginization") of the skin is present. Oral antibiotics such as **cephalexin** or **dicloxacillin** are commonly used. Also, tetracycline derivatives, which may be prescribed in patients over 10 years of age, are effective.
- During flare-ups, the acute, open, weeping, crusted lesions that develop from infection or scratching may be treated with a drying antibacterial agent, such as **Burow's solution,** before topical steroids are applied.
- **Clorox bleach**—1 to 2 teaspoonfuls per tubful of water, which can be increased up to 6 teaspoonfuls added to daily bath water—is a quite effective and inexpensive alternative to topical and oral antibiotics.
- Another topical option is topical 2% mupirocin cream **(Bactroban)** or ointment **(Centany).**

Topical Immunomodulator Therapy

- Currently, these drugs are indicated for the short-term or intermittent treatment of atopic dermatitis and are considered as second-line therapy when conventional therapies are inadvisable, ineffective, or not tolerated. Photoprotection is advised when using these agents, although no evidence so far has implicated them in promoting skin cancer.
- For information regarding the long-term safety of these agents, see "Introduction: Topical Therapy."
- **Protopic ointment** (tacrolimus) is a nonsteroidal immunomodulator that has been shown to reduce the symptoms of atopic dermatitis. It is used as an alternative to topical steroids, particularly when the eruption involves the face or intertriginous areas, such as the axillae and groin, where the long-term use of high-potency steroids is limited. **Protopic** has potential as a topical steroid–sparing agent.
  - When applied twice daily, **Protopic** may cause transient side effects, such as burning and itching. This burning and itching may result in patients' refusal to continue applying the medication.
  - It is available as an ointment in 0.1% and 0.03% concentrations.

continued on page 58

- The 0.1% concentration has been approved for the treatment of atopic dermatitis in adults.
- The 0.03% concentration is designated for short-term and intermittent long-term treatment of atopic dermatitis in children (age 2 years and older) and in adults.
- **Elidel cream (pimecrolimus),** in a 1% cream base, is less likely to be irritating, and it is not as greasy as Protopic ointment.

Other Therapeutic Measures

- Oral H_1 antihistamines such as diphenhydramine (**Benadryl**) and hydroxyzine (**Atarax**) probably do not reduce itching, but they are sometimes useful as inducers of sleep, an unacceptable side effect for many patients.
- Oozing, exudative lesions may be soothed and dried with Burow's solution or by bathing in a tub with antipruritic emollients, such as an Aveeno oatmeal bath preparation.
- Sun exposure, ideally in the early morning and late afternoon—when humidity is lowest—may significantly improve atopic dermatitis in selected patients.
- When a patient does not have access to natural sunlight, phototherapy with ultraviolet B rays and, less commonly, ultraviolet A rays, is often very effective for widespread skin involvement.
- Less commonly used today, tar baths, as well as tar preparations formulated as ointments, pastes, and gels, may be used concurrently with topical steroids or alternated with them. (Before the advent of topical steroids, tar preparations were the mainstay of treatment.)
- Emotional stress in patients or in their families may contribute to atopic dermatitis. Measures to reduce stress include support groups and family psychotherapy.
- Before resorting to systemic steroids, a "soak and smear" regimen may be used. (See Introduction, "Topical Therapy.")
- Systemic steroids, immunosuppressive therapy with systemic agents such as **cyclosporine,** or short-term hospitalization is sometimes necessary in patients with severe unresponsive generalized atopic dermatitis.
- For patients with secondary herpes simplex infection (Kaposi's varicelliform eruption), oral antiviral therapy and possibly hospitalization may be required.

Unsuccessful Treatments

- Treatments that do not seem to improve atopic dermatitis include vitamins, mineral or dietary supplements, and other nutritional supplements.
- Topical ointments that include diphenhydramine and doxepin are potential contact allergens and thus are contraindicated.

General Management
Bathing

How often the person who has atopic dermatitis should bathe has been the subject of controversy and misunderstanding. There are many reasons not to restrict frequent bathing:

- Bathing removes crusts, irritants, potential allergens, and infectious agents.
- Bathing provides pleasure and reduces stress.
- Bathing hydrates the skin and allows better delivery of corticosteroids and moisturizers.
- The addition of **Clorox bleach** to bath water ("bleach baths") can be effective (see earlier discussion) for oozing or infected atopic dermatitis.

Bathing Tips

- Mild, moisturizing soaps such as **Dove** or nonsoap cleansers such as **Cetaphil Lotion** should be used.
- The patient should be cautioned not to use soap on lesional skin (many people are erroneously led to believe that scrubbing with "good soaps" may actually help inflamed skin).
- Excessive bathing that is not followed immediately by application of a moisturizer tends to dry the skin.
- Excessive toweling and scrubbing should be avoided.

Prevention of Atopic Dermatitis

The following measures may help the patient to avoid or reduce exposure to triggers such as dry skin, irritants, overheating and sweating, and allergens.

- **Dry skin:** Moisturizers, particularly in the dry winter months, should be applied immediately after bathing to "trap" water in the skin. However, in warm climates or in the summer, moisturizers may actually be irritating or may interfere with healing.
  - Suggested ointments: **Vaseline Petroleum Jelly, Aquaphor**
  - Suggested creams and lotions: **Eucerin, Cetaphil, Lubriderm, Curel, Moisturel**
- **Barrier repair:** Atopiclair, MimyX, and **Epiceram** are multiple-ingredient prescription, nonsteroidal barrier creams that are applied two or three times per day. Their efficacy as topical steroid–sparing agents has been suggested by several studies. The barrier cream and lotion **CeraVe** can be purchased OTC.
- **Irritants:** Nonirritating fabrics, such as cotton, should be worn. Wool clothing may induce itching.
- **Overheating and sweating:** Excess dryness or humidity should be avoided. An air conditioner or humidifier in a child's bedroom may help to avoid the dramatic changes in climate that may trigger outbreaks.

continued on page 59

MANAGEMENT *Continued*

(Unfortunately, humidifiers do not seem to help very much.)

- **Allergens:** Some evidence indicates that the environmental elimination of certain airborne substances, such as house dust mites, may bring some lasting relief. A great deal of controversy surrounds the influence of dietary manipulation and the value of skin testing and hyposensitization on the course of atopic dermatitis. Although some foods may provoke attacks, elimination of them rarely brings a lasting improvement or cure. Skin tests and allergy shots may actually provoke attacks of atopic dermatitis.

 SEE PATIENT HANDOUTS, "Burow's Solution" and "Soak and Smear Instruction Sheet" ON THE SOLUTION SITE

 POINTS TO REMEMBER

- Topical steroids should be applied only to active disease (inflamed skin).
- When topical steroids are applied immediately after bathing, their penetration and potency are increased.
- Low-potency topical steroids are recommended for use on the face and in skin folds, such as the perineal area and underarms.
- A very small number of children show some clinical improvement after measures to control house dust mites are instituted.
- "Soak and smear" therapy can often be substituted for, or limit the use of, systemic steroids.

 HELPFUL HINTS

- There are primarily two causes of eczema: one comes from the *outside* (contact dermatitis), and the other comes from the *inside* (atopic dermatitis).
- Patients and their parents, caregivers, and teachers should be educated about the manifestations and management of atopic dermatitis.
- The "gooiest" and cheapest moisturizer is petrolatum.
- The National Eczema Association can be contacted at:
  - 415-499-3474 or 800-818-7546
  - 4460 Redwood Highway, Suite 16-D, San Rafael, CA 94903-1953
  - info@nationaleczema.org or http://www.nationaleczema.org

 SEE PATIENT HANDOUT "Atopic Dermatitis" ON THE SOLUTION SITE

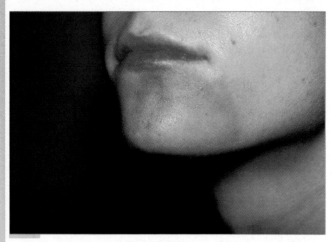

2.23 *Irritant contact dermatitis.* The localized erythema on this boy's face was caused by irritation from benzoyl peroxide in an acne preparation.

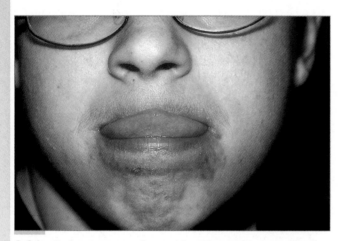

2.24 *Irritant contact dermatitis.* The erythema and scaling are obviously secondary to this child's habit of licking her lips.

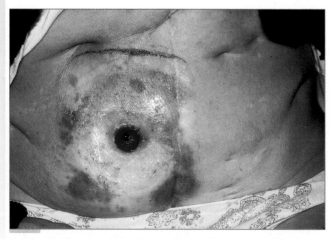

2.25 **Irritant contact dermatitis.** Chronic irritation from a stoma was the cause of this reaction.

Contact dermatitis is an inflammatory reaction of the skin that is caused by an external agent. The appearance of the eruption and a careful history often give clues to the offending agent. The two types of contact dermatitis are *irritant* and *allergic.*

IRRITANT CONTACT DERMATITIS

Also known as nonallergic contact dermatitis, irritant contact dermatitis (ICD) is an erythematous, scaly, sometimes eczematous eruption that is not caused by allergens (Figs. 2.23 and 2.24). A direct toxic reaction to rubbing, friction, or maceration, or to exposure to a chemical or thermal agent, the severity of ICD depends on the concentration of the irritant, its thermal energy, its abrasiveness, and the duration of exposure, among other factors. ICD may occur in anyone.

The eruption of ICD is confined to the areas of exposure, as exemplified by diaper rash, "dishpan hands," and reactions that occur under an adhesive dressing (Fig. 2.25) or where a topical medication was applied. Examples of irritants include alkalis, acids, solvents, soaps, detergents, and numerous chemicals found in the home and workplace that damage the skin after repeated contact. Patients who have atopic dermatitis are more likely to develop ICD as a result of their inherent skin sensitivity and defective barrier function.

Diagnosis, when not clearly evident, is based on a careful history and the ruling out of allergic contact dermatitis (ACD), which is discussed later. Management is fairly simple: Patients should be told to avoid the offending agent or to minimize contact with it.

Diaper Dermatitis (Diaper Rash)

BASICS

- A common example of ICD is diaper dermatitis (diaper rash), referred to as "napkin dermatitis" in the United Kingdom. Diaper dermatitis applies to eruptions that occur in the area covered by a diaper. It can first present as early as the first few weeks of life or occur any time when diapers are worn.
- Irritant diaper dermatitis is by far the most common rash in infancy, but it is not restricted to that age group because it can affect persons of any age group who wear diapers, such as incontinent patients.

Pathogenesis

- Diaper dermatitis is essentially the result of overhydration of the skin that is irritated by chafing, by soaps and detergents, and by prolonged contact with urine and feces. The ammonia that is produced as a breakdown product of urea by bacteria in feces is considered an exacerbating factor.
- Added to this wet, macerated, excrement-laden milieu are the occlusive effect of rubber or plastic diapers and the constant contact with moisture from cloth diapers when they are not changed as soon as possible.

- Diaper dermatitis may also be caused by, or intensified by, the presence of atopic dermatitis, seborrheic dermatitis, or a secondary infection by *Candida albicans*. (*C. albicans* is often isolated from the perineal area in many of these infants; whether it is the cause or effect of the rash is controversial.)

CLINICAL MANIFESTATIONS AND DESCRIPTION OF LESIONS

- Erythema, scale, and possibly papules and plaques are present; occasionally, vesicles and bullae occur.
- With neglect, lesions may erode and ulcerate.
- "Beefy" redness and satellite papules and pustules suggest a primary or secondary infection of diaper dermatitis with *C. albicans*.

DISTRIBUTION OF LESIONS

- Lesions typically spare the creases (genitocrural folds) because such areas do not come into direct contact with the diaper (FIG. 2.26). Primary candidal diaper dermatitis should be considered in an immunocompromised patient, particularly if the creases are involved.
- The eruption may conform to, and be limited to, the diaper area, and it may also affect the lower abdomen, genitalia, perineum, and buttocks.

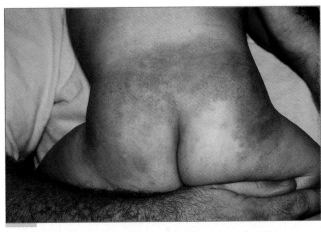

2.26 *Irritant contact dermatitis. Diaper rash.* The eruption conforms to the shape of the diaper.

 DIFFERENTIAL DIAGNOSIS

During infancy, the various causes of diaper dermatitis such as ICD, atopic dermatitis, seborrheic dermatitis, and psoriasis may be indistinguishable.

Atopic Dermatitis

- Atopic dermatitis. In general, patients with atopic dermatitis are more likely to experience ICD; nonetheless, the diaper area is often remarkably spared (FIG. 2.27). Other evidence of atopic dermatitis, such as involvement of the face and extensor areas, may be present, and the patient may have a family history of atopy.

Seborrheic Dermatitis

- Seborrheic dermatitis (intertriginous seborrheic dermatitis) (see "Seborrheic dermatitis" later in this chapter). The creases are involved, and the patient may have lesions elsewhere, such as the axillae or scalp ("cradle cap").

Other less common conditions to consider are tinea cruris, impetigo, child abuse (severe or repeated ulcerations), Kawasaki's disease, and psoriasis, particularly if there is a positive family history or other evidence of psoriasis. In addition, other rare diseases such as Letterer-Siwe disease (a form of Langerhans cell histiocytosis) and acrodermatitis enteropathica (from zinc deficiency) should be considered in recalcitrant cases. Leiner's disease is a very rare eruption resembling seborrheic dermatitis that is associated with diarrhea and a failure to thrive.

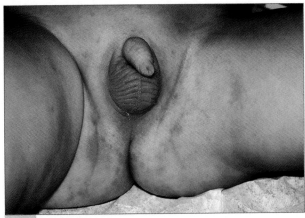

2.27 *Atopic dermatitis.* Note involvement of the inguinal creases.

MANAGEMENT

General preventive measures to minimize friction, absorb moisture, and protect the skin from urine and feces include the following:

- The use of disposable or superabsorbent diapers holds moisture in and keeps it away from the skin.
- The diaper area should be dried gently after changing and aired out.
- Frequent diaper changes should be made promptly after voiding or soiling.
- It is sometimes recommended that the diaper area remain uncovered for long periods of time; however, this is quite impractical for most parents. Such an uncovered approach should be reserved when nonhealing erosions and ulcerations are present.
- Rubber and plastic pants should be avoided.
- Soap-free cleansers such as **Cetaphil Lotion** are recommended.
- Absorbent baby powders such as **Desitin** cornstarch powder, **Zeasorb powder,** and **Johnson's Baby Powder** are useful.
- **Aquaphor ointment** and pure white petrolatum ointment (**Vaseline Petroleum Jelly**) act by trapping water beneath the epidermis.

Specific Treatment Measures
- The first-line therapy is **zinc oxide ointment.** There are many inexpensive OTC products that contain zinc oxide,

such as **Balmex, Desitin,** and **A+D ointment.** They should be applied thickly.
- Petrolatum, zinc oxide, aluminum acetate solution (**1-2-3 Paste**) is a "tried and true" combination product that both protects skin and has a drying effect. It should be applied after each diaper change.
- Low-potency OTC **hydrocortisone 1%** or **0.05% cream** or **ointment** is often all that is necessary for uncomplicated diaper dermatitis.
- Stronger topical steroids (class 6) such as **desonide 0.05%** or **hydrocortisone valerate 0.02%** cream (class 5) or ointment (class 4) may be used for very short periods (1 to 4 days), if necessary.
- **Potent topical steroids, particularly fluorinated preparations such as those contained in Lotrisone, are to be avoided in the diaper area.**
- If the presence of *C. albicans* is suspected, particularly if there is no improvement after several days, a topical antifungal preparation such as the OTC miconazole (**Micatin**) may help; **Vusion ointment** (0.25% miconazole combined with 15% zinc oxide) is another option that is available only with a prescription.
- Consider adding nonabsorbable **oral nystatin** in recalcitrant cases.

 POINTS TO REMEMBER

- Most cases are caused by irritation (ICD).
- Avoid the use of high-potency topical steroids in the diaper area.
- Educate parents and caregivers to change diapers frequently, to wash the patient's genitalia with warm water and mild soap, and to use superabsorbent disposable diapers.
- Consider referral to a dermatologist, particularly in persistent, unresponsive cases.

ALLERGIC CONTACT DERMATITIS

A true allergic reaction that precipitates eczematous dermatitis, ACD is caused by an allergen (antigen) that produces a delayed (type IV) hypersensitivity reaction. It occurs only in sensitized persons. ACD is not dose dependent, and it may spread extensively beyond the site of original contact. ACD is seen less commonly in young children, the elderly, and African-Americans.

Examples of allergic contact sensitizers include jewelry, metal, cosmetics, topical medications, rubber compounds, plants, and the countless chemicals that are found in homes and work environments. The best-known example of ACD is rhus dermatitis, which is caused by poison ivy and poison oak.

Rhus Dermatitis

In the United States, poison ivy and poison oak are the principal causes of rhus dermatitis. Poison ivy is found throughout the country. Poison oak is found more commonly in the western United States. Poison sumac, another cause of rhus dermatitis, is found only in woody, swampy areas.

The three plants belong to the same genus, *Toxicodendron,* which is the "poisonous" branch of the genus *Rhus*. Each of the three plants contains pentadecylcatechol and heptadecylcatechol, the sensitizing allergens, in their resinous oils (urushiol). The plants' invisible oils may reach the skin not only through direct contact but also through garden tools, pet fur, golf clubs, or the smoke of a burning plant. Identical or related antigens are found in the resin of the Japanese lacquer tree, ginkgo trees, cashew nut shells, the dye of the India marking nut (used as a clothing dye in India), and the skin of mangoes. All cause similar skin rashes in sensitized people.

In the eastern United States, rhus dermatitis occurs mainly in the spring and summer. In the western and southeastern United States, where outdoor activity is common all year, rhus dermatitis may occur in any season. Approximately 85% of the population develops a reaction on exposure to one of the plants.

DESCRIPTION OF LESIONS

The characteristic eruptions, which consists of intensely pruritic linear streaks of erythematous papules, "juicy" vesicles, and blisters, appear to be caused by an outside agent (Fig. 2.28). The rash typically occurs 2 days after contact with the plant, but initial reactions have been noted within 12 hours of contact and as long as 1 week later.

Generally, exposed areas of the body are affected first. The rash may later involve covered areas that have come into contact with the plant oil. For example, the external vulva or perianal areas may be affected after women use toilet paper that has been contaminated by plant oil from their hands (Fig. 2.29). In men, involvement of the penis is sometimes a diagnostic sign.

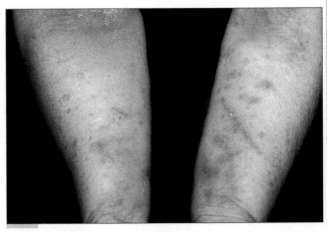

2.28 *Allergic contact dermatitis.* Poison ivy caused this fiery red eruption. Note the "outside job" appearance of the linear streaks of papules and vesicles.

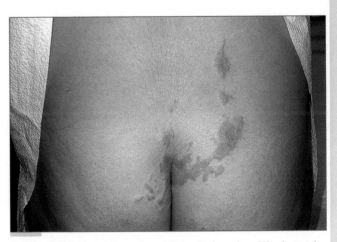

2.29 *Allergic contact dermatitis.* Poison ivy. The buttocks became involved after this patient used toilet paper that had been contaminated by the resin of poison ivy.

DIAGNOSIS

- The diagnosis of rhus dermatitis is based on history of exposure to an antigen and the characteristic distribution of the lesions. Contrary to common belief, the fluid in blisters does not contain the resinous oil, and it cannot transfer the rash to others or cause the rash to spread on the affected person.
- Further dissemination, or autoeczematization, is believed to occur through hematogenous spread and subsequent immune-complex deposition in the skin. This spread may occur within 5 to 7 days after the initial exposure, and the resulting rash may last for 3 weeks or more.

DIFFERENTIAL DIAGNOSIS

Other dermatoses that may resemble rhus dermatitis include:

Plant Dermatitis

- Reactions to meadow grass and other plants may cause atopic dermatitis.

Insect Bite Reactions

- Bites, particularly those from bedbugs, often cause a linear eruption that may occasionally be confused with rhus dermatitis.

Scabies

- In scabietic infestations, other household or family members may report itching. Scabies has its own characteristic distribution of lesions: in the finger webs, wrists, genitals, and axillae.

Herpes Zoster

- Nonpainful herpes zoster, with its linear series of blisters, can cause diagnostic confusion.

 MANAGEMENT

A limited eruption and mild itching may be relieved by the following.

- Cool showers and application of frozen vegetable packages (e.g., frozen peas) may help.
- Cool baths with colloidal oatmeal agents such as Aveeno are recommended.
- Cool compresses of Burow's solution help dry vesicles and bullae.
- Calamine lotion is useful.
- Potent or superpotent topical corticosteroids (class 1), such as **clobetasol cream 0.05%** two or three times daily.
- Oral antihistamines are helpful, particularly at bedtime. In severe cases with widespread eruption and marked pruritus, topical therapy may need to be supplemented with the following:

- Systemic corticosteroids. **Prednisone** is usually used, in a tapering dosage schedule that often starts at 1 mg/kg and decreases by 5 mg every 2 days for at least 2 weeks and for as long as 3 weeks. The dosage may be increased again if flares occur during the tapering regimen. Prednisone tablets should be taken with meals, and the entire daily dose may be taken all at once, rather than in divided doses throughout the day. (Possible side effects of short-term systemic corticosteroids include gastrointestinal upset, sleep disturbances, and mood changes. Hyperactivity, anxiety, depression, and even paranoia have been reported.)
- **Intramuscular corticosteroids. Triamcinolone diacetate** or **hexacetonide** may be used if the patient has gastrointestinal intolerance to oral corticosteroids.

 SEE PATIENT HANDOUT "Burow's Solution" ON THE SOLUTION SITE

 HELPFUL HINTS

To prevent rhus dermatitis, patients can learn to recognize its plants:

- "Leaves of three, let it be." If work or hobbies involve frequent exposure to poisonous plants, a barrier cream may be applied before exposure.
- When people come into contact with the plant or its oil, they should wash with soap and cold water as soon as possible. All exposed clothing should be laundered.
- Vaccines against poison ivy and other immunizations given orally or as injections may result in serious negative side effects and often fail.
- **Medrol Dosepaks** (methylprednisolone) usually do not provide enough days of treatment for most patients with severe rhus dermatitis.

- During the tapering prednisone regimen for treatment of severe rhus dermatitis, patients may experience a rebound of the eruption and itching. When this rebound occurs, it may be suggested that patients increase the dosage back to the one that worked the day before and then titrate downward thereafter.
- There are advantages to prescribing doses consistently in increments of 5 mg. It is easier for the patient and health care provider to keep track of the dosage schedule, and tablets usually do not have to be broken in half to decrease the dose.

Other Forms of Allergic Contact Dermatitis

Other than the poisonous *Toxicodendron* species, the most common contact allergens are nickel, thimerosal (a mercurial preservative), neomycin (a topical antibiotic), formaldehyde (found in shampoo and cosmetics), paraphenylenediamine (found in certain hair dyes), and quaternium-15 (a preservative often found in cosmetics). Patterns of distribution and shapes of the rash may serve as clues to the specific allergen, as in, for example, dermatitis from rubber in underpants (FIG. 2.30), neomycin in eardrops (FIG. 2.31), or nickel in earrings (FIG. 2.32).

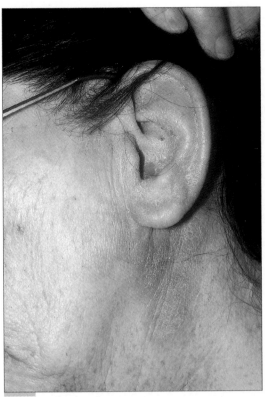

2.31 *Allergic contact dermatitis.* This contact dermatitis was caused by neomycin in this patient's ear drops.

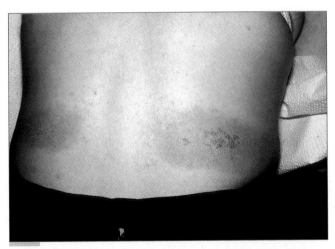

2.30 *Allergic contact dermatitis.* This patient reacted to the rubber in the elastic waistband of her underpants. Note sparing at the sites where the garment did not come into constant contact with the skin.

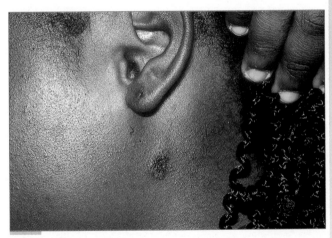

2.32 *Allergic contact dermatitis.* Nickel in earrings caused the dermatitis on the earlobe and neck of this girl, who wore long earrings.

➤ THE TOP TEN ALLERGENS

- **Nickel.** Found in jewelry, clasps, and metal buttons. ACD to nickel is more common in women than in men.
- **Gold.** Found in jewelry.
- **Balsam of Peru.** Included in perfumes and skin lotions.
- **Thimerosal.** Used as a preservative in local antiseptics and vaccines.
- **Neomycin sulfate.** Found in first aid creams and in some cosmetic products.
- **Fragrance mix.** Found in foods, cosmetics, perfumes, insecticides, dental products, etc.
- **Formaldehyde.** A preservative that is included in paper products, dry cleaning solvents, paints, and cosmetic products.
- **Cobalt chloride.** In hair dyes and metals.
- **Bacitracin.** A topical antibiotic.
- **Quaternium-15.** A preservative often found in cosmetics and industrial agents.

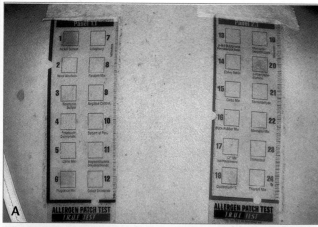

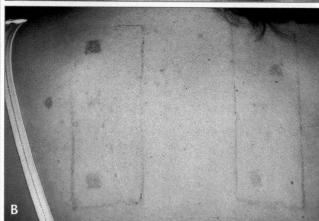

2.33 A and B *Allergic contact dermatitis.* Test patches. **A:** These test patches were removed after 48 hours. **B:** The final reading at 96 hours shows positive reactions to various allergens.

DIAGNOSIS

- Patients should be questioned regarding their daily habits and occupational exposures, so that any possible contactants can be revealed.
- Patch testing is used to identify specific allergens in patients with histories suggestive of ACD (FIGS. 2.33A–B). The allergens most commonly responsible for ACD are standardized and are available commercially. The allergens, which are fixed in dehydrated gel layers, are taped against the skin of the patient's back for 48 hours and are then removed. A final reading is performed after 96 hours. The area is examined for evidence of contact dermatitis. The presence of erythema, papules, or vesicles (i.e., an acute eczematous reaction) is strongly positive. A bullous reaction is extremely positive.
- Interpretation of patch test results and correlation with clinical findings require experience and are generally performed by dermatologists.

 DIFFERENTIAL DIAGNOSIS

Conditions to include in the differential diagnosis are the following:

- ICD
- Other types of acute and chronic eczematous dermatitis (especially atopic dermatitis)
- Systemic drug reactions

 MANAGEMENT

Patients with ACD may be managed with the following:

- Identification and removal of the inciting agent
- Advice on how to avoid the inciting agent
- Treatment with topical or systemic corticosteroids, if necessary

POINT TO REMEMBER

- Patch testing may be the only way to differentiate ACD from ICD.

HELPFUL HINT

- When an immediate reaction to a contactant occurs (i.e., visible hives develop in less than 30 minutes after exposure), this may indicate a contact urticaria (not ACD), particularly if urticarial in appearance and if associated with other symptoms such as distant urticaria, wheezing, angioedema, or anaphylaxis. Rubber latex currently is the most important source of allergic contact urticaria.

Atopic Hand Eczema (Chronic Hand Dermatitis)

BASICS

- When eczema involves the hands and is caused by exposure to an irritant or an allergic contactant, the diagnosis is contact dermatitis (see earlier).
- The onset of atopic hand eczema is uncommon before adolescence. After middle age, the frequency of acute episodes tends to decrease.
- When there is no suggestive history or documentation of an exogenous cause of hand eczema, the diagnosis is most likely atopic hand eczema (also known as chronic hand dermatitis). Most patients with atopic hand eczema report an atopic history, such as a personal or familial atopic diathesis (e.g., asthma, hay fever, sinusitis), or patients may have had a previous episode of atopic dermatitis or a concurrent manifestation elsewhere on the body. Even with these findings, a diligent history must be taken to rule out contactant etiology.
  - In addition, patch testing (see earlier in this chapter) with putative allergens may be performed if an exogenous cause is suspected.
  - It is also common for both exogenous (contact) and endogenous (atopic) factors to be at work in the same patient. Whatever the origin, hand eczema is often a cause of social embarrassment and can result in performance problems in the workplace.

DESCRIPTION OF LESIONS, CLINICAL MANIFESTATIONS, AND DISTRIBUTION OF LESIONS

For descriptive purposes, atopic hand eczema may be divided into two clinical types that may overlap in the same patient: a "wet" type and a "dry," scaly type.

"Wet" Type

Dyshidrotic eczema, the wet type (FIGS. 2.34 and 2.35), was formerly referred to as *pompholyx* (the Greek word for bubble), which describes the following:

- Itchy, clear vesicles.
- The vesicles are typically located on the sides of the fingers, but they can also occur on the palms and, less commonly, on the soles of the feet and the lateral aspects of the toes. The term "dyshidrotic" is a misnomer based on the erroneous assumption that the vesicles were caused by "trapped sweat." We now understand that they result from inflammation and foci of intercellular edema ("spongiosis"), which becomes loculated in the thicker stratum corneum of the palms and soles.
- Initially, the very small and clear vesicles resemble little bubbles.
- Later, as they dry and resolve without rupturing, they generally turn a golden brown color.
- Secondary *impetiginization* may occur.

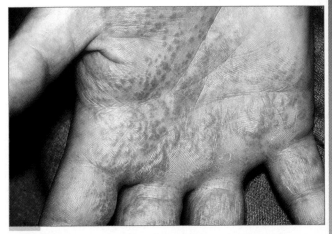

2.34 *Atopic hand eczema, dyshidrotic or "wet" type.* The characteristic vesicles (pompholyx) are apparent in this patient's palm.

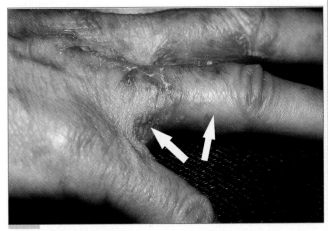

2.35 *Atopic hand eczema, dyshidrotic or "wet" type.* The vesicles on the sides of the fingers (*arrows*) are shown here.

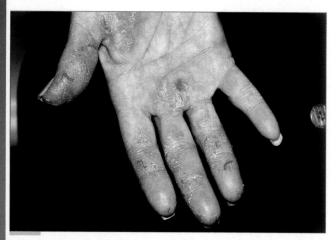

2.36 *Atopic hand eczema ("dry," scaly type).* The fingers have become dry and fragile, with resultant painful fissures.

"Dry," Scaly Type

In nondyshidrotic hand eczema—the dry, scaly type—the following are noted:

- Lesions are scaly and red.
- Scaly, hyperkeratotic, lichenified plaques may arise.
- The fingertips may become dry, wrinkled, red, and fragile, with resultant painful fissures and erosions (FIG. 2.36).
- The central palm or palmar aspect of the hands and fingers is also commonly affected in patients with chronic hand eczema. It is characterized by highly itchy, scaly palms.
- Fissures in the folds of the hands and fingers are painful and can limit the use of the hands.
- As with the dyshidrotic type of hand eczema, oozing and secondary bacterial infection ("honey-crusted" skin) can occur.
- With long-standing disease, patients' fingernails may reveal dystrophic changes (e.g., irregular transverse ridging, pitting, thickening, discoloration) when the nail matrix (root) becomes involved (see FIG. 2.17).

FACTORS THAT MAY TRIGGER RECURRENCES

Many of the triggers that exacerbate eczema are ubiquitous in daily life and in certain work settings. They include the following:

- Emotional stress.
- Environmental conditions (including seasonal changes, hot or cold temperatures, humidity).
- Contact allergens (including nickel, balsams, paraphenylenediamine, chromates) and irritants (including soaps).
- *Staphylococcus aureus.* This microbe is thought to play a role in the exacerbation of eczema because it is virtually omnipresent on the skin of patients with atopic dermatitis. Colonization with *S. aureus* results in the secretion of toxins (superantigens) that promote skin inflammation.

DIAGNOSIS

- The diagnosis of atopic hand eczema is usually made on clinical grounds or when other causes are excluded.

DIFFERENTIAL DIAGNOSIS

Contact Dermatitis
(Fig. 2.37).

- This is suspected, particularly if the eruption is on the dorsum of the hands or feet.
- Contact dermatitis is considered when the patient has a history of exposure to a suspected contactant.
- On occasion, contact allergy to nickel has been shown to cause dyshidrotic eczema.

Tinea Manuum
Figure 2.38.

- This is suggested by well-demarcated plaques on the palms (often on one palm only) and soles or a positive KOH examination or fungal culture.

Psoriasis on the Palms
Figure 2.39.

- This may be indistinguishable from hand eczema.
- Pustular psoriasis of the palms may also, at times, be indistinguishable from pustular dyshidrotic hand eczema.

- The patient may have evidence of psoriasis elsewhere on the body or a personal or family history of psoriasis.

Scabies
(See Chapter 20, "Bites, Stings, and Infestations.")

- This diagnosis should be considered if there is an acute pruritic vesicular eruption in the web spaces of the fingers.

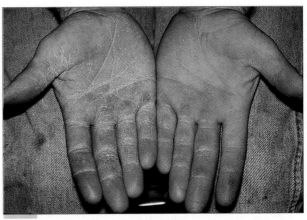

2.38 *Tinea manuum.* Only one palm shows a well-demarcated plaque. The scale of this palm was positive for fungus.

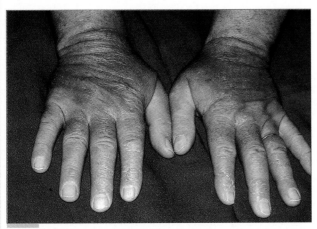

2.37 *Contact dermatitis.* This eczematous dermatitis on the dorsa of the hands was caused by exposure to latex gloves.

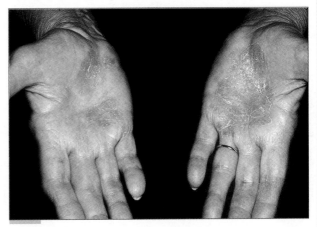

2.39 *Psoriasis of the palms.* These palmar lesions can easily be mistaken for eczema or tinea manuum.

MANAGEMENT

Mild Cases

Patients with mild cases of atopic hand eczema are managed as follows.

- Mild cleansers or soap substitutes are recommended.
- Protective cotton-lined gloves should be used for washing dishes or other similar tasks.
- Fastidious hand protection is necessary, with emollient barrier creams, protective gloves, and the avoidance of irritants and allergens.
- For oozing and infected lesions, compresses with **Burow's solution** (aluminum acetate) are applied. This treatment promotes drying and has an antibacterial effect. The solution is applied in a 1:40 dilution two or three times daily until bullae resolve (usually within a few days).
- Topical corticosteroids are the mainstay of treatment. Ointments penetrate skin better than creams do, but patients may prefer to use creams during the day. Most patients require medium-potency (class 3) corticosteroids (e.g., **triamcinolone 0.1%**), with or without occlusion. However, higher-potency (class 2) corticosteroids (e.g., **fluocinonide 0.05%**) can be used on an as-needed basis. Lower-strength (class 5) corticosteroids (e.g., **hydrocortisone valerate 0.2%**) may sometimes be applied for long-term maintenance.
- Short-term application of **Protopic ointment** (tacrolimus) 0.1% or **Elidel cream** (pimecrolimus) 1% may also be effective.

Severe Cases

Severe atopic hand eczema is often very difficult to manage.

- Application of corticosteroids under occlusion is occasionally effective when it is done early in the course of an eruption. However, potent topical corticosteroids applied under plastic or vinyl occlusion and superpotent topical corticosteroids can be used only intermittently and for short periods, because they increase the risk of atrophy.
- Systemic antibiotics should be administered for obvious or suspected secondary infection.
- Short-term use of systemic corticosteroids may be required for very severe flares. However, they should be given very infrequently.
- Treatment of hyperkeratotic palmar eczema is notoriously difficult. **Acitretin (Soriatane),** an aromatic retinoid, may help control hyperkeratosis.
- Other measures, such as **oral psoralen plus topical ultraviolet A (PUVA), oral cyclosporine, azathioprine,** and low-dose **methotrexate** are used for severe, refractory cases.
- **Superficial X-irradiation** (rarely used today) had been used to treat some patients with resistant chronic hand eczema.

 SEE PATIENT HANDOUTS "Burow's Solution" AND "Hand Eczema" ON THE SOLUTION SITE

Eczema Variants

Numerous common clinical variants of eczema are recognized: nummular eczema, lichen simplex chronicus, prurigo nodularis, asteatotic eczema, neurotic excoriations, hand eczema, and nonspecific eczematous dermatitis. These disorders are usually found in patients with an atopic history. However, on occasion, they manifest in patients without an atopic predisposition; in such instances, a methodic search for an exogenous cause, such as a contact dermatitis, is often necessary. Included here are stasis dermatitis and seborrheic dermatitis, which are also eczematous eruptions that may or may not be related to an atopic history.

Nummular Eczema

DESCRIPTION OF LESIONS

The round lesions of nummular eczema often have the shape of coins. The word "nummular" comes from the same root as "numismatic," meaning "coin-shaped." Lesions are usually itchy eczematous patches and plaques that often occur in clusters (Figs. 2.40 and 2.41). Although this disorder is usually seen in patients who have a history of atopy, it is not uncommon in adult patients who do not have such a history.

DISTRIBUTION OF LESIONS

Lesions are seen mainly on the legs; less commonly, they arise on the arms and trunk. The patches or plaques sometimes clear centrally and resemble tinea corporis ("ringworm"). Healing or resolving lesions often display postinflammatory hyperpigmentation, particularly in dark-skinned patients.

DIAGNOSIS

- The diagnosis of nummular eczema is based on the clinical appearance and, if necessary, negative results of a KOH examination.

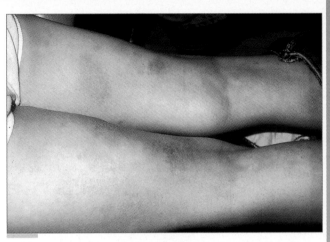

2.40 *Nummular eczema.* Erythematous, coin-shaped lesions are seen in a typical location.

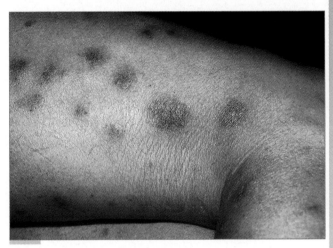

2.41 *Nummular eczema.* These coin-shaped scaly lesions show evidence of postinflammatory hyperpigmentation.

DIFFERENTIAL DIAGNOSIS

Tinea Corporis
FIGURE 2.42.

• Lesions of tinea corporis are often—but not always—clear in the center (annular).

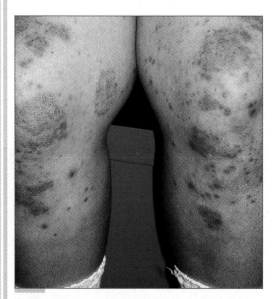

2.42   Tinea corporis (ringworm). Initially treated as nummular eczema, this itchy eruption has a scaly border that demonstrated hyphae on potassium hydroxide examination. Note the resemblance to both nummular eczema and psoriasis. This is often referred to as "tinea incognito."

• In tinea corporis, the KOH examination or fungal culture is positive.
• Nummular eczema is frequently misdiagnosed as tinea corporis ("ringworm").

Psoriasis
FIGURE 2.43.

• Psoriasis is less likely to itch than nummular eczema.
• Psoriatic lesions frequently occur on elbows and knees and may have a whitish or micaceous scale.

Lichen Simplex Chronicus
(See later in this chapter.)

• Focal lichenified plaques are noted.
• Often, a positive atopic history is present.

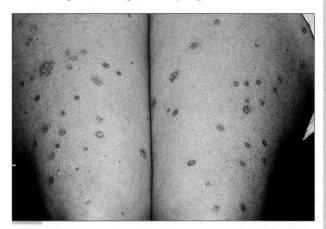

2.43   Psoriasis. This patient has erythematous papules with typical psoriatic scale. Again, note the similarity to nummular eczema.

MANAGEMENT

• Nummular eczema can often be controlled by an intermediate-strength (class 3 or 4) topical corticosteroid, such as **triamcinolone acetonide cream 0.1%,** applied sparingly two to three times daily.
• If necessary, a high-potency (class 1) topical corticosteroid, such as **clobetasol cream 0.05%** once or twice daily, may be used.

• Recalcitrant cases may require occlusion—provided by a polyethylene wrap or **Cordran tape** (flurandrenolide)—or intralesional corticosteroid injections.
• Long-term treatment can be accomplished with less potent topical corticosteroids.

POINT TO REMEMBER

• Nummular eczema is frequently misdiagnosed as tinea corporis ("ringworm") and is often inappropriately treated with topical antifungals as well as combination antifungal/topical steroid combinations.

Lichen Simplex Chronicus

Also known as neurodermatitis, lichen simplex chronicus is a common, chronic, often solitary, pruritic eczematous eruption caused by repetitive rubbing and scratching. It is seen most commonly in adults, particularly in patients with other atopic manifestations, such as asthma and allergic rhinitis.

CLINICAL MANIFESTATION AND DISTRIBUTION OF LESIONS

Patients with lichen simplex chronicus have a focal lichenified plaque or multiple plaques, most often on the nape of the neck, scalp, external ear canals, wrists, extensor forearms, ankles (FIG. 2.44), pretibial areas, or inner thighs. Lichen simplex chronicus may also involve the vulvae, scrotum (FIG. 2.45), intragluteal area (FIG. 2.46), and perianal area (pruritus ani) (FIG. 2.47). Patients often have only one area of involvement. Chronic or paroxysmal pruritus is the primary symptom.

DIAGNOSIS

- The diagnosis is readily apparent and is made on clinical grounds.

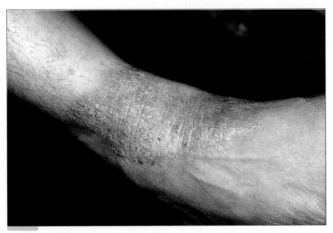

2.44 *Lichen simplex chronicus.* This focal lichenified plaque involves the distal pretibial area and ankle. This patient not only scratched the lesion, but he also persistently rubbed it with his contralateral heel.

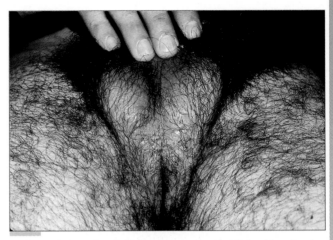

2.45 *Lichen simplex chronicus.* Scrotal lichenification in an atopic patient. This condition is often mistaken for tinea cruris.

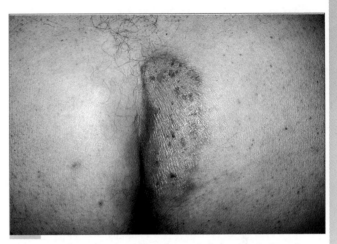

2.46 *Lichen simplex chronicus.* A lichenified gluteal plaque is seen in this atopic patient.

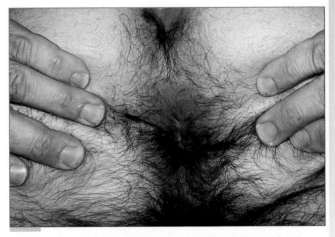

2.47 *Lichen simplex chronicus.* Perianal lichenification in an atopic patient. This is a frequent cause of pruritus ani.

DIFFERENTIAL DIAGNOSIS IN GENITAL AREA

Tinea Cruris and Candidiasis
FIGURE 2.48.

- A chronic itchy vulvar or scrotal rash may also suggest a fungal infection such as tinea cruris or candidiasis.
- KOH examination or fungal culture is positive.

Inverse Psoriasis and Intertrigo
FIGURES 2.49 and 2.50.

- Inverse psoriasis and intertrigo should be considered when lesions involve the inguinal creases and perianal area.

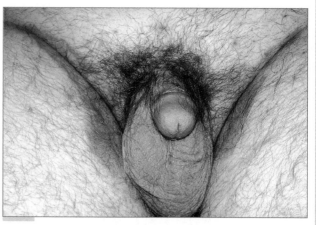

2.49 *Inverse psoriasis.* KOH-negative erythema in a patient who has psoriasis.

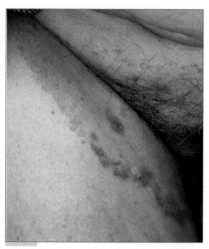

2.48 *Tinea cruris.* This is a typical scaly, KOH-positive example of fungal infection. Note the scalloped shape of the lesions and the "active" scaly border.

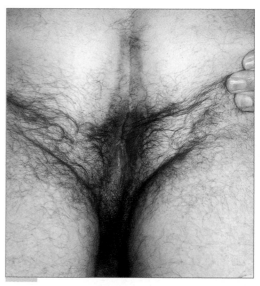

2.50 *Inverse psoriasis.* This is the same patient as in the previous figure.

MANAGEMENT

- The most important aspect of therapy is the elimination of scratching and rubbing. Unfortunately, many patients scratch themselves in their sleep.
- As with nummular eczema, lichen simplex chronicus may be treated with an intermediate-strength (class 3 or 4) topical corticosteroid. If necessary, a high-potency (class 1) topical corticosteroid can be used.
- Occlusion, when required, has the added advantage of preventing patients from scratching or rubbing—or, at least, reminding them not to do so.

- Oral antihistamines may be helpful at bedtime because of their sedative effect.
- **Protopic ointment** (tacrolimus) **0.03%** or **0.1%** may prove beneficial in patients with vulvar or perianal lichen simplex chronicus. (Patients should be warned about the potential for stinging and burning when tacrolimus ointment is applied to these sensitive areas.)
- Alternatively, **Elidel cream 1%** (pimecrolimus) may be effective. It is less irritating than Protopic ointment.

Prurigo Nodularis

Another chronic, but much less common, variant of atopic dermatitis is prurigo nodularis. It is seen in the same clinical context as lichen simplex chronicus and may be considered a papular or nodular form.

DESCRIPTION OF LESIONS

Lesions are reddish, brown, or hyperpigmented dome-shaped papules or nodules that resolve with postinflammatory hyperpigmentation (FIG. 2.51).

CLINICAL MANIFESTATION AND DISTRIBUTION OF LESIONS

- Lesions are most commonly noted on the pretibial shafts and sometimes on the extensor areas of the arms.
- They are often crusted or excoriated—pruritus may be intense.
- Healing generally results in significant postinflammatory hyperpigmentation.

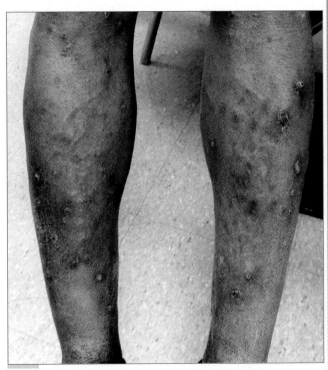

2.51 *Prurigo nodularis.* These intensely pruritic excoriated papules on the pretibial shafts show marked postinflammatory hyperpigmentation.

 MANAGEMENT

- Prurigo nodularis tends to be very resistant to topical corticosteroids.
- Occlusion topical steroid therapy with **Cordran tape** or a class 1 topical steroid are sometimes effective.
- In recalcitrant cases, intralesional corticosteroid injections may be helpful.

- **Thalidomide** has been reported as effective in intractable cases. (Thalidomide should not be used in women who are pregnant. In the United States, only physicians who are part of a special registry are permitted to administer this drug.)

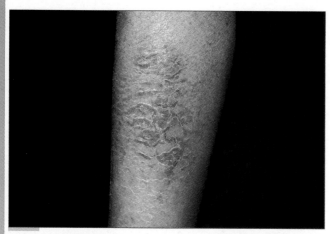

2.52 *Asteatotic eczema (erythema craquelé).* The scaly patches on this patient's shin demonstrate superficial fissures that resemble a cracked antique china vase or a dry riverbed.

 MANAGEMENT

- Asteatotic eczema is usually managed readily by having the patient bathe less frequently and apply moisturizers regularly.
- A very effective treatment is **Lac-Hydrin** (12% ammonium lactate cream or lotion), which is available only by prescription, and the similar preparation, **AmLactin,** which can be obtained without a prescription. These agents are applied immediately after bathing.
- If necessary, pruritic lesions respond readily to low- to moderate-strength (class 3 or 4) topical corticosteroids.

 DIAGNOSIS AND DIFFERENTIAL DIAGNOSIS

- Nonspecific eczematous dermatitis is a diagnosis of exclusion when no underlying cause, such as a contact allergen, scabies, or occult fungal infection (tinea incognito), is found.

Asteatotic Eczema

A common form of dermatitis, asteatotic eczema appears in dry, cold winter months. It is also referred to as winter eczema, and because its lesions consist of scaly patches with superficial fissures that resemble a cracked antique china vase, it is sometimes called *erythema craquelé.* It occurs only in adults.

CLINICAL MANIFESTATION AND DISTRIBUTION OF LESIONS

- The condition may be pruritic.
- Lesions consist of characteristic scaly patches with very shallow erythematous fissures resembling a cracked, dry riverbed (Fig. 2.52).
- They are located most commonly on the shins, arms, hands, and trunk.

 DIFFERENTIAL DIAGNOSIS

- The differential diagnosis of asteatotic eczema includes xerosis (dry skin) and nummular eczema.

"Neurotic" Excoriations and Factitia

Patients with neurotic excoriations, also referred to as neurodermatitis, compulsively pick at their skin. Lesions may accompany or exacerbate atopic dermatitis, or they may have been preceded by atopic dermatitis or an insect bite. Most often, no precipitating cause can be determined.

Nonspecific Eczematous Dermatitis

Many people, particularly the elderly, have chronic, recurrent, itchy, eczematous dermatitis without the typical distribution of atopic dermatitis. These patients may or may not have an apparent atopic history. Frequently, they complain of dry or sensitive skin that tends to become drier and itchier in winter months. The eruption tends to worsen with aging, as the skin loses some of its barrier function and lubrication (asteatosis). Itching with or without specific lesions tends to occur on the arms, legs, and upper back.

 MANAGEMENT

- Treatment consists of an intermediate-strength (class 3 or 4) topical corticosteroid.

- If necessary, a higher-potency (class 1 or 2) topical corticosteroid may be used. Patients with nonspecific eczematous dermatitis should avoid the use of soap on affected areas. In dry winter months, moisturizers may be beneficial.

CLINICAL MANIFESTATION AND DISTRIBUTION OF LESIONS

- Lesions frequently suggest an external cause, often referred to as an "outside job" by dermatologists. Lesions are often noted to be erosions, linear crusts, or ulcerations that suggest manipulation by the patient. Postinflammatory hyperpigmentation and whitish hypopigmented lesions indicate chronicity (Fig. 2.53).
- Deep ulcerations with geometric shapes suggest factitia (Fig. 2.54), a self-induced condition caused by habitual scratching or picking. In factitia, lesions tend to show a wide range of bizarre patterns (Fig. 2.55) uncharacteristic of any specific disease. The presence of factitia may imply that the patient has severe emotional problems.
- The lesions of neurotic excoriation tend to be located on the upper back or ankles—areas that are easily reachable by the patient (see Fig. 2.53).
- Factitial lesions may appear anywhere and often have bizarre shapes.
- Many patients with neurotic excoriations or factitia may also show signs and symptoms of a neurosis (e.g., obsessive-compulsive disorder) or a delusional psychosis that underlies the repetitive self-destructive behavior.

DIAGNOSIS

- The diagnosis is either given by the patient, who readily admits that the lesions are self-created, or the lesions themselves may be indicative.
- Bizarre lesions and a *la belle indifférence* affect on the part of the patient suggest factitial dermatitis as the cause.

 MANAGEMENT

- High-potency topical corticosteroids, topical corticosteroids under occlusion, and intralesional corticosteroids are sometimes useful, but these treatments will be ineffective if the underlying psychologic cause is not addressed.
- Bedtime antihistamines are sometimes helpful.
- Psychotherapy and/or psychopharmacologic drugs should be used, if indicated.

 HELPFUL HINT

- When the diagnosis is in doubt, the lesions may be covered with a thick dressing, and the patient is then instructed not to remove it. Consequently, when the patient cannot access them, the lesions heal rapidly.

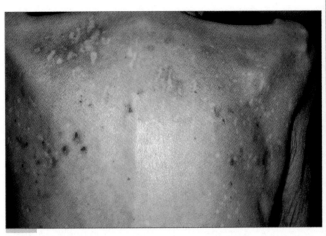

2.53 *Neurotic excoriations (neurodermatitis).* Lesions tend to be located on the upper back or ankles, areas that are easily reachable.

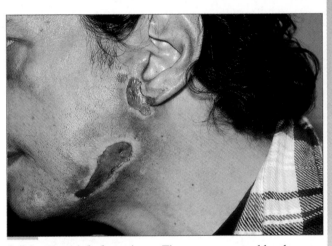

2.54 *Factitial ulcerations.* These were created by the patient. Note their geometric appearance. The patient has a severe psychiatric disorder.

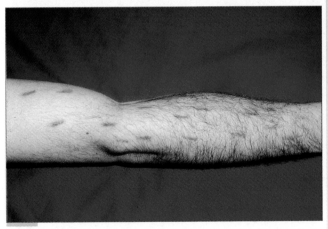

2.55 *Factitial purpura.* These purpuric lesions were obviously self-induced.

Seborrheic Dermatitis ("Seborrheic Eczema")

BASICS

- Seborrheic dermatitis is a very common, chronic inflammatory dermatitis. Its characteristic distribution involves areas that have the greatest concentration of sebaceous glands: scalp, face, presternal region, interscapular area, umbilicus, and body folds (intertriginous areas).
- Many people experience some degree of dandruff—a whitish scaling of the scalp that is sometimes itchy and is fairly easily controlled with dandruff shampoos. When dandruff is accompanied by erythema, a sign of inflammation, it is referred to as seborrheic dermatitis. When seborrheic dermatitis occurs in the body folds, it is called intertrigo, or intertriginous seborrheic dermatitis.
- Seborrheic dermatitis is seen more commonly in male patients and often begins after puberty. There appears to be a hereditary predisposition to its development. When it presents in patients who are infected with the human immunodeficiency virus, seborrheic dermatitis may serve as an early marker of the acquired immunodeficiency syndrome. Seborrheic dermatitis is also seen commonly in patients with Parkinson's disease and in patients taking phenothiazines.
- Seborrheic dermatitis has many features in common with chronic eczema and psoriasis. Typical lesions of seborrheic dermatitis often appear in patients with psoriasis, and the histologic features of the lesions of seborrheic dermatitis resemble those of both eczema and psoriasis. In fact, some dermatologists do not consider seborrheic dermatitis a distinct nosologic entity but instead assign it to various forms of eczema or psoriasis. In the latter case, the term "seborrhiasis" has been used. In the United Kingdom, seborrheic dermatitis is referred to as "seborrhoeic eczema."

Pathogenesis

- Traditionally, seborrheic dermatitis has been described as idiopathic. However, some evidence indicates that *Pityrosporon ovale,* a small yeast, may play a part in its pathogenesis because seborrheic dermatitis occasionally responds to antifungal medications (see following).
- Because seborrheic dermatitis occurs only where the sebaceous glands are found, sebum has also been thought to play a role, although no link has been shown.

DESCRIPTION OF LESIONS

The appearance of the lesions of seborrheic dermatitis varies depending on their location.

- On the face, lesions are red, with or without an overlying whitish scale, or they may appear as orange-yellow greasy patches.
- On the scalp, seborrheic dermatitis may range from a mild erythema and scaling to thick, armorlike plaques that are indistinguishable from psoriasis ("sebopsoriasis") (FIG. 2.56).

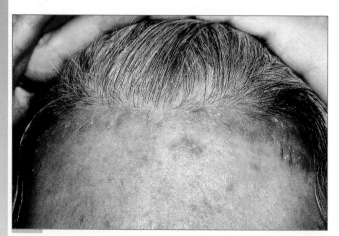

2.56 **Seborrheic dermatitis.** Scale and erythema are evident along the frontal hairline.

- When lesions occur in body folds, they often consist of sharply defined, bright red plaques that may develop fissures.

DISTRIBUTION OF LESIONS

The eruption of seborrheic dermatitis tends to be bilaterally symmetric in its distribution.

- **Scalp, face.** Lesions appear on the forehead, eyebrows, eyelashes, cheeks, beard, and nasolabial folds (FIG. 2.57).
- **Ears.** Lesions occur behind the ears and in the external ear canal (FIG. 2.58).
- **Body folds.** Body folds and anogenital areas are affected—inframammary areas, axillae, inguinal creases, intragluteal crease, perianal area, and umbilicus. In these areas, seborrheic dermatitis is often clinically indistinguishable from tinea cruris and inverse psoriasis.
- Presternal lesions are not unusual and are scaly or papular.

CLINICAL MANIFESTATIONS

- On the scalp, there may be itching and scale with resultant dandruff that, embarrassingly, often falls on clothing.
- Facial seborrheic dermatitis usually flares in the winter and improves in the summer. However, many patients report provocation of the condition *after* sun exposure.
- When fissures develop in the body folds and umbilicus, symptoms may consist of burning, itching, oozing, and pain.

Clinical Variants

Nonspecific vulvitis and balanitis and the interscapular "itchy back syndrome" are considered variants of seborrheic dermatitis by some dermatologists. Seborrheic dermatitis in infants is generally self-limiting and usually disappears by 8 months of age. It presents either as "cradle cap," a buildup of a scaly, greasy adherent plaque on the vertex of the scalp, or as erythematous lesions in body folds. Both these presentations are probably unrelated to adult seborrheic dermatitis.

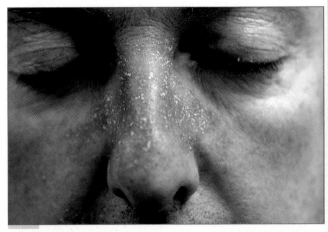

2.57 *Seborrheic dermatitis.* Here we see typical involvement of the cheeks, eyebrows, eyelashes, and nasolabial folds.

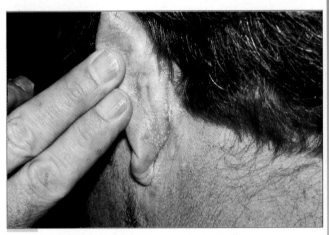

2.58 *Seborrheic dermatitis.* This patient has involvement of the retroauricular area.

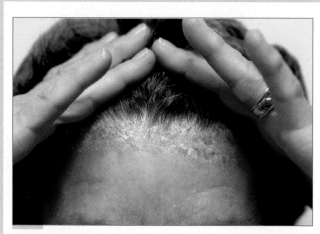

2.59 *Psoriasis.* This is quite similar to seborrheic dermatitis seen in FIG. 2.56.

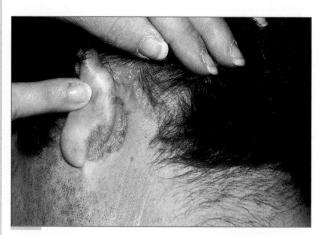

2.60 *Psoriasis.* Note the similarity to FIG. 2.58.

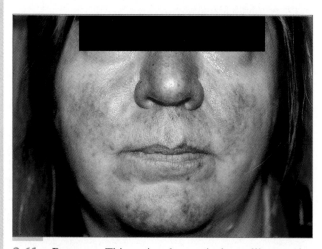

2.61 *Rosacea.* This patient has typical acnelike papules and erythema in the central third of her face. (Note similarity to FIG. 2.57.)

continued on page 81

DIFFERENTIAL DIAGNOSIS

- The differential diagnosis of seborrheic dermatitis varies depending on the age, sex, and ethnic background of the patient and, particularly, on the location of lesions.

Scalp and External Ears
Psoriasis
FIGURES 2.59 and 2.60.

- Psoriatic lesions elsewhere on body
- Family history of psoriasis

Eczematous Dermatitis
- Eczematous lesions elsewhere on body
- Atopic history
- Onset often before adolescence

Tinea Capitis
- Preteen age group
- Prevalent in urban African-American toddlers
- Focal areas of alopecia
- Positive KOH examination or positive fungal culture

Face
Erythrotelangiectatic Rosacea, Rosacea
FIGURE 2.61.

- Telangiectasias
- Acnelike papules and pustules

"Butterfly" Rash of Systemic Lupus Erythematosus
- Positive antinuclear antibody test
- Other features of lupus erythematosus

Tinea Faciale
- Lesions generally annular (ring-shaped) with an asymmetric distribution
- Positive KOH examination or positive fungal culture

Body Folds and Genitalia
Inverse Psoriasis
FIGURES 2.49 and 2.50.

- Often indistinguishable from seborrheic dermatitis (see Chapter 3, "Psoriasis")
- Negative KOH examination
- No growth on fungal culture

DIFFERENTIAL DIAGNOSIS *Continued*

Tinea Cruris
See FIGURE 2.48 and Chapter 7, "Superficial Fungal Infections."

- Arcuate shape with advancing "active border" with central clearing
- Positive KOH examination or fungal culture

Candidiasis
See Chapter 7, "Superficial Fungal Infections."

- "Beefy" red plaques, "satellite pustules"
- Positive KOH examination

- Fungal culture positive for *Candida* species
- Most common in patients with diabetes mellitus

Eczematous Dermatitis, Such as Atopic Dermatitis
- Eczematous lesions elsewhere on the body
- Atopic history
- Marked pruritus

MANAGEMENT

Treatment options for seborrheic dermatitis vary according to the location of the lesions (TABLE 2.1).

Scalp
Mild scalp seborrheic dermatitis generally responds to the numerous commercially available antidandruff, antiseborrheic shampoos that contain one or more of the following ingredients: **zinc pyrithione, coal tar, salicylic acid, selenium sulfide,** and/or **sulfur,** as well as the antifungals **ciclopirox** and **ketoconazole.**

- The shampoos should be left on for at least 5 minutes after lathering.
- For itching and inflammation, a medium-strength (class 3 or 4) topical steroid in a gel or solution, such as betamethasone dipropionate lotion 0.05% (**Diprosone**) or betamethasone valerate foam 0.12% (**Luxiq foam**), may be used, but only if necessary.

Severe scalp seborrheic dermatitis ("sebopsoriasis") is often managed in the same manner as psoriasis of the scalp.

- Potent (class 2) agents such as fluocinonide gel 0.05% (**Lidex**) and superpotent (class 1) clobetasol propionate gel/lotion/foam 0.05% (**Temovate, Olux foam, Clobex lotion**) may be used. These topical steroids are frequently preceded by keratolytic agents to remove thick scale, allowing the medications to penetrate the scalp.
- Scale may be removed with a keratolytic preparation (e.g., **Salex, Keralyt**) as often as necessary, usually two

to three times per week initially and then whenever it builds up again.

Intertriginous Body Fold Areas
- Other areas of the body. Body folds and genital areas are similarly treated with low-potency (class 4, 5, 6, or 7) topical steroids.

Face
- Seborrheic dermatitis of the face responds quickly to topical steroids, but this treatment requires long-term maintenance and vigilance to avoid atrophy, telangiectasias, and rosacealike side effects.
- To minimize these unwanted reactions, low-potency topical steroids may be alternated with antifungals such as ketoconazole cream 2% (**Nizoral**), ketoconazole gel 2% (**Xolegel**), or ciclopirox 0.77% gel (**Loprox**).
- Very low-potency (class 7) topical steroids are used, with caution, when treating seborrheic dermatitis of the eyelid.

"Cradle Cap"
- Minor amounts of scale can be removed with mild antiseborrheic shampoos that contain sulfur and salicylic acid, such as **Sebulex.** Mineral oil or olive oil also help remove scale.
- Stronger keratolytic agents such as **Salex cream** or **lotion** or **Keralyt gel** are used for thick, dense, adherent scale.
- Very mild topical steroids may be applied to reduce inflammation and itching.

continued on page 82

Table 2.1 SEBORRHEIC DERMATITIS FORMULARY

SCALP

Shampoos/gels/lotions

Antiseborrheics	Pyrithione zinc (**Head & Shoulders***) shampoo
	Coal tar (**Neutrogena T/Gel***) shampoo
	Coal tar (**Zetar***) shampoo and emulsion
	1% selenium sulfide (**Selsun Blue***) shampoo
	2.5% selenium sulfide shampoo
	1% ketoconazole shampoo (**Nizoral***)
Antifungals	2% ketoconazole shampoo (**Nizoral**), ciclopirox 0.77% (**Loprox** shampoo and gel)

Keratolytics *(agents that remove excessive scale)*

Sulfur 2%, salicylic acid 2% (**Sebulex***) shampoo, or **Salex** cream or lotion, or **Keralyt** gel
Tar plus salicylic acid (**Neutrogena T/Sal***) shampoo

Topical corticosteroids

Medium potency (class 4)	Betamethasone valerate 0.1% (**Valisone**)
	Desoximetasone (**Topicort**) gel 0.05%, betamethasone valerate 0.12% (**Luxiq Foam**)
	Fluocinolone acetonide (**Capex**†) shampoo 0.01%
High potency (class 2)	Fluocinonide (**Lidex**) gel or solution 0.05%
Superpotency (class 1)	Clobetasol gel, foam, or scalp application 0.05%

FACE AND INTERTRIGINOUS AREAS

Topical steroids

Very low potency (class 7)	Hydrocortisone cream or ointment 0.5% to 1%*
Low potency (class 6)	Desonide (**DesOwen**) cream, lotion 0.05%, desonide 0.05% foam (**Verdeso**)
Medium potency (classes 4 and 5)	Hydrocortisone valerate (**Westcort**) cream, ointment 0.2%

Topical creams/ointments

Antifungals	Ketoconazole (**Nizoral***) 1% cream, ciclopirox 0.77% (**Loprox** gel), and (econazole cream 1% (**Spectazole**)*
	Ketoconazole (**Nizoral**) 2% cream, gel (**Xolegel**), foam (**extina**)
Immunomodulators	Tacrolimus 0.03% and 0.1% (**Protopic**) ointment
	Pimecrolimus 1% (**Elidel**) cream

*Available over the counter.

†This shampoo contains a mid-potent topical steroid. It is used two or three times weekly, as needed.

 POINTS TO REMEMBER

- Seborrheic dermatitis is often confused with psoriasis, rosacea, and fungal infections.
- Topical steroids should be used *only for brief periods* for seborrheic dermatitis, as with all steroid-responsive dermatoses.

 SEE PATIENT HANDOUT "Scalp Psoriasis: Scale Removal" ON SOLUTION SITE

 HELPFUL HINTS

- Seborrheic dermatitis of the scalp is not seen in preadolescent children; therefore, excessive use of shampoos should *not* be encouraged in this age group. The child may actually have atopic dermatitis, which is only aggravated by frequent shampooing.
- The application of topical antifungals may work as well or better than topical steroids in many cases.
- The limited use of **Protopic ointment** (tacrolimus) 0.1% and **Elidel cream** (pimecrolimus) 1% may also be effective in the treatment of facial and intertriginous seborrheic dermatitis.
- OTC ketoconazole (**Nizoral**) 1% cream or shampoo can be very effective for seborrheic dermatitis.

BASICS

- Stasis dermatitis (gravitational dermatitis) is an eczematous eruption that is most commonly located on the lower legs. It often appears on the medial ankles of middle-aged and elderly patients and rarely occurs before the fifth decade of life.
- The dermatitis is a consequence of chronic venous insufficiency ("leaky valves") and is seen more often in women, particularly those with a genetic predisposition to develop varicosities. It may also occur in patients with acquired venous insufficiency resulting from surgery (e.g., vein stripping or harvesting of saphenous veins for coronary bypass), deep venous thrombosis, or other types of traumatic injury to the lower venous system.

Pathogenesis

- Traditionally, the following sequence of events has been proposed to explain the pathogenesis of stasis dermatitis:

> Varicose veins ➤ Reversed flow through incompetent valves ➤ Diminished venous return ➤ Increased hydrostatic capillary pressure ➤ Peripheral edema and relative tissue hypoxia

- The preceding schema may account for the pruritic, eczematous eruption seen in the early stages of stasis dermatitis; however, several other theories offer explanations for the exact mechanism at the tissue level, and the issue is still a topic of debate.

PROGRESSION OF LESIONS

- Lesions begin with erythema and scale (eczematous dermatitis) (FIG. 2.62). Later, the rash may become subacute, with more intense erythema, edema, erosions, crusts, and secondary bacterial infection (FIG. 2.63). The rash may progressively lead to the chronic stages of stasis dermatitis, in which pigmentary changes occur. After an initial redness (from extravasated red blood cells), affected areas turn reddish brown (from iron left from the breakdown of red blood cells).
- Postinflammatory hyperpigmentation (from melanin) also occurs. These colors may overlie a cyanotic background.
- Ultimately, the skin thickens and becomes less supple and nonpitting, and it feels permanently bound down and fibrotic ("woody") on palpation.

DISTRIBUTION OF LESIONS

- Most cases of stasis dermatitis and associated ulcers are located on the medial malleolus. When symptoms progress, lesions may spread to the foot or calf.

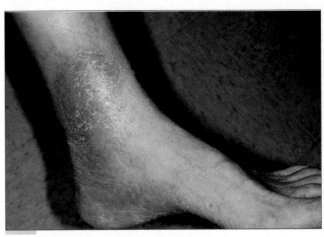

2.62 *Acute stasis dermatitis.* This patient has the earliest signs of stasis dermatitis—pruritus, erythema, scale (eczematous dermatitis), and slight distal hyperpigmentation.

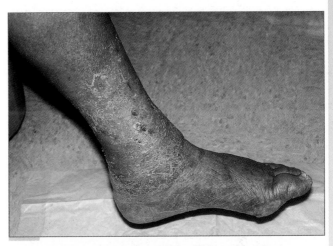

2.63 *Subacute stasis dermatitis.* This patient shows symptoms of more advanced stasis dermatitis—increased scale, peripheral edema, erosions, crusts, and secondary bacterial infection ("impetiginization").

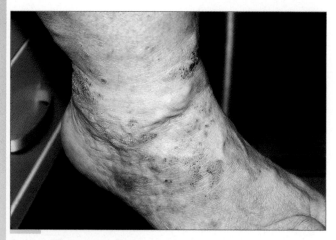

2.64 *Chronic stasis dermatitis.* Large venous varicosities are evident proximal to the eruption, and superficial varicosities surround the affected area.

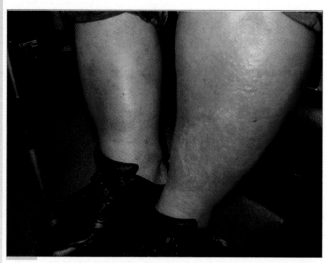

2.65 *Cellulitis.* This patient has a painful, tender, pretibial plaque. Image courtesy of Joseph Eastern, M.D.

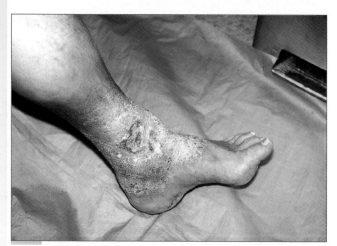

2.66 *Stasis dermatitis with venous stasis ulcer.* Note the eczematous eruption, the nonpitting edema ("woody" fibrosis) surrounding the ulcer (lipodermosclerosis).

CLINICAL MANIFESTATIONS

- Large venous varicosities may be evident proximal to the eruption, and superficial varicosities may surround the affected area (FIG. 2.64).
- Pruritus may occur.
- Ankle edema that is initially pitting later becomes fibrotic and nonpitting.
- Even during inactive periods of the eruption, the skin remains thickened and permanently pigmented.

Possible complications of stasis dermatitis include the following:

- **Venous stasis ulcers** that are presumably caused by microcirculatory abnormalities and the generation of an inflammatory response. The ulcers may be exacerbated by trauma (e.g., scratching), bacterial infection, or improper care of the eczematous rash (FIG. 2.65). Such ulcers sometimes produce a dull pain.
- Induration may progress to **lipodermatosclerosis,** which has a classic "inverted water bottle" appearance (FIGS. 2.66 and 2.67).
- **Autoeczematization** (id reaction) is a widespread, often explosive, acute eczematous eruption that is presumably triggered by secondary bacterial infection (impetiginization) of eczema, with resultant circulating immune complexes released from the site of the stasis dermatitis lesions (FIGS. 2.68A–B). It is hypothesized that patients become sensitized to their own tissue breakdown products.

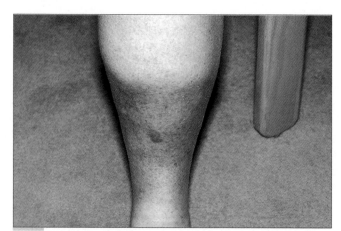

2.67 *Lipodermosclerosis.* Chronic stasis dermatitis has produced a circumferential fibrosis that gives the leg an "inverted water bottle" appearance.

DIFFERENTIAL DIAGNOSIS

Cellulitis

- Typical stasis dermatitis is generally an obvious diagnosis, but it is often confused with cellulitis. Cellulitis (see Fig. 2.65) is an acute infection of skin and soft tissues characterized by localized pain, swelling, tenderness, erythema, and warmth. It is usually caused by gram-positive aerobic cocci (e.g., *S. aureus, S. pyogenes*).

Other Diagnoses

- The presence of ulceration should point to other possible conditions, such as arterial disease, cryoglobulinemia, the antiphospholipid syndrome, protein C deficiency, skin cancer, or pyoderma gangrenosum.

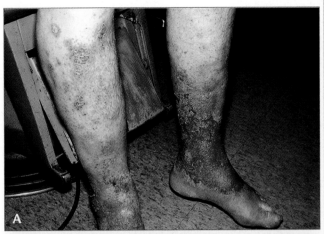

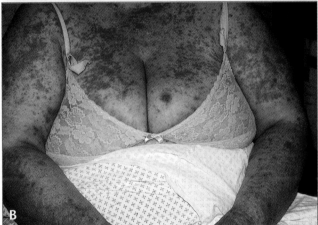

2.68 A and B **Stasis dermatitis with secondary impetiginization. Autoeczematization.** The same patient as in the previous figure. This patient's ankle eruption has become widespread as a result of impetiginization of the eczema on her legs.

MANAGEMENT

Stasis Dermatitis

Diminished Venous Return

- Venous return can be increased by engaging in regular exercise, such as brisk walking and bicycling.
- Furthermore, the affected leg(s) should be elevated **above the level of the heart.** (Sitting with the leg elevated by a stool is inadequate.)
- At night, leg elevation can be accomplished by propping up the foot end of the bed with 1 to 2 inches of plywood or a bedding fabric such as sheets.

Edema

Significant edema may be managed with **compressive therapy,** which augments the "calf pump," the mainstay of therapy for venous insufficiency. However, in the presence of arterial insufficiency, compression is contraindicated.

- **Support hose** help decrease the stretching of blood vessels. Elastic bandages and specialized compression (Jobst-type) stockings that deliver a controlled gradient of pressure are strongly recommended.
- The patient's peripheral arterial circulation should be assessed (clinically or with a Doppler study) before compression is recommended.

Rash

- The eczematous rash (stasis dermatitis) should be carefully managed with topical therapy. **Burow's solution** soaks to help dry oozing or infected areas.
- Twice-daily application of a low- to moderate-strength (class 4, 5, or 6) topical corticosteroid ointment (such as

continued on page 86

MANAGEMENT *Continued*

desonide 0.05%, **hydrocortisone valerate 0.2%**, or, if necessary, **triamcinolone 0.1%**) is usually sufficient to treat the eczematous rash and alleviate any itching.

- Patients should be advised not to apply topical corticosteroid preparations directly to stasis ulcers because the preparations may interfere with healing. Long-term use of potent topical corticosteroids may promote atrophy and should be avoided.
- OTC preparations that contain benzocaine, lanolin, or neomycin should also be avoided, since patients with stasis dermatitis tend to develop contact dermatitis quite easily.

Infection

- Obvious superficial infections (impetiginization) should be treated with systemic antibiotics that have activity against *S. aureus* and *Streptococcus species* (e.g., **dicloxacillin, cephalexin,** or a **fluoroquinolone**).
- A widespread autoeczematized eruption may require treatment with both systemic corticosteroids and oral antibiotics.

Stasis Ulcers

Stasis ulcers are managed by treating the underlying eczematous dermatitis, controlling weight, preventing infection, and using compression dressings. Venous ulcers at times produce a dull pain that is relieved by elevation.

- **Unna's boot** is a commercially available bandage (Dome-Paste bandage, Gelocast bandage) that is impregnated with zinc oxide paste. It is best applied in the morning, before edema progresses. After application, the bandage hardens into a cast. The boot decreases edema, promotes healing, and serves as a barrier from trauma (e.g., scratching). It should be changed weekly until the ulcer heals.
- If feasible, corrective surgery, such as skin grafts or vascular procedures, may be another option.
- The areas surrounding the ulcer may be treated with topical steroids, whereas the ulcer itself can be treated with moist wound healing methods, high-compression therapy, fibrinolytic agents, and newer modalities, such as growth factors, matrix materials, and biologically engineered tissue. (These methods are beyond the scope of this chapter.)

  SEE PATIENT HANDOUT "Burow's Solution" ON THE SOLUTION SITE

 POINTS TO REMEMBER

- Stasis dermatitis is often misdiagnosed as cellulitis.
- Infected stasis dermatitis should be considered in patients who develop a sudden onset of extensive generalized eczematous dermatitis (autoeczematization).
- Contact dermatitis or autoeczematization should be considered in patients who become clinically worse despite appropriate topical treatment.
- Compression is the mainstay of therapy for venous insufficiency and venous leg ulceration.

HELPFUL HINTS

- Sitting in a reclining chair while reading or watching television can help promote venous return.
- Walking regularly at a brisk pace should be encouraged.
- Physical therapy should be considered.
- Smoking and long periods of standing or sitting should be discouraged.

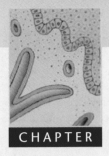

CHAPTER 3 Psoriasis

OVERVIEW

Psoriasis (psoriasis vulgaris) is a red and scaly chronic skin condition of unknown cause. The primary concern to most patients is the unsightly appearance of lesions whose visibility and persistence often lead them to feel self-conscious and unclean. The emotional toll and the personal struggle to come to terms with psoriasis are expressed in an autobiographic short story, "At War with my Skin," by John Updike, an author with severe psoriasis. After undergoing an operation for a broken leg, Updike reflected, "I chiefly remember amid my pain and helplessness being pleased that my shins, at that time, were clear and I would not offend the surgeon."

Psoriasis affects 1% to 2% of the world's population. The condition is much less common in West Africans, African-Americans, Native Americans, and Asiatic people than it is in whites. It is found equally in men and women. Psoriasis most frequently begins in the second or third decade of life, but it can first present in infants or in the elderly. About 30% of patients with psoriasis have a family history of the disease. Patients may also develop psoriatic arthritis, which may precede or follow the onset of skin lesions.

Psoriasis can be a major blow to one's ego. It may stifle social activities and sexual spontaneity, interfere with job opportunities, and inhibit participation in sports and the use of beaches and public swimming pools. Because psoriasis is a visible disease, it may arouse a fear of contagion, as well as repugnance and avoidance, from persons who are not used to seeing it. The young child with psoriasis has the additional burden of embarrassment caused by the undisguised scrutiny and thoughtless remarks of other children. A parent may have to cope with guilt for having genetically passed psoriasis on to his or her child.

A person who has psoriasis often spends an excessive amount of time treating skin lesions and trying to hide them, as well as searching for external causes and possible cures. The National Psoriasis Foundation provides information about psoriasis to educate patients, the public, and health care providers. The contact information is as follows: 6600 S.W. 92nd, Suite 300, Portland, OR 97223; 800-723-9166; www.psoriasis.org.

The clinical presentations of psoriasis listed here create a somewhat artificial classification, which is based on the characteristics or morphology of the predominant type of lesion and its distribution. There may be composites of these different types in a given patient. Because each type is managed somewhat differently and has its own differential diagnosis, each is discussed separately.

➤ LOCALIZED PLAQUE PSORIASIS

➤ GENERALIZED PLAQUE PSORIASIS

➤ ACUTE GUTTATE PSORIASIS (SEE ALSO CHAPTER 27, "SPECIAL CONSIDERATIONS IN THE SKIN OF PEDIATRIC AND ELDERLY PATIENTS")

➤ ERYTHRODERMIC PSORIASIS (EXFOLIATIVE DERMATITIS SECONDARY TO PSORIASIS) (SEE ALSO CHAPTER 25, "CUTANEOUS MANIFESTATIONS OF SYSTEMIC DISEASE")

➤ PSORIASIS IN CHILDREN (SEE ALSO CHAPTER 27, "SPECIAL CONSIDERATIONS IN THE SKIN OF PEDIATRIC AND ELDERLY PATIENTS")

➤ HIV-INDUCED PSORIASIS (SEE ALSO CHAPTER 24, "CUTANEOUS MANIFESTATIONS OF HIV INFECTION")

➤ INVERSE PSORIASIS (ON THE GROIN, PENIS, AXILLAE, AND PERIANAL AND INFRAMAMMARY REGIONS)

➤ PSORIASIS OF THE PALMS AND SOLES

➤ SCALP PSORIASIS

➤ PSORIATIC NAILS (SEE ALSO CHAPTER 13, "DISEASES AND ABNORMALITIES OF NAILS")

➤ PSORIATIC ARTHRITIS

➤ OTHER RARE CLINICAL VARIANTS: LOCALIZED PUSTULAR PSORIASIS (HALLOPEAU) AND THE RARE GENERALIZED PUSTULAR PSORIASIS OF VON ZUMBUSCH

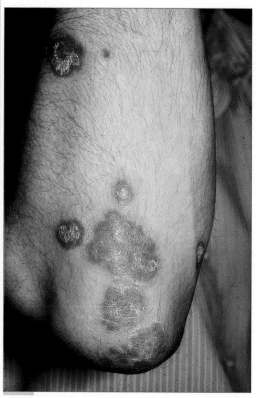

Pathophysiology

- Psoriasis is essentially an inflammatory skin condition with abnormal epidermal differentiation and hyperproliferation. It is suggested that the inflammatory process is immunologically based and most likely set off—and maintained by—T cells in the dermis.
- The lesions of psoriasis result from an increase in epidermal cell turnover. The cell's transit time from the basal layer of the epidermis to the stratum corneum is decreased from the normal 28 days to 3 or 4 days.
- This "turned-on" epidermis, with its rapid accumulation of cells, accounts for the characteristic lesion of psoriasis: a red papule or plaque (FIG. 3.1). It also explains the accumulation of white or silvery (micaceous) scale; the great increase in cellular kinetics does not allow time for shedding (FIGS. 3.2 and 3.3).
- Because psoriasis is now considered to be an immunologic disease, most current therapies, including topical corticosteroids, phototherapy, photochemotherapy, methotrexate, and cyclosporine, are directed at the suppression of responsible T cells.

3.1 *Psoriasis.* This is a typical location for the characteristic lesions of psoriasis. Note the well-circumscribed erythematous plaques surmounted by a fine scale.

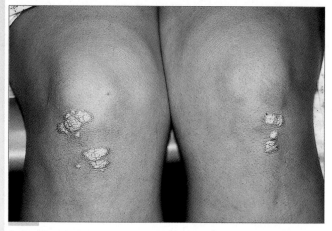

3.2 *Psoriasis.* Here the scale is thicker (hyperkeratotic) and white in color.

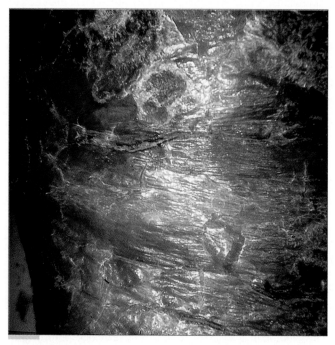

3.3 *Psoriasis.* The silvery, shiny luster of the micaceous scale is obvious.

Histopathology

The histopathologic findings demonstrate the altered cell kinetics of psoriasis (ILL. 3.1):

- Increased mitosis of keratinocytes, fibroblasts, and endothelial cells. Skin biopsies typically show:
  - Marked thickening (acanthosis) and also thinning of the epidermis with resultant elongation of the rete ridges
  - Parakeratosis (nuclei retained in the stratum corneum)
- Inflammatory process:
  - Dermal inflammation (lymphocytes and monocytes)
  - Epidermal inflammation (polymorphonuclear cells) in the stratum corneum that may form the so-called microabscesses of Munro

DISTRIBUTION OF LESIONS

The distribution of thickened, reddened, silvery or whitish, scaly papules or plaques can range from only a few small asymptomatic lesions on the elbows and knees to larger plaques that cover extensive areas of the body.

- Psoriasis tends to be remarkably symmetric. It usually spares the face. Lesions are most commonly located as follows:
  - On large extensor joints (elbows, knees, and knuckles)
  - On the scalp
  - On the anogenital region (perineal and perianal areas, glans penis)
  - On the palms and soles
- Trunk lesions may be small, guttate (teardrop-shaped) plaques or large plaques.
- When psoriasis involves only the scalp and retroauricular areas, it is sometimes referred to as "sebopsoriasis" or "seborrhiasis" (see FIGS. 2.56 and 2.58).
- When the entire body is involved, generalized, disseminated plaques or exfoliative erythroderma may be evident.
- When lesions occur primarily in the intertriginous areas (inguinal creases, axillae, and inframammary, perineal, and perianal areas), this manifestation is referred to as inverse psoriasis.
- Psoriasis is commonly a cause of nail deformity, which is often mistaken for, and treated incorrectly as, a nail fungus infection (onychomycosis).
- Psoriatic arthritis occurs in 5% to 10% of patients who are diagnosed with psoriasis.

CLINICAL MANIFESTATIONS

Pruritus

- Psoriasis generally is asymptomatic, but it can become quite pruritic and uncomfortable, particularly during acute flare-ups or when it involves the scalp or intertriginous regions.

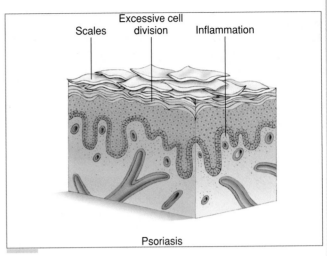

I3.1 *Psoriasis.* Scales, excessive cell division, and inflammation.

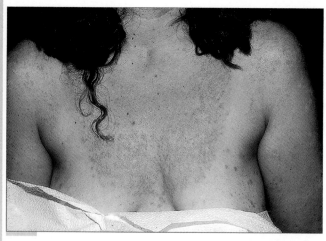

3.4 *Psoriasis.* The Köbner phenomenon is localized to the area of sunburn. The region that had been covered by the patient's bathing suit is almost free of lesions.

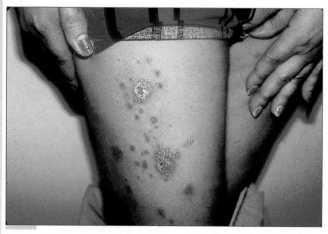

3.5 *Psoriasis.* The Köbner phenomenon is evident in this diabetic patient, who developed psoriatic plaques at the sites of insulin injections.

The Köbner Reaction (Isomorphic Response)
- Patients commonly recognize the phenomenon that new lesions may appear at sites of injury or trauma to the skin.
- Noxious stimuli, such as scratching and rubbing, or a sunburn can elicit a Köbner reaction (Figs. 3.4 and 3.5; see also Fig. 4.16).

Fissuring of Plaques
- Painful fissures may occur when lesions are present over joints, intragluteally, or on the palms and soles.

Psychosocial Problems
The health care provider should be attuned to the psychologic ramifications of psoriasis—anxiety, social isolation, alcoholism, depression, suicidal ideation—as possible associations and outcomes of this essentially benign skin disease. Stress has been implicated in the acute exacerbations and progression of psoriasis. In a vicious cycle, the poor self-image that may be incited by lesions can create more stress. Factors that may adversely influence psoriasis include:

- **Alcohol.** Alcohol overindulgence has been reputed to exacerbate psoriasis, which, once again, can create a vicious cycle of worsening the alcohol overindulgence.
- **Drugs.** Antimalarials, beta-blockers, angiotensin-converting enzyme inhibitors, certain nonsteroidal anti-inflammatory drugs (e.g., indomethacin), systemic interferon, and lithium carbonate have been reported to worsen psoriasis; however, preexisting psoriasis is not necessarily a contraindication to their use. Both systemic and potent topical steroids have been known, albeit rarely, to trigger a severe, acute, potentially fatal pustular psoriasis (pustular psoriasis of von Zumbusch) that tends to occur after withdrawal of the medication.
- **Physical trauma.** Surgery, thermal and chemical burns, and infections potentially exacerbate psoriasis. For example, an increase in psoriasis activity has been observed in patients who are, or become, infected with the human immunodeficiency virus (HIV).
- **Sunlight.** A small minority of patients find that their psoriasis is worsened by strong sunlight, probably via the Köbner reaction (Fig. 3.4), whereas the vast majority of patients generally consider sunlight to be beneficial.
- **Other factors.** There is evidence that psoriasis is associated with smoking, obesity, and dyslipidemia. It has also been noted that severe psoriasis appears to increase the risk of a myocardial infarction.

Course

- Psoriasis is an erratic condition with an unpredictable, waxing-and-waning course. It has no known cure; however, there are many methods of keeping it under control.
- Many patients tend to improve during the summer and worsen during the colder periods of the year. This fluctuation is presumably the result of the positive influence of sunlight on psoriasis.
- There have been anecdotal reports of patients with psoriasis who were "cured," and some patients claim that they "grew out of it." This situation may be explained by either a misdiagnosis of the original skin problem or by cases of acute guttate psoriasis (see later discussion) that resolved without recurrence.

DIAGNOSIS

- The diagnosis of psoriasis is made on clinical grounds.
- A skin biopsy or fungal studies may be performed to rule in or rule out other possible diagnoses.

 DIFFERENTIAL DIAGNOSIS

The differential diagnosis of psoriasis varies, depending on the type and location of lesions. In general, psoriasis most often must be differentiated from the following:

- Eczematous dermatitis
- Superficial fungal infection
- Seborrheic dermatitis
- Pityriasis rosea
- Drug eruption
- Parapsoriasis and mycosis fungoides (cutaneous T-cell lymphoma)
- Secondary syphilis, the "great imitator"

 SEE PATIENT HANDOUT, "Psoriasis" ON THE SOLUTION SITE

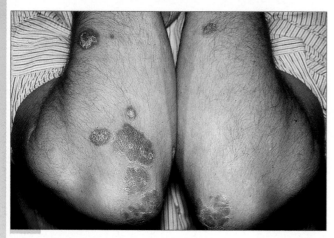

3.6 *Psoriasis.* Note the symmetry of the plaques.

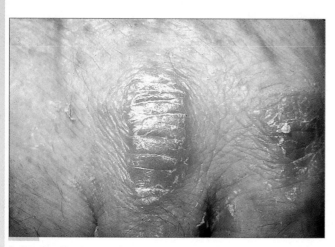

3.7 *Psoriasis.* Typical lesions on knuckles.

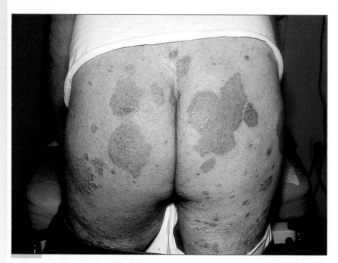

3.8 *Psoriasis.* Widespread plaques on buttocks (compare to FIGS. 3.12 and 3.13).

BASICS

In its mildest manifestation, psoriasis is an incidental finding and consists of mildly erythematous, scaly patches on the elbows or knees. Localized plaque psoriasis, the most common presentation of psoriasis, may remain limited and localized (FIGS. 3.6–3.8), or it may become unstable and become widespread.

DIAGNOSIS

- If the typical well-demarcated whitish or silvery plaque is present in the usual locations, the diagnosis of psoriasis is quite evident.
- Other helpful diagnostic features include a family history of psoriasis and nail findings (see later in this chapter and also Chapter 13, "Diseases and Abnormalities of Nails").
- If necessary, other tests, such as a skin biopsy and fungal examinations, can be performed to rule out other conditions. For example, Bowen's disease, parapsoriasis, and mycosis fungoides are diagnosed by skin biopsy (see FIG. 3.12).

DIFFERENTIAL DIAGNOSIS

Eczematous Dermatitis (Lichen Simplex Chronicus and Atopic Dermatitis)
FIGURE 3.9 and see Chapter 2, "Eczema."

- The patient or a close relative may have a history of atopy.
- Lichenification (an exaggeration of normal skin markings) may be present. Lesions are poorly demarcated; they blend gradually into normal surrounding skin.
- Usually, lesions itch, and crusts and excoriations may be seen.

Nummular Eczema
FIGURE 3.10.

- An atopic history may or may not be present.
- An extensor or flexural distribution is noted, most often on the legs.
- "Coin-shaped" patches and plaques are present.
- Usually, lesions itch (often a major differentiating factor from psoriasis), with possible crusts, excoriations, and lichenification.

Tinea Corporis
FIGURE 3.11.

- Patients may have a history of exposure to fungus.
- Lesions usually are annular ("ringlike")—round and clear in the center but may present a plaques.
- The potassium hydroxide (KOH) examination or fungal culture is positive.
- Lesions usually itch.

Bowen's Disease (Squamous Cell Carcinoma in Situ)
- The solitary lesion may resemble a typical psoriatic plaque.
- The condition is unresponsive to topical steroids.

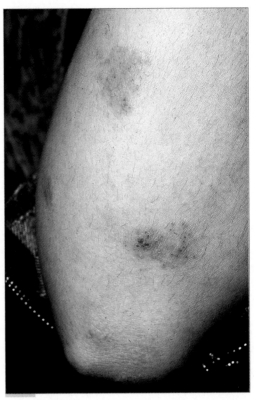

3.10 *Nummular eczema.* Pruritic, round, nummular (coin-shaped), itchy patches with erythema, crusts, and lichenification.

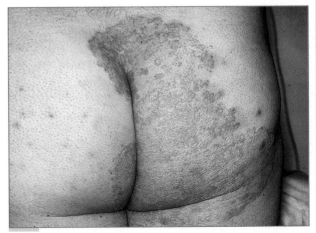

3.11 *Tinea corporis.* Asymmetric erythema and KOH-positive scale ("active border"). This patient has a "psoriasiform" plaque.

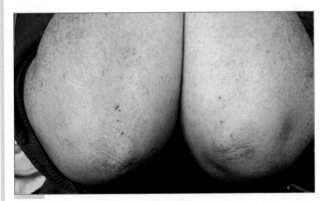

3.9 *Eczema (lichen simplex chronicus).* Note the lichenification and poor demarcation of these lesions (they blend gradually into normal surrounding skin).

continued on page 94

Parapsoriasis

- The term "parapsoriasis" derives from the fact that the condition clinically resembles psoriasis but in fact is a completely different entity.
- Idiopathic multiple, barely elevated patches are usually found on the trunk and arms.
- There are small and large plaque variants.

Mycosis Fungoides (Cutaneous T-Cell Lymphoma)
FIGURE 3.12.

- "Smudgy" patches and plaques or tumors are noted, usually on the buttocks and trunk.
- Lesions are often pruritic.
- A biopsy may demonstrate a cutaneous T-cell lymphoma.

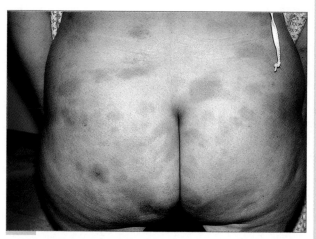

3.12 *Mycosis fungoides (cutaneous T-cell lymphoma).* Lesions have characteristic "smudgy," poorly defined patches and plaques as seen here in a typical location.

 MANAGEMENT

General Principles

- Because psoriasis is a chronic skin condition, any approach to its treatment must be considered for the long term. Treatment regimens must be individualized according to age, sex, occupation, personal motivation, other health conditions, and available resources. Disease severity is defined by the number and extent of plaques present, as well as by the patient's perception and acceptance of the disease. Treatment, therefore, must be designed with the patient's specific expectations in mind.
- Therapy for psoriasis is aimed at decreasing size and thickness of plaques, reducing pruritus, alleviating arthritic symptoms if present, and improving emotional well-being. Ultimately, the determination of successful treatment includes both objective and subjective measures.
- The types of treatment selected are determined by some of the following factors:
  - Age of the patient: Many oral agents that are used to treat severe psoriasis, such as methotrexate and oral retinoids, are less likely to be used in children. Very young children, particularly infants, are not able to cooperate with phototherapy treatment (described later).
  - Type of psoriasis.
  - Site and extent of involvement.
  - Health care provider's experience in managing psoriasis. (Management of mild to relatively moderate psoriasis can be performed by primary care clinicians.

Moderate to severe psoriasis is best treated by dermatologists.)
  - Availability of facilities, such as a phototherapy unit.
  - Presence of psychosocial problems, such as anxiety, depression, alcoholism, and substance abuse.
- Three basic treatment modalities are available for the overall management of psoriasis: (a) topical agents, (b) phototherapy, and (c) systemic agents, including biologic therapies. These treatments may be used alone or in combination.
- Topical therapy is the first-line approach in the treatment of plaque psoriasis (TABLES 3.1 and 3.2). A number of topical treatments are available (e.g., corticosteroids, coal tar, anthralin, calcipotriene, tazarotene). No single topical agent is ideal, and many are often used concurrently in a combined approach. Auxiliary agents such as scale-removing keratolytics can often be added to these preparations.
- Phototherapy and systemic therapy are initiated only after topical treatments have been unsuccessful (see also the later section titled "Generalized Plaque Psoriasis"). These treatments are considered for patients with very active psoriasis or patients who have disease that is physically, psychologically, or socially disabling.

Specific Treatment of Localized Plaque Psoriasis
Topical Corticosteroids
The use of a potent topical steroid for a limited period, followed by a less potent topical steroid for maintenance, is

continued on page 95

the most common method for treating psoriasis and many inflammatory dermatoses (see "Introduction").

Advantage
- Rapid onset in decreasing erythema, inflammation, and itching

Disadvantages
- Drug tolerance (tachyphylaxis) is not uncommon
- Expensive and time consuming, especially when large areas are treated

Occlusion of Topical Steroids

Generally a medium- or high-potency agent is applied and then covered with polyethylene wrap (e.g., Saran Wrap) for several hours or overnight, if tolerated. **Cordran tape** (see "Introduction: Topical Therapy") is similarly effective (see also Chapter 2, "Eczema").

Advantage
- Increases the absorption, and thus potency, of topical steroids

continued on next page

Table 3.1 SHORT LIST OF TOPICAL STEROIDS

POTENCY	GENERIC NAME	BRAND NAMES
Class I	Clobetasol propionate cream/gel/ointment/foam, lotion 0.05%	Temovate, Olux foam, Clobex lotion, Cormax scalp solution
	Flurandrenolide (small and large rolls)	Cordran tape small roll, large roll
Class II	Desoximetasone/0.05% gel	Topicort
	Fluocinonide cream/ointment/solution/gel 0.05%	Lidex
Class III	Fluticasone ointment 0.005%	Cutivate
Class IV	Triamcinolone acetonide ointment 0.1%	Kenalog
	Betamethasone valerate 0.12%	Luxiq foam
	Hydrocortisone valerate cream 0.2%	Westcort
Class V	Triamcinolone acetonide cream 0.1%	Kenalog
	Desonide ointment 0.05%	DesOwen
Class VI	Desonide cream 0.05%, foam	DesOwen, Verdeso foam
Class VII	Hydrocortisone cream/ointment/lotion 0.5%, 1.0%*	Hytone, Cortizone-10, and many other brands

Most preparations are available in tubes of 15, 30, or 60 g. Lotions and solutions are available in bottles of 20 to 60 mL.
*Available over the counter.

Table 3.2 OTHER TOPICAL AGENTS

GENERIC NAME	BRAND NAME	GENERIC NAME	BRAND NAME
Keratolytic agents		*Topical immunomodulators*	
Salicylic acid 6%	Keralyt gel (1 oz)	Tacrolimus ointment 0.03%, 0.1%	Protopic ointment
Salicylic acid 6%	Salex cream (400 g) and lotion (441 mL)	Pimecrolimus 1% cream	Elidel
		Anthralin preparations	
Topical vitamin D₃		Anthralin 0.1%, 0.25%, 0.5%	Drithocreme
Calcipotriene 0.005%	Dovonex cream, scalp solution	Anthralin 0.25%, 0.5%	Dritho-Scalp
		Anthralin 1% cream	Psoriatec
Topical vitamin D₃–topical steroid combination		*Tar preparations*	Estar*
Calcipotriene–betamethasone dipropionate 0.064%	Taclonex		PsoriGel*
			Balnetar*
Topical retinoids			Doak tar oil*
Tazarotene 0.05%, 0.1%, cream/gel	Tazorac cream/gel		

Note: All tar preparations (except liquor carbonis detergens) must be used in grease- or oil-based vehicles. Tar is commonly available in shampoos and is often combined with salicylic acid. Liquor carbonis detergens is an alcohol-extracted tar.
*Available over the counter.

continued on page 96

MANAGEMENT *Continued*

Disadvantage
- Side effects of topical steroids (described previously) are more common.

Additional Suggestion
- A plastic shower cap can be used during treatment of the scalp with topical steroids; the resultant occlusion increases efficacy.

Intralesional Steroids

Intralesional **triamcinolone acetonide (Kenalog,** 2.5 to 5 mg/mL) is delivered intradermally with a 30-gauge needle. The plaque is infiltrated until it blanches. This procedure may be repeated at 4- to 6-week intervals.

Advantages
- Useful with limited number of lesions
- Acts rapidly
- Provides longer period of remission

Disadvantages
- Painful
- Possible local atrophy and telangiectasias
- Requires office visits to administer injections

Topical Vitamin D$_3$ (Dovonex)
- Calcipotriene is a form of synthetic vitamin D$_3$. It slows down the rate of skin cell growth, flattens psoriasis lesions, and removes scale.
- Dovonex is available as a cream, ointment, and scalp solution in a 0.005% strength.

Advantages
- Dovonex is used in combination with many other treatments.
- Unlike topical steroids, Dovonex has few side effects.
- Dovonex scalp solution is a water- and alcohol-based formulation specifically designed for treating scalp psoriasis.
- Combining Dovonex with topical steroids may help. For example, a combined maintenance treatment of daily Dovonex plus weekend use of a superpotent topical steroid (called **pulse therapy**) may prolong remissions.
- Dovonex increases the effectiveness of ultraviolet treatments.

Disadvantages
- Dovonex is not very effective at decreasing inflammation and does not work as quickly as superpotent topical steroids.
- The most common minor side effect is skin irritation, usually in the form of stinging or burning.

- The face, genitals, and skin folds can be sensitive to Dovonex irritation.
- The active ingredient in Dovonex is easily inactivated, particularly by acidic compounds such as salicylic acid.

Topical Vitamin D$_3$–Potent Steroid Combination
- Calcipotriene and betamethasone dipropionate; **Taclonex ointment**

Advantages
- The calcipotriene slows down the rate of skin cell growth, flattens psoriasis lesions, and removes scale.
- The steroid helps reduce inflammation and itching.
- The preparation is applied once a day.

Disadvantages
- Because Taclonex contains a potent topical steroid, it should not be applied to the face, armpits, groin, or other skin folds.
- The preparation is expensive.

Topical Tar Preparations
- Before the advent of topical steroids, tar preparations such as crude coal tar were the mainstay of therapy for psoriasis as well as most inflammatory dermatoses. Currently, they are used much less often.
- Agents such as liquor carbonis detergens, **Balnetar, Doak Tar oil, Estar gel, PsoriGel,** and **T/Derm tar oil** are the traditional tar preparations.

Topical Anthralin
- Anthralin is a coal tar derivative that evolved as an answer to many of the side effects of crude coal tar. It may be used for shorter periods than coal tar, such as for half an hour.
- This short-term anthralin treatment is referred to as short-contact anthralin therapy (**SCAT**). Its major drawbacks are the possible occurrence of skin irritation and a reversible brownish purple staining of the skin.

Innovative Management Strategies
Rotational Therapy
- An innovative approach to the management of psoriasis consists of cycling or rotating different treatment modalities. This strategy presumably decreases cumulative side effects and drug tolerance (tachyphylaxis), and it often allows for lower dosages and shorter durations of therapy for each agent.
- For example, a superpotent (class 1) topical steroid, such as **clobetasol,** may be applied for 2 weeks, discontinued for 1 or 2 weeks, and then restarted. Alternatively, clobetasol may be used on weekends only, and **Dovonex ointment** can be used during the week.

Exfoliative Dermatitis (Exfoliative Erythroderma)

BASICS

Rarely, a patient may develop a sudden or subacute appearance of generalized scaling and erythema (FIG. 3.14), often with accompanying fever and chills. This condition, exfoliative dermatitis, can be the presenting symptom of psoriasis or a subsequent complication of limited psoriatic disease (see Chapter 25, "Cutaneous Manifestations of Systemic Disease," for a discussion of exfoliative dermatitis).

Some of the trigger factors that may lead to exfoliative dermatitis in patients with psoriasis are as follows:

- Administration of systemic or superpotent topical corticosteroids in patients with preexisting psoriasis
- Topical therapy that is irritating or produces severe contact dermatitis
- High levels of emotional stress
- Medical procedures (e.g., surgery) or certain conditions (e.g., infections)

Alternatively, psoriasis may initially present as exfoliative dermatitis.

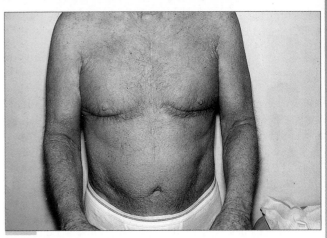

3.14 *Psoriasis.* Erythrodermic variant of exfoliative dermatitis.

 MANAGEMENT

Treatment of exfoliative dermatitis secondary to psoriasis may involve some of the measures used for generalized plaque psoriasis (e.g., UV light therapy, oral agents) in addition to the following:

- Bed rest
- Cool compresses
- Lubrication with emollients
- Antipruritic therapy with oral antihistamines
- Low- to moderate-strength topical corticosteroids
- Hospitalization in extreme cases

Acute Guttate Psoriasis

See also Chapter 27, "Special Considerations in the Skin of Pediatric and Elderly Patients."

BASICS

This type of psoriasis refers to the sudden onset of multiple guttate (teardrop-shaped) lesions (FIG. 3.15). It is often the initial presentation of psoriasis in children or young adults.

Acute guttate psoriasis is occasionally preceded by a group A beta-hemolytic streptococcal pharyngitis (positive throat culture or serologic evidence of antistreptolysin O). These patients should be treated promptly with appropriate antibiotic therapy, because it has been reported that some of these patients have self-limited cases of psoriasis. Long-term follow-up has indicated that many of these patients with "one-time" cases of psoriasis eventually proved to have recurrences, suggesting typical psoriasis.

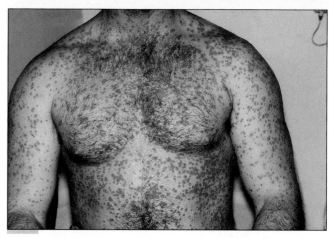

3.15 *Psoriasis (acute guttate).* This patient had a recent group A beta-hemolytic streptococcal pharyngitis.

 DIFFERENTIAL DIAGNOSIS

- Pityriasis rosea (FIG. 3.16)
- Drug eruption
- Parapsoriasis
- Secondary syphilis

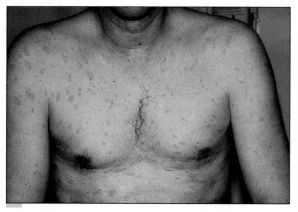

3.16 *Pityriasis rosea.* Typical distribution of elliptic, scaly lesions (see also Chapter 4, "Inflammatory Eruptions of Unknown Cause").

 MANAGEMENT

- UVB phototherapy or natural sunlight exposure
- Appropriate antibiotic therapy, such as penicillin or erythromycin for group A beta-hemolytic streptococcus
- High-potency (class 1, 2, or 3) topical steroids or SCAT (described earlier)

See also Chapter 27, "Special Considerations in the Skin of Pediatric and Elderly Patients."

BASICS

In approximately 10% of patients, psoriasis begins before the age of 10 years. An early onset portends more severe disease, and there is often an associated family history of the disease.

In some infants, psoriasis begins as a diaper rash, which may be difficult to distinguish from irritant dermatitis, atopic dermatitis, or cutaneous candidiasis. The rash may clear; however, the child may later develop psoriasis. Conversely, psoriasis may present with typical plaques, such as those seen in adults.

Infantile or childhood psoriasis deserves particular attention. It requires intensive educational guidance and counseling of the patient and family.

 MANAGEMENT

Many of the treatments that are used in adults, such as superpotent topical steroids, phototherapy, methotrexate, and retinoids, are generally avoided in children. Low- to medium-potency topical steroids, SCAT (described earlier), and natural sunlight, if available, are also used in children. All of these treatments should be administered with caution.

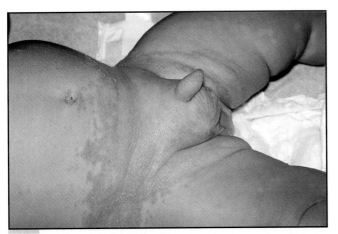

3.17 *Psoriasis in an infant.* This eruption was initially considered to be a simple diaper rash.

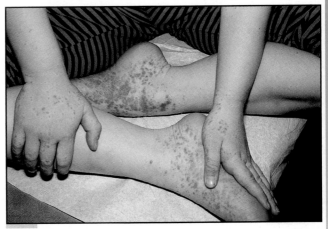

3.18 *Acute guttate psoriasis.* This child also had a streptococcal throat infection.

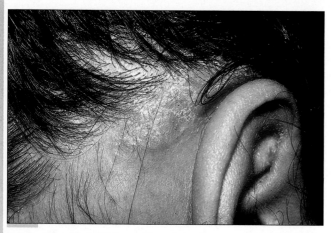

3.19 *Psoriasis of the scalp.* This discrete, scaly plaque is one of many this patient has on her scalp.

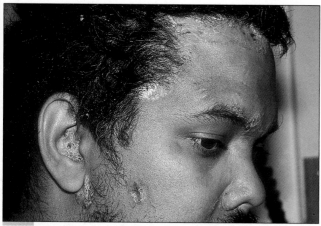

3.20 *Psoriasis of the scalp and ears.* Note the crusted excoriations behind this patient's ear and along his hairline.

BASICS

Psoriasis may involve the scalp alone, or the scalp may be affected along with other areas of the body. The plaques are often thick and well demarcated with a whitish scale (FIG. 3.19). They are frequently hidden in the scalp or behind the ears, but often they extend beyond the hairline and become more obvious when the hair is held back and when the retroauricular area is examined. Often, the external ears and ear canals are involved (FIG. 3.20).

Features of scalp psoriasis include:

- Pruritus and scratching, which may exacerbate the condition (Köbner reaction).
- Lesions that range from flaky dandruff to thick, extensive, armorlike plaques.
- Possibly problematic management. When severe, it is particularly difficult to treat because hair blocks UV light as well as the topical application of psoriatic medications.

 DIFFERENTIAL DIAGNOSIS

Adults
Seborrheic Dermatitis and Eczematous Dermatitis of Scalp
FIGURES. 3.21 and 3.22.

- Both conditions are very common and may be clinically indistinguishable from scalp psoriasis.
- Both conditions may be present elsewhere on the body.

Eczematous Dermatitis of Scalp
- Eczematous lesions may be present elsewhere on the body.
- An atopic history is usually present.

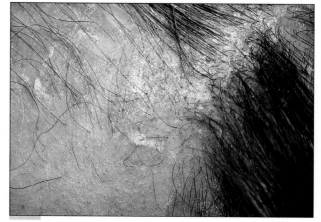

3.21 *Seborrheic dermatitis.* Finer, thinner scale than is shown in FIGURES. 3.19 and 3.20.

continued on page 105

Children
Tinea Capitis
- A KOH test and/or fungal culture may be positive.

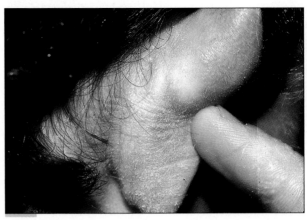

3.22 *Seborrheic dermatitis.* Retroauricular erythema and scale. Compare to FIGURE. 3.20. (See also Chapter 2, "Eczema.")

 ## MANAGEMENT

Mild Cases
- In patients with minimal scaling and thin plaques (similar to what is seen in seborrheic dermatitis (see Chapter 2, "Eczema"), the psoriasis can often be managed with anti-dandruff shampoos and a mid-potency (class 3 or 4) topical steroid, used as needed for itching.
- Over-the-counter options include shampoos that contain tar (**Zetar, T/Gel**), selenium sulfide (**Selsun Blue, Head & Shoulders**), or **salicylic acid (T/Sal).**

Topical Steroids
- Low-potency (class 6) topical steroids include preparations such as **Capex** shampoo or **Verdeso foam**. Gel, foam, or solution preparations reach the scalp more readily than do ointments or creams.

Antifungals
- Shampoos containing the antifungals **ketoconazole 2% (Nizoral)** and **ciclopirox (Loprox)** are available by prescription.

Severe Cases
- In patients with thick scales and plaques, the scale must be removed before the plaques can be treated effectively. Scale removal is accomplished by applying either **Keralyt gel** or **Salex cream** or **lotion** one to three times per week. This regimen may be sufficient to keep scale under control, thus allowing penetration of a topical steroid.
- After the scale is removed, a medium- to high-potency (class 2, 3, or 4) topical steroid is used. For example, **fluocinonide solution** or **gel** or **desoximetasone (Topicort)** gel can be applied once or twice daily as needed, under shower cap occlusion overnight, or for 3 to 4 hours during the day. If necessary, a superpotent (class 1) topical steroid such as **clobetasol propionate lotion, foam,** or **gel** can be used without occlusion. In recalcitrant situations, the superpotent topical steroid can be applied under occlusion once or twice per week.
- **Dovonex lotion** can be used as maintenance or rotational therapy (see earlier section).
- Injections of **intralesional triamcinolone** (3 to 5 mg/mL) in a limited amount (1 to 2 mL or less per treatment) every 4 to 8 weeks are used to target particularly itchy areas and may bring longer remissions.

 SEE PATIENT HANDOUT, "Scalp Psoriasis: Scale Removal" ON THE SOLUTION SITE

Inverse Psoriasis

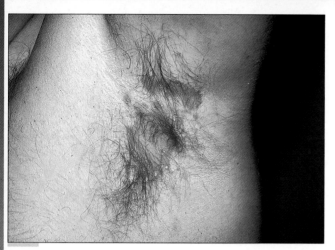

3.23 *Inverse psoriasis.* Axillary involvement is shown here. Both axillary psoriasis and inframammary psoriasis are often misdiagnosed as cutaneous candidiasis. (Compare to Fig. 3.28)

BASICS

- Psoriasis seen in intertriginous areas such as the axillae, inframammary folds, perineal and perianal areas, scrotum, glans penis, and inguinal creases is referred to as inverse psoriasis (Figs. 3.22–3.27).
- Typically, lesions are red, glistening, well-demarcated plaques that generally lack scale. This manifestation is seen when two apposing surfaces of skin rub together, such as under the breasts. Such constant rubbing does not allow scale to build up.
- Fissures may occur in the groin and gluteal creases.

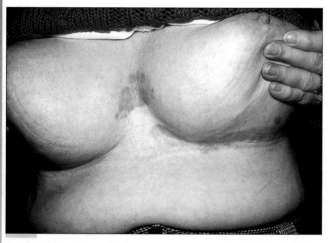

3.24 *Inverse psoriasis.* Well-demarcated inframammary lesions. (Compare to Fig. 3.29)

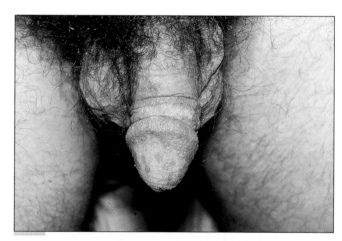

3.26 *Inverse psoriasis.* Typical psoriatic lesions on the penis are not unusual.

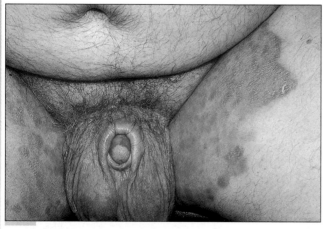

3.25 *Inverse psoriasis.* Note involvement of the scrotum, foreskin, and glans. This is often misdiagnosed as cutaneous candidiasis or tinea cruris. (Compare to Fig. 3.30)

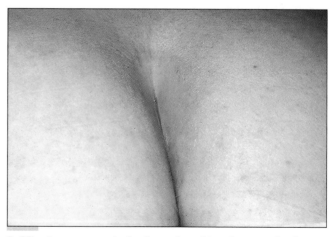

3.27 *Inverse psoriasis.* Intragluteal involvement is also not unusual. Note the painful fissure.

- Inverse psoriasis is commonly misdiagnosed by nondermatologists as tinea or candidiasis. Accordingly, it is often incorrectly treated with topical antifungal agents.

Intertrigo or Contact Dermatitis

A common inflammatory condition of skin folds (FIG. 3.28), intertrigo occurs when opposing skin surfaces rub against each other, such as seen in diaper dermatitis (see also Chapter 27, "Special Considerations in the Skin of Pediatric and Elderly Patients"). Common features include:

- Induction or aggravation by heat, hyperhidrosis, moisture, maceration, and friction
- May be caused by contactants such as antiperspirants or dry cleaning solvents
- Location in the axillae and inguinal and intragluteal creases; often occurs under pendulous breasts and abdominal folds
- Possible colonization by secondary infection such as *Candida albicans*, particularly in patients with diabetes (FIG. 3.29)
- Often complicates obesity

Tinea Cruris

- Lesion with a scalloped, active border (FIG. 3.30)
- Generally spares the scrotum and penis
- Positive KOH examination and fungal cultures for dermatophytes

Cutaneous Candidiasis

- "Beefy red" color to the lesions
- Satellite pustules seen beyond the border of the plaques
- Positive KOH examination for budding yeast
- Positive culture for *Candida* species

Atopic Dermatitis

- Eczematous lesions that occur elsewhere on the body
- Patients have an atopic history

Seborrheic Dermatitis

- May be indistinguishable from inverse psoriasis (intertriginous seborrheic dermatitis)

Other Considerations

- When lesions are present on the glans penis, **nonspecific balanitis** (more commonly seen in elderly men) and balanitis from candidal species should be considered in the differential diagnosis.
- **Pruritus ani** also may be confused with inverse psoriasis.
- Secondary overgrowth with *Candida* species and tinea must also be considered.

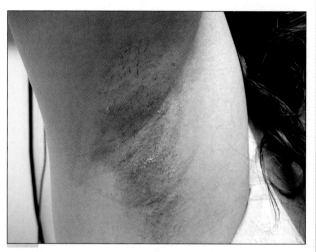

3.28 *Irritant intertrigo.* This patient's eruption is caused by irritation from antiperspirants used to treat hyperhidrosis. This problem is common when opposing skin surfaces rub against each other.

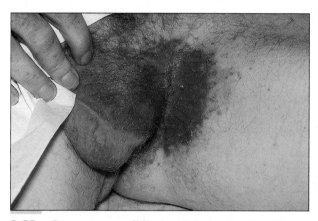

3.29 *Cutaneous candidiasis.* Note the "beefy red" plaque and "satellite pustules" in this diabetic patient.

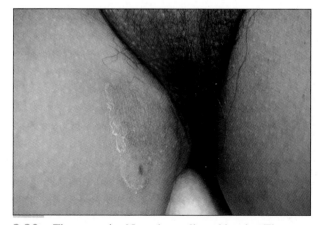

3.30 *Tinea cruris.* Note the scalloped border. The KOH examination is positive. The scrotum is spared in most cases.

MANAGEMENT

- The lowest-potency nonfluorinated topical steroids are used to avoid atrophy and striae.
- To achieve rapid improvement, treatment may be initiated with a higher-potency (class 5) steroid that is used for several days before it is changed to a lower-potency (class 6 or 7) agent.
  - **Dovonex cream** or **ointment** may be used primarily (if it is not irritating) or in rotation with a mild topical steroid.
  - **Tacrolimus (Protopic) ointment** 0.03% or 0.1% can be applied once or twice daily.
  - **Pimecrolimus (Elidel) cream** 1% may be used once or twice daily.

 POINT TO REMEMBER

- Intertriginous areas are moist and occluded; therefore, the penetration and efficacy of topical agents are increased in these regions; consequently, topical steroids are more likely to produce striae (linear atrophy).

BASICS

Psoriasis that manifests on the palms and soles presents a difficult therapeutic challenge. The palms or soles alone may be affected, or these areas may be a part of more extensive psoriasis on the body. As with inverse psoriasis (see earlier), palmoplantar psoriasis, by virtue of its location, cannot benefit from UV light therapy. There are two variants:

- **Hyperkeratotic.** Like its counterparts elsewhere, this form of psoriasis is characterized by well-demarcated, scaly plaques (FIGS. 3.31 and 3.32). The location of these lesions presents additional problems such as pain, impairment of function, fissuring, bleeding, and embarrassment.
- **Pustular.** This rare form of psoriasis has historically had many clinical descriptions and eponyms. It is most commonly seen in adults, and lesions tend to be symmetric and well defined. It favors the insteps of the feet, the heels, and the thenar and hypothenar eminences. Less commonly, it appears on the palms (FIG. 3.33).

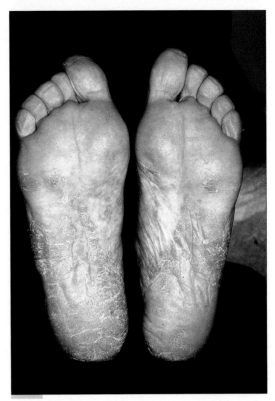

3.32 **Psoriasis.** Note the clear demarcation between involved and uninvolved skin. Similar lesions were present on this patient's palms.

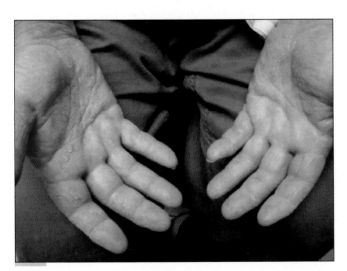

3.31 **Psoriasis.** This patient's lesions are symmetric and well-demarcated.

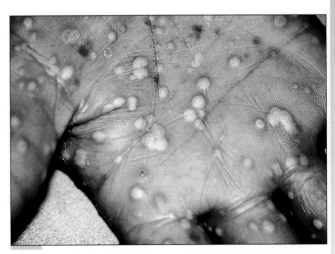

3.33 **Psoriasis.** This is the pustular variant of psoriasis.

DIFFERENTIAL DIAGNOSIS

Contact Dermatitis

- This is suspected, particularly if the eruption is on the dorsum of the hands or feet.
- The patient has a history of exposure to a suspected contactant.

Hand Eczema or Dyshidrotic Eczema

See Chapter 2, "Eczema."

- "Sago-grain" vesicles are visible.
- Pruritus is present.
- The patient has evidence of eczema elsewhere on the body or a personal or family history of atopy.
- May be indistinguishable from palmoplantar psoriasis.

Tinea Manuum and Pedis

- A "two-feet, one-hand" presentation is noted (see Chapter 7, "Superficial Fungal Infections").
- The KOH examination or fungal culture is positive.

MANAGEMENT

Topical treatment is the first line of therapy. Because of their thick stratum corneum, the palms and soles present the greatest barrier to cutaneous penetration; potent topical steroids are used, often under occlusion. Treatment options include the following:

- Superpotent (class 1) topical steroids, such as **clobetasol propionate,** are first tried without occlusion, but occlusion (under vinyl or rubber gloves) may be used if necessary.
- Salicylic acid preparations such as **Keralyt gel** or **Salex cream** or **lotion** may be used to remove scale, if necessary.
- **Calcipotriene (Dovonex)** ointment or cream can be used.

- **Anthralin,** overnight or as SCAT, may be useful.
- Emollients may be useful.

When a patient is not responding to topical therapies, treatment options can include:

- **PUVA** (see earlier discussion): **topical UVA** therapy using a "hand-foot box"
- **Oral retinoids,** such as etretinate
- **RePUVA** (low-dose etretinate combined with PUVA)
- **Oral methotrexate**
- **Oral cyclosporine**
- Biologics (see earlier discussion). **Raptiva** is increasingly considered the biologic of choice for hand–foot disease. Raptiva plus low-dose acitretin has been shown to be an excellent regimen for severe, disabling hand–foot disease.

BASICS

Involvement of nails is very common in patients with psoriasis (see also Chapter 13, "Diseases and Abnormalities of Nails"). Psoriatic nail dystrophy is a chronic, primarily cosmetic condition. However, in some instances, thickened psoriatic toenails can become painful, and psoriatic fingernail deformities may result in interference with function. Psoriatic nail dystrophy is more commonly noted in patients who have psoriatic arthritis.

Typical nail changes may involve:

- **Pitting**, which is the most characteristic nail finding in psoriasis. It is produced by tiny punctate lesions that arise from the nail matrix (nail root) and appear on the nail plate as it grows (FIG. 3.34).
- **Onycholysis**, which represents a separation of the nail plate from the underlying pink nail bed. The separated portion is white or yellow-white and opaque, in contrast to the pink translucence of the attached portion (FIG. 3.35).

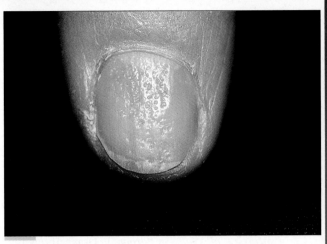

3.34 *Psoriasis (pitting).* The result of tiny punctate lesions that arise from the nail matrix, pitting appears on the nail plate as it grows.

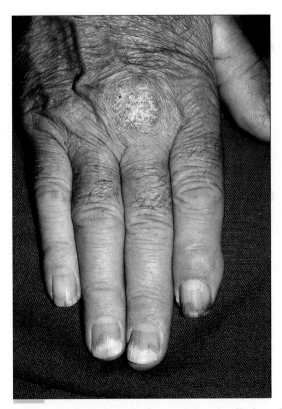

3.35 *Psoriasis (onycholysis).* Several nail plates have separated from the underlying pink nail bed. The separated portion is white or yellow-white and opaque, in contrast to the pink translucence of the attached portion. Note the typical psoriatic plaque on this patient's knuckle.

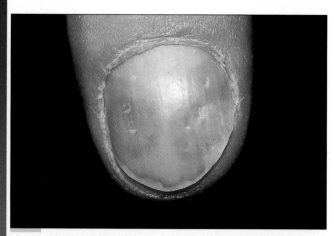

3.36 *Psoriasis ("oil spots" or "drops").* Orange-brown coloration appears under the nail plate, presumably the result of psoriasis of the nail bed. Onycholysis is also evident.

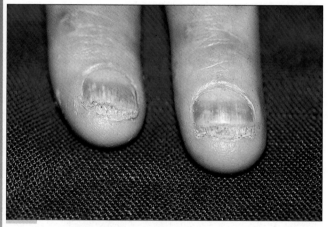

3.37 *Psoriasis (subungual hyperkeratosis).* A buildup of scale beneath the nail plate resembles onychomycosis. Also note in this figure "oil spots" and onycholysis.

- **"Oil spots"** or **"drops,"** which are orange-brown colorations appearing under the nail plate. They are presumably the result of psoriasis of the nail bed (FIG. 3.36).
- Thickening, or **subungual hyperkeratosis**, which is a buildup of scale beneath the nail plate. It resembles onychomycosis, with which it is often confused and may coexist, particularly in toenails (FIG. 3.37).

 DIFFERENTIAL DIAGNOSIS

Onychomycosis
- In onychomycosis, the KOH examination or fungal culture is positive (FIG. 3.38).

Eczematous Dermatitis
- Eczematous dermatitis with secondary nail dystrophy lacks subungual hyperkeratosis. Eczema is noted in the area of the proximal nail fold (see FIG. 2.17).

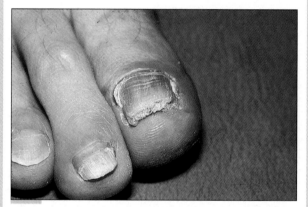

3.38 *Onychomycosis.* The subungual hyperkeratosis is similar to psoriasis; however, a fungal culture grew a dermatophyte.

 MANAGEMENT

Treatment is generally unrewarding, but some measures can be helpful:

- Careful trimming and paring of the nails are recommended.
- The application of a super-potent (class 1) topical steroid to the proximal nail folds is followed by covering with plastic wrap, **Cordran tape**, or a plastic glove.
- **Tazarotene (Tazorac) gel** 0.01%, applied to the proximal nail fold nightly, has been shown to reduce onycholysis and pitting of psoriatic nails. (It has no effect on thickening and severe dystrophy.)

- **Intralesional corticosteroids** can be injected into the nail matrix. The proximal and/or lateral nail fold is sprayed first with a refrigerant spray for anesthesia, and 2.5 mg/mL is injected with a 30-gauge needle every 4 to 6 weeks.
- At present, three systemic medications are most commonly used to treat psoriasis and nail psoriasis: **methotrexate, retinoids,** and **cyclosporine.** All have potential serious side effects and toxicities, and, in most cases, the psoriatic nail disease recurs after the systemic therapy is stopped.
- Systemic agents such as **biologics** are reserved for intractable cases, particularly when psoriatic arthritis is also present.

BASICS

Although psoriatic arthritis can be seen at any age, it most often begins between the ages of 35 and 45 years. It develops before or, more often, after the outbreak of skin manifestations of psoriasis. Overexpression of TNF alpha is thought to play a key role. Multiple human leukocyte antigen associations are known.

An earlier onset of psoriatic arthritis in adulthood can portend a worse prognosis that may include destructive arthropathy. Psoriatic arthritis has the following clinical features:

- A test for the rheumatoid factor is usually negative.
- It is seen in 5% to 10% of patients with psoriasis.
- It is more likely seen in patients with severe cutaneous disease.
- Nail involvement is more frequently noted.
- Peripheral psoriatic arthritis may be indistinguishable from Reiter's syndrome.

There are five clinical patterns of psoriatic arthritis:

- Asymmetric involvement of one or several small or medium-sized joints is the most common initial presentation of psoriatic arthritis. If a finger joint is affected initially, the result is sometimes referred to as a "sausage finger deformity" (FIG. 3.39).
- Mild involvement of the distal interphalangeal joints is considered the classic form of psoriatic arthritis. It is often accompanied by nail disease.
- Symmetric joint involvement is difficult to distinguish from rheumatoid arthritis. (However, a test for rheumatoid factor is negative.)
- Involvement of the joints in the axial skeleton that resembles, and may overlap with, ankylosing spondylitis can occur.
- Mutilating, grossly deforming, arthritis mutilans may occur (FIG. 3.40).

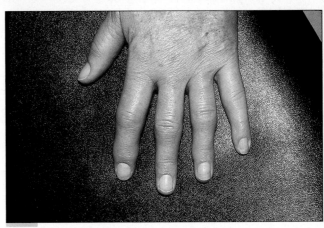

3.39 **_Psoriatic arthritis._** "Sausage finger deformity" of the distal interphalangeal joint.

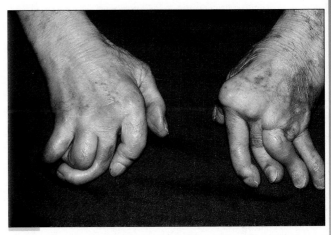

3.40 **_Psoriatic arthritis ("arthritis mutilans")._** This patient has severe psoriatic arthritis with marked deformities and subluxations of the small bones of the hands. Note also the characteristic onycholysis on the nails.

 MANAGEMENT

- Treatment consists of analgesics, primarily non-steroidal anti-inflammatory drugs, and methotrexate.
- Biologics may also be helpful (see earlier discussion).

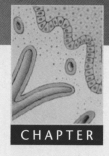

Inflammatory Eruptions of Unknown Cause

➤ **PITYRIASIS ROSEA**

- Classic
- Atypical or inverse
- Pityriasis rosea-like eruption in association with various drugs

➤ **GRANULOMA ANNULARE**

- Childhood
- Adult
- Subcutaneous
- Disseminated

➤ **LICHEN PLANUS**

- Hypertrophic
- Atrophic
- Erosive (mucosal)
- Follicular (lichen planopilaris)

Other eruptions resembling lichen planus are seen in the following conditions:

- Drug-induced
- Lichenoid reactions associated with graft-versus-host disease
- LP associated with hepatitis C

OVERVIEW

Pityriasis rosea, granuloma annulare, and lichen planus are unique inflammatory conditions of unknown etiology. Each has various clinical presentations, and distinctive patterns of anatomic distribution. Most often the diagnosis can be readily made based upon the typical signs and symptoms of these curious dermatioses.

There are conflicting reports about the association of these entities with certain infectious and metabolic conditions. For example, pityriasis roses is thought to represent a viral exanthem possibly caused by a herpesvirus. An association has been noted between lichen planus and hepatitis C, chronic active hepatitis, and primary biliary cirrhosis and widespread granuloma annulare is considered by some investigators to be associated diabetes mellitus.

BASICS

Pityriasis rosea (PR), which means "fine pink scale," is an acute, benign, self-limiting eruption with a characteristic clinical course. PR tends to occur in the spring and fall, and although it may occur at any age, it is seen mostly in young adults and older children. The cause is unknown; however, the occasional clustering of cases and seasonal appearances suggest an infectious, transmissible origin. A single outbreak tends to elicit lifelong immunity, although repeat cases have reportedly been observed.

Pathogenesis

A viral etiology has been suggested, but this has not been confirmed. Despite the prevailing opinion that PR is caused by an infectious agent, it does not appear to be contagious; household contacts and schoolmates usually do not develop the eruption.

DESCRIPTION OF LESIONS

- The typical course of PR often begins with the larger herald patch (FIG. 4.1), a 2- to 5-cm, scaly lesion that may exhibit central clearing and therefore may mimic, and often be confused with, tinea corporis.
- The herald patch is followed in several days to 2 weeks by multiple characteristic oval or elliptic erythematous patches with fine, thin scale on their surfaces (FIG. 4.2).
- Individual lesions often develop a thin, circular, collarette of scale (see "Introduction: Reaction Patterns, Shapes, and Configurations"). Lesions in very dark-skinned patients may lack the typical pink color of PR and may appear darker than the surrounding skin.

DISTRIBUTION OF LESIONS

- The initial lesion, the herald patch, is most commonly observed on the trunk, neck, or extremities (FIG. 4.3). The absence of the herald patch does not necessarily rule out the diagnosis; it may be absent or hidden in an obscure location such as the scalp or groin.
- Subsequent lesions appear on the trunk, neck, arms, and legs in an "old-fashioned bathing suit" distribution.

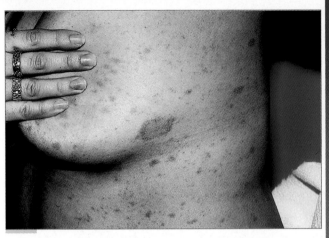

4.1 *Pityriasis rosea.* This patient has a herald patch on her chest. Other, smaller, elliptical lesions can be seen.

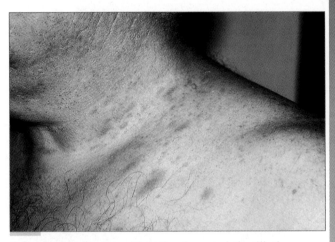

4.2 *Pityriasis rosea.* Note the characteristic elliptic ("football") shape of lesions.

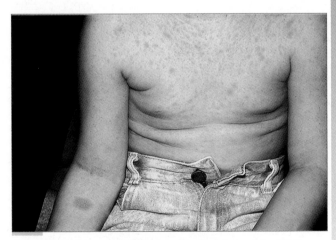

4.3 *Pityriasis rosea.* The herald patch is on this child's flexor forearm.

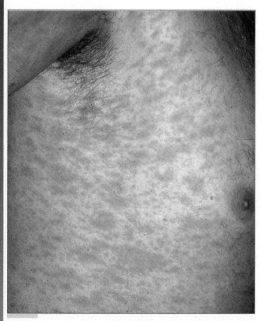

4.4 Pityriasis rosea. Here the lesions are more exuberant and the "Christmas tree" pattern is evident.

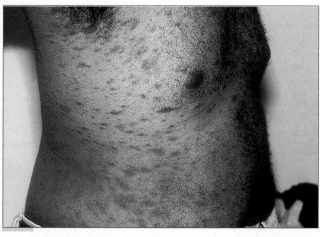

4.5 Pityriasis rosea. Note the hyperpigmented lesions in this African-American patient.

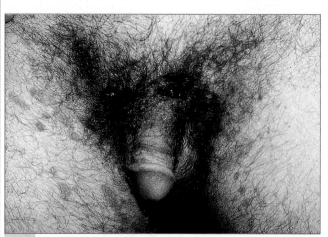

4.6 Pityriasis rosea. Atypical (inverse). The larger herald patch is present in the left inguinal area.

- The long axis of the lesions runs parallel to skin tension lines. This gives a so-called "Christmas tree" pattern on the trunk (FIG. 4.4).

CLINICAL MANIFESTATIONS

- Itching is usually absent or mild but may be severe in a minority of patients.
- PR is a self-limiting, benign disorder; it usually lasts for 6 to 8 weeks.
- On resolution, postinflammatory pigment changes (hyperpigmentation) can occur, particularly in dark-skinned people (FIG. 4.5).
- Recurrences are rare.

CLINICAL VARIANTS

- PR can occur with less typical presentations such as those in which the herald patch is not noted by the patient or clinician. Moreover, in dark-skinned patients, the lesions may be vesicular and uncharacteristically pruritic.
- The eruption may be limited in its distribution, or it may present in an inverse fashion involving the groin (FIG. 4.6), axillae, or distal extremities (inverse PR).
- Infrequently, eruptions resembling those of PR also can occur in association with many drugs. These include barbiturates, bismuth, captopril, clonidine, diphtheria toxoid, gold, isotretinoin, ketotifen, levamisole, metronidazole, and D-penicillamine.

DIAGNOSIS

The diagnosis is made clinically in most cases. In general, laboratory tests are not necessary or helpful, with the following exceptions:

- A potassium hydroxide (KOH) examination may be helpful when only the herald patch is present, to help rule in or rule out tinea corporis; similarly, a KOH examination may be used to distinguish tinea versicolor (see Chapter 7, "Superficial Fungal Infections") from PR.
- A rapid plasma reagin (RPR) or venereal disease research laboratory (VDRL) test should be performed in all patients with PR.
- A skin biopsy may be performed when the eruption is atypical, the diagnosis is uncertain, or the disease has not resolved after 3 to 4 months.

DIFFERENTIAL DIAGNOSIS

Guttate Psoriasis
FIGURE 4.7.

- Guttate psoriasis often follows streptococcal pharyngitis, and its abrupt onset and appearance can easily be confused with PR.
- Scale is generally thicker than that of PR.

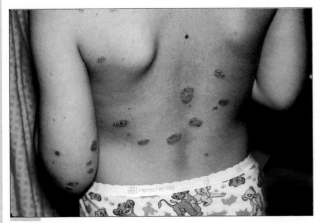

4.7 *Guttate psoriasis.* Here the plaques are thicker and more round or oval in shape than those seen in PR.

Tinea Versicolor
FIGURE 4.9.

- Round or oval macules or patches are present.
- Pigmentation may be varied ("versicolor").
- The KOH examination is positive.

Drug Eruption or Viral Exanthem
- Lesions are redder, less scaly, and tend to be itchier than in PR.
- There may be other symptoms (e.g., fever).

Nummular Eczema
- "Coin-shaped" patches and plaques are present.
- Lesions tend to be on the legs; they are less common on the arms.
- This condition generally itches.

Parapsoriasis
- Lesions may be similar to those of PR.
- Despite its similar name, parapsoriasis is unrelated to psoriasis.

Secondary Syphilis
FIGURE 4.8.

- Lesions are often seen on the palms, soles, and face, as well as the trunk, and may be indistinguishable from PR.
- The RPR or VDRL test is positive.

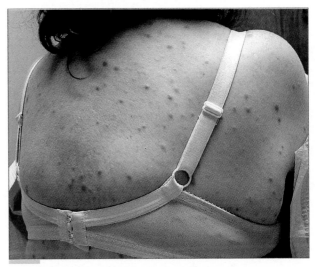

4.8 *Secondary syphilis.* Papulosquamous lesions appear on the trunk, similar to PR. (Image courtesy of Ed Zabawski, D.O.).

- Parapsoriasis should be considered in PR that persists for longer than 8 weeks.

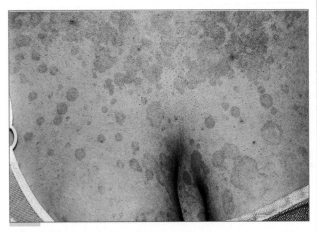

4.9 *Tinea versicolor.* The oval, tan patches are positive on KOH examination.

MANAGEMENT

- Treatment is often unnecessary, because PR is usually a self-limiting, asymptomatic condition with no sequelae.
- All that is usually necessary is to advise the patient about the usual course of the rash and its noncontagious nature.
- Exposure to sunlight or administration of ultraviolet B by a dermatologist may speed resolution of the eruption.

- Follow-up or referral to a dermatologist should be made if the rash persists more than 8 weeks.
- In cases of severe pruritus, oral antihistamines or topical steroids may help alleviate the itching. The sedative effect of the antihistamines may help the patient sleep better at night. On occasion, systemic steroids (prednisone, 0.5 to 1 mg/kg/day for 7 days) can be used in patients with severe pruritus.

 POINTS TO REMEMBER

- Lesions characteristically appear "from the neck to the knees."
- PR is observed in otherwise healthy people, most frequently in children and young adults.
- Patients should be told that PR is a benign condition that will resolve over 6 to 8 weeks without treatment.
- Secondary syphilis should be considered in the differential diagnosis, especially when lesions are present on the palms and soles.

BASICS

Granuloma annulare (GA) is an idiopathic, generally asymptomatic, ring-shaped grouping of dermal papules. The papules are composed of focal granulomas that coalesce to form curious circles or semicircular plaques, which are often misdiagnosed as "ringworm." Familial cases of GA in identical twins and siblings suggest the possibility of a hereditary component.

- In very young children, GA is often self-limiting.
- In adults, GA tends to be a chronic condition that occurs in women (2.5:1 female-to-male ratio).

GA has been associated with diabetes mellitus based on an increased number of GA patients in a small case series.

Pathophysiology

Proposed pathogenic mechanisms include cell-mediated immunity (type IV), immune complex vasculitis, and an abnormality of tissue monocytes. None of these theories has convincing supporting evidence.

DESCRIPTION OF LESIONS

- Lesions are skin-colored or red firm dermal papules, with no epidermal change (scale).
- The lesions may be individual, isolated papules, or they may be joined in annular or semiannular (arciform) plaques with central clearing (FIGS. 4.10 and 4.11). The centers of the lesions may be slightly hyperpigmented and depressed relative to their borders.
- Occasionally, GA may present as subcutaneous nodules that are similar to rheumatoid nodules.

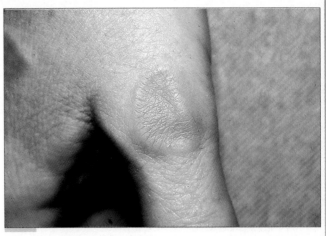

4.10 *Granuloma annulare.* These dermal plaques are typical ringlike lesions.

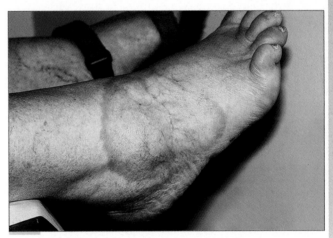

4.11 *Granuloma annulare.* An annular plaque of the dorsal foot.

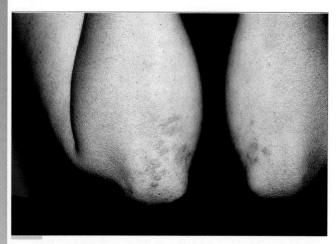

4.12   *Granuloma annulare.* Papules of granuloma annulare are located below the elbows in this middle-aged woman.

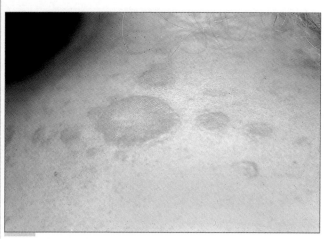

4.13   *Granuloma annulare.* Note the similarity of these annular lesions to FIGURES 4.14 and 4.15.

DISTRIBUTION OF LESIONS

- Although any part of the cutaneous surface may be involved, lesions are most often distributed symmetrically on dorsal surfaces of hands, fingers, and feet (acral areas).
- In adults, lesions may also be found around the elbows (FIG. 4.12) and on the trunk (FIG. 4.13).
- Subcutaneous nodules may be seen on the arms and legs.

CLINICAL MANIFESTATIONS

- GA is generally asymptomatic and is primarily a cosmetic problem, although many patients tend to find it alarming.

DIAGNOSIS

- The diagnosis is most often made on clinical grounds.
- GA has a characteristic histopathologic appearance. It consists of foci of altered collagen and mucin surrounded by granulomatous inflammation of histiocytic and lymphocytic cells. The degenerative collagen is referred to as necrobiosis.

DIFFERENTIAL DIAGNOSIS

Tinea Corporis ("Ringworm")
- Scale is present at the "active border" (FIG. 4.14).
- Lesions tend to be "ringlike" (clear in the center), and they are not firm and infiltrated as seen in GA.
- An asymmetric distribution of lesions is apparent.
- The KOH examination or fungal culture is positive.
- Lesions are often pruritic.

Erythema Migrans Rash of Lyme Disease
(See also Chapter 20, "Bites, Stings, and Infestations.")
- Lesions of erythema migrans are larger than those associated with GA (FIG. 4.15).
- They are often associated with a history of tick bite.
- The rash is self-limited.
- Lesions are not as firm to palpation as in GA.

Cutaneous Sarcoidosis
- This condition is most commonly seen in black and Scandinavian adults.
- Lesions often appear around orifices (e.g., the mouth, nose, ocular orbits) or develop in scars (see FIGS. 25.35 and 25.36).
- Other diagnostic features of sarcoidosis are usually present.
- Annular sarcoidosis may be indistinguishable from GA.

Rheumatoid Nodules
- These may be indistinguishable from subcutaneous nodules of GA.

Necrobiosis Lipoidica Diabeticorum
- Necrobiosis lipoidica diabeticorum (NLD) is characterized by yellow-red to brown, translucent plaques, with epidermal atrophy and telangiectasia (see FIGS. 25.1 and 25.2).
- NLD is seen more frequently in people with type 1 diabetes and may occur before the onset of clinical diabetes.
- A minority of patients have no clinical evidence or family history of diabetes; in these patients, the term necrobiosis lipoidica is used.

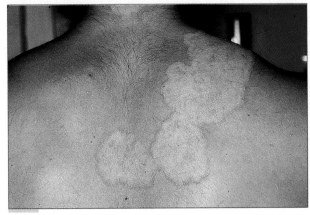

4.14 *Tinea corporis.* KOH-positive scale is present at the "active border."

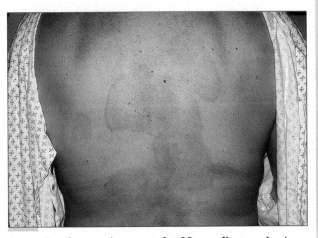

4.15 *Erythema migrans rash of Lyme disease.* Lesions tend to be larger than those associated with GA.

MANAGEMENT

- The patient should be reassured of the benign nature of this condition but advised that it may be a harbinger of diabetes mellitus particularly in case of disseminated granuloma annulare.
- Localized lesions on nonvisible skin in children are best left untreated.
- Topical steroids such as class 2 high-potency **fluocinonide 0.5% cream (Lidex)** or super-potent class 1 **clobetasol 0.05% cream** may be applied. **Cordran tape** is another option (see "Introduction: Topical Therapy").
- Intralesional **triamcinolone acetonide (Kenalog),** in a dose of 2.5 to 5 mg/mL, is injected directly into the elevated border of the lesions with a 30-gauge needle. The plaque is infiltrated until it blanches.
- This may be repeated at 4- to 6-week intervals.

Lichen Planus

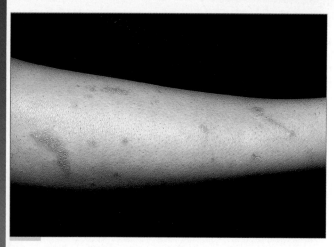

4.16 *Lichen planus.* The Köbner phenomenon (isomorphic response) results from scratching.

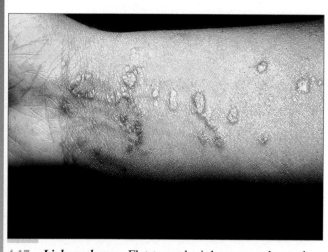

4.17 *Lichen planus.* Flat-topped, violaceous, polygonal papules on the flexor wrists are present. There are active and resolving lesions. Note the postinflammatory hyperpigmentation.

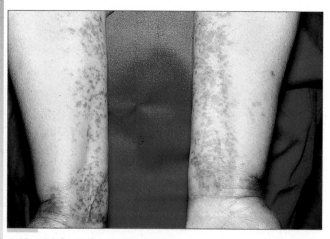

4.18 *Lichen planus.* Postinflammatory hyperpigmentation in a characteristic distribution.

BASICS

Lichen planus (LP) is a relatively uncommon cutaneous inflammatory disorder. "Classic" (idiopathic) LP is a pruritic, idiopathic eruption with characteristic shiny, flat-topped (Latin *planus,* "flat") papules on the skin, often accompanied by mucous membrane lesions. The papules are characterized by their violaceous color, polygonal shape, and, sometimes, fine scale. LP is most commonly found on the extremities, genitalia, and mucous membranes. Less commonly lesions can also involve the hair and nails.

LP is seen predominantly in adults and occurs in women more often than men. More than two-thirds of patients are between 30 and 60 years of age; however, the condition can occur at any age. LP is rare in children and the geriatric population.

Pathophysiology

LP is a cell-mediated immune response of unknown origin. An association is noted between LP and hepatitis C infection, chronic active hepatitis, and primary biliary cirrhosis.

DESCRIPTION OF LESIONS

The "Seven Ps"
1. Lesions are often **pruritic,** but they may be asymptomatic.
2. Lesions are often **purple** (actually red to violet).
3. Lesions tend to be **planar** (flat-topped) (FIG. 4.16).
4. Lesions form **papules** or **plaques.**
5. Lesions may be **polygonal** (FIG. 4.17).
6. Lesions may be **polymorphic** in shape and configuration—that is, oval, annular, linear, confluent (plaquelike), large, and small, even on the same person.
7. Lesions tend to heal with residual **postinflammatory hyperpigmentation,** leaving darkly pigmented macules in their wake (FIG. 4.18).

Other Clinical Findings Associated with Lichen Planus

- New lesions may be noted at sites of minor trauma such as scratches or burns (the Köbner reaction [isomorphic response]; see FIG. 4.16). See also Chapter 3, "Psoriasis," for another example of this phenomenon.
- Wickham's striae are characteristic white, lacelike streaks that are best visualized on the surfaces of lesions after mineral oil is applied. If present, they are virtually pathognomonic of LP.
- Mucous membrane lesions may be characterized by white lacy streaks in a netlike pattern (FIG. 4.19) or by atrophic erosions or ulcers (see Chapter 12, "Disorders of the Mouth, Lips, and Tongue").

DISTRIBUTION OF LESIONS

- The flexor areas such as the wrists, forearms, dorsa hands, dorsa feet, pretibial shafts, scalp, trunk, sacrum, glans penis, and labia minora are most often affected. Hypertrophic (verrucous) lesions tend to occur on the lower legs. Lesions may also become generalized.
- Mucous membrane involvement is common and may be found without skin involvement. Lesions are most commonly found on the tongue and buccal mucosa but may also be noted on the gingiva, palate, or lips.
- Genital involvement is common in men with cutaneous disease. Typically, an annular configuration of papules is seen on the glans penis (FIG. 4.20). Less commonly, linear white streaks (Wickham's striae) can be seen on male genitalia. Vulvar involvement can range from reticulate papules to severe erosions.

CLINICAL MANIFESTATIONS

- Pruritus, which may be severe, and the cosmetic appearance of lesions are the major concerns to patients.
- The course of LP is unpredictable. The onset may be abrupt or gradual. The lesions may resolve spontaneously, recur intermittently, or be chronic for many years. Chronicity is especially likely when hypertrophic lesions appear.
- Mucous membrane involvement may become erosive and painful, particularly if ulcers are present. Rarely, malignant transformation to squamous cell carcinoma has been documented.
- Vulvar lesions can result in dyspareunia, burning, and pruritus.
- Nail lesions may exhibit symptoms ranging from a mild dystrophy to a total loss of the nails.
- Scalp lesions result in a permanent, patchy, scarring follicular alopecia (lichen planopilaris, see Chapter 10, "Hair and scalp Disorders.").

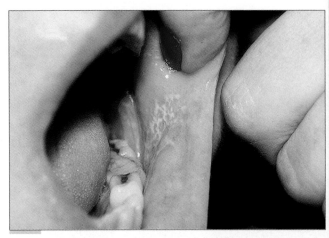

4.19 *Lichen planus.* Oral lesions, with a white, lacy, reticulated, pattern on the buccal mucosa.

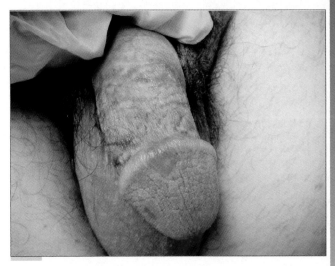

4.20 *Lichen planus.* Typical flat-topped papules are noted on the glans and the distal shaft of this patient's penis (compare to psoriasis of penis in FIGURE 4.24).

Clinical Variants

Variations in LP include the following:

- **Hypertrophic:** These extremely pruritic lesions are most often found on the extensor surfaces of the lower extremities (FIG. 4.21), especially around the ankles. Hypertrophic lesions are often chronic; residual pigmentation and scarring can occur when the lesions eventually clear.
- **Atrophic:** Atrophic LP is characterized by a few lesions, which often develop into hypertrophic lesions.
- **Erosive:** These lesions are found on the mucosal surfaces.
- **Follicular:** Lichen planopilaris is characterized by keratotic papules that may coalesce into plaques. Scarring alopecia may result.

Other eruptions resembling LP are seen in the following conditions:

- Drug-induced LP, associated with gold, thiazides, captopril, and antimalarials
- Lichenoid reactions associated with graft-versus-host disease
- LP associated with hepatitis C

DIAGNOSIS

- LP is often very easy to diagnose by its appearance, despite its range of clinical presentations.
- The presence of Wickham's striae is diagnostic.
- Characteristic oral lesions are helpful in making the diagnosis.
- Skin biopsy is performed, if necessary.
- Serology for hepatitis B and C should be obtained if history is suggestive.

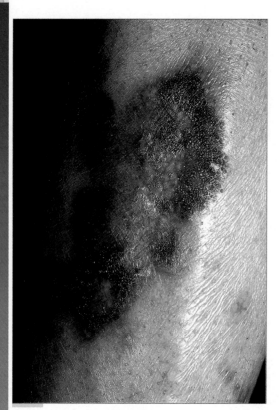

4.21 *Lichen planus, hypertrophic.* Darkly pigmented hypertrophic lesions are present on the pretibial shaft.

 DIFFERENTIAL DIAGNOSIS

Lichen Simplex Chronicus and Other Variants of Eczematous Dermatitis
See Chapter 2, "Eczema," and FIGURE 4.22.

- Lichenification may be present.
- Condition may be clinically indistinguishable from LP.
- Patient often has a positive atopic history.

Drug-Induced or Chemically Induced Lichenoid ("Lichen Planus–Like") Eruptions
- Causal drugs include thiazides, furosemide, beta-blockers, sulfonylureas, antimalarials, penicillamine, gold salts, and angiotensin-converting enzyme inhibitors.
- Rarely, photodeveloping chemicals, dental materials, and tattoo pigments are involved.
- There is generally a latent period of several months between drug introduction and the appearance of lesions.

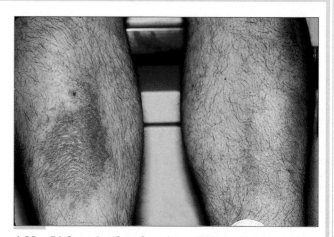

4.22 *Lichen simplex chronicus.* This patient has itchy pretibial hypertrophic plaques.

continued on page 125

- Lesions resolve when the inciting agent is discontinued, often after a prolonged period.
- Skin lesions are indistinguishable from those of classic LP.
- Oral lesions are lacking.

Other Diagnoses to Consider

- Pityriasis rosea
- Drug eruption
- Guttate psoriasis
- Tinea corporis
- Discoid lupus erythematosus
- Lichen nitidus
- **Oral mucous membranes** (see Chapter 12, "Disorders of the Mouth, Lips, and Tongue")
  - Normal bite line (FIG. 4.23)
  - Leukoplakia
  - Oral hairy leukoplakia
  - Candidiasis
  - Squamous cell carcinoma (particularly in ulcerative lesions)
  - Aphthous ulcers
  - Herpetic stomatitis
  - Secondary syphilis
- **Genital mucous membranes**
  - Psoriasis (penis and labia) (FIG. 4.24)
  - Lichen sclerosis
  - Fixed drug eruption (penis)
  - Candidiasis (penis and labia)
- **Hair and scalp**
  - Scarring alopecia (pseudopelade)
  - Folliculitis decalvans

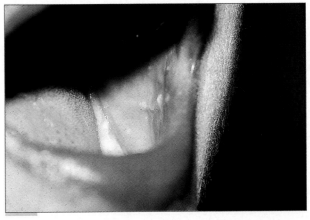

4.23 *Normal bite line.* This is a common finding on the buccal mucosa that is often confused with oral lichen planus.

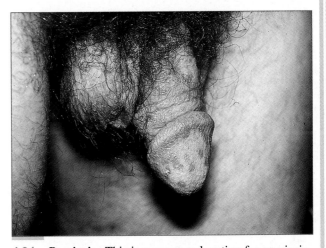

4.24 *Psoriasis.* This is a common location for psoriasis. There are typical psoriasiform papules and plaques on this patient's penis.

 MANAGEMENT

- Mild cases can be treated symptomatically with **potent topical steroids.** Patients with more severe cases, especially those with scalp, nail, and mucous membrane involvement, may require systemic therapy.
- High-potency (class 2) or super-potent (class 1) topical steroids may be used alone or with polyethylene occlusion, or with **Cordran tape** (see "Introduction: Topical Therapy").

- The first-line treatments of cutaneous LP are potent topical steroids.
- **Systemic steroids** (e.g., prednisone beginning at 0.5 to 1 mg/kg daily) in short, tapering courses may be necessary for symptom control and possibly more rapid resolution.
- Oral acitretin (**Soriatane**) has been occasionally helpful.
- For symptomatic LP of the oral mucosa, topical steroids are usually tried first. Alternatively, topical tacrolimus (**Protopic**) ointment 0.1% has been tried with some success.

 POINT TO REMEMBER

- Serial oral or genital examinations are indicated for erosive/ulcerative lesions to rule out squamous cell carcinoma.

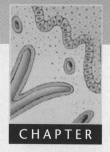

CHAPTER 5
Superficial Bacterial Infections, Folliculitis, and Hidradenitis Suppurativa

➤ **IMPETIGO**

➤ **FOLLICULITIS**

- Staphylococcal folliculitis
- Pseudomonas (hot tub) folliculitis

➤ **FOLLICULITIS: OTHER TYPES**

- Irritant, frictional, or chemical folliculitis
- Steroid-induced acne and rosacea (see also Chapter 1, "Acne and Related Disorders")
- Eosinophilic pustular folliculitis (see also Chapter 24, "Cutaneous Manifestations of HIV Infection").
- Pityrosporum folliculitis
- Majocchi's granuloma
- Viral folliculitis: herpes virus folliculitis (see Chapter 6, "Superficial Viral Infections")

➤ **FURUNCULOSIS ("BOILS")**

➤ **HIDRADENITIS SUPPURATIVA (ACNE INVERSA)**

OVERVIEW

Bacteria such as Corynebacterium, Brevibacterium, Acinetobacter, and some Staphylococcus species, are commonly found on normal skin and are not pathogenic. Propionibacterium bacteria reside in hair follicles and contribute to acne.

The two gram-positive cocci, *Staphylococcus aureus* and the group A β-hemolytic streptococci, account for the vast majority of cutaneous infections. They may colonize normal skin or be secondary invaders of cutaneous ulcers, surgical or traumatic wounds, as well as in eczematous dermatitis, a skin disorder in which the barrier function of the skin is defective.

Methicillin resistant *Staphylococcus aureus* (MRSA) is the term used for bacteria of the *S. aureus* group that are resistant to the traditional antibiotics used against them. Problems arise because antibiotic choice becomes very limited.

BASICS

Impetigo is a primary superficial bacterial infection of the superficial layers of the epidermis. Traditionally, impetigo has been divided into two forms—bullous and nonbullous (crusted). These conditions are clinically more or less indistinguishable; therefore, it is probably less confusing to use the term impetigo to describe both of them.

Impetigo is a common, highly contagious finding in preschoolers. The incidence of impetigo in children younger than 6 years of age is higher than it is in adults; however, the condition may occur in persons of all ages. Impetigo rarely progresses to systemic infection, although poststreptococcal glomerulonephritis is a rare complication.

Impetigo is caused most often by *Staphylococcus aureus;* less often, group A beta-hemolytic streptococci (GABHS) may be the primary pathogen. In fact, both organisms can be present at the same time in the affected sites. In recent years, methicillin-resistant *S. aureus* (MRSA) has been noted as a cause of impetigo; this infection is observed more commonly with the nonbullous form of impetigo than the bullous form.

Secondary Impetigo (Impetiginization)

Impetigo can, and often does, emerge as a secondary infection of preexisting skin disease or traumatized skin; it is then referred to as secondary impetiginization. Examples include impetiginized eczema. Patients who have atopic dermatitis or other inflammatory skin conditions often have skin colonized by *S. aureus.*

Other conditions that may lead to impetiginization include the following:

- Stasis dermatitis
- Herpes simplex and varicella infections
- Scabies and insect bites
- Lacerations and burns

DESCRIPTION OF LESIONS

- Impetigo begins as a crust or thin-roofed, fragile vesicle or bulla that ruptures and often leaves a peripheral collarette of scale or a darker, hemorrhagic, crusted border. Intact bullae are not usually present because they are very fragile; rather, they often demonstrate a collarette of scale or the flaccid remains of bullae (FIGS. 5.1 and 5.2).
- Oozing serum dries and gives rise to the classic golden-yellow, "honey-crusted" lesion. Lesions appear to be stuck on (FIG. 5.3).

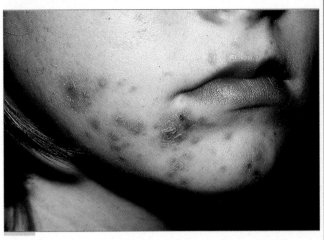

5.1 *Impetigo.* This child has a mixture of intact bullae and drying crusts.

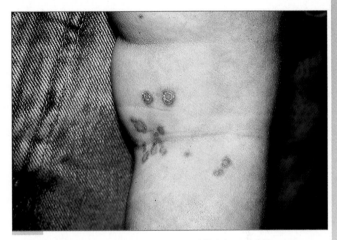

5.2 *Impetigo.* In this 2-year-old child, intact blisters are not present; only the flaccid remains (scaly collarettes) of bullae are seen.

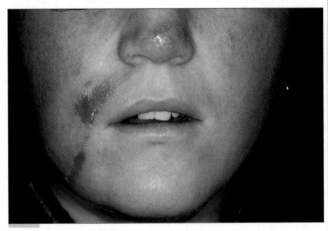

5.3 *Impetigo.* Oozing "honey-crusted" lesions in a typical location.

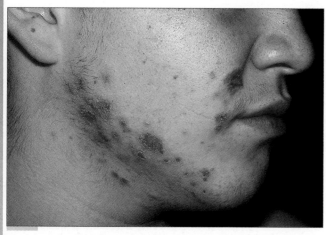

5.4 *Impetigo (gladiatorum).* This is a college wrestler (see also discussion of herpes gladiatorum in Chapter 6).

- In time, a varnishlike crust (Fig. 5.4) develops centrally that, if removed, reveals a moist red base.

DISTRIBUTION OF LESIONS

- In children, the face is commonly involved, particularly in and around the nose and mouth, along with other exposed parts of the body (e.g., arms, legs), sparing the palms and soles.
- In adults, lesions may occur anywhere on the body.

CLINICAL MANIFESTATIONS

Spread of lesions is by autoinoculation.

- Lesions are usually asymptomatic; occasionally they may itch.
- The infection is self-limiting—even without treatment—and generally spontaneously resolves after a few weeks. It also typically clears with topical or oral antibiotics; only rarely do serious complications occur (see below).
- Healing takes place without scarring, but it may cause temporary postinflammatory hyperpigmentation in dark-skinned persons.
- Recurrent or persistent impetigo may indicate a carrier state in the patient or the patient's family.

DIAGNOSIS

- Diagnosis is usually made on clinical grounds.
- Bacterial culture and sensitivity testing are recommended if standard topical or oral treatment does not result in improvement.
- A bacterial culture of the nares may be obtained to determine whether a patient is a carrier of *S. aureus.*
- Urinalysis is necessary to evaluate for acute poststreptococcal glomerulonephritis if the patient develops edema or hypertension. Hematuria, proteinuria, and cylindruria are indicators of renal involvement.

DIFFERENTIAL DIAGNOSIS

Tinea Corporis

FIGURE 5.5.

- The potassium hydroxide examination or fungal culture is positive.
- Central clearing of lesions is noted.
- Honey-colored crusts are absent.

Other Diagnoses

- Rare considerations include primary bullous diseases such as bullous dermatosis of childhood and bullous pemphigoid.

RARE COMPLICATIONS

- Cellulitis, lymphangitis, scarlet fever, erysipelas, bacteremia with subsequent pneumonitis, septic arthritis, and septicemia may develop; rarely, bacterial endocarditis may also occur.
- Staphylococcal scalded skin syndrome occurs more commonly in younger children. (See Chapter 9, "Bacterial Exanthems")
- Acute glomerulonephritis develops in 2% to 5% of individuals with impetigo caused by GABHS, most often in

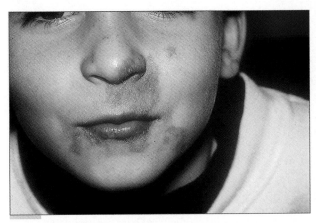

5.5 *Tinea corporis (faciale).* This young boy was initially treated with topical antibiotics for presumptive impetigo.

children aged 2 to 4 years. The onset is usually 10 days after the lesions of impetigo first appear, but it can occur from 1 to 5 weeks later. Transient proteinuria and hematuria may occur during impetigo and resolve before renal involvement develops.

- Ecthyma, a deep dermal infection, can result, after which subsequent scarring can occur.

MANAGEMENT

- Antibacterial soaps such as povidone-iodine (**Betadine**) or chlorhexidine (**Hibiclens**) are used twice daily.
- Gentle débridement of lesional crusts is done with a washcloth and the antibacterial soap.
- Mupirocin 2% (**Bactroban, Centany**) ointment or cream applied three times daily may be used alone to treat very limited cases of impetigo. It is used until all lesions are cleared. Topical application of these preparations has been shown to be as effective as oral antibiotics.
- For widespread involvement, an oral staphylocidal penicillinase-resistant antibiotic, such as cephalosporin,

dicloxacillin, or erythromycin, may be used alone or in conjunction with topical antibiotics.

- If bacterial cultures reveal MRSA, **tetracyclines, trimethoprim/sulfamethoxazole** (**Bactrim**), **clindamycin,** or **linezolid** are effective oral antibiotics.
- In patients who have been determined to be chronic nasal carriers and have recurrent impetigo, and for those with MRSA, mupirocin 2% cream or ointment can be applied inside the nostrils three times daily for 5 days each month to reduce bacterial colonization in the nose.
- Patients who are chronic nasal carriers also can be treated with **rifampin** (see later in this Chapter).

POINTS TO REMEMBER

- Rarely, poststreptococcal glomerulonephritis (but not rheumatic fever) has been reported to follow impetigo caused by certain strains of streptococci.
- Family members should be evaluated as potential nasal carriers of *S. aureus* and treated, if necessary.

HELPFUL HINTS

- Chronic or recurrent impetigo should alert the clinician to the possibility of an impaired immune status.
- Strains of *S. aureus* are usually resistant to penicillin and may be resistant to erythromycin.
- An emerging problem is MRSA, which may appear in both immunocompromised and immunocompetent patients. If infectious skin lesions do not improve during treatment intended for methicillin-sensitive *S. aureus*, the diagnosis of MRSA should be considered, and definitive antibacterial therapy should be determined on the basis of in vitro antibiotic sensitivity.

Folliculitis

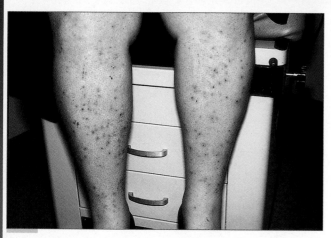

5.6 *Folliculitis.* This woman had a leg waxing. Note the crusted papules.

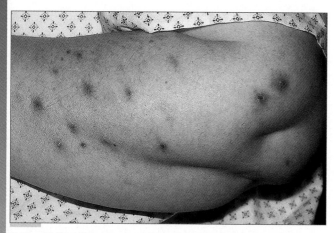

5.7 *Folliculitis.* Intact follicular pustules and crusted papules.

BASICS

Folliculitis, in its broadest sense, may be defined as a superficial or deep infection or inflammation of the hair follicles. It has multiple causes: various infections, physical or chemical irritation, occlusive dressings or clothing, and the use of topical or systemic steroids. Hereditary forms of folliculitis such as follicular eczema are generally classified as atopic dermatitis (see Chapter 2, "Eczema"). The deeper forms of inflammatory folliculitis that involve the entire follicular structure, such as folliculitis decalvans, occur most commonly in black men and women (see Chapter 10, "Hair and Scalp Disorders Resulting in Hair Loss").

Folliculitis may also be seen as a secondary infection in conditions such as eczema, scabies, and excoriated insect bites. It is more commonly found in patients who are diabetic, obese, or immunocompromised. Viral folliculitis may be seen in patients with herpes simplex infections, particularly in patients with human immunodeficiency virus (HIV) infection.

Staphylococcal Folliculitis

Coagulase-positive *S. aureus* is the responsible pathogenic bacterium in most cases of infectious folliculitis.

CAUSES AND PRECIPITATING FACTORS

As in cases of inflammatory folliculitis (see Chapter 2, "Eczema"), bacterial folliculitis may be seen after the following:

- Repeated trauma (such as waxing, plucking, and shaving of the face, legs, and pubic areas)
- Wearing of restrictive clothing, such as tight jeans
- Excessive sweating

DESCRIPTION OF LESIONS

- A pustule or papule with a central hair is the primary lesion in folliculitis. The central hair shaft may not always be visible.
- Follicular lesions tend to manifest a gridlike pattern on hair-bearing areas of the body (FIGS. 5.6 and 5.7).
- Lesions are often polymorphic, displaying a mixture of papules and pustules, or they may be monomorphic and consist solely of papules.
- In darkly pigmented patients, primary lesions may consist of obvious papules or pustules; alternatively, only secondary, hyperpigmented lesions arranged in a follicular pattern may be all that is clinically visible.

DISTRIBUTION OF LESIONS

- Lesions occur on hair-bearing areas—the face, scalp, thighs, and body folds.
- The axillae, groin, and legs are particularly prone to folliculitis when they are regularly shaved.

CLINICAL MANIFESTATIONS

- Lesions of folliculitis elicit mild discomfort and cosmetic concern.

CLINICAL VARIANTS

- Tender, painful, folliculitis involving an eyelash is called a hordeolum, or "sty."
- Similarly, folliculitis may affect a single nasal hair follicle and may produce a tender erythematous papule or pustule in or on the distal nose or near the tip of the nose (FIG. 5.8).

DIAGNOSIS

This is generally diagnosed by clinical findings. In cases that are resistant to treatment, the following procedures may be performed:

- Gram stain and bacterial culture. In typical cases, a Gram stain shows gram-positive cocci, and culture grows *S. aureus*.
- Nasal culture. The patient and, if necessary, the patient's family members may require a nasal culture to look for *S. aureus*.

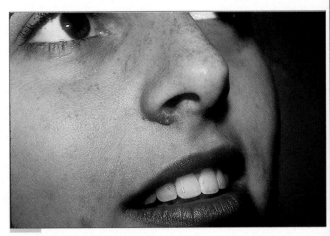

5.8 *Folliculitis.* This patient has a tender papule that originated in a nasal hair follicle.

 DIFFERENTIAL DIAGNOSIS

Acne Vulgaris and Other Acnelike Conditions
- Keratosis pilaris is frequently confused with acne and folliculitis (see Chapter 2, "Eczema").
- Because keratosis pilaris involves the hair follicles, it manifests in a gridlike pattern, similar to that of folliculitis.
- Lesions have a rough texture and are persistent.

Insect Bite Reactions
- Lesions are grouped in a nonfollicular pattern (see Chapter 20, "Bites, Stings, and Infestations").

MANAGEMENT

Mild Cases

- Mild cases of bacterial folliculitis can sometimes be prevented or controlled with antibacterial soaps.
- In addition, topical antibiotics, such as **erythromycin** 2% topical solution or clindamycin (**Cleocin**) 1% solution, may be applied once or twice a day to the affected areas.

Chronic and Recurrent Cases

Chronic and recurrent cases of bacterial folliculitis present a difficult therapeutic problem.

- If staphylococcal colonization is present, mupirocin 2% (**Bactroban**) ointment should be applied to the nasal vestibule twice a day for 5 days to eliminate the *S. aureus* carrier state.
- Family members may be treated similarly, if necessary. **Rifampin** (600 mg/day for 10 to 14 days) may also eliminate the carrier state.
- Even in cases of negative bacterial cultures, a systemic antibiotic is often needed for coverage of *S. aureus* because it is the most common pathogen. This organism is often resistant to penicillin, and thus dicloxacillin (250 to 500 mg four times a day) or a **cephalosporin,** such as **cephalexin** (1 to 4 g/day in two doses) is generally the first choice. **Minocycline** (50 to 100 mg twice a day) is sometimes used for MRSA.

 POINTS TO REMEMBER

- Bacterial cultures should be considered for cases that are resistant to therapy.
- Culturing and treating of family members should be considered in cases of chronic bacterial folliculitis.

Pseudomonas (Hot Tub) Folliculitis

Pseudomonas folliculitis, which may be acquired from communal hot tubs, is caused by *Pseudomonas aeruginosa* infection. Although hot tubs have increased the incidence of folliculitis, they are often overlooked as a cause. Jacuzzis, therapeutic whirlpools ("whirlpool folliculitis"), public swimming pools, and the use of loofah sponges can be sources of *Pseudomonas* infection. *Pseudomonas* folliculitis has been found to occur under diving areas and after wax depilation.

DESCRIPTION OF LESIONS

- Lesions of hot tub folliculitis consist of intensely pruritic or tender follicular papules or pustules that are most often found on the trunk, particularly on areas covered by a bathing suit (FIG. 5.9).

CLINICAL MANIFESTATIONS

- Pruritic lesions occur 1 to 3 days after bathing in a hot tub, whirlpool, or public swimming pool.

DIAGNOSIS

- The diagnosis is based on a history of exposure.
- *Pseudomonas* organisms can be isolated in patients with this condition.

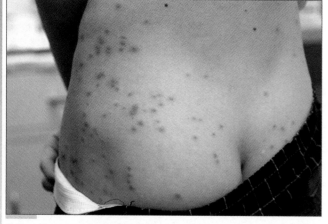

5.9 *Hot tub folliculitis ("hot tub buns").* Multiple pruritic follicular papules and pustules occurred on the buttocks of this young man 3 days after he had bathed in a hot tub. Bacterial culture grew *Pseudomonas aeruginosa.*

 MANAGEMENT

- Hot tub folliculitis usually resolves spontaneously, but it may not if it is very extensive or symptomatic.
- If necessary, it may be treated with oral **ciprofloxacin** (500 mg twice a day for 5 days).

Folliculitis: Other Types

Irritant, Frictional, or Chemical Folliculitis

Nonbacterial, or sterile, folliculitis can arise from physical or chemical irritation. Such irritants include leg waxing, leg shaving, axillary shaving, and hair plucking. Chemical depilatories, electrolysis, occlusive dressings, and excessive sweating can also contribute to this problem, as well as wearing tight clothing. Nonbacterial folliculitis may also be related to working conditions, such as the use of greases or oils, and to the application of various cosmetics. Bacteria such as *S. aureus* are not infrequent secondary invaders.

Steroid-Induced Acne and Rosacea

Topical or systemic steroid treatment may lead to steroid-induced acne, which is actually a form of folliculitis. Diagnosis of these conditions is aided by a history of potent topical or systemic steroid use (FIG. 5.10 and also see Chapter 1, "Acne and Related Disorders").

Eosinophilic Pustular Folliculitis

Eosinophilic pustular folliculitis, another form of sterile folliculitis, has intensely pruritic lesions that resemble urticaria papules. It is seen in patients with acquired immunodeficiency syndrome (see Chapter 24, "Cutaneous Manifestations of HIV Infection").

Fungal Folliculitis

Pityrosporum Folliculitis

This acnelike eruption, seen on the trunk, is caused by *Malassezia furfur,* which is a lipophilic yeast. Lesions are chronic, erythematous, pruritic papules and pustules that usually appear on the back and chest of young adults. The eruption appears in a follicular pattern. This condition is seen more frequently in the summer. *Pityrosporum* folliculitis should be considered as a diagnosis when folliculitis resists antibiotic treatment. It looks like acne, but it does not respond to acne therapy (See Chapter 7, "Superficial Fungal Infections").

Majocchi's Granuloma

Tinea corporis of the lower legs may produce tinea folliculitis in women who shave their legs. The organism is introduced into the hair follicle by shaving.

Viral Folliculitis: Herpes Virus Folliculitis

This form of folliculitis is caused most often by an infection by herpes simplex virus type 1. It is found in areas adjacent to a primary cold sore and is spread by shaving. See also Chapter 6, "Superficial Viral Infections."

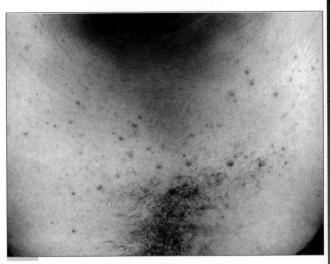

5.10 *Systemic steroid-induced folliculitis.* This patient is taking long-term oral prednisone for sarcoidosis.

 POINTS TO REMEMBER

- Bacterial, fungal, or viral cultures should be considered in cases that are resistant to therapy.
- In HIV-positive patients, a skin biopsy should be performed for suspected cases of eosinophilic pustular folliculitis.

Furunculosis ("Boils")

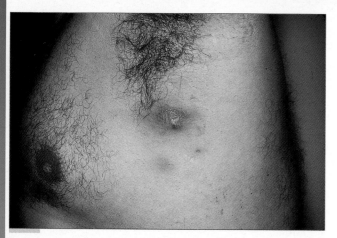

5.11 *Furuncle.* This patient has a tender "boil" located in his axilla.

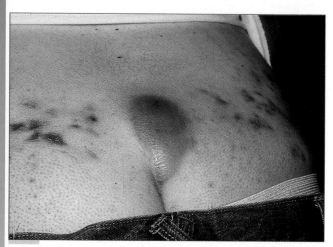

5.12 *Abscess.* This patient has the **follicular occlusion triad** ("tetrad" in this case), which consists of hidradenitis suppurativa, acne conglobata, and dissecting cellulitis of the scalp. This walled-off lesion began as a pilonidal sinus that later developed into an abscess. Note the older violaceous scars from previous furuncles and cystic acne lesions.

BASICS

Folliculitis may evolve into a furuncle ("boil"), which is a deeper infection; the term *carbuncle* refers to an aggregation of furuncles. *S. aureus* is the customary responsible pathogenic bacterium. Furuncles are painful nodules or abscesses (walled-off collections of pus) in an infected hair follicle; they are more common in boys and young adults.

Chronic or recurrent furunculosis is a difficult therapeutic problem that is often the result of nasal carriage of *S. aureus*. Like folliculitis, furunculosis is more common in diabetic patients and in obese persons.

DESCRIPTION OF LESIONS

- A furuncle is a tender, painful nodule with overlying erythema (FIG. 5.11).
- As the lesion evolves, a fluctuant abscess may form (FIG. 5.12).
- If untreated, it may rupture and drain spontaneously.

DISTRIBUTION OF LESIONS

- Hair-bearing areas are commonly involved, with body folds the preferred sites.
- The scalp, face, buttocks, thighs, axillae, and inguinal areas are affected.
- Furuncles are often seen in the axillae, groin, posterior neck, thighs, and buttocks. When they occur in a contiguous cluster on the occipital scalp, they are referred to as **carbuncles.**

CLINICAL MANIFESTATIONS

- Furuncles can cause throbbing pain and can be quite tender.

DIAGNOSIS

- This is based on the clinical presentation.
- Gram stain generally reveals gram-positive cocci; culture often grows *S. aureus*.

 DIFFERENTIAL DIAGNOSIS

Hidradenitis Suppurativa
See the following section.

- Abscesses resembling furuncles are noted.
- Bacteria are secondary invaders.
- The condition is more common in women.
- It may be indistinguishable from furunculosis in its early stages.

 MANAGEMENT

- Furuncles come to a "head" with warm compresses, or they may be incised and drained.
- Systemic staphylocidal antibiotics such as **dicloxacillin**, **erythromycin**, or **cephalosporin** may be added. **Minocycline** is sometimes used for MRSA.
- The daily coating of the distal nasal mucosa with **mupirocin** should be considered in carriers or recurrent cases.

BASICS

Hidradenitis suppurativa (HS) should not be classified as an infection; rather, it is a chronic, recurrent, scarring, inflammatory disease that affects the regions of the skin-bearing apocrine sweat glands: the axillae, inguinal folds, suprapubic area, anogenital area, buttocks, areola, and under the female breasts. Bacterial involvement is not a primary pathogenic event. Autosomal-dominant inheritance has been described.

HS appears after puberty, and most cases develop during the second and third decades of life. It is seen mostly in women and only rarely before puberty. When HS occurs in African-American women, it tends to be more severe.

Pathophysiology

The exact cause of HS is unknown. Traditionally, it had been considered a primary inflammatory disorder of the apocrine glands (and was sometimes referred to as *apocrinitis* or *apocrine acne*). The current hypothesis suggests that poral occlusion of the hair follicle leads to retention of the secretory products and subsequent inflammation. This hypothesis is supported by the finding that in most biopsy specimens, the apocrine glands are intact and unaffected, and follicular occlusion is constant. Inflammation of the apocrine glands is thus considered to be secondary or incidental. Bacterial involvement is also considered a secondary pathogenic event. The plugged structure dilates, ruptures, becomes infected, and progresses to abscess formation, draining, and fistulous tracts.

In the chronic state, secondary bacterial infection probably is a major cause of exacerbations.

Like acne vulgaris, HS is related to androgen excess and often flares with menstruation. Symptoms often improve during the estrogen-elevation phases of the menstrual cycle. Moreover, HS frequently improves during pregnancy, only to flare during the postpartum period.

DESCRIPTION OF LESIONS AND CLINICAL MANIFESTATIONS

- Initially, HS presents with nodules and abscesses that may be indistinguishable from furunculosis or common "boils."
- Lesions are painful and tender, and they often become infected secondarily and exude a serosanguineous or foul-smelling purulent material that may stain clothing.
- HS is often a cause of embarrassment and, possibly, social isolation.
- Lesions recur, new lesions crop up, and old lesions scar in a frustrating, unrelenting process.
- Frequently there is a menstrual flare.
- Chronic HS is indicated by the appearance of sinus tract and fistula formation, ulcerations, and, eventually, hypertrophic, ropelike linear bands of scars and dermal contractures (FIG. 5.13).
- Characteristic multiple open comedones ("blackheads") develop in long-standing cases.

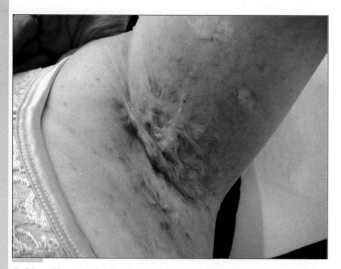

5.13 *Chronic hidradenitis suppurativa.* This patient has involvement of the axilla with bandlike hypertrophic scars and draining abscesses.

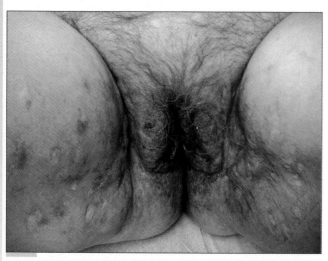

5.14 *Hidradenitis suppurativa.* This patient has involvement of the inguinal areas, labia majora, and mesial thighs.

DISTRIBUTION OF LESIONS

- The most common area of involvement is the axillary area (Fig. 5.13); the groin is also frequently involved (Fig. 5.14).
- However, lesions may also be seen on the perineum, inframammary areas, the buttocks, and, rarely, the neck and scalp.

DIAGNOSIS

- The multiple lesions of HS that scar and form sinus tracts should be easily distinguishable from other conditions.

DIFFERENTIAL DIAGNOSIS

In its early stages, HS is most often confused with the following:

- **Recurrent folliculitis** and **furunculosis** (FIGS. 5.15 and 5.16). Solitary lesions resemble a furuncle, lymphadenitis, or an infected epidermoid cyst.

- In the vaginal area, an infected Bartholin's cyst may resemble a solitary lesion of HP.

Other conditions appear to be related to HS and may coexist in the same patient. The so-called follicular occlusion triad, which consists of HS, acne conglobata, and dissecting cellulitis of the scalp, has been well documented. Pilonidal sinus was later added to the triad, making it a tetrad (see FIG. 5.12).

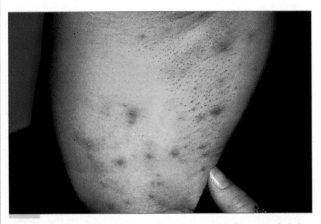

5.15 *Folliculitis.* This patient has multiple superficial papules and pustules in her axillary vault.

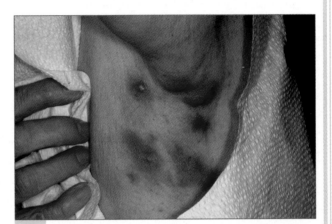

5.16 *Furunculosis.* This patient has multiple painful, "pointing" furuncular papules and nodules in her axilla.

MANAGEMENT

- HS is a difficult, frustrating condition to control.
- Large cysts should be incised and drained. Smaller cysts respond to intralesional injections of triamcinolone acetonide (**Kenalog**, 2.5 to 10 mg/mL).
- Weight loss helps reduce the activity and severity of HS.
- Actively discharging lesions should be cultured. Repeated bacteriologic assessment is advisable in all cases.
- Antibiotics are the mainstay of treatment, especially for the early stages of the disease. Long-term oral antibiotics such as **tetracycline** (500 mg twice daily), **erythromycin** (500 mg twice daily), **doxycycline** (100 mg twice daily), or **minocycline** (100 mg twice daily) may prevent disease activation. Lower doses may be effective for maintenance once control is established. **Topical clindamycin** may also be effective.

Preventive Measures During Remissions

- Wearing of ventilated cotton clothing is advised.
- Other therapeutic measures involve the use of absorbent powders and bacteriostatic soaps.

Topical Therapy

- Limited and very early disease may be helped somewhat by the daily use of topical antibiotics, such as **clindamycin** or **erythromycin.**
- **Intralesional corticosteroid injections** inserted directly into painful lesions are used to treat limited acute exacerbations.

Systemic Therapy

- **Prednisone** can be used in short courses, particularly if inflammation is severe. A short course of prednisone, 40 to 60 mg daily, to be tapered over 2 to 3 weeks is often quite effective.
- Prednisone may be given alone or, most often, in combination with oral antibiotics, such as minocycline, erythromycin, ciprofloxacin, cephalosporins, or semisynthetic penicillin, given in the usual doses used for soft tissue infections. For example, **minocycline,** in doses ranging from 50 to 100 mg twice a day, may be used on an episodic basis for weeks or, if necessary, months at a time and then tapered to the lowest dosage that relieves

continued on page 138

symptoms. Long-term administration of an antibiotic, such as minocycline, can also be used to prevent episodic flares. The efficacy of minocycline seems to be attributable to its anti-inflammatory action rather than its antibiotic effect.

- Alternative antibiotics that can be helpful include **erythromycin** (250 to 500 mg three or four times a day), **ciprofloxacin** (500 mg twice a day), **cephalexin** (250 to 500 mg four times a day), and **dicloxacillin** (250 to 500 mg twice a day).
- Systemic retinoids, such as oral isotretinoin (**Accutane**), have been used with limited benefit in early disease that has not yet produced significant scarring. The systemic retinoids are not as effective in treating HS as they are in treating severe nodular acne; moreover, relapses are very common after seemingly effective treatment is stopped.
- Certain oral contraceptives, such as cyproterone acetate (which is not available in the United States), have been reported to be helpful in some cases. **Cyclosporine** has also been reported to be of some value.
- Infliximab (**Remicade**) is a monoclonal antibody that targets tumor necrosis factor alpha and inhibits its activity that is used in the treatment of psoriasis (see Chapter 3, "Psoriasis"). It has been anecdotally reported to be effective in some severe cases of HS; however, toxic events and lack of efficacy have been demonstrated in one recent series.

Surgical Measures
- **Incision and drainage** are performed only on fluctuant lesions. This approach affords short-term relief of troublesome, painful abscesses. Repeated incision and drainage may lead to more scarring and sinus tract formation.
- Severe refractory HS is best treated with **wide, complete surgical excision** of the involved area, which may produce a definitive cure.
- A narrow excision of inflamed areas may help temporarily, but this method has a high recurrence rate.
- **Ablation techniques** using a carbon dioxide laser that spares normal tissue have been tried successfully. These techniques may become the standard of surgical treatment.

Prognosis
The course of HS varies.

- Some patients have very mild disease that may be indistinguishable from chronic furunculosis.
- Remissions may occur more frequently as the patient ages or as more scar tissue develops; however, total spontaneous resolution is rare. More commonly reported is a decline in severity at or after menopause.

 POINTS TO REMEMBER

- Recurrent tender furuncles or sterile abscesses in the axillae or groin, on the buttocks, or below the breasts suggest the diagnosis of HS.
- Many cases, especially of the thighs and vulva, are mild and misdiagnosed as recurrent furunculosis.
- Chronic disease is indicated by the presence of old scars, sinus tracts, and open comedones.

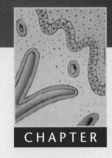

Superficial Viral Infections

OVERVIEW

Viruses are capable of causing a wide variety of disorders of the skin and mucous membranes. Specific skin lesions vary greatly and include vesicles, pustules, papules, ulcers, and tumors. Cutaneous viral infections present in various reaction patterns, most commonly, vesicobullous, vascular (viral exanthems), or papulosquamous (pityriasis rosea).

Certain viral infections—warts in particular—vary greatly in their gross clinical manifestations despite all being caused by the same, albeit different subtypes, of human papilloma virus (HPV). For example, the clinical appearances of warts often differ markedly and manifest as papillomatatous (common warts), threadlike (filiform warts), flat (planar warts), to exuberant moist papules (condyloma acuminata), or tumors (giant condyloma acuminatum of Buschke-Löwenstein). See Chapter 19, "Sexually Transmitted Diseases." In contrast, lesions of molluscum contagiosum tend to be quite monomorphic and uniform in appearance and vary primarily by size.

The virus of varicella-zoster (VZV) may produce the clinical syndrome of either chickenpox or herpes zoster. Herpes simplex virus (HSV) lesions may manifest in ways that produce systemic problems, whereas the virus of warts and molluscum contagiosum are entirely localized to the skin (dermatotrophic) and do not cause systemic symptoms. Systemic viral disorders such as varicella are discussed in Chapter 8, "Viral Exanthems."

> ➤ **WARTS (NONGENITAL)**

- Common warts
- Plantar warts
- Flat warts
- Filiform warts

> ➤ **MOLLUSCUM CONTAGIOSUM**

> ➤ **HERPES SIMPLEX (NONGENITAL)**

- Primary orolabial herpes simplex
- Recurrent orolabial herpes simplex
- Clinical variants of herpes simplex infections

> ➤ **HERPES ZOSTER**

- Disseminated herpes zoster
- Post herpetic neuralgia

Warts (Nongenital)

BASICS

The emergence of common warts (verrucae vulgaris) and other forms of cutaneous warts is extremely common, particularly in children and young adults. An estimated 20% of school-age children will at some time have at least one wart. In children, warts tend to regress spontaneously. In many adults and in immunocompromised patients, however, warts often prove difficult to eradicate.

All warts are caused by the human papillomavirus (HPV); to date, more than 150 different subtypes have been identified. The virus infects epidermal keratinocytes, which stimulates cell proliferation. Viral transmission occurs primarily through skin-to-skin contact such as handshaking or kissing. The recently shed virus can also be found on almost anything in a moist, warm environment, including doorknobs, hand railings, and floors of locker rooms, as well as around swimming pools. Contact with any of these surfaces is another means of viral transmission; the virus is virtually impossible to avoid. Often, several family members develop warts. Whether this reflects a genetic susceptibility or is simply a result of the ubiquitous nature of the contagion has not been determined.

Factors that Predispose to Human Papillomavirus Infection

- Infection with the human immunodeficiency virus (HIV) or the presence of other immunosuppressive diseases, such as lymphomas, can predispose one to become infected.
- Taking drugs that decrease cell-mediated immunity (e.g., prednisone, cyclosporine, chemotherapeutic agents) is another predisposing factor. Transplant recipients who, by necessity, use such medications on a long-term basis have warts that can be very resistant to treatment.
- Handling raw meat, fish, or other types of animal matter in one's occupation (for example, butchers) increases susceptibility.

DESCRIPTION OF LESIONS

- Warts are most often diagnosed based on their clinical appearance, but a biopsy can be performed if the diagnosis is in doubt. A typical wart is a papillomatous, corrugated, hyperkeratotic growth that is confined to the epidermis. Despite a common misconception, warts have no "roots," and there is no "mother wart."
- Warts may be skin colored to tan and measure 5 to 10 mm in diameter. However, they may coalesce into clusters (mosaic warts) that can be up to 3 cm in diameter.
- Warts often vary widely in shape, size, and appearance. The different names for warts generally reflect their clinical appearance, location, or both. For example, filiform warts are threadlike, planar warts are flat, and plantar warts are located on the plantar surface of the feet.
- Genital warts (condyloma acuminata) may be large and cauliflowerlike, or they may consist of small papules.

DISTRIBUTION OF LESIONS

- Warts may develop anywhere on the body, but they are most often found at sites subject to frequent trauma, such as the hands and feet.
- The distribution is generally asymmetric, and lesions are often clustered.
- Viral protein and infectious particles have been detected in the absence of visible skin surface lesions using electron microscopy, polymerase chain reaction, and DNA hybridization techniques. Thus, it is well documented that HPV can exist in a subclinical or latent state.
- This latency explains the not infrequent recurrence of warts at the same site or at an adjacent site, even when they had been apparently "cured" many years before.

CLINICAL VARIANTS
Common Warts

- Verrucae vulgaris, or common warts (FIG. 6.1), occur most often on the hands and fingers and in the nail area—both around (periungual) and under (subungual) nail areas (FIGS. 6.2 and 6.3). They are frequently seen on the knees and elbows, especially in children.
- Their distribution is generally asymmetric, and lesions are often grouped.

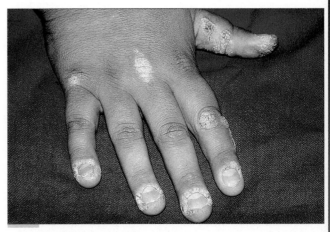

6.1 ***Common warts (verruca vulgaris).*** This young boy has multiple common warts.

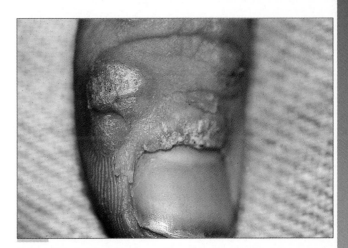

6.2 ***Common warts (verruca vulgaris).*** Periungual warts.

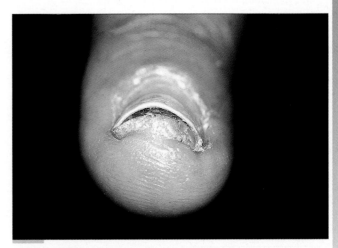

6.3 ***Common wart (verruca vulgaris).*** This subungual lesion could easily be mistaken for onychomycosis, and, in rare instances, prove to be a squamous cell carcinoma (when only one nail is involved).

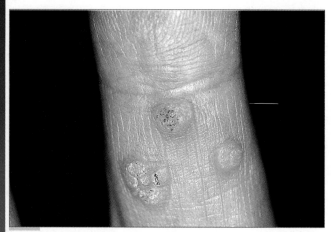

6.4 *Common warts (verruca vulgaris).* These lesions demonstrate loss of normal skin markings, and "black dots," or thrombosed capillaries, are pathognomonic.

DESCRIPTION OF COMMON WARTS

- Common warts generally have a verrucose, or vegetative, appearance.
- Lesions show loss of normal skin markings (e.g., finger-prints and handprints).
- "Black dots," or thrombosed capillaries, are pathognomonic (FIG. 6.4).
- Usually warts are asymptomatic, but they can be tender and often cause embarrassment.

 DIFFERENTIAL DIAGNOSIS OF COMMON WARTS

Pediatric
- Molluscum contagiosum (see FIG. 6.15)

Adult/Elderly
- Seborrheic keratosis
- Acrochordon (skin tag)
- Solar keratosis and cutaneous horn
- Squamous cell carcinoma
- Keratoacanthoma

Seborrheic Keratosis
See Chapter 21, "Benign Skin Neoplasms."

- These benign lesions occur in middle-aged and older people.
- They are most often seen along the frontal hairline, face, and trunk.
- They have a "stuck-on" appearance.
- They may be clinically indistinguishable from warts.

Solar Keratosis (Actinic Keratosis)
See Chapter 22, "Premalignant and Malignant Skin Neoplasms."

- These lesions occur in elderly, fair-complexioned persons, and they are sometimes associated with a cutaneous horn.
- They are rough-textured papules that appear in sun-exposed areas.
- Biopsy may be necessary to distinguish these lesions from squamous cell carcinoma.

Squamous Cell Carcinoma Under the Nail
- Biopsy is necessary.
- This lesion can easily be misdiagnosed as a subungual wart.

Onychomycosis
See Chapter 7, "Superficial Fungal Infections."

- The potassium hydroxide examination or fungal culture is positive.

Plantar Warts

- Plantar warts are seen on the plantar surface of the feet and occur mostly in children and young adults.
- They usually appear on the metatarsal area, heels, insteps (FIG. 6.5), and toes in an asymmetric distribution.

DESCRIPTION AND DISTRIBUTION OF PLANTAR WARTS

- Plantar warts may be painful and can impair ambulation, particularly when present on a weight-bearing surface, such as the sole of the foot during walking.
- Lesions may be solitary or multiple, or they may appear in clusters (mosaic warts) (FIG. 6.6).
- There is loss of normal skin markings (dermatoglyphics). Often, there are pathognomonic "black dots" (thrombosed dermal capillaries) and punctate bleeding that become evident after paring with a no. 15 blade (FIG. 6.7).

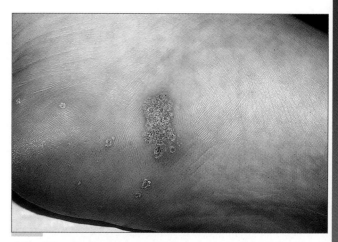

6.5 *Mosaic plantar warts.* Characteristic "black dots" are seen in this cluster of plantar warts.

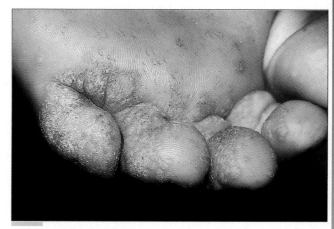

6.6 *Mosaic plantar warts.* Note the clustering, "kissing lesions" on this patient's toes.

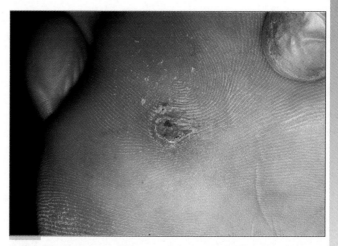

6.7 *Plantar wart.* Characteristic punctate bleeding is present after paring. Note the loss of skin markings.

- **Corns** (clavi) are sometimes difficult to distinguish from warts. Similar to calluses, corns are thickened areas of the skin that form in response to excessive pressure and friction.
- They are usually hard and circle-shaped, with a polished or central translucent core, like the kernel of corn from which they take their name (FIG. 6.8).
- Corns do not have "black dots," and skin markings are retained, except for the area of the central core.
- Corns most commonly develop on the tops and the tips of toes and along the sides of the feet. Lesions are also typically seen between the fourth and fifth toes ("kissing corns").
- Wearing high-heeled shoes—particularly shoes that shift the body weight into a narrow, tapering toe box—can produce corns.

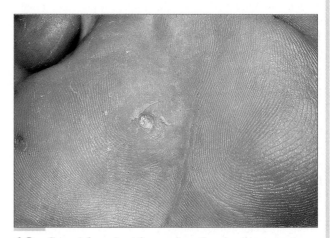

6.8 ***Corn (clavus).*** After paring, the circular central translucent core resembles a kernel of corn.

Flat Warts

Verrucae planae, or flat warts, are commonly found on the face (FIGS. 6.9 and 6.10), arms (FIG. 6.11), dorsa of hands, and the shins (women), where lesions are often spread by leg shaving.

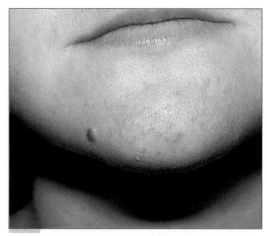

6.10 ***Flat warts (verruca planae).*** Very subtle, flesh-colored papules are present on this woman's chin.

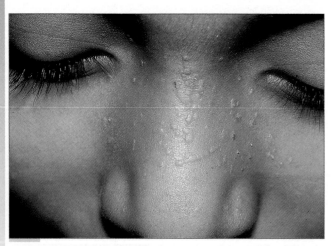

6.9 ***Flat warts (verruca planae).*** Lesions are slightly elevated papules the color of the patient's skin. Note the linear configuration resulting from autoinoculation of lesions on the bridge of this child's nose.

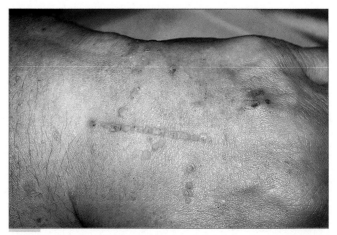

6.11 ***Flat warts (verruca planae).*** Lesions are slightly elevated, flat-topped papules. Linear autoinoculation is apparent.

DESCRIPTION OF FLAT WARTS

- These small, flat-topped, papular warts are slightly elevated and well-defined.
- Papules are skin-colored or tan to brown in color, and they range in size from 1 to 5 mm. Side lighting may be necessary to see them.
- Sometimes, flat warts show a linear configuration caused by autoinoculation.
- In men, flat warts are spread by shaving. Flat warts tend to resolve spontaneously, sometimes after a sudden increase in number, size, and inflammation.

 DIFFERENTIAL DIAGNOSIS OF FLAT WARTS

- Flat warts may resemble **molluscum contagiosum** (see later text), which manifests as shiny, waxy, dome-shaped papules with a central white core.

Filiform Warts

These tan, slender, delicate, fingerlike growths that emanate from the skin, filiform warts, are most commonly seen on the face (FIG. 6.12)—usually around the ala nasi, mouth, eyelids—and on the neck.

 DIFFERENTIAL DIAGNOSIS OF FILIFORM WARTS

- These finger-like papules that are seen in the elderly, usually on sun-exposed areas, may overlie a wart or a squamous cell carcinoma.

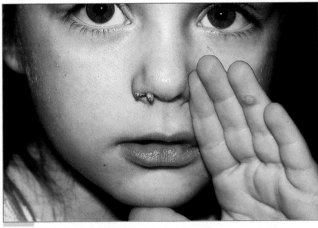

6.12 Filiform and common warts. This child has filiform warts on her nose and a common wart on her finger.

 MANAGEMENT

General Principles

The management of warts is often challenging, and there is no ideal treatment. The abundance of therapeutic modalities described in this chapter is a reflection of the fact that none of them is uniformly effective (see also TABLE 6.1). The method of treatment depends on the following:

- The age of the patient
- The patient's pain threshold
- The type of wart
- The location of the lesion

Providing no treatment at all may be safe and cost effective, because many warts resolve on their own. Painful, aggressive therapy should be avoided, unless there is a pressing need to eliminate the wart.

Children

- In children, most warts tend to regress spontaneously, which is probably related to a host immune response.
- Social factors are also important. For example, a 2-year-old child with a filiform wart located near the ala nasi, or with multiple hand warts, should warrant less aggressive

continued on page 146

Table 6.1 TOPICAL WART MEDICATIONS FORMULARY

AGENT	APPLICATION	FORMS
Topical Agents: Over-the-Counter		
DuoFilm solution	Apply daily under occlusion	17% salicylic acid
DuoFilm patch	Apply daily	40% salicylic acid in rubber-based vehicle
Dr. Scholl's Callus Removers	Apply daily	40% salicylic acid in rubber-based vehicle
Occlusal-HP solution	Apply daily	17% salicylic acid in polyacrylic solution
Compound W gel	Apply daily	17% salicylic acid in flexible collodion
Topical Agents: Prescription		
Aldara	Nightly as tolerated	5% imiquimod cream; 12 packets in a box

treatment than a 6-year-old child with similar lesions who may suffer from the teasing of other children.

Duct Tape ("Ducto-Therapy")

For stubborn common warts around and under the fingernails, the patient (or parent) is instructed in the following safe, easy, painless, inexpensive method that has been reported to help promote wart resolution:

- Cut a roll of shiny, electrical (duct) tape into 1-inch strips.
- Completely wrap the affected area with two "layers" of the tape (ILL. 6.1), making it airtight. Do not wrap the tape too tightly.
- Leave the tape on for 6 days, and then remove it for half a day. Leave the tape on during bathing, working, school, and all activities.
- Repeat this procedure (6 days on, 6 days off).

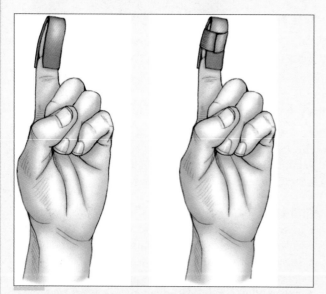

I6.1 *Treating warts using "ducto-therapy."* (Modified courtesy of Jerome Z. Litt, M.D.).

- Treat one digit at a time.
- Expect that after several weeks, the wart will become smaller, soft, and macerated and hopefully disappear.

Adults and Immunocompromised Patients

- In many adults and immunocompromised patients, warts often prove difficult to eradicate.
- It is necessary to explain to patients that there is no known practical way actually to kill HPV, and in many patients, when warts regress it is not because they have been "cured" but because the infection has become latent.
- Patients may also be reminded that so far there are no cures for acquired immunodeficiency syndrome (AIDS) or the common cold—both of which are caused by viruses—so it is not surprising that the virus that causes warts is difficult to eradicate. Treatment often takes numerous sessions, and, on occasion, warts fail to resolve.
- In short, the immune system apparently plays the most significant role in the expression of HPV. Treatment merely prompts or stimulates the immune system into dealing more effectively with the virus.
- The following treatment suggestions are given in a stepwise fashion, beginning with the least painful methods. (Note: The use of many of the following topical chemical approaches may be contraindicated during pregnancy or in women who are likely to become pregnant during the treatment period.)

Home Treatment: Topical Salicylic Acid

- **Salicylic acid** is a keratolytic (peeling) agent that can be self-administered. It has a role in exfoliating the hyperkeratotic "dead skin" of warts and inducing inflammation.
- Salicylic acid is available in numerous over-the-counter (OTC) trade name preparations such as **Compound W** gel and solution and **Duofilm** gel, patch, and solution.

continued on page 147

- For best results with any keratolytic agent, the affected area should be hydrated first by soaking it in warm water for 5 minutes before application of the agent.

Advantages
These preparations provide the best treatment for small children in whom warts are usually self-limiting.

- Usable on periungual warts
- Nonscarring
- Painless to apply
- Relatively inexpensive
- Do not require office visits

Disadvantages
- Slow response
- Often no response
- Time-consuming

Cryotherapy with Liquid Nitrogen
- Liquid nitrogen (LN_2) may be applied with a cotton swab or with a cryotherapy gun (Cryogun) (see Chapter 26, "Diagnostic and Therapeutic Procedures"). The goals are a rapid freeze and a slow thaw. Repeated freeze–thaw cycles increase cell damage. Cryotherapy is best for warts on hands.
- Regardless of whether LN_2 is applied with a saturated cotton swab or with a cryotherapy gun, one should aim to create a 2- to 3-mm zone of freeze around the lesion for a total of 4 to 5 seconds. The time of application varies, depending on the thickness of the lesion.
- If possible, an attempt should be made to freeze lesions at a right angle; this approach may lessen the patient's pain and may minimize collateral damage to normal surrounding skin.
- The procedure is repeated at 2- to 3-week intervals, based on patient tolerance or on previous treatment results, degree of pain, and posttreatment morbidity.

Advantages
- Treatment is rapid.
- Many lesions can be treated during a single office visit.
- It works well for hand warts.

Disadvantages
- This approach necessitates the availability of an LN_2 unit and holding tank.
- Treatment is painful and must be used cautiously on fingertips and on periungual lesions.

- This treatment can cause painful blisters.
- On darkly pigmented skin, cryotherapy can result in hypopigmentation or hyperpigmentation, or even depigmentation, because LN_2 destroys melanocytes.
- Overaggressive treatment may cause scarring.
- Treatment often requires multiple office visits.

Electrocautery and Blunt Dissection
- In electrosurgical procedures, the wart is burned by an electrical current that uses heat conduction from a hot probe heated by a direct current.
- These methods are best for warts on the knees, elbows, and dorsa of hands. They are also effective for filiform warts.

Advantages
- Treatment is tolerable in most adults.
- Warts are removed on the day of treatment.

Disadvantages
- Local anesthesia is required. Treatment sometimes necessitates a digital block, which can be painful, especially on the fingers and the soles of the feet.
- Treatment may cause scarring.
- It can cause nail deformity after injury to the nail matrix.

Laser Ablation
- Laser destruction of warts is reserved only for large or refractory lesions.
- This method is expensive and requires local anesthesia.
- One study concluded that laser ablation is no more effective in eradicating recalcitrant warts than are the less costly conventional methods described herein.

Immunotherapy
Interferon Induction
- **Aldara cream 5%** (imiquimod), a local inducer of interferon that stimulates immune up-regulation, may be applied at home by the patient. It is available as a 5% cream that is approved for the treatment of genital warts (condyloma acuminatum) (See Chapter 19, "Sexually Transmitted Diseases").
- There have been numerous anecdotal reports of the successful off-label use of imiquimod on common warts and plantar warts. It is applied under duct tape occlusion after hydrating the area to be treated. This is best done at bedtime and washed off after 6 to 10 hours. It is applied to facial flat warts without occlusion (see later discussion).

continued on page 148

MANAGEMENT *Continued*

Sensitizing Agents

- The deliberate induction of allergic reactions by injecting or applying sensitizing agents is sometimes used to treat warts.
- Intralesional injection of the *Candida* skin test antigen has been associated with some reports of total clearance of warts in sites that were remote from the location of injection.
- There are other contact (applied) immunotherapy agents, such as diphencyprone, dinitrochlorobenzene (DNCB), and squaric acid dibutylester (SADBE), that produce a delayed-type hypersensitivity reaction; however, there are possible mutagenic and side effects with these agents.

Oral Therapy

- The results in treating recalcitrant warts with high-dose oral cimetidine (**Tagamet**) have been disappointing in most placebo-controlled studies. However, this agent may at times to be effective in children.

Vesicants

- Cantharidin (**Cantharone**), or "bug juice," a vesicant (blister-producing agent), is a chemical that was originally derived from the green blister beetle. It is applied in an office setting.
- The preparation is applied to individual warts in a thin coat, using a cotton-tipped applicator or a toothpick. A waterproof bandage is used to cover the lesion(s). The procedure is painless. The occlusive dressing is left in place for 4 to 6 hours, and the skin is washed with soap and water.
- The cantharidin causes the skin under the wart to blister, and the wart is thus lifted off the skin. When the blister dries, the wart—if treatment is successful—detaches with the blistered skin.
- There usually is no scarring. Although cantharidin does not hurt when it is applied, the resulting blister can be painful.
- The combination of cantharidin, salicylic acid, and podophyllin in flexible collodion (**Cantharone Plus**) is a very potent alternative to the use of Cantharone alone; this approach may cause severe blisters and pain and should be used with caution.

Caustic Agents

- **Dichloroacetic acid, trichloroacetic acid, podophyllin, formic acid, 5-fluorouracil, formaldehyde,** and **glutaraldehyde** have all been used, with varying results.
- Intradermal injections of **bleomycin,** a chemotherapy agent that inhibits cell division, is another treatment for highly resistant warts. This agent is expensive and causes severe pain and possible tissue necrosis.

- Topical benzoyl peroxide and retinoids are sometimes used for facial flat warts (see below).

Treatment of Specific Types of Warts

Common Warts

- LN$_2$ or electrosurgery is effective.
- Topical cantharidin (**Cantharone**) when LN$_2$ fails or is not tolerated; this is an excellent treatment for periungual lesions.

Plantar Warts

- Paring with a no. 15 blade parallel to the skin surface often immediately relieves pain on walking.
- Instruct the patient to apply salicylic acid preparations between visits, as well as to perform "sanding" with an emery board, a foot file such as **Dr. Scholl's Callous Removers,** or a pumice stone, which keeps the wart flat and thus painless. Application of OTC **Salactic film** (17% salicylic acid solution) or **Mediplast,** a 40% salicylic acid plaster cut to the size of the wart, follows. The patient should leave the solution on overnight; he or she may leave the plaster on for 5 to 6 days or use a pumice stone.
- LN$_2$, blunt dissection, electrodesiccation, and curettage are reserved for more recalcitrant warts or when patients insist on aggressive therapy.
- **Aldara cream** under occlusion may be used (see earlier discussion).

Flat Warts

- Cautious application of LN$_2$ therapy (e.g., with a cotton-tipped applicator) or light (low-intensity) electrocautery are appropriate treatment options.
- These destructive measures may be used in combination with the daily application of imiquimod cream (**Aldara cream**), which may hasten resolution of lesions. When applied to the face, imiquimod cream is used without occlusion.
- Benzoyl peroxide and retinoids are applied topically.
- Topical retinoids such as tretinoin (**retinoic acid, Retin-A**) are used; there is less scarring than with cryotherapy or surgery, and these may be best for warts on the face. Instruct patients to apply them twice daily for 4 to 6 weeks.
- Lactic-salicylic acid (**Duofilm**) or **Occlusal-HP,** a salicylic acid, requires daily treatment for about 3 months.
- Salicylic acid (**Trans-Ver-Sal**) in a transdermal delivery system requires daily treatment for about 6 weeks.
- Flat warts are notoriously recalcitrant to therapy.

continued on page 149

Filiform Warts

- A virtually painless method is to dip a mosquito hemostat into LN$_2$ for 10 seconds and then gently grasp the wart for about 4 to 5 seconds (FIG. 6.13 A and B).
- The frozen wart is generally shed in 7 to 10 days (see also Chapter 21 and FIG. 21.24). This method often requires multiple office visits.
- A "snip excision" or electrocautery may be used following local anesthesia.

Alternative Treatments

- Hypnosis has been used to treat refractory warts. Several published studies have documented the success of hypnotherapy.
- Hyperthermia involves immersing the involved surface in hot water (113°F) for 30 to 45 minutes, two to three times per week.
- An OTC freezing device is now sold in many drug counters. It consists of a canister filled with a liquid mixture of the compressed gases dimethyl ether, propane, and isobutane. No success with this device has been documented.
- Raw garlic cloves have been demonstrated to have antiviral activity. This can be rubbed onto the wart nightly, followed by occlusion.
- Vaccines are currently in development.

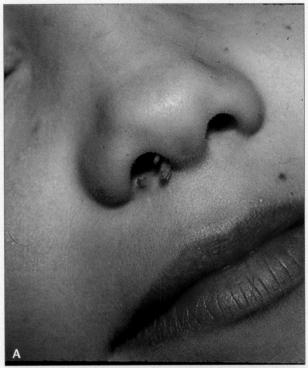

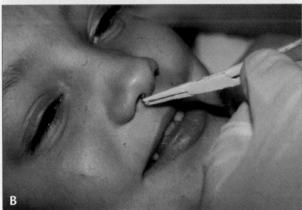

6.13 A and B *Filiform wart treatment.* A relatively painless method is to dip a mosquito hemostat into LN$_2$ for 10 seconds and then gently grasp the wart for about 4 to 5 seconds. This treatment is repeated four to five times during each visit as tolerated.

POINTS TO REMEMBER

- Freezing and other destructive treatment modalities do not kill the virus but merely destroy the cells that harbor HPV. In other words, when you treat a wart, only the "host" is destroyed, not the virus itself.
- Because HPV persists after therapy, some degree of infectivity and the potential for recurrence may remain, even in the absence of clinical lesions.
- Patients always ask, "How do you know when the warts are gone?" Answer: "When they don't recur."
- How to avoid getting warts? *Never shake hands. Never kiss anyone. Never walk barefoot. Never share towels. Live in a bubble . . . and there's still a good chance you'll get one.*

- No single therapy for warts is uniformly effective or superior; thus, treatment involves a certain amount of trial and error.
- Conservative, nonscarring treatments are preferred. Each treatment is associated with a 60% to 70% cure rate. A clinical "cure" is achieved when the skin lines are restored to a normal pattern and there is no recurrence.

Important Information About Plantar Warts Only

- **Melanoma** can mimic a plantar wart.
- **Verrucous carcinoma,** a slow-growing, locally invasive, well-differentiated squamous cell carcinoma, may also be easily mistaken for a plantar wart.

➤ **WART HEROES**

The hero of successful wart treatment is usually the last person to treat the wart, or the last person to recommend a treatment, before the wart regresses. The "wart hero" may have been a wart charmer, a dermatologist, a hypnotist, or a person who recommends a folk medicine remedy, such as the application of garlic or aloe vera. More often than not, warts tend to "cure" themselves over time, especially in immunocompetent patients. This outcome should be borne in mind and explained to patients early in the course of therapy.

 SEE PATIENT HANDOUT "Warts" ON THE SOLUTION SITE

BASICS

Molluscum contagiosum (MC) is a common superficial viral infection of the epidermis. It is spread by skin-to-skin contact and is caused by a large DNA-containing poxvirus. It is seen most often in three clinical contexts:

- It occurs in young, healthy children (infants and preschoolers), in whom the incidence decreases after the age of 6 or 7 years. Most often it arises in young children who have atopic dermatitis.
- It occurs in HIV-positive patients.
- It occurs in young adults who are sexually active and not HIV seropositive.

DESCRIPTION OF LESIONS

- MC lesions are dome-shaped, waxy or pearly papules with a central white core (FIG. 6.14). Less frequently, the papules are the color of the patient's skin.
- Lesions are generally 1 to 3 mm in diameter, but they may coalesce and become giant mollusca.
- Frequently, the lesions are grouped.
- The number of lesions varies from 1 to 20 up to hundreds.

DISTRIBUTION OF LESIONS

- Lesions of MC most often appear on the face and eyelids (FIG. 6.15), the trunk, the axillae, genitalia, and the extremities.
- Usually, lesions are asymmetric in distribution, depending on the sites of initial inoculation.
- They are spread by autoinoculation from picking and rubbing.
- MC can appear in areas of the skin that are traumatized or inflamed, as seen in the flexural creases and axillae in children who have underlying atopic dermatitis at these sites (FIG. 6.16).

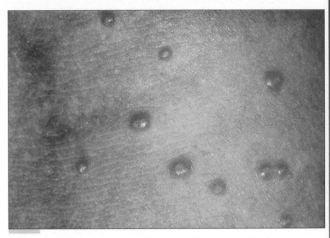

6.14 *Molluscum contagiosum.* Characteristic dome-shaped, shiny, waxy papules have a central white core.

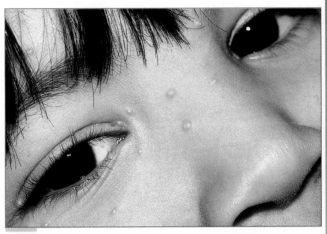

6.15 *Molluscum contagiosum.* This is a typical distribution of lesions on a child's face. Note the eyelid lesions.

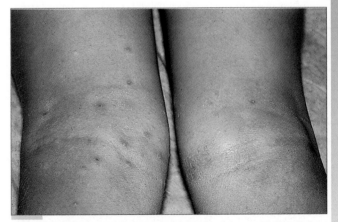

6.16 *Molluscum contagiosum.* Lesions are present on a background of atopic dermatitis of the flexural creases.

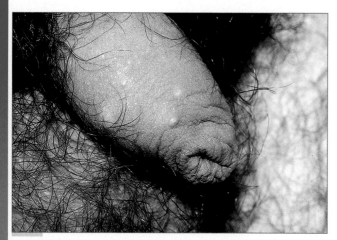

6.17 *Molluscum contagiosum.* Characteristic dome-shaped, shiny, waxy papules are present on the penis.

- Lesions may be seen on the external genitalia (FIG. 6.17), on the lower abdominal wall, on the inner thighs, and on the pubic area.
- Such lesions are often spread sexually in adults, and their presence in these locations may—in rare occasions—be considered a sign of sexual abuse in children.

CLINICAL MANIFESTATIONS

- Generally asymptomatic, MC may itch slightly, may be scratched, and may become secondarily infected.
- In children, the course is self-limiting; 70% of the time lesions of MC resolve within 6 to 8 months. Recurrences are rare in immunocompetent persons.
- MC in HIV-positive patients is common (see Chapter 24, "Cutaneous Manifestations of HIV Infection").
  - More than 100 lesions may be seen.
  - They appear most commonly on the face and are spread by shaving (FIG. 6.18).
  - The giant molluscum or coalescent double or triple lesions are frequently seen in these patients.
  - The lesions are often chronic and are difficult to eradicate.

DIAGNOSIS

- Typical papules are easily recognized.
- Inspection with a handheld magnifier often reveals the central core.
- A short application of cryotherapy with LN_2 accentuates the central core (FIGS. 6.19 A and B).

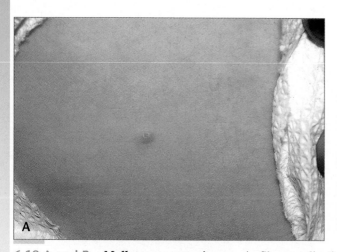

6.18 *Molluscum contagiosum.* Note the double and "giant lesions" on the face of a patient with acquired immunodeficiency syndrome.

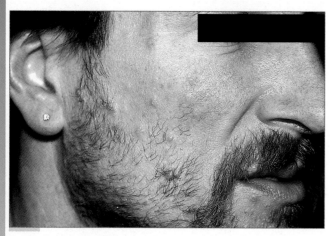

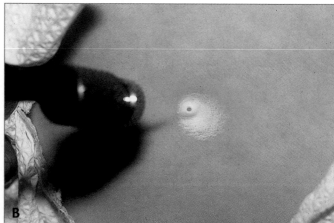

6.19 A and B *Molluscum contagiosum.* A: Short application of liquid nitrogen (LN_2). B: LN_2 accentuates the central core.

- A direct microscopic smear of a lesion (crush preparation) demonstrates characteristic "molluscum bodies" (FIG. 6.20).
- A shave biopsy is performed, if necessary. Identification of characteristic intracytoplasmic inclusion bodies in histologic or cytologic preparations is made by hematoxylin and eosin staining of biopsy sections.

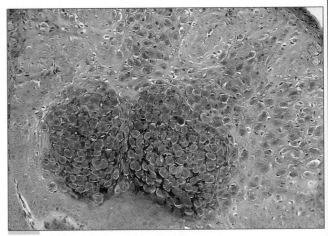

6.20 *Molluscum contagiosum.* "Molluscum bodies" (hematoxylin and eosin stain).

 DIFFERENTIAL DIAGNOSIS

Warts (Nongenital), Especially Small Flat Warts
Distinguishing features are as follows:

- Warts are not waxy.
- They are tan or brown.
- They have no central white core.

Warts (Genital)
- **Condyloma acuminatum** appears on the inner thighs, pubic area, vulvae, and penis.

- A biopsy may be necessary to differentiate these lesions from molluscum contagiosum.

Other Diagnoses
- Disseminated cryptococcosis, toxoplasmosis, and histoplasmosis in HIV-infected patients should also be considered.
- A biopsy may be necessary to differentiate these infections from MC.

 MANAGEMENT

Home Treatment
Lesions may be ignored until they resolve spontaneously, or MC may be treated by the patient or caregiver with:

- A topical OTC antiwart preparation, such as liquid salicylic acid in a rubber-based vehicle (**DuoFilm**), which is applied daily to the core of each lesion with a toothpick.
- Imiquimod 5% cream (**Aldara cream**) available only by prescription, is applied three times per week at bedtime. It is very expensive.

Office Treatment
If MC lesions cause social embarrassment and exclusion from activities (e.g., school, day care, swimming), the following treatments are available:

Cryotherapy
- In adults and older children, the lesions may be frozen lightly for 3 to 5 seconds with LN$_2$ applied with a cotton swab or a Cryogun (see FIG. 6.19).

Cantharidin Therapy
- In young children, a topical vesicant (blistering agent), such as cantharidin (**Cantharone**), is daubed on carefully with a toothpick or the wooden end of a cotton swab to each lesion and allowed to dry. This is done every 3 to 4 weeks, or until lesions are resolving.
- This method is less painful and better tolerated than LN$_2$. Care should be taken to avoid applying the agent to the uninvolved surrounding skin. Treated areas should not be occluded.

continued on page 154

MANAGEMENT *Continued*

- Parents should be instructed to wash off the agent with soap and water 2 to 4 hours later. In axillary and other skin-to-skin areas, the Cantharone should be washed off in 2 hours.
- The face should not be treated with Cantharone.

Other Treatments

- **Electrodesiccation and curettage** may be necessary for patients with refractory lesions.

- **Trichloroacetic acid peels** have been performed with some success in HIV-infected patients with extensive lesions.
- For refractory lesions in HIV-infected patients, highly active antiretroviral therapy has been very effective in reducing the incidence of MC in recent years.
- Systemic treatment with agents such as **griseofulvin** and **cimetidine** has been anecdotally reported to be effective in the treatment of MC; however, no controlled studies have been performed to confirm this.

 POINTS TO REMEMBER

- Lesions on an infant or a young preschool child should not be treated aggressively. The pain and emotional trauma associated with curettage and cryotherapy make them undesirable treatments in this age group.
- MC—particularly if it is located on the face of an adult—should alert the clinician to the possibility of HIV infection.
- MC in healthy, immunocompetent persons generally is self-limiting and heals after several months or longer.

 HELPFUL HINTS

- For anxious children, a topical anesthetic such as **EMLA** (eutectic mixture of local anesthetics) cream can be applied under occlusion 1 hour before treatment to decrease the discomfort associated with procedures such as curettage, local anesthetic injections, or cryosurgery.
- Because many children with MC also have atopic dermatitis, further spread of the MC lesions is perpetuated by itching and scratching. Consequently, it is best to treat and control all eczematous lesions before the lesions of MC are addressed.

SEE PATIENT HANDOUT "Molluscum Contagiosum" ON THE SOLUTION SITE

Herpes Simplex (Nongenital)

BASICS

Herpes simplex virus (HSV) infections are caused by two virus types: HSV-1 and HSV-2. HSV-1 causes most nongenital infections. These highly contagious viruses are spread by direct contact with the skin or mucous membranes. After the primary infection resolves, the virus retreats to a dorsal root ganglion, where it becomes incorporated into the genetic material of the cell. The virus remains latent until it is reactivated by precipitating factors or triggers, such as sunlight exposure, menses, fever, common colds, and, possibly, stress.

Primary infections are acquired in infancy and early childhood; most are subclinical. Patients who have AIDS or who are under treatment with immunosuppressants for organ transplantation or cancer chemotherapy are at greatest risk for contracting severe recalcitrant HSV infections.

Nongenital HSV infection is extremely common. In fact, herpes-specific antibody (for type 1 and, less commonly, type 2) can be found in the serum of many lesion-free adults. Asymptomatic shedding probably accounts for the widespread transmission of this ubiquitous virus.

Since the 1980s, the public attention that genital herpes has attracted has led to misconceptions about HSV infection and to its overdiagnosis, especially in regard to lesions that occur within the oral cavity. For example, many people who suffer from recurrent nonherpetic painful intraoral mouth sores (aphthous stomatitis, or canker sores) are given a diagnosis of "herpes," and thus they may feel the stigma associated with sexually transmitted diseases. Because recurrent aphthous stomatitis—which has no known viral association—has a clinical appearance and course similar to those of recurrent herpes labialis, the two conditions are often confused by patient and clinician alike. HSV lesions, particularly recurrent ones, occur inside the mouth very infrequently, unless the virus is a primary infection or occurs in immunocompromised patients.

Pathophysiology

Intimate contact between a susceptible person (without antibodies against the virus) and an individual who is actively shedding the virus or with body fluids containing the virus is required for transmission of HSV infection to occur. Contact must involve mucous membranes or open or abraded skin.

HSV invades and replicates in neurons as well as in epidermal and dermal cells. Virions travel from the initial site of infection on the skin or mucosa to the sensory dorsal root ganglion, where latency is established. Viral replication in the sensory ganglia leads to recurrent clinical outbreaks. These outbreaks can be induced by various stimuli, such as trauma, ultraviolet radiation, extremes in temperature, stress, immunosuppression, or hormonal fluctuations. Viral shedding, leading to possible transmission, is most likely to occur during the period of primary infection, during subsequent recurrences, and during periods of asymptomatic viral shedding.

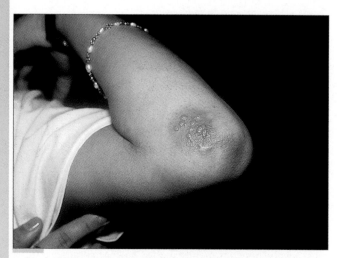

6.21 ***Herpes simplex virus.*** In this typical grouping, umbilicated vesicles overlie an erythematous base.

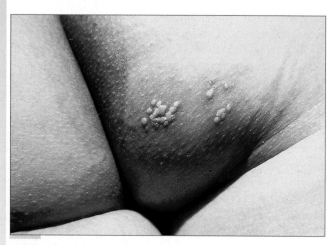

6.22 ***Herpes simplex virus.*** Here, most vesicles have evolved into pustules.

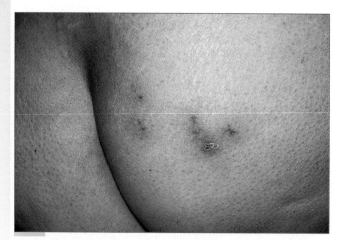

6.23 ***Herpes simplex virus.*** The presacral and gluteal areas are common locations of herpes simplex type 2 in women. This patient shows drying crusts (scabs) and erosions.

DESCRIPTION OF LESIONS

The following sequence of events describes the easily recognizable evolution of HSV "cold sores" or "fever blisters":

- A single vesicle or a group of vesicles overlies an erythematous base (Fig. 6.21). Vesicles may sag in the center (umbilicate).
- The vesicles may become pustules (Fig. 6.22), or they may dry and become crusts or erosions (Fig. 6.23).
- The lesions generally heal without scarring (because they are intraepidermal).

Primary Orolabial Herpes Simplex

Herpes labialis is most commonly associated with HSV-1 infection. It often occurs in childhood and is usually asymptomatic.

DISTRIBUTION OF LESIONS

When symptoms are present during a primary HSV infection, the oral cavity (the lips, gums, buccal mucosa, fauces, tongue, and hard palate) is the area generally affected (Fig. 6.24).

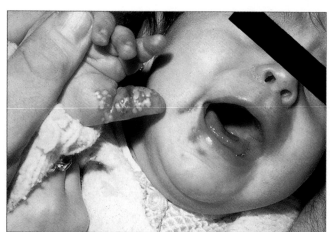

6.24 ***Primary herpes simplex virus infection.*** This infant has multiple vesicles and pustules as well as gingivostomatitis.

CLINICAL MANIFESTATIONS

Most cases of primary HSV are subclinical.

- Symptomatic primary HSV infections tend to be more severe than those of recurrent disease; they include gingivostomatitis, fever, sore throat, and submandibular or cervical lymphadenopathy.
- Distinguishing primary HSV infection from severe cases of recurrent HSV can be difficult.
- Painful vesicles develop on the lips, the gingiva, the palate, or the tongue and are often associated with erythema and edema. Lesions tend to ulcerate and heal within 2 to 3 weeks.
- Encephalitis and aseptic meningitis are rare complications.

Recurrent Orolabial Herpes Simplex

DISTRIBUTION OF LESIONS

- Lesions tend to recur at or near the same location within the distribution of a sensory nerve.
- Recurrences are most often seen on or near the vermilion border of the lip (herpes labialis) (FIG. 6.25).

CLINICAL MANIFESTATIONS

- Symptoms are generally milder and the number of lesions fewer than those associated with primary HSV.
- Patients commonly experience a prodrome of itching, pain, or numbness.
- The recurrent vesicular lesions eventually ulcerate or form a crust.
- Infrequently, regional lymphadenopathy occurs.
- Over time, recurrences decrease in frequency and often stop altogether.
- Persistent ulcerative or verrucous vegetative lesions may be seen in immunocompromised patients.
- Most cases of recurrent erythema multiforme minor accompany, and appear to be caused by, recurrent (both clinical and subclinical) HSV episodes (see Chapter 18, "Diseases of Vasculature").

DIAGNOSIS OF HERPES SIMPLEX

The diagnosis of HSV is usually based on clinical appearance and history. At the time of an office visit, patients often present with only nonspecific crusted lesions or merely with a history consistent with recurrent HSV. When necessary, the following tests may be administered on fresh lesions:

- A Tzanck preparation, if positive, suggests HSV or varicella-zoster virus (VZV) infection. This test is used to rapidly determine the presence of HSV or VZV; it does not distinguish between these two viruses (FIG. 6.26) (see the description of the Tzanck procedure in the sidebar).

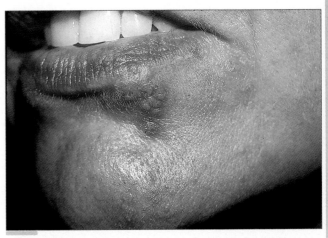

6.25 *Recurrent herpes simplex virus infection (herpes labialis).* Lesions are evident on the vermilion border of the lip and beyond.

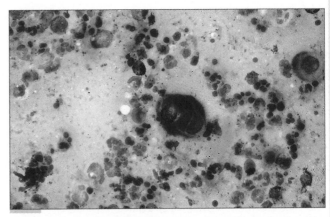

6.26 *Positive Tzanck preparation.* Note the typical multinucleated giant cells with large nuclei. This test does not distinguish between herpes simplex and herpes zoster. Note the presence of nuclei of normal-sized keratinocytes, which are the size of neutrophils.

TZANCK PREPARATION

A Tzanck preparation is used to aid in the diagnosis of HSV, herpes zoster, and VZV. This technique furnishes an inexpensive, efficient provisional diagnosis, but it does not enable one to distinguish HSV from VZV.

1. For best results, a fresh, intact vesicle or bulla usually present for less than 24 hours is preferred.
2. After the lesion is swabbed with an alcohol preparation, the blister is unroofed by piercing it with a no. 11 blade or a needle, followed by blotting with a sponge.
3. The underlying moist base of the lesion is then scraped with a no. 15 scalpel blade, and a thin layer of material is spread onto a glass slide.
4. The specimen is then air dried and is stained with a supravital stain such as Giemsa, Wright's, or methylene blue, which is left on for 1 minute.
5. The specimen is then gently flooded with tap water for 15 seconds to remove any remaining stain.
6. Examination, initially under 40-power magnification and then 100-power oil immersion, helps identify the characteristic multinucleated giant cells (see FIG. 6.26).

- Detection and typing of HSV are performed by obtaining a culture from intact vesicles, ideally early in the course of the infection, but the false-negative rate increases after 48 hours of lesion onset.
- HSV tissue culture using monoclonal antibodies requires only 24 hours. The test is 90% sensitive, but it is expensive.
- Polymerase chain reaction for HSV DNA detection can be conducted; however, like the monoclonal antibody method, it is expensive.
- Serologic tests for HSV are generally not very useful because so much of the general adult population has antibodies to herpes simplex; however, primary HSV infection can be documented by demonstration of seroconversion, high titers, or rising titers.

DDx DIFFERENTIAL DIAGNOSIS: OROLABIAL HERPES SIMPLEX

Aphthous Stomatitis
- Lesions of aphthous stomatitis are small, punched-out erosions that occur on the tongue and on the buccal, labial, and gingival mucosa (see Chapter 12, "Disorders of the Mouth, Lips, and Tongue") (FIG. 6.27).
- Lesions typically consist of painful, shallow, gray or yellow 2- to 3-mm erosions.

Hand-Foot-and-Mouth Disease
- Oval erythematous erosions are most often seen on the soft palate and uvula (see Chapter 8, "Viral Exanthems").
- Lesions are asymptomatic.
- Lesions may also appear on the hands and feet.
- Lesions are shallower than those of primary HSV.

Herpangina
- Small, painful vesicular or ulcerative lesions occur on the roof of the mouth and in the throat.
- Lesions have a white to whitish-gray base and a red border.
- The condition is usually caused by coxsackie virus, typically coxsackie group A viruses.
- Typically, it occurs during the summer and frequently affects children, but it also may occur in young adults.

- Mouth ulcers, a high fever, sore throat, and headache are characteristic.
- Symptoms may precede the appearance of lesions.

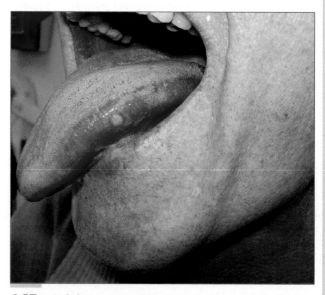

6.27 *Aphthous stomatitis.* This shallow erosion is surrounded by a ring of erythema.

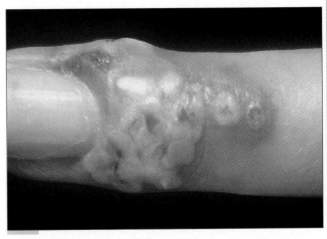

DIFFERENTIAL DIAGNOSIS: EXTRAOROLABIAL HERPES SIMPLEX

- Although HSV infections may occur anywhere on the body, 70% to 90% of HSV-1 infections occur above the umbilicus.
- In contrast, 70% to 90% of HSV-2 infections occur below the umbilicus. Lesions also tend to occur on the presacral area in women, but they may be found anywhere on the cutaneous surface (see Chapter 19, "Sexually Transmitted Diseases").

Herpes Zoster

- Lesions of herpes zoster are unilateral, dermatomal, and often painful (see the discussion of herpes zoster later in this chapter).
- Lesions are also grouped but tend to vary in size.
- The condition may be clinically indistinguishable from HSV when lesions are located in a single focus.

6.28 Herpes whitlow. This infection in a health care worker was caused by a needle puncture.

Clinical Variants of Herpes Simplex Infections

Herpetic Whitlow

- Painful herpetic whitlow results from the direct inoculation of the virus to the fingertip (Fig. 6.28).
- Before the current stringent infection control measures and the widespread use of gloves by health care providers, herpetic whitlow was an occupational hazard among dental and medical health care personnel whose fingertips came in contact with infected oral or respiratory excretions.

Eczema Herpeticum

FIGURE 6.29.

- Also known as Kaposi's varicelliform eruption, eczema herpeticum is an uncommon disseminated form of HSV infection caused by HSV-1. It occurs mainly in children who have severe atopic dermatitis, burns, or other inflammatory skin conditions.

Herpes Gladiatorum

- This is caused by HSV-1 and is seen as papular or vesicular eruptions on the torsos of athletes in sports involving close physical contact (classically, wrestling).

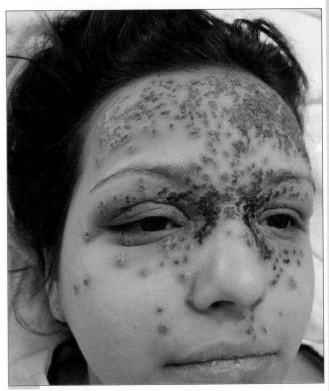

6.29 Eczema herpeticum (Kaposi's varicelliform eruption). This patient has an uncommon disseminated form of HSV infection. She has underlying atopic dermatitis. (Image courtesy of Joseph Eastern, M.D.).

Disseminated Herpes Simplex

- Infection can occur in individuals who are immunocompromised.
- These patients may present with atypical signs and symptoms of HSV, and the condition may be difficult to diagnose. Larger lesions or necrotizing ulcers may occur, and widespread areas may be involved.

Neonatal Herpes Simplex

- Newborns are exposed to HSV-2 via the birth canal of an actively infected mother.
- Infection occurs most often peripartum, although in utero transmission also occurs.

Herpetic Sycosis

- This follicular infection with HSV may present as a vesiculopustular eruption in the beard area in men.
- It often results from autoinoculation after shaving through a recurrent herpetic outbreak.

Ocular Herpes Simplex

- Herpes conjunctivitis, keratitis, uveitis, optic neuritis, and retinitis are possible sequelae of HSV.

 MANAGEMENT

Topical Therapy

Skin symptoms may be eased by soaking in **Burow's solution** (aluminum acetate or aluminum sulfate) two to three times daily. Alternatively, soaks with water or saline may help dry the eruption and may prevent secondary infection.

- Topical acyclovir 5% (**Zovirax**) ointment, penciclovir 1% (**Denavir**) cream, and docosanol 10% (**Abreva**) cream are not very effective treatments, but they may help reduce healing time.
- Patients in whom sun exposure incites recurrent HSV of the lips can apply an opaque sun-blocking agent before sun exposure.
- Patients can lessen the discomfort of oral HSV lesions by applying viscous lidocaine applications or OTC "caine" products, taking oral analgesics, or sucking on ice cubes.

Systemic Therapy

Pharmacologic agents used for the treatment of HSV include acyclovir, valacyclovir, and famciclovir. Valacyclovir is rapidly converted to acyclovir, and its bioavailability is three to five times greater than that of acyclovir. Similarly, famciclovir is converted to the more bioavailable penciclovir. For these reasons, acyclovir has been supplanted by valacyclovir and famciclovir in the treatment of HSV in adults.

- Dose reduction is recommended for patients who have renal impairment.

- The use of valacyclovir is contraindicated in some patients (e.g., in some renal and bone marrow transplant recipients and in those infected with HIV) because of reports of thrombotic thrombocytopenic purpura and hemolytic-uremic syndrome.

Treatment with Antiviral Agents

Primary Herpes Simplex

- Valacyclovir (**Valtrex**) (1 g twice daily for 7 to 10 days)
- Famciclovir (**Famvir**) (250 mg three times daily for 7 to 10 days)
- **Acyclovir** (200 mg five times daily or 400 mg three times daily for 10 days)

Recurrent Herpes Simplex

This treatment should be initiated at the first sign of prodrome, because it can often abort the lesions. Following are treatment options:

- Valacyclovir (Valtrex) (2 g twice daily for 1 day taken about 12 hours apart). This is a shorter, more economical course.
- Famciclovir (Famvir) (single-day therapy; 1,000 mg in the morning and 1,000 mg in the evening, or 125 mg twice daily for 5 days). In HIV-positive patients, 500 mg twice a day is given for 7 days.
- Acyclovir (200 mg twice daily or 400 mg three times daily for 5 days).

continued on page 161

MANAGEMENT *Continued*

For frequent recurrences (more than six recurrences per year), persistent HSV, severe disease, or recurrent erythema multiforme minor, **long-term suppressive oral therapy** may be used. After 1 year of treatment with these agents, the medication should be discontinued to determine the recurrence rate, and the dosage can be adjusted as needed.

- Valacyclovir (1 g daily for 6 to 12 months; afterward, the clinician should attempt to taper the dose to 500 mg or to discontinue the agent)
- Famciclovir (250 mg twice daily for 12 months)
- Acyclovir (400 mg twice daily for 12 months)

Immunocompromised hosts, those with Kaposi's varicelliform eruption, or those with HSV encephalitis often require intravenous acyclovir therapy.

 SEE PATIENT HANDOUT "Herpes Simplex" ON THE SOLUTION SITE

 POINTS TO REMEMBER

- Intraoral ulcers in immunocompetent patients are most likely canker sores (aphthous stomatitis).
- Recurrent HSV attacks can be aborted by treatment on a short-term basis with oral antivirals administered during the prodromal stage.
- Frequent recurrences can be aborted by treatment with suppressive oral antivirals.
- A truly effective topical treatment for HSV has yet to be found.
- Pregnant women with active genital HSV may need a cesarean section to prevent neonatal HSV, a potentially fatal disease.

Herpes Zoster

BASICS

- Herpes zoster ("shingles") is caused by the same herpesvirus that causes varicella, or chickenpox. The virus first manifests as varicella (see Chapter 8, "Viral Exanthems"), a primary infection usually seen in childhood. Subsequently, when the same latent virus is reactivated, its second episode manifests as herpes zoster.
- The risk of herpes zoster increases with age and is 8 to 10 times more likely to develop in people 60 years of age or older as in younger people.
  - The disease also develops frequently in immunocompromised patients, such as transplant recipients and those with HIV infection or malignant disease, particularly lymphoproliferative malignancies (e.g., Hodgkin's disease).
  - Elderly persons and immunocompromised patients also tend to have more severe disease, with complications such as postherpetic neuralgia (PHN), disseminated zoster, and chronic zoster.

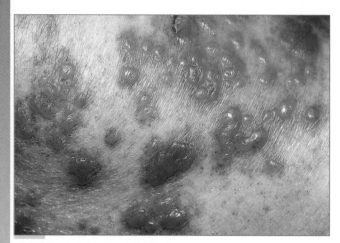

6.30 Herpes zoster. These umbilicated vesicles of various sizes are grouped on an erythematous base.

- The infectious course of herpes zoster infection, or VZV infection, is similar to that of HSV infection.
  - After the primary infection resolves, the virus retreats to the dorsal root ganglion, where it remains in a dormant state. Reactivation—into dermatomal "shingles"—may be caused by severe illness or infection with HIV, but most often it occurs spontaneously, without an obvious precipitating cause. It is most likely a sign that immunity to VZV, which most people acquire in childhood, has decreased.
  - The reemergence as a local vesicobullous eruption derives from the anterograde migration of virions through the axon to the skin of a single dermatome or several adjacent ones. In immunocompetent patients, recurrent or bilateral herpes zoster episodes are extremely uncommon; immunity to the virus is presumably boosted by the initial episode of herpes zoster.
- The pain of herpes zoster is thought to result from nerve damage caused by the spread of the virus to the skin through the peripheral nerves. An inflammatory reaction leads to scarring of the peripheral nerves and dorsal root ganglia. PHN presumably results from the consequent hyperexcitability of neurons, which tend to discharge spontaneously.
- VZV infection occurs occasionally in pregnant women. A primary VZV infection (varicella) may result in severe fetal abnormalities; however, the development of herpes zoster during pregnancy does not appear to harm the developing fetus.

DESCRIPTION OF LESIONS

The following sequence of events describes the evolution of herpes zoster:

- Lesions begin as "juicy" erythematous papules that rapidly mature into clustered vesicles or bullae on top of an erythematous base. They tend to vary more in size than do the lesions of HSV (Fig. 6.30).

- Successive crops continue to appear for 6 to 8 days. The blisters sometimes umbilicate (sag in the middle); occasionally, they become pustular and hemorrhagic.
- In time, lesions dry into crusts or erosions that may heal and disappear completely or resolve with postinflammatory hyperpigmentation or hypopigmentation and, possibly, scarring.
- Lesions of herpes zoster in HIV-infected patients tend to be more verrucous and ulcerative, and they often heal with scars.
- Infrequently, dermatomal neuralgia may be accompanied or followed by nonbullous or urticarialike lesions (FIG. 6.31). Rarely, skin lesions are absent ("zoster sine herpete").

DISTRIBUTION OF LESIONS

- Lesions of herpes zoster occur in a characteristic unilateral dermatomal ("zosteriform") distribution.
- Occasionally, lesions involve contiguous dermatomes or extend beyond the midline.
- Although it can affect any dermatome, herpes zoster is most commonly found on the thoracic (FIG. 6.32), trigeminal, lumbosacral (FIG. 6.33), and cervical areas.
- Immunocompromised patients have a greater risk of multidermatomal zoster, recurrent zoster, and dissemination beyond the skin (e.g., into the eyes or the lungs) (see FIG. 24.6).

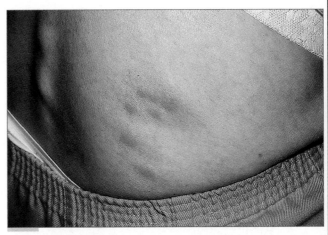

6.31 *Herpes zoster.* "Juicy," erythematous, urticarialike papules are seen here in a "zosteriform" distribution.

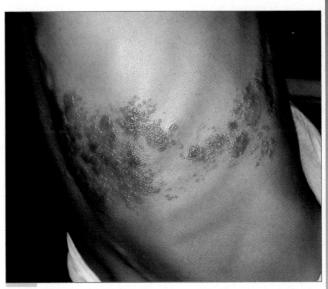

6.32 *Herpes zoster.* Drying hemorrhagic crusts appear in a "zosteriform" distribution. In this immunocompromised patient, the lesions will probably heal with scars.

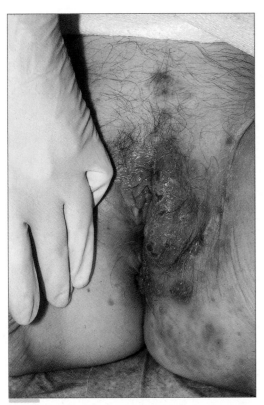

6.33 *Herpes zoster.* This patient has painful lesions of the vulva and perineum in a dermatomal distribution.

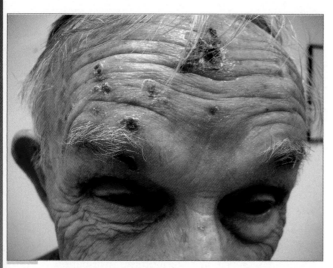

6.34 *Herpes zoster ophthalmicus.* This condition affects the first branch of the fifth cranial nerve.

Disseminated Herpes Zoster

See FIGURE 24.6.

- In immunocompromised patients, the eruption usually begins with typical dermatomal herpes zoster. The lesions may then become widespread, with 25 or more lesions found outside the primary dermatome.
- The condition can become chronic and indistinguishable from varicella.

DIAGNOSIS

- Herpes zoster can most often be diagnosed on the basis of clinical appearance and the presence of pain in a dermatomal distribution.
- If necessary, a Tzanck smear should be obtained from the base of a fresh lesion (see the discussion of Tzanck preparation earlier in this chapter). A positive result suggests either HSV or VZV infection.
- A skin biopsy is generally unnecessary, but it can help to confirm the diagnosis.

CLINICAL MANIFESTATIONS

Several days before the cutaneous eruption, patients may experience the following focal (dermatomal) symptoms: pain, numbness, pruritus, paresthesia, and skin tenderness or sensitivity (tactile allodynia).

- In children, herpes zoster is often asymptomatic.
- In contrast to the disease in children, both the likelihood and severity of pain (acute and chronic) associated with herpes zoster are significantly increased in patients older than 50 years.
- Second episodes of herpes zoster in immunocompetent people are rare, probably because of the immunologic "boosting" effect of the first episode.
- Pain and paresthesia in the affected dermatome may accompany the eruption or may precede it by 1 to 2 weeks. The neuropathic pain of some patients has been described as "boring," "burning," "crushing," or "stabbing." Some patients presenting with such pain have been thought to have a myocardial infarction or pleurisy, until the characteristic eruption of herpes zoster establishes the diagnosis.

Complications

- PHN is defined as pain persisting for more than 1 month after the eruption of the initial herpes zoster lesions. The pain may also develop after a pain-free interval. The frequency of PHN increases with age. It occurs more commonly in people with compromised immune systems, such as HIV-infected patients.
- In many elderly patients, PHN can cause chronic depression, anxiety, and social isolation.
- When herpes zoster occurs in the ophthalmic division of the fifth, or trigeminal, nerve, it is called **herpes zoster ophthalmicus** (FIG. 6.34). Eye involvement, such as conjunctivitis, acute retinal necrosis, uveitis, and retinal arteritis, can lead to blindness. Ophthalmic zoster warrants an immediate ophthalmologic consultation.
- VZV involvement of the geniculate ganglion is called the **Ramsay Hunt syndrome.** This condition results in motor and sensory neuropathy of the seventh cranial nerve.

DIFFERENTIAL DIAGNOSIS

Herpes Simplex Virus Infection

- When HSV presents in a site usually occupied by herpes zoster, or when it occurs in a semidermatomal distribution, it may be clinically indistinguishable from herpes zoster.
- The vesicles of herpes simplex, however, tend to be more uniform in size and are much less painful than those seen in herpes zoster.
- Recurrence strongly suggests HSV infection.

Poison Ivy

- Also known as rhus dermatitis, poison ivy often occurs in a linear distribution of blisters that corresponds to, or suggests, a dermatome.
- Rhus dermatitis, however, is pruritic and painless. Most patients with rhus dermatitis offer a history of contact with poison ivy or poison oak.

 MANAGEMENT

Topical Therapy

For the acute episode of herpes zoster, the following treatments are available without a prescription:

- **Burow's solution.** Wet dressings with Burow's solution (aluminum acetate or aluminum sulfate) are soothing and drying; so are moist soaks with water or saline.
- **Topical anesthetic "caines"** such as benzocaine may be helpful.

Systemic Therapy

Pain control is generally the paramount concern in herpes zoster.

- Oral analgesics, such as **acetaminophen, aspirin,** and other **nonsteroidal anti-inflammatory drugs,** as well as mild **narcotics,** are helpful in mild, self-limited cases.
- Both **valacyclovir** and **famciclovir** are most effective when they are given within 72 hours of the appearance of the zoster rash. They are equally effective in accelerating cutaneous healing, in shortening the duration of acute episodes, and in decreasing the chronic pain of PHN.
- Valacyclovir is much less expensive than famciclovir; however, its use is contraindicated in HIV-infected patients. Both valacyclovir and famciclovir are superior to acyclovir, which is reserved for use in children and for intravenous administration.

Regimens

Following are the treatment options for immunocompetent adult patients with herpes zoster:

- Valacyclovir (**Valtrex**) 1 g (two 500-mg caplets) three times daily for 7 days
- Famciclovir (**Famvir**) 500 mg three times daily for 7 days
- **Acyclovir** 800 mg five times daily for 7 days

Immunocompromised patients may require intravenous acyclovir. **Intravenous foscarnet** is used for acyclovir-resistant VZV infection.

Corticosteroids

- The use of systemic corticosteroids in combination with oral acyclovir, valacyclovir, or famciclovir has been controversial. Anecdotal reports claim a faster resolution of acute pain and a decreased incidence of PHN. The rationale for adding corticosteroids is that they may decrease nerve inflammation. However, no double-blind studies demonstrate the efficacy of systemic corticosteroids, and the theoretical risk of dissemination of the virus is an issue.
- Elderly patients, in whom PHN more often occurs, are more likely to experience significant adverse side effects from systemic corticosteroids than are younger patients. Potential relative contraindications to the use of corticosteroids include hypertension, diabetes, glaucoma, and peptic ulcer disease.

continued on page 166

Chronic Pain

Treatment of PHN is problematic. The following measures have met with varying degrees of success. Their great number reflects the finding that none of them appears to be totally satisfactory. Optimally, the acute episode of herpes zoster should be treated as quickly as possible after onset to decrease the risk of PHN.

- **Lidocaine** patches. These bandages, impregnated with lidocaine, are the only treatment for PHN approved by the United States Food and Drug Association.
- Capsaicin (**Zostrix**). The active molecule in hot chili peppers, capsaicin depletes substance P, a pain impulse transmitter. It is available OTC and is applied three to five times daily. Unfortunately, many patients cannot tolerate the burning sensation that occurs after application.
- Low-dose tricyclic antidepressants. These agents (e.g., **amitriptyline**) may be helpful. Higher doses of tricyclic antidepressants—used alone or in combination with **phenothiazines**—may also be tried.
- **Neurontin** (gabapentin), an antiseizure drug, has been helpful in some patients.
- **Neurosurgical procedures** include nerve blocks with local anesthetics.
- **Intralesional corticosteroids** may be given as subcutaneous injections.

- **Transcutaneous electrical nerve stimulation** may be useful.
- **Acupuncture** may be tried.
- **Biofeedback** may be helpful.

Prevention

Vaccination

The recent introduction of the vaccine **Zostavax** promises to reduce the risk of developing herpes zoster and result in less frequent, less painful, and shorter courses of PHN episodes. The preventive effect of the vaccine is thought to be a result of its boosting effect on an older person's cell-mediated immunity to VZV.

- Zoster vaccination (a single dose of the vaccine) is approved for everyone older than 60 years of age who has had chickenpox. Zostavax contains the same attenuated virus as the varicella vaccine but is far more potent.
- Zoster vaccination is contraindicated in people with active, untreated tuberculosis and in pregnant women. Whether to vaccinate immunocompromised persons is a controversial issue that is important to resolve because of increased risk of herpes zoster in this population, because the vaccine is a live attenuated virus, it is contraindicated.

Tai Chi

A recent study suggests that tai chi may help prevent shingles. Further studies are necessary to confirm these findings.

 POINTS TO REMEMBER

- Herpes zoster, particularly if it is recurrent or disseminated, may be an early indicator of an immunosuppressive disorder or a lymphoproliferative disease.
- An evolving herpes zoster eruption should be treated with antiviral drugs as early as possible.
- PHN is unusual in people younger than 50 years.
- Patients with herpes zoster can transmit the virus as chickenpox to persons who have not already been infected with this virus.

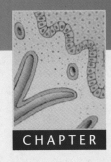

Superficial Fungal Infections

OVERVIEW

Superficial fungi are capable of germinating on the dead outer horny layer of skin. They produce enzymes (keratinases) that allow them to digest keratin, with resulting epidermal scale (e.g., **tinea pedis, tinea versicolor**); thickened, crumbly nails (**onychomycosis**); and hair loss (**tinea capitis**). In the dermis, an inflammatory reaction may result in erythema, vesicles, and, infrequently, a more widespread autoeczematous eruption known as an "id" reaction.

Infection may be acquired by the following means:

- Person-to-person contact
- Animal contact, especially with kittens and puppies
- Contact with inanimate objects (fomites)

Environmental and hereditary factors leading to fungal infections are as follows:

- Warm, moist, occluded environments such as the groin, axillae, and feet
- Family history of tinea infections
- Lowered immune status of the host, such as seen in patients with acquired immunodeficiency syndrome (AIDS), diabetes, collagen vascular diseases, or long-term systemic steroid therapy
- Diagnosis can often, but not always, be made on clinical grounds.
- A direct potassium hydroxide (KOH) examination or a fungal culture is necessary to make a definitive diagnosis.
- Periodic acid–Schiff stain on biopsy specimens can be helpful.
- Wood's lamp examination may be useful in some cases of tinea capitis and tinea versicolor.

> **DERMATOPHYTE INFECTIONS**

The term *tinea* refers to an infection by dermatophytes. Tinea is named according to the location on the body:

- **Tinea pedis and tinea manuum** (feet and hands)
- **Tinea cruris** (inguinal folds)
- **Tinea capitis** (scalp)
- **Tinea corporis and tinea faciale** (body and face)
- **Tinea unguium (onychomycosis)** (nails)

> **YEAST INFECTIONS**

- *Tinea versicolor*

Tinea versicolor is an exception; in fact, it is not caused by a dermatophyte but rather by a yeastlike organism. Tinea versicolor is referred to as pityriasis versicolor by many authors.

- *Candidiasis*

Cutaneous candidiasis is also caused by yeast.

Tinea Pedis ("Athlete's Foot")

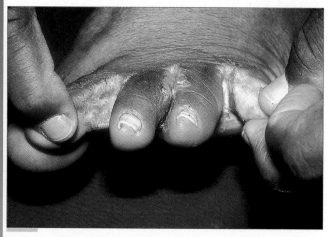

7.1 *Interdigital tinea pedis (toe web infection).* Note fissuring and maceration.

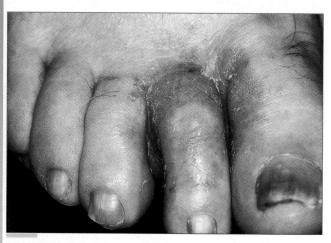

7.2 *Interdigital tinea pedis.* Here the lesions are more inflammatory.

BASICS

Tinea pedis is an extremely common problem seen mainly in young men. Ubiquitous media advertisements for athlete's foot sprays and creams are testimony to the commonplace occurrence of this annoying dermatosis.

Most cases are caused by *Trichophyton rubrum,* which evokes a minimal inflammatory response, and less often by *T. mentagrophytes,* which may produce vesicles and bullae; less frequently, *Epidermophyton floccosum* may be responsible. There are three clinical types of tinea pedis: type 1: interdigital; type 2: chronic plantar; and type 3: acute vesicular.

Type 1: Interdigital Tinea Pedis

BASICS

This is the most common type of tinea pedis. It is seen predominantly in men between the ages of 18 and 40 years.

DESCRIPTION OF LESIONS

- Scale, maceration, and fissures are characteristic (FIG. 7.1).

DISTRIBUTION OF LESIONS

- Toe web involvement is seen, especially between the third and fourth and the fourth and fifth toes; however, any web space may be involved (FIG. 7.2).

CLINICAL MANIFESTATIONS

- It is often asymptomatic; however, it may itch intensely.
- Marked inflammation and fissures suggest secondary bacterial superinfection.
- There may be coexistent yeast or saprophytic fungi present.

DIAGNOSIS

- A positive KOH examination or fungal culture is diagnostic.

Atopic Dermatitis
FIGURE 7.3.

- Atopic dermatitis and dyshidrotic eczema may be clinically indistinguishable from tinea pedis (see Chapter 2, "Eczema").

- There is a positive atopic history.
- It is seen especially in children on the dorsal or plantar surface of the feet (tinea pedis is unusual in preteens).

Contact Dermatitis (FIG. 7.4)
- This occurs most often on the dorsum of the feet.

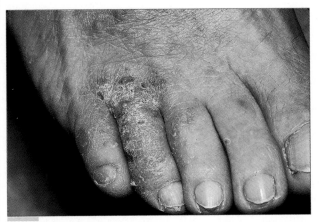

7.3 *Atopic dermatitis.* Note the lichenification on the dorsal toes. The distinction from tinea pedis was based on a negative KOH and a positive atopic history.

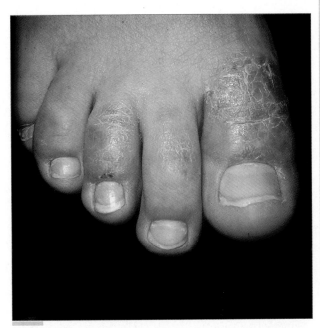

7.4 *Contact dermatitis.* In this case it was determined that the patient was allergic to a component of his shoe leather.

MANAGEMENT

- For acute oozing and maceration, **Burow's solution** compresses are used two to three times daily. (See handout Burow's Solution)
- Broad-spectrum topical antifungal agents such as ketoconazole (**Nizoral**), ciclopirox (**Loprox**), or clotrimazole (**Lotrimin**) are applied once or twice daily. (See TABLE 7.1.)

Prevention consists of maintaining dryness in the area by:

- Using a hairdryer after bathing.
- Applying powders, such as **Zeasorb-AF,** that contain miconazole as an active ingredient.

Table 7.1 ANTIFUNGAL DRUG FORMULARY

AGENT	APPLICATION	FORMS	COMMENTS
Topical agents: over-the-counter			
Terbinafine 1% (**Lamisil**)	1 to 4 weeks, twice daily	Cream, solution, spray	Tinea (not indicated for *Candida*)
Clotrimazole 1% (**Lotrimin**)	Twice daily	Cream, lotion, solution	Tinea, *Candida,* tinea versicolor
Miconazole 2% (**Micatin**)	Twice daily	Cream, lotion, spray	Tinea, *Candida,* tinea versicolor
Tolnaftate 1% (**Tinactin**)	Twice daily	Cream	Tinea
Selenium sulfide 1% (**Selsun Blue**)	Apply daily to wide area for 10 minutes, followed by a shower	Shampoo	Tinea versicolor
Miconazole 2% (**Zeasorb-AF powder**)	As needed	Powder	Tinea, *Candida,* tinea versicolor; antifungal, antifriction/drying agent
Topical agents: prescription			
Ketoconazole 2% (**Nizoral**)	Once daily	Cream	Tinea, *Candida,* tinea versicolor
Econazole 1% (**Spectazole**)	4 weeks, once daily	Cream	Tinea, *Candida,* tinea versicolor, Gram-positive bacteria
Ciclopirox 0.77% (**Loprox**)	4 weeks, as needed	Cream, lotion, shampoo	Lotion preferred for nail penetration
Naftifine 1% (**Naftin**)	Once daily	Cream, gel	Tinea; has anti-inflammatory activity
Sulconazole (**Exelderm**)	4 weeks, twice daily	Cream, solution	Tinea, *Candida,* tinea versicolor
Miconazole (**Monistat-Derm**)	4 weeks, twice daily	Cream	Tinea, *Candida,* tinea versicolor
Oxiconazole 1% (**Oxistat**)	4 weeks, once to twice daily	Cream, lotion	Tinea, *Candida,* tinea versicolor
Systemic antifungal agents			
Griseofulvin (**Fulvicin, Grisactin, Gris-PEG**)		Microsized: 250-, 500-mg tablets; ultramicrosized: 125-, 250-, 333-mg tablets. Pediatric: Microsized: 125 mg/tsp pediatric suspension	Effective only against dermatophytes Contraindicated in pregnancy Fungistatic Take with fatty meals Alcohol should be avoided Occasional headache Gastrointestinal upset Photosensitivity Elevation of liver function tests Significant drug interactions (phenobarbital, warfarin, other drugs metabolized in liver)
Terbinafine (**Lamisil**)		250-mg tablets 125-mg oral granules 187.5-mg oral granules	Side effects minimal; include rare hepatotoxicity, reversible taste loss Many fewer drug interactions than with itraconazole; blood levels decreased by cimetidine and terfenadine and increased by rifampin; lowers cyclosporine levels

continued on page 171

Table 7.1 ANTIFUNGAL DRUG FORMULARY *(Continued)*

AGENT	APPLICATION	FORMS	COMMENTS
			Severe hepatotoxicity including liver failure has been reported in patients with no pre-existing liver disease. A baseline hepatic profile (alanine and aspartate aminotransferase) levels is recommended for all patients before initiating therapy with this agent. These tests should be monitored in patients receiving continuous treatment for more than 1 month or patients who develop signs or symptoms suggestive of liver disease.
Itraconazole (**Sporanox**)		100-mg capsules	Side effects minimal; rare hepatotoxicity
		Oral solution (10 mg/mL)	Significant drug interactions and contraindications: drugs not to be taken with itraconazole include astemizole, cisapride, terfenadine, triazolam, midazolam, lovastatin, and simvastatin
			Studies report a risk for developing congestive heart failure (CHF) from negative inotropic effects of this drug. Because of this risk, itraconazole should not be used in the treatment of onychomycosis in patients with ventricular dysfunction such as CHF or a history of CHF.
Fluconazole (**Diflucan**)		50-, 100-, 150-, 200-mg tablets; oral solution 10 mg/mL, 40 mg/mL	Side effects minimal; rare hepatotoxicity Liver toxicity must be monitored if used long term Not to be taken with cisapride

SEE PATIENT HANDOUT "Athlete's Foot (Tinea Pedis)" ON THE SOLUTION SITE

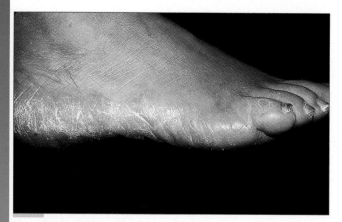

7.5 *Tinea pedis.* Chronic scaly infection of the plantar surface of the foot in a "moccasin" distribution. Note involvement of the nails.

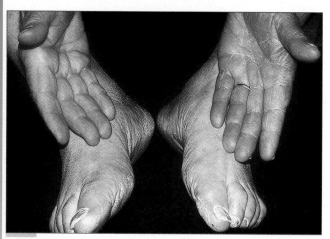

7.6 *"Two feet, one hand" variant of tinea pedis.* The scale is present on one hand only. Note the nail involvement. These findings are pathognomonic.

Type 2: Chronic Plantar Tinea Pedis

BASICS

• Tinea pedis ("moccasin" type) is relatively common.

DESCRIPTION OF LESIONS

• Lesions consist of diffuse scaling of the soles (FIG. 7.5).

DISTRIBUTION OF LESIONS

• The entire plantar surface of the foot is usually involved.
• Borders are distinct along the sides of the feet.
• There is often nail involvement.

CLINICAL MANIFESTATIONS

• Symptoms are minimal, unless painful fissures occur.

DIAGNOSIS

• The KOH examination or fungal culture is positive.

"Two Feet, One Hand" (Palmar/Plantar) Tinea

• Tinea can present on one or both palms (tinea manuum). Not infrequently, it appears in a "two feet, one hand" distribution. This is pathognomic for tinea (FIG. 7.6).
• Management is similar to that for chronic tinea pedis.

 DIFFERENTIAL DIAGNOSIS

Psoriasis
• Psoriasis has sharply demarcated plaques (FIG. 7.7).

Atopic Dermatitis
• Atopic dermatitis usually is pruritic, whereas chronic plantar tinea pedis is generally asymptomatic.
• There is a positive atopic history.

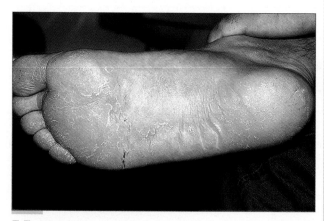

7.7 *Psoriasis.* A well-demarcated plaque that spares the instep is seen here.

MANAGEMENT

This is the most difficult type of tinea pedis to cure, because topical agents do not effectively penetrate the thickened epidermis. Treatment generally requires oral antifungal agents such as the following (TABLE 7.1):

- Terbinafine (**Lamisil**) 250 mg once daily for 30 days or longer, if necessary

- Itraconazole (**Sporanox**) 200 mg once daily for 30 days or longer, if necessary
- Fluconazole (**Diflucan**) 150 to 200 mg once daily for 4 to 6 weeks, if necessary

Nail involvement requires longer treatment because nails may serve as a reservoir for reinfection and take much longer to grow out normally (see later in this chapter).

Type 3: Acute Vesicular Tinea Pedis

BASICS

This is the least common clinical variant.

DESCRIPTION OF LESIONS

- Vesicles and bullae generally occur on the sole, great toe, and instep of the foot.

CLINICAL MANIFESTATIONS

- Acute vesicular tinea pedis is pruritic (FIG. 7.8).

DIAGNOSIS

- For diagnosis, the specimen should be obtained from the inner part of the roof of the blister for KOH examination or culture.

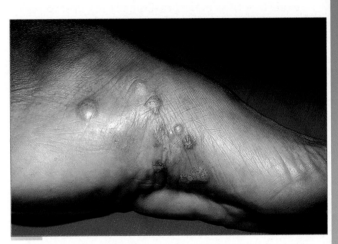

7.8 *Acute vesicular tinea pedis.* A KOH culture specimen is obtained from under the roof of a vesicle.

 DIFFERENTIAL DIAGNOSIS

Dyshidrotic eczema is easily confused with acute tinea pedis (FIG. 7.9).

- Patients often have a positive atopic history.
- It is KOH negative.

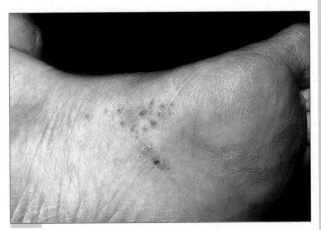

7.9 *Dyshidrotic eczema.* Note the small vesicles and the similarity to acute tinea pedis.

MANAGEMENT

See TABLE 7.1.

- For symptomatic relief of severe inflammation and itching, a potent topical steroid, such as **triamcinolone acetonide cream**, may be used for 4 to 5 days. The resultant anti-inflammatory effect also helps to increase the yield of obtaining organisms on KOH examination or culture.
- Treatment is similar to that of type 1, although **systemic** as well as **topical antifungals** are often necessary.
- Prevention involves decreasing wetness, friction, and maceration. Absorbent powders, such as miconazole (**Zeasorb-AF**) powder, should be applied after the eruption clears to prevent recurrence.

Clinical Variant

Uncommonly, an id reaction (dermatophytid) may occur. This is considered to be a hypersensitivity to fungal elements. Clinically, lesions consist of itchy, sterile (KOH and culture negative) vesicles on the hands similar to dyshidrotic eczema; this resolves when the primary acute process on the feet resolves.

 POINT TO REMEMBER

- Not all rashes of the feet are fungal. In fact, if a child younger than 12 years has what appears to be tinea pedis, it is probably another skin condition, such as eczema.

 HELPFUL HINTS

- When the diagnosis is in doubt, a potent topical steroid may be applied—for a week or so only—to relieve the acute itch and burning.
- To increase positive yields, KOH examination or fungal cultures should be obtained only after the patient has not used topical therapy for at least 24 to 48 hours.
- Positive results of KOH examination and fungal cultures are not necessarily proof of pathogenesis, because some organisms, especially yeasts and molds, may be saprophytes, or "contaminants."
- When there is a rash on the palms, the feet should *always* be examined.

- A common error is automatically to assume that a rash of the feet, or "athlete's foot," is fungal in origin. Often, these conditions are mistakenly treated with topical antifungal preparations alone or in combination with topical steroids with a "shotgun" approach. Careful observation and a positive KOH examination reveal the true nature of the problem. This caveat also applies to tinea cruris (see following section).

Type 2 (Chronic Plantar and/or Palmar) Only:

- In patients in whom oral antifungal agents are contraindicated, a keratolytic agent such as Salex cream or lotion can be used to remove scale, followed by a topical antifungal agent such as ketoconazole cream.

BASICS

Tinea cruris ("jock itch") is a common infection of the upper inner thighs that most often occurs in postpubertal male patients. It is generally caused by the dermatophytes *T. rubrum* and *E. floccosum.* In contrast to candidiasis and lichen simplex chronicus, it generally spares the scrotum.

DESCRIPTION OF LESIONS

• Lesions are bilateral, fan-shaped, or annular plaques (plaques with central clearing), with a slightly elevated scaly "active border" (FIG. 7.10).

DISTRIBUTION OF LESIONS

• Lesions may involve the upper thighs, the crural folds, and possibly the pubic area and buttocks (see FIG. 3.12).
• It generally spares the scrotum and penis.

CLINICAL MANIFESTATIONS

• Generally, the lesions are pruritic, "burning," or irritating.
• Frequently, the patient also has tinea pedis.
• The condition may be chronic or recurrent, depending on environmental factors and exercise.
• The likelihood of the spread of tinea cruris between sexual partners appears to be very small.

DIAGNOSIS

• A positive KOH examination or fungal culture is found most easily by sampling from the borders of the lesions.

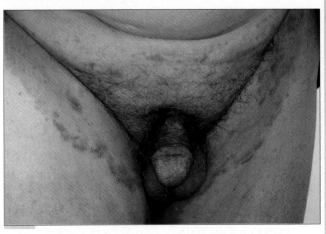

7.10 *Tinea cruris.* Note the scalloped shape with an "active border."

DIFFERENTIAL DIAGNOSIS

Lichen Simplex Chronicus (Eczematous Dermatitis)
FIGURE 7.11 (see also FIG. 2.45).

• It often involves the scrotum.
• KOH examination and fungal cultures are negative for fungus.
• Often, there is an atopic history.
• Lesions are confluent (no central clearing).
• Lichenification occurs as the condition becomes chronic.

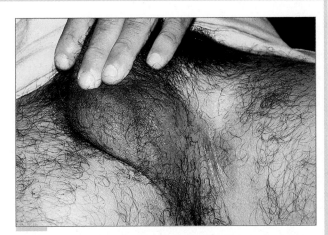

7.11 *Lichen simplex chronicus (chronic eczematous dermatitis).* Lichenification of scrotal and inguinal skin results from relentless scratching and rubbing.

continued on page 176

DIFFERENTIAL DIAGNOSIS *Continued*

Inverse Psoriasis
FIGURE 7.12 (see also FIG. 3.24.)

- It often involves the scrotum.
- Evidence of psoriasis may be noted elsewhere.
- KOH examination and fungal cultures are negative for fungus.
- Lesions are confluent (no central clearing).

OTHER DIAGNOSES

Seborrheic Dermatitis, Candidiasis, Intertrigo, and Irritant Dermatitis
- All of these conditions may be clinically indistinguishable from one another.

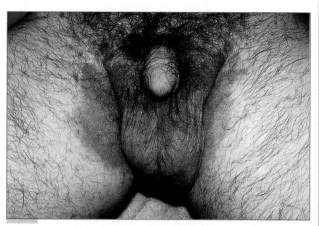

7.12 *Inverse psoriasis.* Note the well-demarcated plaques with no "active border."

 MANAGEMENT

See TABLE 7.1.

- Topical antifungal creams, applied once or twice daily, are often effective in controlling, and sometimes curing, uncomplicated, localized infections. Over-the-counter (OTC) preparations of miconazole (**Micatin**), terbinafine (**Lamisil**), and clotrimazole (**Lotrimin**) are available.
- For severe inflammation and itching, a mild OTC **hydrocortisone 1%** preparation or moderate-strength hydrocortisone valerate 0.2% (**Westcort**) may be used for 4 to 5 days for symptomatic relief.

- Systemic antifungal therapy may be necessary in cases that do not respond to topical therapy and cases of chronic recurrent tinea cruris, particularly in immunocompromised patients.

    Prevention aims toward decreasing wetness, friction, and maceration by:

- Using an absorbent powder such as miconazole (**Zeasorb-AF**).
- Drying the area with a hairdryer after bathing.
- Wearing loose clothing; briefs are less frictional than boxer shorts.

 SEE PATIENT HANDOUT "Tinea Cruris (Jock Itch)" ON THE SOLUTION SITE

BASICS

Tinea capitis, or "ringworm," most commonly occurs in pre-pubertal children. In the United States, African-American children are disproportionately affected by this superficial fungal infection of the hair shaft. The incidence of tinea capitis has been increasing and presents a growing public health concern, especially in overcrowded, impoverished inner-city communities.

T. tonsurans is, by far, the most common etiologic agent; more than 90% of cases are caused by it. Other species, such as *Microsporum audouinii*, which is spread from human to human, and *M. canis,* which is spread from animals (cats and dogs), are more often seen in white children. Patients frequently have a family member, pet, or playmate with tinea.

Tinea capitis is quite contagious and is generally spread by person-to-person contact. Studies have demonstrated a 30% carrier state of adults exposed to a child with *T. tonsurans*. The organism has also been isolated from such inanimate objects as hairbrushes and pillows.

DESCRIPTION OF LESIONS

Clinical Types

There are essentially five clinical expressions of tinea capitis, with some overlapping physical presentations:

- **Inflamed, scaly,** often alopecic patches, mimicking seborrheic dermatitis, are especially common in infancy until the age of 6 to 8 months (FIG. 7.13).
- A diffuse scaling is seen with multiple round areas, characterized by alopecia that occurs secondary to broken hair shafts, leaving residual black stumps (**"black dot"** ringworm) (FIG. 7.14). It is seen uncommonly and is often mistaken for alopecia areata.
- The **"gray patch"** type (FIG. 7.15) consists of round, scaly plaques of alopecia in which hairs are broken off close to the surface of the scalp.
- Tender pustular nodules or plaques called kerions may occur.
  - A **kerion** is a boggy, pustular, indurated, tumorlike mass, which represents an inflammatory hypersensitivity reaction to the fungus. A kerion can result in localized scarring.

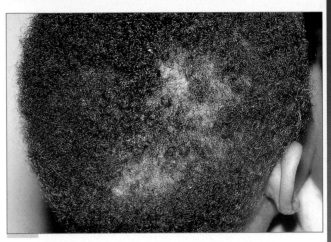

7.13 *Tinea capitis.* Scaly, alopecic patches mimic seborrheic dermatitis.

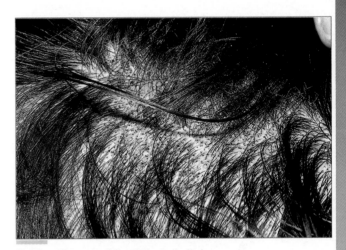

7.14 *Tinea capitis.* "Black dot" ringworm.

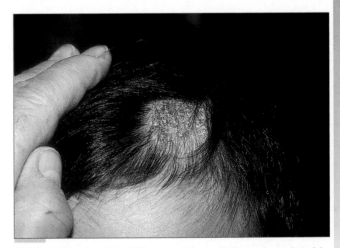

7.15 *Tinea capitis.* "Gray patch type." Note alopecia with broken off hairs close to scalp surface. *Microsporum canis* was found on culture, and the area fluoresced green with a Wood's lamp.

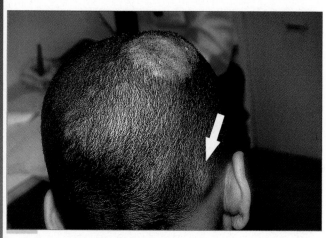

7.16 *Tinea capitis with kerion.* There is also a palpable, asymptomatic, nontender right occipital lymph node (*arrow*).

- Secondary bacterial invaders such as *Staphylococcus aureus* and some gram-negative organisms may sometimes be recovered from a kerion. Often, there is accompanying nontender regional adenopathy (FIG. 7.16).
- Occasionally, a pustular variety, with or without alopecia, can mimic a bacterial infection.

DIAGNOSIS

- A KOH preparation or fungal culture confirms the diagnosis.
  - When in doubt, or when a KOH preparation is negative, a fungal culture placed on Sabouraud's agar should be done. This can be performed by obtaining broken hairs and scale by stroking the affected area with a sterile toothbrush, a familiar object to a child and one that is less frightening than a surgical blade or forceps (see Chapter 26, "Diagnostic and Therapeutic Procedures"). The collected material is then tapped onto the surface of Sabouraud's agar.
  - An alternative method of harvesting broken hairs is by rubbing a moistened gauze pad on the involved area of scalp and then using forceps to place the hairs on the culture medium or slide. Pustules generally are sterile or grow bacterial contaminants.
- A biopsy is rarely necessary.
- In the past, Wood's light examination was a valuable screening tool to diagnose tinea capitis easily (because *Microsporum* species are usually fluorescent), but it has largely lost its usefulness because most cases are caused by the nonfluorescing *T. tonsurans.*

 DIFFERENTIAL DIAGNOSIS

Alopecia Areata
FIGURE 7.17.

- This has a well-demarcated, symmetric patch of alopecia.
- It is smooth and free of scales.
- The KOH test is negative

Atopic Dermatitis
- This is a common cause for an itchy, scaly scalp in children
- No hair loss is noted

Seborrheic Dermatitis
- Infants show "cradle cap" with thick scale.
- Alopecia is absent in adults who have scalp involvement.

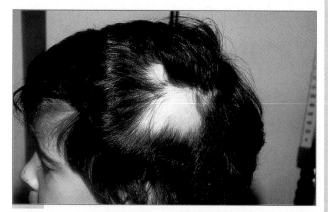

7.17 *Alopecia areata.* This child has smooth, well-demarcated, noninflammatory, asymptomatic patches of alopecia.

continued on page 179

Other Diagnoses

- Psoriasis
- Trichotillomania (a self-induced cause of hair loss) (see Chapter 10, "Hair and Scalp Disorders Resulting in Hair Loss")
- Tinea amiantacea (Fig. 7.18), which is a KOH-negative local patch or plaque of adherent scale ("tinea" is a misnomer for this condition, See Chapter 27, "Special Considerations in Pediatric and Elderly Skin")
- Bacterial scalp infection
- Secondary syphilis
- Acute and chronic cutaneous discoid lupus erythematosus

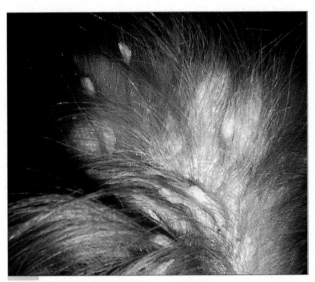

7.18 *Tinea amiantacea.* An inflammatory condition of the scalp in which heavy white or yellow (from sebum) scales extend onto the hairs and bind the proximal portions together; it is not caused by a fungus despite its name. "Pityriasis amiantacea" is probably a better name for this condition.

 ## MANAGEMENT

See TABLE 7.1.

- **Topical therapy** is of little or no value in treating tinea capitis, although an adjunctive antifungal shampoo such as ketoconazole 1% to 2% (**Nizoral**) or selenium sulfide 1% to 2.5% (**Selsun**) may be used by the infected person and contacts to prevent reinfection and spread.

Systemic Therapies

Griseofulvin

- In children, systemic therapy with a **liquid suspension of griseofulvin** has been the mainstay of therapy.
  - The dosage of **microsized griseofulvin** is 20 to 25 mg/kg/day and is sometimes as high as 25 mg/kg/day in divided doses. Ultramicrosized griseofulvin is given as a dosage of 15 to 20 mg/kg/day. It should be given with milk or food, which increases its absorption. It should be continued until the patient is clinically cured, generally 6 to 8 weeks. Some patients may require longer therapy.
  - Occasionally, an "idlike" reaction occurs shortly after the initiation of griseofulvin therapy. This consists of multiple small sterile papules on the face or body, and it probably represents a hypersensitivity response.
  - Treatment failure, which is uncommon with griseofulvin, may indicate inadequate doses or duration of therapy, drug resistance, reinfection from another family member, poor compliance, or immune incompetence.
  - It is also believed that resistance to griseofulvin is currently rising.
- Itraconazole, terbinafine, and fluconazole are newer and more efficacious agents. They have been used in some cases of griseofulvin treatment failure.
- Pediatric dosages are as follows:
  - Itraconazole (**Sporanox**) (5 mg/kg/day). This drug is available as 100-mg capsules or as an oral solution (10 mg/mL).
  - Terbinafine (**Lamisil**). Dosage should be reduced according to weight: Children weighing less than 20 kg should receive one fourth of a tablet (62.5 mg) per day; children 20 to 40 kg are given 125 mg/day; children weighing more than 40 kg receive 250 mg/day (the medication is available as 250-mg tablets only). Formerly, children reluctant to swallow tablets were given terbinafine by crushing a tablet and mixing it in their food. Currently, there is a new Food and Drug

continued on page 180

MANAGEMENT *Continued*

Administration–approved formulation of "child-friendly" **Lamisil granules**. The formulation has been approved for use by children 4 years of age and older. The amount of granules corresponds to 125 mg and 187.5 mg of terbinafine. Parents are instructed to sprinkle it on the food of a child who may not like to take medicine.

- Fluconazole (**Diflucan**) (6 mg/kg/day for 2 weeks; repeat at 4 weeks if indicated). This drug is available in 100-mg, 150-mg, and 200-mg tablets and as an oral solution (10 and 40 mg/mL).

HELPFUL HINTS

- The pustular variety of tinea capitis can mimic a bacterial infection, and antibiotics are sometimes given before the correct diagnosis is made.
- When a child has scaling alopecia and enlarged lymph nodes in the posterior auricular or occipital area, obtain a fungal culture and consider starting empiric antifungal treatment.
- In many instances, therapy may have to be initiated in a patient with negative KOH examination and fungal cultures, based solely on clinical appearance.
- Siblings of tinea capitis patients should be evaluated, or else the infection might be "ping-ponged " back and forth within the family.
- Occasionally, concomitant systemic steroid therapy is warranted in addition to griseofulvin when the patient is experiencing a severe, tender, or painful kerion. A very short course (usually 3 or 4 days) of **oral prednisone,** 1 mg/kg/day, is sufficient.

POINTS TO REMEMBER

- The current standard of diagnosis is a positive KOH examination or culture.
- Topical therapy does not work.
- Systemic therapy must be in an adequate dosage and duration.

BASICS

Tinea corporis is commonly referred to as "ringworm," a term used by laypersons, and, frequently, many in the health care community, to describe practically any annular or ringlike eruption on the body. In fact, there are many nonfungal conditions that assume an annular "ringwormlike" configuration: granuloma annulare, erythema multiforme, erythema migrans (seen in acute Lyme disease), and figurate erythemas such as urticaria.

Tinea corporis (described as tinea faciale if it is located on the face) is most often acquired by contact with an infected animal, usually kittens and occasionally dogs. It may also spread from other infected humans, or it may be autoinoculated from other areas of the body that are infected by tinea such as tinea pedis or tinea capitis. Another common method of transmission of tinea corporis is noted in wrestlers (**tinea gladiatorum,** see FIG. 5.4). *M. canis, T. rubrum,* and *T. mentagrophytes* are the usual pathogens.

DESCRIPTION OF LESIONS

- Lesions are generally annular, with peripheral enlargement and central clearing. Odd gyrate or concentric rings may appear (FIGS. 7.19 and 7.20).
- The scaly, "active border" can sometimes be pustular or vesicular.
- Lesions are single or multiple.

DISTRIBUTION OF LESIONS

- If multiple lesions are present, their distribution is typically asymmetric.
- Lesions are found most often on the extremities, face, and trunk.

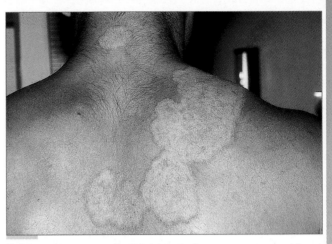

7.19 *Tinea corporis.* Multiple lesions are present, with a border of scale.

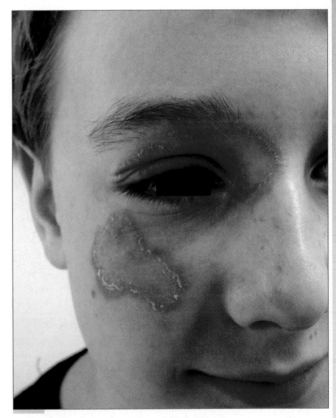

7.20 *Tinea faciale.* Two erythematous, scaly, annular lesions are noted on this child's face.

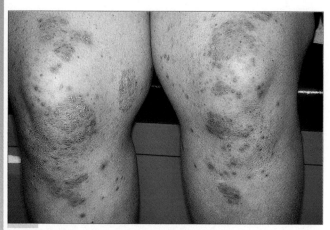

7.21 *Tinea corporis ("tinea incognito").* This patient was treated with topical steroids for months until the correct diagnosis was made. The topical steroids modified the typical clinical appearance of tinea corporis; in fact, her lesions look more like psoriasis.

CLINICAL MANIFESTATIONS

- Lesions may be pruritic or asymptomatic.
- **Majocchi's granuloma** is a follicular deep form of tinea corporis. It may result when inappropriate therapy, such as topical steroids, or shaving drives the fungi into hair follicles.
- Tinea corporis is very often misdiagnosed and treated with topical steroids ("tinea incognito") (FIG. 7.21).

DIAGNOSIS

- Diagnosis is confirmed by a positive KOH examination or fungal culture (it is especially easy to find hyphae in those patients who have been previously treated with topical steroids).
- A skin biopsy may be necessary for diagnosis.
- A history of a newly adopted kitten, or of another infected contact, is helpful.

 DIFFERENTIAL DIAGNOSIS

Urticaria
FIGURE 7.22.

- Erythema with no scale (i.e., epidermal involvement)

Acute Lyme Disease (Erythema Migrans)
FIGURE 7.23.

- Erythema with no scale
- Characteristic targetlike appearance

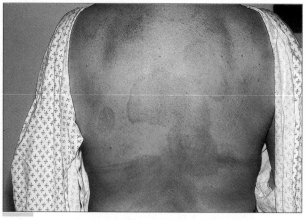

7.22 *Urticaria.* Dermal vasodilatation occurs, with no epidermal change (scale).

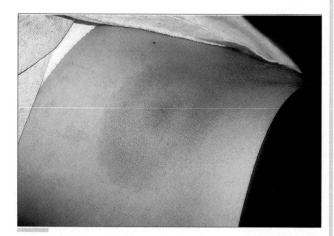

7.23 *Acute Lyme disease (erythema migrans).* Note the targetlike concentric rings with no scale.

continued on page 183

DIFFERENTIAL DIAGNOSIS *Continued*

Granuloma Annulare
FIGURE 4.10.

- Skin-colored or red firm papules
- Absence of scale
- Symmetric distribution of lesions
- Lesions slightly firm to palpation

Other Diagnoses
- Atopic dermatitis
- **Psoriasis** (FIG. 7.24)
- Subacute lupus erythematosus
- Mycosis fungoides (cutaneous T-cell lymphoma)

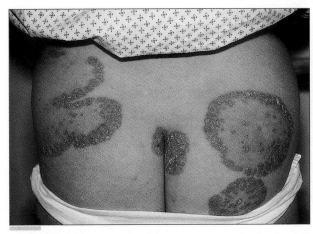

7.24 ***Psoriasis.*** Extensive annular, serpiginous lesions are present in this patient.

 MANAGEMENT

See TABLE 7.1.

- Topical antifungal agents are useful.
- Systemic antifungal agents (see the earlier discussion of tinea cruris) are sometimes necessary when multiple lesions are present or in areas that are repeatedly shaved, such as men's beards (tinea barbae) or, especially, women's legs, in which granulomatous lesions (Majocchi's granuloma) may appear.
- If pets appear to be the source of infection, they may also need antifungal treatment after evaluation by a veterinarian.

 POINT TO REMEMBER

- Inquire about sports activities, such as wrestling.

Onychomycosis (Tinea Unguium)

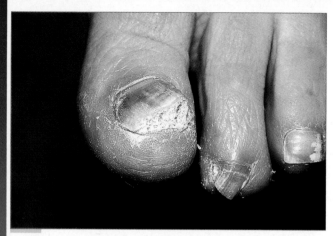

7.25 Distal subungual onychomycosis. The nail is dystrophic and discolored, and there is a buildup of keratin underneath it (subungual hyperkeratosis).

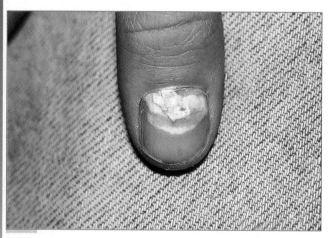

7.26 Superficial white onychomycosis. A KOH specimen was easily obtained from the surface of this lesion.

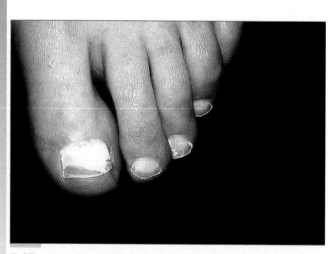

7.27 Proximal white subungual onychomycosis. HIV infection should be suspected in this patient.

BASICS

The term *onychomycosis* refers to an infection of the fingernails or toenails caused by various fungi, yeasts, and molds. In contrast, the term *tinea unguium* refers specifically to nail infections caused by dermatophytes. Onychomycosis is uncommon in children, but its prevalence increases dramatically with advancing age, with prevalence rates as high as 30% in those 70 years and older.

The major causes of onychomycosis are as follows:

- The dermatophytes *E. floccosum, T. rubrum,* and *T. mentagrophytes*
- Yeasts, mainly *Candida albicans*
- Molds, such as *Aspergillus, Fusarium,* and *Scopulariopsis* species

DESCRIPTION OF LESIONS

Distal subungual onychomycosis (Fig. 7.25) accounts for more than 90% of all cases of onychomycosis. It is usually characterized by the following:

- Nail thickening and subungual hyperkeratosis (scale buildup under the nail)
- Nail discoloration (yellow, yellow-green, white, or brown)
- Nail dystrophy
- Onycholysis (nail plate elevation from the nail bed)

CLINICAL MANIFESTATIONS

- Aside from footwear causing occasional physical discomfort and the psychosocial liability of unsightly nails, onychomycosis is usually asymptomatic.
- Left untreated, onychomycotic nails, can, however, infrequently act as a portal of entry for more serious bacterial infections of the lower leg, particularly in patients with diabetes.
- Distal subungual onychomycosis is sometimes associated with chronic palmoplantar tinea (i.e., "two feet, one hand" variant of tinea).

Clinical Variants

- In superficial white onychomycosis (Fig. 7.26), the fungus is superficial, and material for scraping may be obtained from the dorsal surface of the nail.
- Proximal white subungual onychomycosis (Fig. 7.27) may be seen in persons with human immunodeficiency virus (HIV) infection.

DIAGNOSIS

- A positive KOH examination or growth of dermatophyte, yeast, or mold on culture is diagnostic.

DIFFERENTIAL DIAGNOSIS

See also Chapter 13, "Diseases and Abnormalities of Nails."

Psoriasis of the Nails
FIGURE 7.28.

- This may be indistinguishable from, or coexist with, ony-chomycosis.
- Usually, evidence of psoriasis is found elsewhere on the body.
- The KOH examination is generally, but not always, neg-ative.
- Characteristic nail pitting and nail discoloration ("oil spots," yellowish brown pigmentation) may be present.

Chronic Paronychia
FIGURE 7.29.

- This is seen in patients with an altered immune status (e.g., diabetic patients) and in people whose hands are constantly in water.
- Erythema and edema of the proximal nail fold are noted.
- The cuticle is absent.
- There is nail dystrophy.
- Culture may be positive for *Candida* and/or bacteria.

Pseudomonas Infection of the Nail (Green Nail Syndrome)
FIGURE 7.30.

- Onycholysis occurs, with secondary bacterial (pseudo-monas) colonization.
- A distinctive green coloration is apparent.
- This is usually found in women with long finger nails.

Other Diagnoses
Onycholysis unrelated to a fungus or psoriasis can be idio-pathic or associated with nail trauma, thyroid disease, use of nail polish or nail hardeners, and oral tetracyclines, especially demeclocycline (Declomycin), coupled with sun exposure.

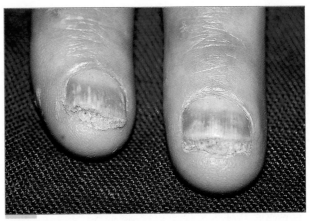

7.28   *Psoriasis of nails.* Subungual hyperkeratosis and "oil spots" are noted.

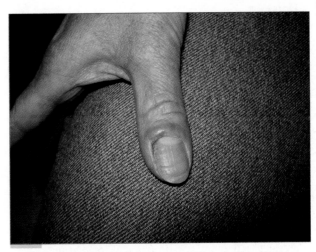

7.29   *Chronic paronychia.* Note the swelling of the proximal nail fold, the loss of the cuticle, and the dystrophy of the nail plate.

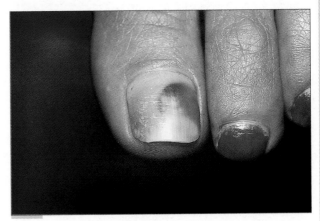

7.30   *Green nail, onycholysis.* The green color is the result of a secondary infection with *Pseudomonas.*

MANAGEMENT

Media attention has brought scores of patients to their health care providers to have their unsightly nails treated with the oral antifungal agent terbinafine (**Lamisil**). Lamisil and itraconazole (**Sporanox**) have replaced griseofulvin, which is less effective and is associated with a high recurrence rate (TABLE 7.1).

Oral Therapy

Important factors to consider before starting oral therapy:

- Diagnostic confirmation by KOH examination or fungal culture
- Patient motivation and compliance
- Family history of onychomycosis
- Patient's age and health
- Drug cost
- Possible drug interactions and side effects (see TABLE 7.1)

Terbinafine (Lamisil) Tablets

- It is fungicidal, especially against dermatophytes.
- Long-term cure rate is probably no greater than 40% to 50%.
- Side effects are infrequent. However, baseline liver function tests are performed, and the tests are repeated in 4 to 6 weeks.
- This drug has a reservoir effect. Because it persists in the nail for up to 4 to 5 months, there is no need to wait until the nail appears clinically normal; there is continued clearing even after cessation of therapy. Baseline liver function tests should be done, and the tests should be repeated in 6 to 8 weeks if therapy is long term.

Dosage

- Adults: 250 mg/day for 6 weeks for fingernails; 250 mg/day for 12 weeks for toenails
  - Alternatively, pulse dosing with 250 mg/day for 1 week monthly for 4 months
- Children: weight 20 to 40 kg: 125 mg/day; weight more than 40 kg: 250 mg/day for 6 to 12 weeks

Itraconazole (Sporanox) Capsules

- This is a broad-spectrum fungistatic agent.
- The primary drawback to the use of this drug is the risk for significant drug interactions.
- Long-term cure rate is probably no greater than 40% to 50%.

- Side effects are infrequent. However, liver function tests should be performed at baseline and repeated in 4 to 6 weeks.
- This drug also has a reservoir effect.

Dosage

- 200 mg/day for 6 weeks for fingernails; 12 weeks for toenails
  - Alternatively, pulse dosing with 200 mg twice daily, taken with full meals, for 7 days of each month (3 months for fingernails, 4 months for toenails)

Fluconazole (Diflucan) Tablets

- This is a broad-spectrum fungistatic agent.
- It is more extensively used in patients with HIV infection.
- It has many fewer drug interactions than itraconazole.
- Side effects are minimal. Liver toxicity must be monitored if the drug is used long term.

Dosage

- 150 to 400 mg daily for 1 to 4 weeks or 150 mg once per week for 9 to 10 months

Other Treatment Methods

Other treatments include the following:

- Surgical ablation of nails is rarely indicated and is generally ineffective.
- Topical agents are generally ineffective because of poor nail penetration. In early distal subungual and superficial white onychomycosis, these drugs may be used as adjuvant therapy or to prevent recurrences after clearing with oral agents.
  - One such preparation is **Carmol 40 Gel,** which contains 40% urea, a keratolytic agent; this is applied once daily to thickened nails. It may be used in conjunction with other topical antifungal agents.
  - **Penlac Nail Lacquer Topical Solution** 8% is a topical nail lacquer containing the antifungal agent ciclopirox; it is used in conjunction with oral antifungal agents or alone for the prevention of recurrent infection. The overall efficacy of this agent remains to be determined.
  - **Amorolfine nail lacquer** (available in Europe) is reported to be effective when it is applied for at least 12 months.

POINTS TO REMEMBER

- Onychomycosis should be confirmed with a positive KOH test or culture before initiating oral therapy.
- Nails that appear abnormal do not always have a fungal infection.
- Onychomycosis is generally asymptomatic, and treatment with the newer systemic antifungal agents is expensive and not always curative.
- Pre-existing liver disease is a relative contraindication to the use of antifungal agents for onychomycosis.
- A patient with a family history of onychomycosis is less likely to have a successful treatment outcome than a person without such a history.

 HELPFUL HINTS

The following important questions must be answered before oral therapy is prescribed:

- What are the patient's age and health status?
- Can the patient afford the cost of the drug?
- Is the patient taking any other medications that could interact adversely with the antifungal agent?

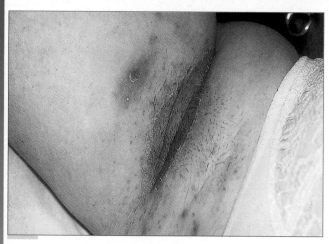

7.31 *Cutaneous candidiasis of the axillae*. This patient has diabetes. Note the satellite pustules.

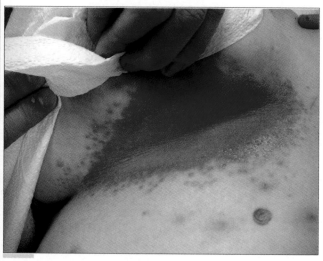

7.32 *Cutaneous candidiasis of skin folds*. This patient with pendulous breasts has rheumatoid arthritis and is on immunosuppressive therapy. Note the "beefy red" plaque and satellite pustules.

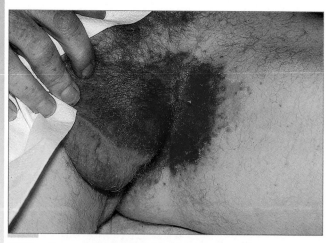

7.33 *Cutaneous candidiasis of the groin*. The characteristic "beefy red" plaque and satellite pustules are seen here.

BASICS

Cutaneous candidiasis is a superficial fungal infection of the skin and mucous membranes caused by *Candida albicans*. It is seen much less commonly than tinea infections. *C. albicans* thrives on moist, occluded sites, particularly as a secondary invader. It occurs in the following:

- People who continually expose their hands to water (e.g., dishwashers, health care workers, florists)
- Obese persons
- Infants (in the diaper area or mouth)

It is also found in persons with an altered immune status, such as:

- Patients with diabetes
- Patients taking long-term systemic steroid therapy
- Patients with AIDS
- Patients with polyendocrinopathies

DESCRIPTION OF LESIONS

- The appearance of lesions varies according to the location.

Candidal Intertrigo

- Initially, pustules appear, followed by well-demarcated erythematous plaques with small papular and pustular lesions at the periphery ("satellite pustules").
- Erythematous areas later become eroded and "beefy red" (Figs. 7.31 and 7.32).
- Lesions are not annular (they have no central clearing), as seen in tinea infections.

DISTRIBUTION OF LESIONS

- Lesions are seen in intertriginous areas, such as under pendulous breasts (see Fig. 7.32), the axillae, the groin, the intergluteal fold, the perineal region including the scrotum (Fig. 7.33), and at the corners of the mouth (perlèche).

Other Locations and Descriptions of Clinical Variants

- **"Erosio interdigitalis blastomycetes."** Superficial interdigital scaly, erythematous erosions or fissures occur in the web spaces of the fingers.
- **Candidal diaper dermatitis** occurs in the area occluded under diapers.
- **Candidal folliculitis** is characterized by follicular pustules.
- **Candidal balanitis** is seen in men with diabetes. Erythema, edema, and moist curdlike accumulations occur on the glans penis, with possible fissuring and ulceration of the foreskin.
- **Candidal vulvitis/vulvovaginitis** consists of erosions, pustules, and erythematous plaques.

- **Candidal paronychia** is characterized by edema, erythema, and purulence of the proximal nail fold with secondary nail dystrophy (see Chapter 13, "Diseases and Abnormalities of Nails").
- **Oral candidiasis ("thrush")** is characterized by white, creamy exudate or plaques, which, when removed, appear eroded and beefy red. Oral candidiasis appears in infants ("thrush") and in the clinical settings of immunosuppression and diabetes (see Chapter 24, "Cutaneous Manifestations of HIV Infection").

CLINICAL MANIFESTATIONS

- Cutaneous candidiasis is characterized by itching and burning.

DIAGNOSIS

- The organism is KOH positive for pseudohyphae, budding yeast, or mycelia (see Chapter 26, "Diagnostic and Therapeutic Procedures").
- Fungal culture on Sabouraud's media reveals creamy, dull-white colonies.

 MANAGEMENT

See TABLE 7.1.

- **Burow's solution** in cool wet soaks two to three times daily is helpful. This solution can be applied to decrease moisture and maceration.
- The intertriginous area should be kept dry with powders, such as miconazole (**Zeasorb-AF**) powder, and by drying with a hairdryer after bathing.
- Topical broad-spectrum antifungal creams, such as prescription ketoconazole (**Nizoral**) cream or the over-the-counter preparations of clotrimazole (**Lotrimin**) and miconazole (**Micatin**), can be applied.
- Systemic antifungal agents, such as **itraconazole** or **fluconazole**, are used for widespread involvement or recalcitrant infections.

 POINT TO REMEMBER

- Cutaneous candidiasis is frequently confused with inverse psoriasis and irritant intertrigo; thus, documentation of candidal organisms should be made.

 DIFFERENTIAL DIAGNOSIS

- Inverse psoriasis
- Tinea infections
- Irritant intertrigo (FIGS. 7.34 and 7.35)
- Atopic dermatitis
- Seborrheic dermatitis

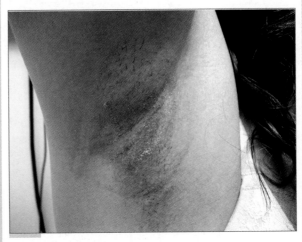

7.34 *Irritant intertrigo.* This itchy eruption was caused by the patient's deodorant.

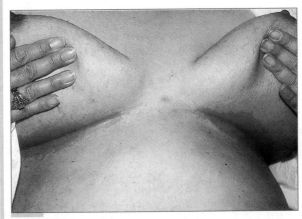

7.35 *Irritant intertrigo.* This is often mistaken and treated for candidiasis. The maceration and pendulous breasts are the cause of this woman's problem.

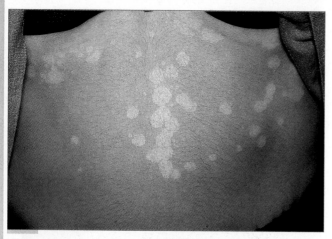

7.36 *Tinea versicolor.* This patient has hypopigmented lesions. Note the similarity to vitiligo.

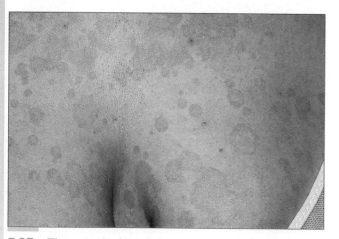

7.37 *Tinea versicolor.* This patient has light tan (faun-colored) tinea versicolor.

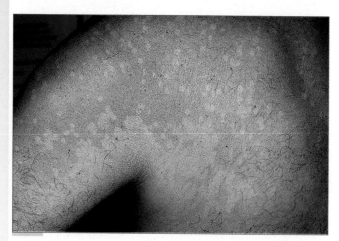

7.38 *Tinea versicolor.* Here the lesions are dark brown and confluent.

BASICS

Tinea versicolor, also known as pityriasis versicolor, is a very common superficial yeast infection caused by the hyphal form of *Pityrosporum ovale.* The organism is also known as *P. orbiculare* and *Malassezia furfur.* Seen mostly in young adults, it is unusual in very young and elderly persons. Tinea versicolor is primarily of cosmetic concern and is generally asymptomatic. The term "versicolor" refers to the varied coloration that tinea versicolor can display. The color of the lesions may vary from whitish to pink to tan or brown (Figs. 7.36–7.38). It is a chronic relapsing condition because the causative fungus is part of the skin's normal flora. It is ubiquitous in tropical and subtropical countries.

DESCRIPTION OF LESIONS

- The primary lesions are well-defined round or oval macules with an overlay of fine scales; the lesions often coalesce to form larger patches.
- The condition is more common in consistently hot climates and recurs during the summer in more temperate zones.

DISTRIBUTION OF LESIONS

- Lesions are most often distributed on the trunk, upper arms, and neck; however, they may also be seen on the face.

DIAGNOSIS

- If scale is present, KOH examination is positive, and the typical "spaghetti and meatball" hyphae are abundant and easily found (FIG. 7.39; see FIG. 26.7), diagnosis is positive.
- Wood's light examination is used to demonstrate the extent of the infection and may help to confirm the diagnosis, because lesions often fluoresce an orange-mustard color when the Wood's light is held close to lesions in a dark room.

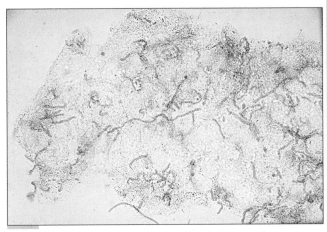

7.39 **_Tinea versicolor._** In this photomicrograph of a KOH examination, note the short, wavy hyphae ("spaghetti") and several clusters of spores ("meatballs").

 DIFFERENTIAL DIAGNOSIS

Vitiligo

- The whitish (hypopigmented) variety of tinea versicolor is frequently mistaken for vitiligo (FIG. 7.40)

Pityriasis rosea

- A **Pityriasis rosea** may also be a cause of diagnostic confusion (see Chapter 4, "Inflammatory Eruptions of Unknown Cause").

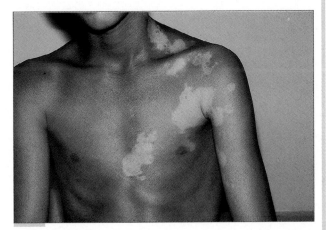

7.40 **_Vitiligo._** Note the complete depigmentation and the lack of scale.

MANAGEMENT

See TABLE 7.2.

Topical Agents

- For mild, limited tinea versicolor, topical therapy is applied in the shower. Daily applications of selenium sulfide (**Selsun Blue**) shampoo, pyrithione zinc (**Head & Shoulders**) shampoo, and ketoconazole 1% (**Nizoral**) cream or shampoo are inexpensive OTC methods that often clear the eruption.
- In addition, application of topical antifungals such as miconazole (**Micatin**), clotrimazole (**Lotrimin**), or terbinafine (**Lamisil**) sprays (Micatin and Lamisil sprays allow for easy application on the back) is useful. The topical agents are used once or twice daily.

- Alternatively, topical ciclopirox (**Loprox**) **gel** or **shampoo,** which is available only by prescription, may be applied.
- This treatment regimen may be repeated for 3 or 4 weeks. It is also a good idea to repeat this regimen before the next warm season or before a tropical vacation.

Systemic Therapy

- For stubborn or widespread disease, systemic therapy with **ketoconazole,** itraconazole (**Sporanox**) or fluconazole (**Diflucan**) may be prescribed (see formulary in TABLE 7.2).
- Although administered for a very short term (3 to 5 days), systemic therapy should not be given routinely for this essentially cosmetic problem.

Table 7.2 FORMULARY FOR TINEA VERSICOLOR

AGENT	DOSAGE
Topical agents: over-the-counter	
Selenium sulfide 1% (**Selsun Blue**) shampoo	Apply daily to wide area for 10 minutes, followed by a shower
Selenium sulfide 1%, zinc pyrithione (**Head & Shoulders**) shampoo	Apply daily to wide area for 10 minutes, followed by a shower
Miconazole 2% (**Micatin**) spray	Spray on once daily for 2 weeks
Clotrimazole (**Lotrimin**) 1% cream	Apply once daily for 2 weeks
Terbinafine (**Lamisil**) 1% cream	Apply 1 to 4 weeks, twice daily
Topical agents: prescription required	
Ketoconazole 2% gel (**Xolegel, foam [extina]**)	
Ketoconazole 2% (**Nizoral**) shampoo	Apply daily to wide area for 10 minutes, followed by a shower
Selenium sulfide 2.5% (**Selsun 2.5%**) shampoo	Apply daily to wide area for 10 minutes, followed by a shower
Ciclopirox shampoo	Apply daily to wide area for 10 minutes, followed by a shower
Ciclopirox (**Loprox**) gel	Apply 1 to 4 weeks, twice daily
Systemic agents	
Ketoconazole (**Nizoral**)	200 mg for 5 days
Itraconazole (**Sporanox**)	100 mg for 5 days
Fluconazole (**Diflucan**)	150 mg for 5 days

 POINTS TO REMEMBER

- Patients should be advised that the uneven coloration of the skin may take several months to disappear after the fungus has been successfully eliminated.
- Recurrences are very common, especially in warm weather.

 HELPFUL HINTS

- Prophylactic application of ketoconazole cream or shampoo once or twice weekly may prevent recurrences.
- Topical therapy can be repeated 1 week before the next exposure to warm weather.

 SEE PATIENT HANDOUT "Tinea Versicolor" ON THE SOLUTION SITE

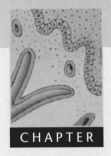

8

Viral Exanthems

Kenneth Howe

OVERVIEW

Viral exanthems are the cutaneous manifestation of an acute viral infection. In most exanthems, viral particles are present within the visible lesions, having reached the skin through the bloodstream. It is unclear whether the observed exanthem results from active viral infection of the skin, the immune response to the virus, or a combination of these two.

Most common in children, viral exanthems may present as distinct, clinically recognizable illnesses such as measles or chickenpox. More frequently, however, a nonspecific eruption is seen that makes an exact diagnosis elusive. More than 50 viral agents are known to cause exanthems, and many of these rashes are indistinguishable from one another. Because most viral illnesses are benign and self-limited, a specific diagnosis is often not made.

In some situations, however, determining the precise etiology may be of vital importance. Examples include the appearance of a viral exanthem during pregnancy or in an immunocompromised patient. It is also important to distinguish viral exanthems from rashes caused by treatable bacterial or rickettsial infections and from hypersensitivity reactions to medications.

- ➤ VARICELLA (CHICKENPOX)
- ➤ HAND-FOOT-AND-MOUTH DISEASE
- ➤ ERYTHEMA INFECTIOSUM (FIFTH DISEASE)
- ➤ ROSEOLA INFANTUM
- ➤ RUBELLA (GERMAN MEASLES)
- ➤ RUBEOLA (MEASLES)

Varicella (Chickenpox)

BASICS

- Varicella, or chickenpox, is an infection caused by the varicella-zoster virus (VZV). Transmission occurs by aerosolized droplet spread, with initial infection occurring in the mucosa of the upper respiratory tract. Traveling through the blood and lymphatics (primary viremia), a small amount of virus reaches cells of the reticuloendothelial system, where the virus replicates during the remainder of the incubation period. Nonspecific host defenses contain the incubating infection at this point, but in most cases these defenses are eventually overwhelmed, and a large secondary viremia results. It is through this secondary viremia that VZV reaches the skin. The viremia occurs cyclically over a period of approximately 3 days and results in successive crops of lesions.
- Most cases occur during childhood, and half of the patients are younger than 5 years of age.
- Epidemics have a peak incidence during late winter and spring.

DESCRIPTION OF LESIONS

- The characteristic lesions begin as red macules and progress rapidly from papules to vesicles to pustules to crusts. The entire cycle may occur within 8 to 12 hours. The typical vesicles are superficial and thin walled, and they are surrounded by an irregular area of erythema, giving them the appearance of "a dewdrop on a rose petal" (FIG. 8.1).
- The lesions are usually pruritic.
- Involvement of the oral mucous membranes (enanthem) occurs as well, most commonly on the palate. Because vesicles in these sites quickly rupture, it is common to observe shallow erosions.
- Because the lesions appear in successive crops, a characteristic feature of varicella is the simultaneous presence of lesions in varying stages of development. In any given area, macules, vesicles, pustules, or crusts may be seen.
- Crusts usually fall off within 1 to 3 weeks, depending on the depth of involvement.
- Large blisters can also be seen in varicella, often resulting from superinfection with *Staphylococcus aureus*. Hemorrhagic lesions may occur in patients with thrombocytopenia.
- Scarring is not unusual in uncomplicated varicella. Facial "punched-out" scars are common.

DISTRIBUTION OF LESIONS

- The eruption typically begins on the face, scalp, and trunk and then spreads to involve the extremities.
- Successive crops appear over 3 to 5 days, resulting in a diffuse, widespread eruption of discrete lesions (FIG. 8.2).

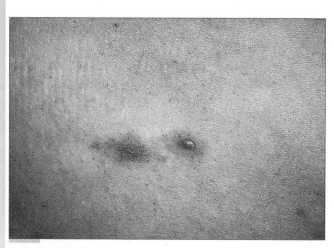

8.1 *Varicella.* "Dewdrops on rose petals."

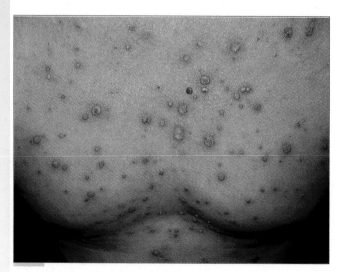

8.2 *Varicella.* Vesicles and crusts.

CLINICAL MANIFESTATIONS

Incubation Period
- The duration typically is 2 weeks (range, 10 to 21 days).
- During this period, children are usually asymptomatic, with the onset of the rash being the first sign of illness.
- In older children and adults, symptoms are typically more severe. The rash is frequently preceded by 2 to 3 days of fever and flulike symptoms, which often persist during the acute illness.

Complications
- Complications in healthy children are rare; complications are more common in infected adults.
- Varicella pneumonia is a relatively uncommon complication that usually occurs in adults and immunocompromised children. It begins 1 to 6 days after onset of the rash, with pulmonary symptoms such as cough, dyspnea, and pleuritic chest pain. The severity of the symptoms is out of proportion to the findings on physical examination. Chest radiographs typically reveal diffuse nodular densities.

DIAGNOSIS
- The diagnosis of varicella is usually straightforward, based on the characteristic presentation and clinical findings.
- A Tzanck smear can be helpful in confirming the diagnosis (see Chapter 6, "Superficial Viral Infections"). When the test is positive, it reveals characteristic multinucleated giant cells. Identical findings are seen in herpes zoster virus or herpes simplex virus (HSV) infections.

Laboratory Testing
- Smears obtained from active lesions can be tested by the direct immunofluorescence technique, which uses fluorescent-labeled antibodies to detect the presence of VZV. This technique has a sensitivity and specificity nearly equal to those of culture, with the advantage of providing rapid results.
- Active lesions can also be cultured for VZV. Culturing of the VZV virus is technically difficult and positive less than 40% of the time.

 DIFFERENTIAL DIAGNOSIS

Other Viral Exanthems
- Vesicular exanthems of coxsackievirus and echovirus infections may be mistaken for varicella.
- These exanthems may show a characteristic distribution, as in hand-foot-and-mouth disease.

Disseminated Herpes Zoster
See FIGURE 24.6.

- Patients have a previous history of primary varicella.
- There is often a typical vesicular eruption accentuated in one unilateral dermatome in a typical "zosteriform" pattern. This is seen in addition to a widespread rash that is indistinguishable from varicella.
- The patient is generally immunocompromised, secondary to medications, malignant disease, or human immunodeficiency virus infection.

Eczema Herpeticum
(Kaposi's Varicelliform Eruption)
See FIGURE 6.29.

- Preexisting skin disease such as atopic dermatitis becomes secondarily infected with HSV.

- Direct immunofluorescence or culture results indicative of HSV infection.

Atypical Measles
- This occurs in adults who received killed measles virus vaccine between 1963 and 1967.
- The eruption begins on the palms and soles and then spreads proximally.
- Pneumonia is a common feature.
- The diagnosis can be confirmed by a rise in measles antibody titers.

Impetigo
- The patient generally feels well.
- Typical moist, honey-colored crusts are present, often in a periorificial distribution (See Chapter 5, "Superficial Bacterial Infections").

MANAGEMENT

Acute Varicella

- Uncomplicated varicella in otherwise healthy children is generally treated with supportive care such as antipruritics and antipyretics. Aspirin should be avoided because of the risk of Reye's syndrome.
- **Oral acyclovir** is warranted in patients who are at an increased risk of complications, and, in general, it should be started within 24 hours of the onset of the rash. These patients include:
  - Otherwise healthy, nonpregnant patients 13 years of age or older.
  - Children older than 12 months of age with chronic skin or pulmonary conditions or who are receiving long-term salicylate therapy.
  - Children receiving short, intermittent, or aerosolized courses of corticosteroids.
- **Intravenous acyclovir** is indicated in immunocompromised patients or in patients with virally mediated complications of varicella.

Varicella Vaccine

The VZV vaccine (**Varivax**) is recommended for universal immunization in all children.

- It is optimally given between 12 and 18 months of age; it may be administered in a single dose at any time before 13 years of age.

- In older adolescents or adults, two doses of vaccine should be administered 4 to 8 weeks apart.
- The appearance of breakthrough varicella, seen in previously immunized persons, has indicated that the effectiveness of the vaccine wanes over time. Consequently, a revaccination booster immunization is now recommended for children between 4 and 6 years of age.

Varicella and Pregnancy

- Peripartal maternal varicella poses a particular risk to the newborn. Neonates born 2 days before or 5 days after the onset of maternal varicella should be given **varicella immunoglobulin (VZIG)**. Those newborns who develop varicella should be treated with intravenous acyclovir.
- **Oral acyclovir** is not recommended in pregnant women with uncomplicated varicella because the risks and benefits to the fetus are unknown.
- Pregnant patients who develop varicella in the first trimester have a 2.3% to 4.9% risk of delivering a child with the **fetal varicella syndrome.**
  - This syndrome is a congenital malformation complex with features such as intrauterine growth retardation, prematurity, cicatricial lesions in a dermatomal distribution, limb paresis and hypoplasia, chorioretinitis, and cataracts.
- It is not known whether the administration of acyclovir prevents these complications.

 POINT TO REMEMBER

- Patients remain contagious until all cutaneous lesions are crusted.

Hand-Foot-and-Mouth Disease

BASICS

- Hand-foot-and-mouth disease is an acute viral infection that manifests as a vesicular eruption with a characteristic distribution. The infection is caused by enteroviruses, most commonly coxsackievirus A16. The virus is spread from person to person by the fecal-oral route.
- Outbreaks are typically in the summer or early fall, and epidemics may occur. Transmission is more likely in crowded environments.
- Young children (1 to 5 years of age) are most commonly infected.
- The incubation period ranges from 4 to 6 days.

DESCRIPTION OF LESIONS

- Oral lesions (enanthem) are the first manifestation of hand-foot-and-mouth disease. Although initially vesicular, it is more common to see multiple shallow erosions, because the vesicles are very fragile.
- Individual lesions may range in size from 1 to 5 mm in diameter, and they may exhibit a rim of erythema. These oral lesions may be painful, and they frequently interfere with eating (FIG. 8.3).
- The exanthem consists of round or angulated, grayish white vesicles that are typically 3 to 7 mm in diameter.
- These vesicles, which are located on the palms and soles, have a characteristic oval or linear shape and tend not to rupture (FIG. 8.4).

DISTRIBUTION OF LESIONS

- The enanthem appears most commonly on the tongue and buccal mucosa and occasionally on the lips, palate, and gums.
- The exanthem is characteristically present on the hands and feet. Lesions occur on the dorsal or lateral aspects of the fingers and toes and on the palms and soles. All three sites may not be involved at the time of presentation.
- The diaper area in infants may show a greater concentration of lesions.
- Occasionally, an eruption of erythematous papules on the proximal extremities may occur, in addition to the acral lesions.

CLINICAL MANIFESTATIONS

- The illness most frequently begins as a sore throat or mouth. In young children, refusal to eat is often a presenting sign.
- Occasionally, a 1- to 2-day prodrome of fever and abdominal pain may be seen.
- The acral eruption follows the development of oral lesions. It is usually not pruritic, although it may be painful.

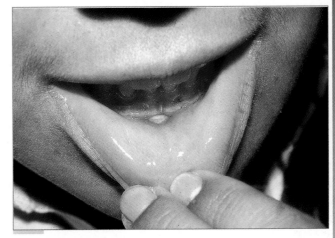

8.3 *Hand-foot-and-mouth disease.* Oral lesion. Note the oval shape and rim of erythema.

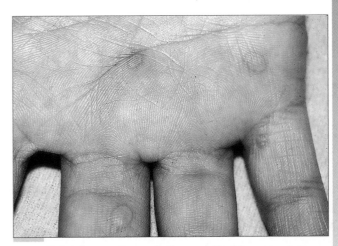

8.4 *Hand-foot-and-mouth disease.* Oval intact vesicles are noted on the palm.

DIFFERENTIAL DIAGNOSIS

Primary Oral Herpes Simplex
(See also Chapter 12, "Disorders of the Mouth, Lips, and Tongue)
- Usually, the lips and gingiva are affected, and the back of the throat is spared.
- There are recurrent outbreaks.
- The Tzanck smear and culture are positive for HSV.

Aphthous Ulcers
- Lesions are painful.
- As with herpes simplex, the lips and gingiva are usually affected, and the back of the throat is spared.

- In contrast to most viral illnesses, lymphadenopathy is absent to minimal.
- Although in general complications are rare, the one seen most frequently is aseptic meningitis.

DIAGNOSIS

- Diagnosis is made on the basis of the characteristic clinical presentation.
- Although not routinely indicated, laboratory testing can confirm the diagnosis. Virus can be cultured from throat washings or stool, with the latter giving a higher yield. Acute and convalescent sera show an elevation in antibody titer to the causative virus.

POINT TO REMEMBER

- The course of the illness is self-limited, lasting less than a week in most cases.

 MANAGEMENT

- Treatment is with supportive care. Antipyretics and a clear liquid diet while the throat is sore are typically all that is necessary.

BASICS

- Erythema infectiosum is a common viral illness caused by infection with parvovirus B19. Transmission is from person to person, probably through respiratory secretions.
- It occurs most commonly in the late winter and spring. Epidemics are frequently seen, particularly among school-age children.
- The incubation period lasts 4 to 14 days, but it may be as long as 3 weeks.
- By the time the characteristic exanthem appears, the patient is unlikely to be infectious.

DESCRIPTION OF LESIONS

- Erythema infectiosum is most commonly identified in children by its characteristic facial erythema. Bright red and tending to involve the malar surfaces, this eruption is described as having a "slapped cheek" appearance (Fig. 8.5A).
- A photosensitive exanthem also appears on the extremities and trunk. This develops 1 to 4 days after the facial erythema, and it begins as a macular or macular and papular erythema that later clears centrally to produce a characteristic reticular ("lacy") pattern (Figs. 8.5B and C).
- Although the exanthem usually resolves in 1 to 2 weeks, the reticular erythema may show a recrudescent course in some patients. In these cases, the erythema tends to flare in response to physical stimuli, such as exercise, excitement, sunlight, or warm baths.

DISTRIBUTION OF LESIONS

- The facial erythema favors the malar surfaces. The "slapped cheek" appearance is further accentuated by a tendency to spare the nasal bridge and the periorbital and perioral areas.
- The reticular erythema most commonly affects the extensor surfaces of the extremities and the buttocks. The palms and soles are usually spared.

CLINICAL MANIFESTATIONS

- Although facial erythema is the most common initial presentation, some patients experience a mild prodrome of low-grade fever, malaise, upper respiratory or gastrointestinal symptoms, and myalgias.
- It can be associated with joint symptoms in adults, particularly in women. A symmetric polyarthropathy develops, involving the hands, feet, elbows, and knees.
- The illness is benign and self-limited, with the exanthem resolving within 1 to 2 weeks.
- Although joint symptoms generally resolve within 2 to 3 weeks, it is not uncommon for them to persist for several months.

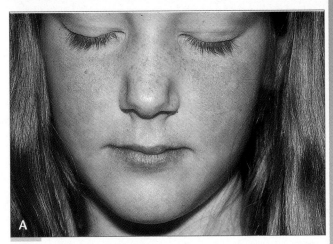

8.5A *Erythema infectiosum.* "Slapped cheeks": The erythema favors the malar surfaces. The slapped cheek appearance is further accentuated by a tendency to spare the nasal bridge and the periorbital and perioral areas.

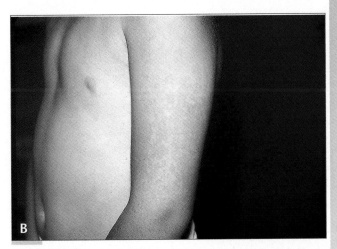

8.5B *Erythema infectiosum.* This child has the characteristic reticular ("lacy") pattern of lesions on her arms.

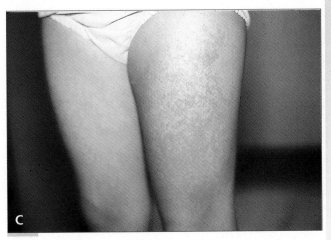

8.5C *Erythema infectiosum.* Similar lesions on legs.

DIFFERENTIAL DIAGNOSIS

Systemic Lupus Erythematosus
- This may be difficult to differentiate from erythema infectiosum with associated joint symptoms.
- The patient often has history of photosensitivity.
- Positive antinuclear antibodies are present.
- Other signs of systemic involvement such as serositis, renal disease, and central nervous system symptoms are noted (See Chapter 25, "Systemic Cutaneous Manifestals).

 POINTS TO REMEMBER

- Facial erythema is often absent in infected adults.
- Because they are at risk for aplastic crisis, all patients with erythema infectiosum who have chronic anemia should have a complete blood cell count.

- Erythema infectiosum during pregnancy may result in fetal death because of the development of hydrops fetalis. The risk of fetal death with maternal infection is estimated at 4.2% to 9%, with greater risk when the infection occurs during the first 20 weeks of pregnancy.
- Infection with parvovirus B19 can lead to aplastic crisis in patients with chronic anemias such as sickle cell disease, hereditary spherocytosis, and thalassemia intermedia.
- Immunocompromised patients who develop chronic parvovirus B19 infection are at risk of chronic red cell aplasia or more generalized bone marrow failure.

DIAGNOSIS

- The diagnosis is based on the characteristic clinical presentation.
- Although usually unnecessary, serologic testing is the most accurate method of confirming infection. The presence of immunoglobulin M (IgM) antibodies to parvovirus B19 is indicative of recent infection. These antibodies appear approximately 3 days after the onset of the exanthem and begin to decline 1 to 2 months later.

MANAGEMENT

- Supportive care is all that is required for uncomplicated cases.
- No effective antiviral therapy exists for parvovirus B19.

BASICS

- Roseola infantum, or exanthem subitum, is an acute viral illness marked by a high fever that characteristically resolves with the onset of the rash (FIG. 8.6).
- It is caused by infection with herpesvirus type 6 (HHV-6).
- Although the exact route of transmission is not known, it is probably spread through oral or respiratory secretions.
- After HHV-6 exposure, there is an incubation period of 7 to 15 days before the onset of symptoms.
- As with other herpesvirus infections, it is likely that HHV-6 establishes a latent infection after the acute illness. The isolation of HHV-6 from the saliva of healthy adults supports this view.

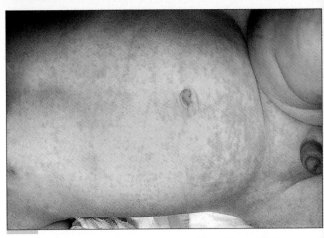

8.6 **Roseola.** (Courtesy of Bernard A. Cohen, M.D.; http://dermatlas.org.)

DESCRIPTION OF LESIONS

- The exanthem appears 1 day before to 1 day after defervescence.
- It consists of discrete macules or papules, 1 to 5 mm in diameter, often with a surrounding rim of pallor. The color of these lesions has been described as "rose pink." Frequently, the individual lesions coalesce to form areas of confluent erythema.
- The exanthem typically clears within 1 to 2 days, although it may persist for up to 10 days.

DISTRIBUTION OF LESIONS

- A widespread distribution is seen, with lesions appearing on the trunk, buttocks, neck, and, occasionally, the face and limbs.

CLINICAL MANIFESTATIONS

- A febrile illness typically precedes the exanthem by 3 to 5 days. Characteristically, this prodrome is marked by a high fever in an otherwise well child.
- On occasion, the fever is accompanied by coryza, cough, headache, or abdominal pain.
- Occipital, cervical, and postauricular lymphadenopathy is commonly present.
- Complications are uncommon and include seizures, encephalitis, and thrombocytopenia.

MANAGEMENT

- During the prodromal phase of illness, antipyretics are often useful, particularly because they may reduce the risk of febrile seizures.

 POINT TO REMEMBER

- Infection with HHV-6 is one of the most common causes of febrile illness in young children.

DIAGNOSIS

- The characteristic clinical presentation is usually sufficient for diagnosis.
- Although rarely necessary, the diagnosis can be confirmed by laboratory studies demonstrating either the presence of IgM to HHV-6 or a fourfold rise in IgG titers to the virus.

DDx **DIFFERENTIAL DIAGNOSIS**

Other Febrile Viral Exanthems
Other conditions such as enterovirus, rubella, and measles must be excluded.

Scarlet Fever
- This has severe constitutional symptoms and characteristic oral changes. It resolves with acral desquamation (See Chapter 9, "Bacterial Exanthems").

Drug Reaction
- This is typically not preceded by high fever.
- The rash is usually of longer duration. (See Chapter 17, "Drug Eruptions")

Rubella (German Measles)

BASICS

- Rubella is a mild viral illness that, because of its devastating effects on the developing human fetus, is recognized as a major public health issue.
- Maternal infection may lead to fetal death or permanent damage. The consequences are more severe when the infection occurs during the first 8 weeks of gestation. Fetal damage is rare after 5 months of gestation.
- Sensory neural hearing loss, cataracts, and cardiac anomalies are the most common defects of congenital rubella.
- The rubella virus is an RNA virus of the Togaviridae family. Humans are the only known natural hosts. The initial infection occurs in the nasopharyngeal mucosa.
- The incidence of rubella has declined markedly since mass immunization for rubella began in 1969.

DESCRIPTION OF LESIONS

- The eruption consists of pink to red macules with faint pinpoint papules.
- Initially discrete, the lesions may coalesce to form an erythematous rash reminiscent of scarlet fever.
- The eruption may be pruritic, particularly in adults.

DISTRIBUTION OF LESIONS

- The eruption begins on the face and spreads within 24 hours to the trunk and extremities (FIG. 8.7).
- The exanthem of rubella is characteristically short-lived, with resolution beginning on the first or second day of the rash. Resolution proceeds in a cephalocaudad direction, and it may be accompanied by fine, branny desquamation.

CLINICAL COURSE

- A mild prodromal illness is the earliest clinical feature of infection.
- A mild fever develops, accompanied by lymphadenopathy. The lymphadenopathy, which most commonly affects the postauricular, suboccipital, and posterior cervical lymph nodes, may be impressive.
- In older patients, the prodrome may be longer and more severe.
- Constitutional symptoms usually resolve within 24 hours of the onset of the rash. In some cases, however, the lymphadenopathy persists for weeks.
- Complications are rare.

DIAGNOSIS

- The clinical features of rubella are not distinctive enough to allow one to make the diagnosis with certainty based on the clinical presentation alone.
- Acute and convalescent antibody titers can confirm the diagnosis. Although unnecessary in most cases, these tests are important in pregnant women who may have been exposed to rubella.

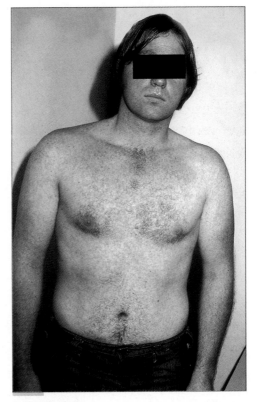

8.7   *Rubella.*

DIFFERENTIAL DIAGNOSIS

Measles

- Prodromal symptoms are of greater severity.
- Koplik's spots are present.
- The rash lasts longer.

Roseola

- A high prodromal fever occurs in the absence of other symptoms.
- The morphologic appearance and duration of the exanthem are similar to those of rubella.

Mononucleosis

- Prominent lymphadenopathy, hepatosplenomegaly, and exudative pharyngitis are noted.
- Atypical lymphocytes and heterophile antibodies are found in the blood.

Erythema Infectiosum

- Patients have a distinctive "slapped cheek" erythema.
- A lacy, reticular eruption occurs on the extremities.
- The exanthem lasts longer than in rubella.

Enterovirus Infection

- This is distinguished by a prominent enanthem.

Scarlet Fever

- Severe constitutional symptoms and pharyngitis are noted.
- Patients have a "strawberry tongue."
- A "sandpapery" exanthem occurs.
- Marked desquamation is associated with resolution (See Figs. 9.1 A and B).

Drug Reaction

- It may be associated with marked pruritus.
- The exanthem lasts longer than in rubella.

 POINT TO REMEMBER

- **Rubella immunization** should be well documented in young women; if antirubella antibiotic titers are negative, rubella immunization should be given.

 MANAGEMENT

- No specific therapy is available. When necessary, supportive care should be provided. Such care includes antipyretics or anti-inflammatory medications for arthralgias.
- Infected patients should be isolated from susceptible persons.

BASICS

- Measles is a viral illness characterized by a distinctive exanthem and enanthem. The primary site of infection is the respiratory epithelium of the oropharynx.
- The measles virus is a single-stranded RNA virus of the Paramyxoviridae family. Humans are the natural host for the virus, although other primates may be infected as well.
- Transmission occurs by the respiratory aerosol route. The incubation period lasts from 9 to 11 days.
- The incidence of measles in the United States has decreased dramatically since the introduction of the measles vaccine.
- Measles has been all but eradicated in the Western Hemisphere. Almost all the cases most recently reported in the United States can be traced to immigrants from nations where measles is more common.
- The disease still rages outside the West. It kills more than 800,000 children worldwide each year, more than half of them in central Africa.

DESCRIPTION OF LESIONS

- The exanthem appears 3 to 5 days after the onset of the prodromal illness. Lesions begin as discrete erythematous macules and papules, which soon coalesce into areas of confluent erythema. Pruritus is usually absent. The rash lasts 4 to 7 days before resolving, often with fine desquamation.

- A characteristic enanthem known as Koplik's spots appears 2 days before the onset of the exanthem. The lesions are 1-mm, bluish white macules that develop on a background of erythematous oral mucosa. These lesions are pathognomonic for measles and, because they develop before the rash, they provide an opportunity for early diagnosis.

DISTRIBUTION OF LESIONS

- The rash most characteristically begins on the forehead or behind the ears. It then spreads to involve the remainder of the face, the trunk, and the arms and legs over 2 to 3 days. It follows a cephalocaudad order in its development, and it later resolves in the same direction.
- Koplik's spots are most prominent on the buccal mucosa opposite the molars, although they may appear on the labial and gingival mucosa as well.

CLINICAL MANIFESTATIONS

- The illness begins with a 2- to 4-day prodrome of fever; hacking, barklike cough; coryza; conjunctivitis; and photophobia. These patients appear acutely ill, and they often have cervical and preauricular lymphadenopathy on examination.
- In most cases, measles is a benign and self-limited infection. Recovery is usually complete within 14 days of the onset of the prodrome.

DIFFERENTIAL DIAGNOSIS

- Atypical measles
- Rubella
- Erythema infectiosum
- Scarlet fever
- Roseola
- Drug hypersensitivity reaction

Complications

- Pneumonia is the most common complication. In children, this most frequently takes the form of primary measles pneumonitis, whereas in adults, secondary bacterial pneumonias are more common. Measles pneumonia is particularly severe in immunosuppressed patients.
- Encephalitis occurs in 1 to 2 patients per 1,000 cases of measles.
- Patients vaccinated with the killed virus vaccine, which was in use from 1963 to 1967, are at risk of developing atypical measles. After a 2- to 3-day prodrome of fever, dry cough, headache, and abdominal pain, a macular and papular exanthem appears. In contrast to classic measles, this eruption begins on the palms and soles and then spreads proximally. Pneumonia is often present in these patients as well.

DIAGNOSIS

- The diagnosis of measles is usually made on clinical grounds.
- Although usually unnecessary, serologic testing is available. A fourfold or greater rise in antibody titers between acute and convalescent sera confirms the diagnosis.

 MANAGEMENT

- No specific therapy for measles virus infection exists. Supportive care should be provided, and patients should be isolated from susceptible persons.
- Passive immunization should be given to pregnant women, infants younger than 1 year, and immunocompromised patients who lack antibodies to the measles virus. Immunoglobulin preparations containing a high antimeasles titer should be administered within 6 days of exposure.
- Routine immunization is recommended for all children 15 months of age or older.

POINTS TO REMEMBER

- A patient with measles becomes contagious 3 days before onset of the rash and remains so until desquamation of the rash.
- All cases should be reported to local public health officials.

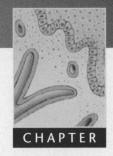

Bacterial Exanthems

Kenneth Howe and Herbert P. Goodheart

OVERVIEW

The term *exanthem* refers to a widespread, symmetric, erythematous rash that begins with macules and papules that remain discrete or become confluent. The eruption may or may not be pruritic and is usually accompanied by systemic symptoms such as fever, malaise, and headache. In pediatric populations exanthems are usually caused by infectious agents such as viruses and bacteria; infrequently, they may be due to a drug reaction.

Bacterial exanthems represent either a reaction to a bacterial toxin, direct injury to the skin by the organism itself, or an immune response. Many common childhood bacterial exanthems have characteristic features, distributions, durations, and systemic symptoms. As with viral exanthems (see Chapter 8, "Viral Exanthems"), when there are no typical lesions or distinctive prodromal signs or symptoms, a specific diagnosis is often difficult, if not impossible, to make. However, a definitive diagnosis may be critical, particularly if a pregnant woman or an immunocompromised patient has been exposed to an infected individual. Furthermore, some of these conditions can become life threatening if not treated promptly with appropriate medications, e.g., Kawasaki's disease.

> ➤ **SCARLET FEVER**
>
> ➤ **TOXIN-MEDIATED STREPTOCOCCAL AND STAPHYLOCOCCAL DISEASE**
>
> ➤ **KAWASAKI'S SYNDROME**

Scarlet Fever

BASICS

- Scarlet fever (SF) is a streptococcal infection of the pharynx associated with widespread mucocutaneous changes that are caused by an erythrogenic exotoxin-producing strain of group A beta-hemolytic streptococci. Less commonly, SF may follow streptococcal wound infections or burns, as well as upper respiratory tract infections.
- In the past, SF was a major public health threat. However, its morbidity, mortality, and incidence have declined markedly, both because of the development of antibiotics and because of a reduction in the virulence of the streptococci causing the condition.
- The cutaneous manifestations of SF represent a delayed hypersensitivity response to streptococcal products. Thus, prior exposure to streptococci is a necessary precondition for SF.

Etiology

- Usually, group A beta-hemolytic *Streptococcus pyogenes* is the pathogenic organism. Uncommonly, exotoxin-producing *Staphylococcus aureus* may be responsible.

DESCRIPTION OF LESIONS

- A finely papular erythematous rash appears on the trunk and extremities. This rash may be referred to as "sandpapery" or "scarlatiniform."
- The skin around the mouth may show a characteristic pallor (circumoral pallor). Linear streaks of petechiae called Pastia's lines may develop in flexural areas such as the antecubital fossae, the axillae, and the inguinal region.
- Mucosal findings include erythema and edema of the pharyngotonsillar area, punctate erythematous macules and petechiae on the palate, and "strawberry tongue." The last is a characteristic finding and is caused by prominence of the papillae on the surface of the tongue.
- During the convalescent phase of the illness, the skin of the palms and soles frequently desquamates. This desquamation may be sheetlike, and the original infection may have passed unnoticed. In such instances, the patient may seek medical attention solely for the desquamation (Figs. 9.1 A and B).

DISTRIBUTION OF LESIONS

- The scarlatiniform eruption is widespread and symmetric, primarily affecting the trunk and extremities.

CLINICAL MANIFESTATIONS

- SF typically begins with the abrupt onset of fever, sore throat, headache, and chills.
- Complications are uncommon but may include pneumonia, pericarditis, meningitis, hepatitis, glomerulonephritis, and rheumatic fever. Erythema nodosum and acute guttate psoriasis may also follow or accompany an infection with group

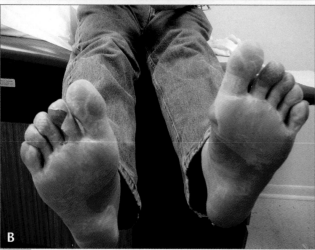

9.1 A and B *Scarlet fever.* Skin peeling from this patient's palms and soles during the convalescent phase of his illness. This exuberant desquamation occurred two weeks after he had fever and a truncal exanthem that began as a streptoccocal throat infection.

A beta-hemolytic streptococci (see Chapter 25, "Cutaneous Manifestations of Systemic Disease," and Chapter 3, "Psoriasis").

- SF can recur, with reported recurrence rates as high as 18%.

DIAGNOSIS

- The diagnosis of SF is often made on clinical grounds.
- The isolation of group A streptococci from the pharynx, or the presence of serologic tests such as an elevation of anti-streptolysin-O titers, can help confirm the diagnosis.

 MANAGEMENT

- First-line treatment is with **penicillin.** Alternatives include **erythromycin, cephalosporins, ofloxacin, rifampin,** and newer **macrolide antibiotics.**
- Emollients can be used to soothe the scarlatiniform eruption.

 DIFFERENTIAL DIAGNOSIS

- **Streptococcal** or **staphylococcal toxic shock syndromes** are distinguished by hypotension and multi-organ system involvement.
- **Kawasaki's syndrome** (see discussion later in this chapter) is characterized by prominent lymphadenopathy.
- **Febrile drug reactions** cause a blotchy, erythematous rash. Pastia's lines and strawberry tongue are not present.
- **Viral exanthem** is a possible diagnosis.
- Flaccid bullae are the predominant feature of **staphylococcal scalded-skin syndrome,** which occurs in newborns and in infants younger than 2 years (see Chapter 27, "Special Considerations in Pediatric and Elderly Skin.")

BASICS

Some streptococcal and staphylococcal species are capable of producing circulating toxins. Patients infected with these toxin-producing bacteria exhibit clinical manifestations distant from the site of local infection. Several distinct syndromes related to these toxins have been recognized, including toxic shock syndrome (TSS) and, rarely, streptococcal toxic shock syndrome (STSS). The principal features of STSS are the same as those of classic TSS: a local infection leads to various clinical manifestations in distant organ systems, resulting from the action of a toxin produced by the infecting bacteria. In most cases of STSS, group A streptococci are isolated from the local infection.

The responsible toxins act as superantigens, bypassing the normal sequence of immune system activation, to stimulate an immune response in a general, nonspecific manner. This nonspecific immunologic activation leads to damage in various organ systems. Certain physical signs—such as strawberry tongue, acral erythema with subsequent desquamation, and an erythematous eruption with perineal accentuation—are shared in common by several of the toxin mediated syndromes.

Toxic Shock Syndrome

BASICS

- TSS is a systemic illness caused by infection with toxin-producing strains of *S. aureus*. Originally described in association with tampon use, TSS now occurs more commonly with a local wound infection, particularly in the postoperative setting.

DESCRIPTION OF LESIONS

- A diffuse macular erythema is often present, which may be scarlatiniform (i.e., "sandpapery" to the touch) and may show accentuation in the flexures.
- Erythema and edema of the palms and soles are often seen.
- Desquamation of the palms and soles, as seen in many bacterial toxin-mediated disorders, occurs 1 to 2 weeks after the onset of illness (see Figs. 9.1 A and B).
- Hyperemia of the conjunctiva and mucous membranes and "strawberry tongue" are often present (see Fig. 9.3).

DISTRIBUTION OF LESIONS

- The erythematous eruption is diffuse, with accentuation in flexures such as the antecubital folds.
- The mucous membranes, palms, and soles are also sites of characteristic changes.

CLINICAL MANIFESTATIONS

- Patients with TSS have a high fever.
- Multiorgan involvement is a hallmark of this condition. Systemic manifestations may include hypotension, elevated blood urea nitrogen and creatinine levels, abnormal liver function test results, leukocytosis and thrombocytopenia, and increased serum creatine kinase levels.
- In nonmenstrual TSS, the classic signs of erythema, tenderness, and purulence may be absent in the local infection, thereby making its identification difficult.

DIAGNOSIS

- Diagnosis is made when the characteristic clinical findings of fever, rash, and hypotension are present in patients who have an infection with *S. aureus* or in menstruating women who use tampons.
- Diagnosis also is made when laboratory tests such as Gram's stain and cultures of vaginal exudate or wounds are positive for *S. aureus* or, rarely, group A streptococci.

 DIFFERENTIAL DIAGNOSIS

- Hypotension does not occur in **scarlet fever.**
- A **febrile drug reaction** is not associated with hypotension.
- **Kawasaki's syndrome** (see following section) usually occurs in children and causes prominent lymphadenopathy.
- **Staphylococcal scalded-skin syndrome** occurs in newborns and in infants younger than 2 years.

 MANAGEMENT

- Treatment of TSS includes the administration of **penicillinase-resistant antibiotics** and drainage of any abscesses.
- Supportive care may include **hydration** and **vasopressors** for hypotension.
- Management of STSS is similar to that of classic TSS.
- **Intravenous gamma globulin** has been reported to be effective in treating STSS, but it is not yet in widespread use.

 HELPFUL HINTS

- Look for a cutaneous site of infection or for a forgotten or retained vaginal tampon.
- STSS may be clinically identical to TSS, but it is usually distinguished by a more marked soft tissue infection at the site of origin, with localized pain in an extremity the most frequent initial complaint.
- Blood cultures are positive in more than 50% of patients with STSS.
- Antibiotic coverage for both staphylococci and penicillin-resistant streptococci should be given.

BASICS

- Kawasaki's syndrome (KS), also known as mucocutaneous lymph node syndrome, is an acute, febrile, multisystem illness that primarily affects young children. Its most serious complications are the result of systemic vasculopathy.
- In fact, KS is best regarded as a generalized vasculitis that involves small to medium-sized arteries. The extent of the coronary vascular involvement is so significant that KS has now surpassed rheumatic fever as the leading cause of acquired heart disease in children from developed nations.
- The peak incidence of KS is between 1 and 2 years of age. It is more common in boys.
- In the United States, children of Asian ancestry are affected six times more often than are white children.
- KS occurs sporadically and in epidemics. A seasonal predilection has been observed, with cases occurring more often in the winter and spring.
- Although the exact cause of KS is unknown, it is most likely the result of a superantigen produced by an infectious agent such as *S. aureus,* resulting in massive cytokine release.

DESCRIPTION OF LESIONS

- The truncal rash of KS is polymorphous and can be macular, papular, urticarial, erythrodermatous, targetoid, or composed of fine micropustules, but it is never vesicular or bullous. The eruption is usually pruritic.
- Changes of the hands and feet are distinctive. An intense erythema appears on the palms and soles on days 3 to 5 of the illness, followed by an indurated edema. A sharp demarcation may be seen at the wrists and the sides of the hands and feet. As noted in SF, during the convalescent phase of the illness, the skin of the fingertips and toes peels off in sheets (FIG. 9.4).

- The presence of scarlatiniform erythema in the perianal or inguinal area (FIG. 9.2) may be a useful diagnostic sign. The rash in this area progresses to desquamation before the palms and soles begin to peel.
- Characteristic findings are present in the mouth, on the lips, and on the tongue. The earliest manifestations are seen on the lips, with bright red erythema accompanied by fissuring and swelling. Prominent papillae create the appearance of a "strawberry tongue" (FIG. 9.3). Examination of the oropharynx reveals a diffuse erythema without vesicles, erosions, or ulcers.

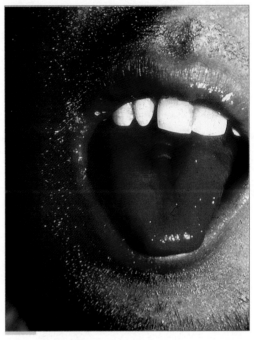

9.3 *Kawasaki's syndrome.* "Strawberry tongue."

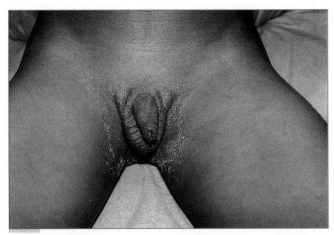

9.2 *Kawasaki's syndrome.* Desquamation in the genital area. This sheetlike desquamation occurred 2 weeks after the original infection.

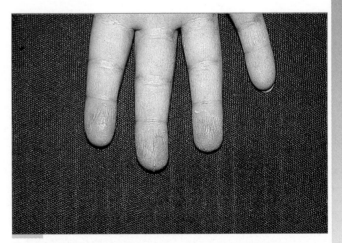

9.4 *Scarlet fever.* Skin peeling from fingertips. This desquamation occurred during the convalescent phase of the illness. It can be a useful diagnostic sign.

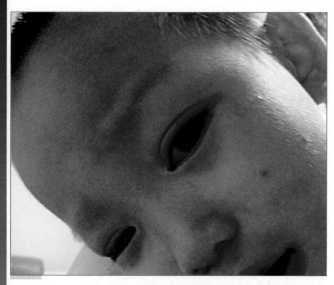

9.5 *Kawasaki's syndrome.* Ocular involvement.

• Eye involvement (FIG. 9.5) consists of bilateral, nonpurulent conjunctival injection. Patients may exhibit signs of photophobia.

DISTRIBUTION OF LESIONS

• The polymorphic eruption favors the trunk and proximal extremities, but it may be generalized.

CLINICAL MANIFESTATIONS

• Fever usually marks the onset of KS. Elevated temperature shows a remittent pattern, with spikes to 103°F and even up to 105°F. The average duration of the fever is 11 days.
• Seen in 75% of patients, cervical lymphadenopathy is the least common diagnostic feature of KS. It usually manifests as a single, enlarged, nonsuppurative lymph node on the side of the neck.
• Cardiac involvement is the most worrisome complication of KS. During the acute phase of the illness, tachycardia may develop, with gallop rhythm, subtle electrocardiographic changes, pericardial effusion, tricuspid insufficiency, or mitral regurgitation. Coronary artery aneurisms have been reported to occur in approximately 25% of untreated patients and may result in thrombosis with subsequent infarction.

DIAGNOSIS

The diagnosis of KS is based on recognition of its clinical features and is supported by compatible laboratory findings; however, laboratory findings are nonspecific. None of the following diagnostic guidelines are in themselves diagnostic, but their presence may be helpful:

• Fever persisting 5 days or more
• Polymorphous rash
• Bilateral conjunctival injection
• Oral mucous membrane changes
• Cervical lymphadenopathy
• Changes of peripheral extremities: erythema of palms and soles, indurative edema of the hands and feet, desquamation of the fingertips

Laboratory Findings
• During the acute phase of the illness, leukocytosis with a predominance of immature and mature granulocytes is common, with 50% of patients having a white blood cell count >15,000/mL.
• Nonspecific abnormalities of acute phase reactants, such as the erythrocyte sedimentation rate and C-reactive protein levels are usually present.

DIFFERENTIAL DIAGNOSIS

- **Staphylococcal TSS** or **STSS** (see earlier section)
- **SF** (see earlier section)
- **Rubella** and **rubeola**
- **Febrile viral exanthems**
- **Mononucleosis**
- **Hypersensitivity reactions** (including Stevens-Johnson syndrome)
- **Drug eruptions** with accompanying fever
- Infantile **polyarteritis nodosum**

MANAGEMENT

- Most children with KS must be hospitalized for a complete workup and supportive care. Because high temperatures and irritability make feeding difficult, intravenous fluids are often needed for hydration.
- The initial goals of therapy are to reduce the fever and the inflammation of the myocardium and to prevent subsequent cardiac sequelae.
- Children with evidence of cardiac disease may require intensive support.
- Once the diagnosis of KS has been established, therapy with intravenous immune globulin (IVIG), or gamma globulin, and aspirin should be started.
- The current recommended therapy for KS in the acute phase includes a single infusion of intravenously administered IVIG and aspirin.

- **High-dose aspirin** at a dose of 80 to 100 mg/kg/day PO in four equally divided doses is continued during the acute phase for its anti-inflammatory effects. It is continued at this dose until day 14 of the illness or until the patient has been afebrile for 48 to 72 hours.
- **IVIG** has a synergistic effect with aspirin and reduces acute inflammation, with the maximal benefits seen when it is given within the first 10 days of the illness. IVIG has been shown to reduce the rate of coronary aneurysms from greater than 25% in untreated patients to 1% to 5% in treated patients. IVIG may decrease autoantibody production and increase solubilization and removal of immune complexes.

POINTS TO REMEMBER

- All patients with KS should have an echocardiogram during the acute illness and 3 to 6 weeks after the onset of fever.
- Prompt treatment with aspirin and IVIG significantly decreases the risk of cardiac complications.
- Although most patients recover with little to no limitations on physical activity, a delay in diagnosis results in a greater likelihood of coronary lesions and related complications.

HELPFUL HINTS

- KS should be considered in children with an unexplained fever lasting more than 5 days who have a polymorphous rash that may look like SF or measles and conjunctivitis without pus.
- Some children may present with an incomplete clinical picture and may not exhibit sufficient clinical signs to fulfill the diagnostic criteria; therefore, a high level of suspicion is required to recognize these patients.

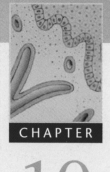

10 Hair and Scalp Disorders Resulting in Hair Loss

Herbert P. Goodheart and Hendrik Uyttendaele

➤ **ANDROGENIC ALOPECIA**

➤ **ALOPECIA AREATA**

➤ **DIFFUSE ALOPECIA**

- Telogen effluvium
- Anagen effluvium
- Senescent alopecia

➤ **SCARRING ALOPECIA**

- Chronic cutaneous lupus erythematosus
- Lichen planopilaris
- Central centrifugal cicatricial alopecia
- Traction alopecia
- Sarcoidosis
- Folliculitis decalvans

➤ **PSEUDOFOLLICULITIS BARBAE AND ACNE KELOIDALIS**

OVERVIEW

Hair has great social and cultural significance in all human societies. It is found on most areas of the human body, except on the palms of the hands, the soles of the feet, and mucous membranes.

TYPES OF HAIR

- **Lanugo,** the fine hair that covers nearly the entire body of fetuses.
- **Vellus,** the short, fine, "peach fuzz" body hair that grows in most places on the body. Vellus hairs are soft and short. It is seen in areas of male pattern baldness.
- **Terminal,** the fully developed hair, which is generally longer, coarser, thicker, and darker than vellus hair and does not appear until puberty.

HAIR TEXTURE AND SHAPE

Hair texture and shape is genetically determined to be straight, curly or wavy, and it can change over time. It can also be affected by hair styling practices such as chemical straighteners, braiding, or curlers.

Whether hair is curly or straight is determined by the shape of the follicle itself and the direction in which each strand grows out of its follicle. For example, curly hair is shaped like an elongated oval and grows at a sharp angle to the scalp (see ILL. 10.1).

CYCLES OF HAIR GROWTH

Hair grows in long cycles over many months: a growth (anagen) phase (see ILL. 11.1) is followed by degenerative (catagen) phase, then a resting (telogen) phase, with different hairs alternating phases.

HAIR LOSS

Some degree of scalp hair loss or thinning generally accompanies aging in both sexes, and it's estimated that half of all men are affected by male pattern baldness by the time they are 50 years of age.

Drugs used in cancer chemotherapy frequently cause a temporary loss of hair, because they affect all rapidly dividing cells, not just the malignant ones. Certain diseases and traumas can cause temporary or permanent loss of hair (e.g., systemic lupus erythematosus, thyroid disease).

BASICS

Androgenic alopecia (AGA), also known as common baldness (male- or female-pattern baldness), is an extremely common, noninflammatory type of alopecia whose incidence increases greatly with advancing age. AGA is not a disease but a normal consequence of aging. In most, if not all, cultures, hair plays a powerful role in a person's psychosexual identity and self-image. It is not surprising that in our youth- and image-driven society, hair replacement and retention methods have taken on almost the status of a subspecialty in health care.

- AGA is seen more frequently in men than it is in women because women's hair loss tends to be less apparent, is less extensive, and generally begins at a later age than it does in men.
- The condition is genetically determined (autosomal dominant with variable penetrance). The incidence and severity of AGA tend to be highest in white men, followed by white women; it is second highest in Asians and African-Americans and lowest in Native Americans and Eskimos.

Pathogenesis

- AGA is caused by an androgenic action on hair follicles that shortens the anagen (growth) phase of the hair cycle, thus producing thinner, shorter hairs in a process known as miniaturization.
- It occurs through the gradual conversion of terminal hairs into indeterminate hairs and finally to short, wispy, nonpigmented vellus hairs.
  - In men, this type of alopecia usually begins in late adolescence, with hair loss often starting at the parietal hairline.
  - In women, the onset is more gradual and the loss of hair is more subtle, and it tends to become obvious later (most often after menopause, but occasionally in the third or fourth decade). This produces a thinning of the hair rather than areas of marked baldness. It is thought that estrogen protects against androgen-mediated miniaturization, which explains both the reduction in severity and the increase in incidence after menopause.

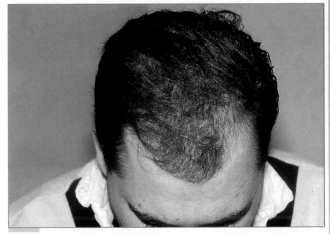

10.1 *Male-pattern alopecia.* This is characterized by an M-shaped pattern of hair loss on the front and vertex of the head.

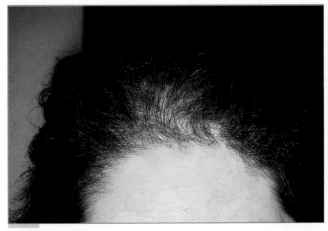

10.2 *Female-pattern alopecia.* A midparietal pattern of decreasing hair loss is noted here. The integrity of the frontal hairline is maintained.

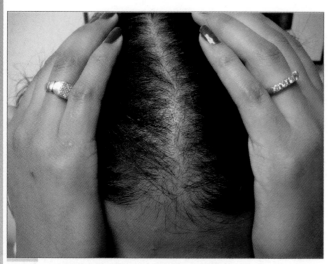

10.3 *Female-pattern alopecia.* The characteristic "widened part" in a "Christmas-tree" pattern toward the vertex is seen in this patient.

 DIFFERENTIAL DIAGNOSIS

- It should be kept in mind that the following conditions are not only independent causes of hair loss but may coexist and exacerbate AGA; they are discussed later in this chapter.
  - **Telogen effluvium** (shedding of resting hairs)
  - **Anagen effluvium** (shedding of growing hairs)
  - **Hair loss from thyroid disease**
  - Hair loss caused by **iron-deficiency anemia** and **insufficient calories, protein,** or **vitamins**
  - Hair loss caused by **androgen excess** in women
- Blood tests and other laboratory studies are necessary only when the diagnosis is in doubt, or other coexisting reasons to explain alopecia are warranted by the history or physical examination (see later section, "Diffuse Alopecia").

CLINICAL MANIFESTATIONS

- AGA usually produces a patterned type of hair loss. In men and women, hair loss is mostly restricted to the vertex and frontal scalp; hair density on the occipital scalp remains unaffected.
  - **In men,** this type of alopecia usually begins in late adolescence, with hair loss often starting at the parietal hairline (FIG. 10.1).
  - **In women,** the loss of hair is more subtle, and it tends to begin later in life (FIG. 10.2).

DESCRIPTION AND DISTRIBUTION OF LESIONS

- Androgenic alopecia produces two typical patterns of hair loss.
  - **In men,** the process usually begins in an M-shaped pattern on the front and vertex of the head (this is often referred to as male-pattern baldness).
  - **In women,** a thinning of the crown in a "Christmas-tree," midparietal pattern (female-pattern baldness) is usually noted initially (FIG. 10.3).
- Hair loss may progress in both sexes but is often more extensive in men. Thus, in the end stages of androgenic alopecia, many men have only a fringe of remaining hair, whereas women tend to maintain the frontal hairline and do not become frankly bald (see earlier section on "Pathogenesis").

DIAGNOSIS

- The diagnosis of AGA is generally based on the clinical pattern of baldness coupled with an absence of clues pointing to a specific disease that may cause hair loss.

MANAGEMENT

Women

- **Minoxidil** (2% solution, applied twice daily) may reduce shedding and may possibly contribute to some regrowth. (The 5% solution of minoxidil may be more effective, but it has not yet been approved for use in women.) The mechanism of action is unknown; however, minoxidil appears to lengthen the duration of the anagen phase, and it may increase the blood supply to the hair follicle. Regrowth is more pronounced at the vertex than in the frontal areas and may not be noted for at least 4 months. Continuing topical treatment with the drug is necessary indefinitely because discontinuation of treatment produces a rapid reversion to the pretreatment balding pattern. The incidence of facial hair growth appears to be increased with the use of the higher-concentration formulation. Patients who respond best to this drug are those who have a recent onset of AGA and small areas of hair loss. In general, women respond better to topical minoxidil than men.
- Women with excess androgen may benefit from **systemic antiandrogen therapy** with agents such as **spironolactone, flutamide,** or **oral contraceptives** that decrease ovarian and adrenal androgen production, especially agents that contain a nonandrogenic progestin.

Men

- Minoxidil 5% solution and foam (**Rogaine**), applied twice daily, may reduce shedding and may possibly contribute to some regrowth.
- Finasteride (**Propecia**), 1 mg/day, is an antiandrogen that acts by inhibiting type II 5-alpha reductase, the enzyme that converts testosterone to dihydrotestosterone.
  - In much higher doses, finasteride is used as a treatment for benign prostatic hyperplasia and prostate cancer.
  - Recognized side effects include erectile dysfunction and, less often, gynecomastia. It is teratogenic and has not been approved by the U.S. Food and Drug Administration for the treatment of AGA in women.

Men and Women

- **Hair transplantation** is performed by harvesting hairs from donor sites such as the occipital scalp. Hair transplantation, which uses a micrografting technique in which a small incision is used to insert one or more donor hairs, is particularly effective in women, because unlike men, women rarely become completely bald.

 POINTS TO REMEMBER

- A patient's anxiety regarding hair loss should be taken seriously by his or her health care provider. Hair loss should not simply be "brushed off" as an insignificant cosmetic complaint. The time spent listening to the patient may be helpful in uncovering other emotional or physical problems.
- Evaluation of a female patient with AGA may include a complete blood count and testing of thyroid-stimulating hormone and serum iron levels.

- Women with symptoms or signs of virilization should undergo a careful history and evaluation for an androgen-excess syndrome. These patients require hormonal studies and may need referral to an endocrinologist.
- AGA is very common; therefore, it may coexist with other forms of hair loss. Consequently, a search for treatable causes of telogen effluvium (e.g., anemia, hypothyroidism), especially in patients with an abrupt onset or a rapid progression of their disease, is indicated.

 SEE PATIENT HANDOUT "Hair Loss" ON THE SOLUTION SITE

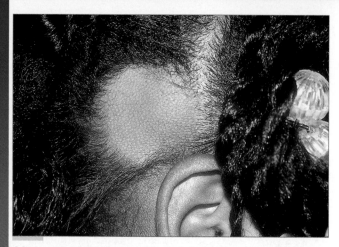

10.4 *Alopecia areata.* The hair is lost in a round patch. Note the absence of scales or inflammation.

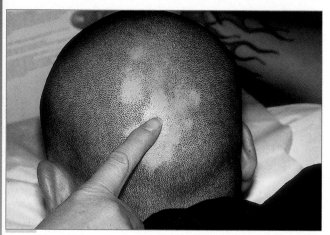

10.5 *Alopecia areata.* Increased friction is noted on palpation of lesional skin as a result of the loss of vellus hairs.

BASICS

- A common, noninflammatory, idiopathic disorder, alopecia areata (AA) is characterized by well-circumscribed round or oval areas of nonscarring hair loss. **Alopecia totalis** is a loss of all or almost all scalp hair and eyebrows. **Alopecia universalis** refers to a total loss of body hair.
- AA most commonly affects young adults and children. Occasionally, a family history of AA exists; often, onset is attributed to recent stress or a major life crisis.

Pathogenesis

The origin of AA is generally considered autoimmune, because biopsy findings demonstrate T-cell infiltrates surrounding the hair follicles and because AA is sometimes associated with other putative autoimmune disorders, such as the following:

- Vitiligo
- Thyroid disease (Hashimoto's disease)
- Pernicious anemia

DESCRIPTION OF LESIONS

- AA most commonly presents as oval, round, or geometric patches of alopecia (FIG. 10.4).
- On occasion, a hand lens may reveal tiny "exclamation mark" hairs at the periphery of lesions.
- Increased friction (not the expected smoothness) is felt on palpation of lesional skin because of the loss of vellus hairs (FIG. 10.5).

DISTRIBUTION OF LESIONS

- Lesions are most often found on the scalp, eyebrows, eyelashes, and areas of the face that bear hair, such as the beard (FIG. 10.6) or mustache on men.
- The entire scalp (alopecia totalis) may rarely be involved, or even the entire body (alopecia universalis), including pubic, axillary, and nasal hair (FIG. 10.7).
- Infrequently, nails may demonstrate a characteristic pitting ("railroad tracks").

CLINICAL MANIFESTATIONS

- There is usually asymptomatic shedding of hair, which is often discovered by the patient's hairdresser or a family member.
- Frequently, hair spontaneously regrows; however, a recurrence of hair loss may be seen in 30% of patients who had experienced regrowth. Regrowing hair is initially thin and sometimes white (vitiliginous) (FIG. 10.8).
- A poorer prognosis is associated with extensive alopecia, an atopic history, and chronicity. Also, when bands of alopecia occur along the hairline margins (**ophiasis**), (FIG. 10.9) that partially or completely encircle the head, a poorer prognosis is also probable.
- Both alopecia universalis and alopecia totalis are generally refractory to therapy and usually last a lifetime; spontaneous regrowth is rare.

DIAGNOSIS

- The diagnosis of AA is generally based on its clinical appearance; however, a scalp biopsy may be performed if the diagnosis is in doubt.
- A potassium hydroxide (KOH) test and fungal culture to rule out tinea capitis is negative.

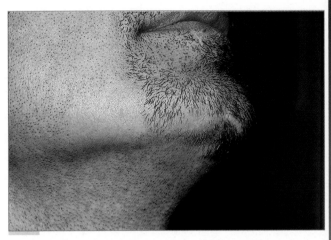

10.6 *Alopecia areata.* This man's AA is limited to his beard.

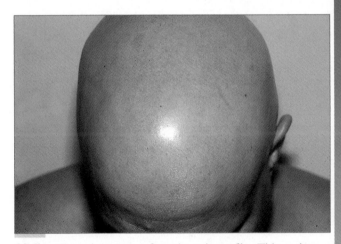

10.7 *Alopecia areata, alopecia universalis.* This patient has lost all of his hair. He has no eyelashes, intranasal hair, pubic hair, or axillary hair; he also has no hair on his extremities.

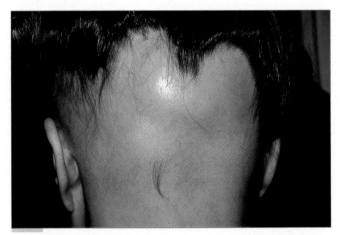

10.9 *Alopecia areata, ophiasis pattern.* A band of alopecia occurs along the hairline margins encircling the head.

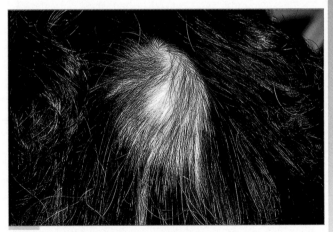

10.8 *Alopecia areata, regrowing hair.* In this patient with AA, clusters of hair regrew after intralesional triamcinolone acetonide injections. Some of the regrown hairs are white (vitiliginous).

DIFFERENTIAL DIAGNOSIS

Tinea Capitis

See Chapter 7, "Superficial Fungal Infections."

- This is seen most frequently in African-American children and uncommonly in African-American adults.
- The scalp is often scaly, itchy, and inflamed.
- The diagnosis is confirmed when the KOH examination is positive for hyphae or when a fungus grows on Sabouraud medium.

Telogen Effluvium

See also later section.

- The hair loss is diffuse.
- There is often a history of antecedent illness or childbirth, for example.

Traction Alopecia and Hot-Comb Alopecia

See later discussion.

Other Diagnoses

Trichotillomania

Trichotillomania is also known as compulsive hair pulling (FIG. 10.10).

- This is seen most often in young girls.
- Hairs tend to be broken at different lengths.
- There is an asymmetric loss of scalp hair.

Secondary Syphilis

Secondary syphilis should always be considered in cases of unexplained patchy hair loss (see FIG. 19.19).

- The hair loss is referred to as "moth-eaten" in appearance.
- Serologic tests for syphilis are generally reactive.

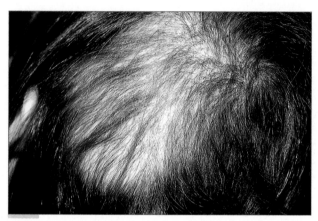

10.10 *Trichotillomania.* This condition is seen most often in young girls. Hairs tend to be broken at different lengths. The areas of alopecia are not completely devoid of hair.

Rx MANAGEMENT

- Because mild cases of AA often show spontaneous regrowth, therapy is often unnecessary.
- The daily application of superpotent **topical steroids,** such as clobetasol cream 0.05%, may speed hair regrowth. To increase drug penetration, potent topical steroids, such as fluocinonide cream 0.05%, may be applied, occluded with a plastic shower cap, and left on overnight.
- If necessary, **intralesional steroid injections** into the alopecic patches with triamcinolone acetonide may be administered every 6 to 8 weeks.

Further Treatment Modalities

The numerous treatment modalities for severe extensive AA that have been tried over the years reflect the fact that few are very effective. The success rates associated with the following measures have ranged from no response to varying degrees of partial success:

- **Irritant therapy** involves using a topical anthralin (a coal tar derivative) preparation.
- **Topical minoxidil** in a 2% or 5% concentration, scalp massage, heat, aloe vera, vitamins, hypnotherapy, oral psoralens combined with exposure to ultraviolet light in the A range (PUVA), topical cyclosporine, and immunotherapy by induction of contact dermatitis with chemical compounds have all been tried.
- The most important part of widespread AA management is providing **emotional support** to the patient.

POINTS TO REMEMBER

- Alopecia totalis and universalis, the most severe forms of AA, generally spark great emotional problems in patients and their families.
- Consider workup for other diseases (e.g., thyroid disease) that may be suggested by the history or examination.

 HELPFUL HINT

- The National Alopecia Areata Foundation is an excellent resource for information and can direct patients to AA support groups and information about wigs, for example. It can be reached at: National Alopecia Areata Foundation, 14 Mitchell Boulevard, San Rafael, CA 94903; phone number: 415.472.3780; Web site: http://www.naaf.org/default2.asp.

 SEE PATIENT HANDOUT "Alopecia Areata" ON THE SOLUTION SITE

Diffuse Alopecia

POINTS TO REMEMBER

- The evaluation of diffuse hair loss in women—and in men—should be a careful, thoughtful, and sympathetic process.
  - Excessive hair loss should not be dismissed as simply a cosmetic issue.
  - History taking should include questions about the patient's physical and mental health status, antecedent illnesses, medications, traumatic events (e.g., loss of a loved one), hairstyling techniques, and family history.
  - In addition, masculinizing signs or symptoms should be noted.

BASICS

- Diffuse alopecia is defined as a uniform, generally nonscarring reduction in hair density over all portions of the scalp. In contrast, a patterned alopecia such as AGA or alopecia caused by androgen excess has a characteristic presentation of hair loss in specific locations that typically spares the temples and occipital regions.
- A large majority of patients who complain about diffuse hair loss are women.
- Unfortunately, the explanation for such hair loss frequently presents a confusing and frustrating challenge for primary care providers as well as for dermatologists. The diagnosis of the manifestations of telogen and anagen effluvium (described later) is made on the basis of history. In many cases, the hair loss may not be apparent to the examiner and at times the cause may be difficult, if not impossible, to determine.

Telogen Effluvium

- This disorder refers to the shedding of hairs from telogen follicles.
  - Hair follicles show intermittent activity that cycles between a growing anagen phase (lasting approximately 3 years) and a resting telogen phase (lasting about 3 months).
  - Each hair grows to a maximum length and is retained for a period without further growth (telogen). It then goes through a catagen phase, is shed, and is replaced by a growing anagen hair (see Ill. 11.1).
  - At the end of the telogen phase, the hair is lost, and a new hair starts growing within the follicle in a new anagen phase.
  - The normal scalp contains approximately a 100,000 hairs, and about 10% to 15% of follicles are in the telogen phase. Hence, it is normal to shed about 100 hairs per day.
- A telogen effluvium occurs when a large number of hairs (greater than 15%) enter the telogen phase at one time, which results in a sudden and increased number of shedding hairs.
- The precipitating event usually precedes hair loss by 6 to 16 weeks, which is the time required for a catagen hair to become a telogen hair. The marked loss of hair can manifest as a blockage of a bathtub drain, or it may be more subtle and chronic.

Acute Telogen Effluvium

- The acute type lasts for 3 to 6 months.
- The hair shedding is typically sudden, rather than a gradual thinning. The patient may state that the shedding hair may be seen on pillows, on combs and brushes, and in the bathtub, and she or he may bring in a plastic bag full of hair as proof of the dramatic alopecia (Fig. 10.11).

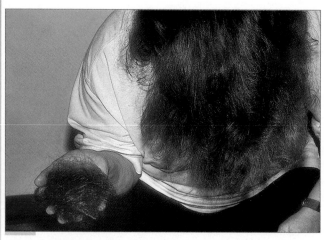

10.11 *Telogen effluvium, acute.* This patient presented with a plastic bag full of hair that had been shed over the course of 1 month.

- The possible causes of acute telogen effluvium include medications, major illness, fever, physical trauma, surgery, general anesthesia, significant weight loss such as that caused by "crash" dieting, or severe emotional stress. The patient may describe a recent history of such an event that typically occurred 3 to 4 months before the onset of alopecia.
- The medications that are most often implicated in acute telogen effluvium are anticoagulants, beta-blockers, cholesterol-lowering medications, antidepressants, angiotensin-converting enzyme inhibitors, propylthiouracil (which induces hypothyroidism), carbamazepine, oral retinoids, and immunizations.
- When an acute telogen effluvium occurs in women in their childbearing years, it may be associated with giving birth (**postpartum effluvium** and **post-breastfeeding effluvium**), aborted pregnancy, or the discontinuation of oral contraceptives.

Chronic Telogen Effluvium

- The chronic type lasts for more than 6 months.
- This type may be caused by the persistent presence of a trigger (such as medications) or by a rapid succession of several acute telogen effluviums. Chronic telogen effluvium may also have metabolic causes, such as **iron** or **zinc deficiency,** or result from low-protein diets, thyroid disease, or chronic systemic illnesses such as systemic lupus erythematosus or syphilis.
- The patient may complain of both increased shedding, albeit less severe than in acute telogen effluvium, and hair thinning is manifested by a more visible scalp.

DESCRIPTION OF LESIONS AND CLINICAL MANIFESTATIONS

- This diffuse (nonpatterned) hair shedding involves the entire scalp and is usually not obvious to the clinician. Scarring and inflammation of the scalp are not seen.
- Occasionally, patients state that the scalp hair simply feels less dense, that more of the scalp seems to be visible, and that the hair has changed in texture. This is often seen in chronic telogen effluvium. Complete alopecia is not seen.
- If the precipitating event is removed, it usually takes about 1 year to completely return to the pre-effluvium hair volume, but hair may not grow back completely.

DIAGNOSIS

- The diagnosis is more often based on history, because the diffuse loss of telogen effluvium is more often barely perceptible to the clinician.
- There is a loss of 400 or more hairs per day (normal shedding is 40 to 100 hairs a day). A gentle hair pull (of approximately 20 hairs) often yields more than four hairs per pull. The lost hairs are telogen hairs that can be identified by having a small white "bulb" at their proximal ends.
- A scalp biopsy reveals an increased telogen-to-anagen ratio (above 15%).

Laboratory Tests

When the cause of telogen effluvium is not apparent, the following laboratory tests should be assessed when warranted by the history or physical examination:

- Baseline chemistries and liver function tests may detect a systemic cause of hair shedding.
- A complete blood count, sexually transmitted disease testing, and antinuclear antibody tests should be performed.
- Thyroid-stimulating hormone level should be determined.
- Serum ferritin and erythrocyte sedimentation rate (ESR) levels should be tested, because both ESR and ferritin determinations can be elevated as acute-phase reactants. A ferritin value greater than 50 μg/L is optimal.
- Serum dehydroepiandrosterone-sulfate (DHEA-S), free testosterone, prolactin, and morning cortisol levels should be obtained if virilization is evident.
- When diffuse AA is suspected, or an inflammatory or scarring alopecia is present, a scalp biopsy may be necessary to make the diagnosis.

MANAGEMENT

- The patient should be reassured that, most often, hair tends to grow back normally.
- The management of telogen effluvium often involves treating or eliminating the underlying cause. Once the trigger is removed, it may be sufficient simply to wait for the hair to grow back.
- Consultation with a dietitian may sometimes be necessary to ensure adequate caloric, vitamin, iron, zinc, and protein intake.
  - Iron supplementation and correction may reverse the chronic telogen effluvium caused by this deficiency.
  - However, correction of thyroid function unfortunately does not always result in a reversal of the effluvium.

 DIFFERENTIAL DIAGNOSIS

Androgenic Alopecia
See earlier discussion of AGA.

- This has a patterned distribution.

Anagen Effluvium Secondary to Drugs
See discussion later in this chapter.

- It is more diffuse and more rapid than telogen effluvium.
- Cancer chemotherapy and immunotherapy drugs are causes.

 POINTS TO REMEMBER

- A careful history should be taken to look for antecedent illness, recent childbirth, ingestion of drugs, or trauma 3 to 4 months before the onset of rapid alopecia.
- In women with AGA, there is usually a positive family history of patterned alopecia. However, because AGA is quite prevalent, it should also be kept in mind that a diffuse alopecia may coexist with AGA.

Anagen Effluvium

BASICS

- In comparison with telogen effluvium, anagen effluvium produces a more extensive and a more rapid and dramatic hair loss.
- At any given time, 80% to 90% of hair follicles on the scalp are in the anagen stage; hence a tremendous amount of shedding may occur.

Pathogenesis

- Anagen effluvium is usually precipitated by a toxic event, such as a reaction to certain drugs. However, an acute and severe systemic illness such as systemic lupus erythematosus (SLE) may also result in an anagen effluvium. The dramatic hair loss usually starts 1 to 2 weeks after the precipitating event.
- Among the agents that have been commonly associated with anagen hair loss are:
  - Drugs used for cancer chemotherapy (e.g., doxorubicin, nitrosoureas, cyclophosphamide)
  - Immunotherapeutic medications (cyclosporine, methotrexate, colchicine)
  - Intoxication of thallium or mercury
  - Radiation therapy

CLINICAL MANIFESTATIONS

- Anagen effluvium presents as a diffuse, nonscarring, noninflammatory type of hair loss (FIG. 10.12). Hence, the presence of scale, pustules, or scars indicating inflammation may suggest a different cause for the hair loss.
- The hair pull is grossly positive, pulling more than four hairs per pull. In contrast to telogen effluvium, pulled hairs have a tapered end that is caused by the sudden cessation of hair shaft production.

DIAGNOSIS

- The diagnosis tends to be straightforward because of an obvious triggering event, such as chemotherapy.

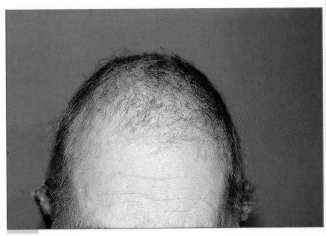

10.12 *Anagen effluvium.* This patient's alopecia resulted from chemotherapy for lung cancer. Her hair loss was diffuse, and her hair is now regrowing.

 MANAGEMENT

- Management of anagen effluvium simply involves the identification and removal, if feasible, of the precipitating cause.
- Laboratory tests are not necessary unless causes of telogen effluvium or intoxication are suspected.
- Local cooling of the scalp has been proposed to prevent hair loss during chemotherapy.

Prognosis

- Anagen effluvium is entirely reversible, and patients should be reassured that the hair loss is temporary. New hair growth starts a few weeks after the termination of treatment. However, the color and texture of the new hair may be different.

MANAGEMENT

- No treatment has been shown to be effective for this condition.
- Patient education and reassurance that this type of hair loss is part of the normal process of aging may be helpful.

Senescent Alopecia

BASICS

- Aging results in a gradual decrease of scalp hair density. Whereas a newborn has about 1,100 hairs per square centimeter, by age 30 this has decreased to about 600 hairs per square centimeter, and by age 50 this has further decreased to about 500 hairs per square centimeter.
- This type of alopecia affects men and woman equally and is seen in patients 50 years and older.

CLINICAL MANIFESTATIONS

- Patients generally complain of thinning of the scalp and do not report increased shedding.
- Senescent alopecia is a diffuse, nonscarring, noninflammatory type of hair loss. It represents a diagnosis of exclusion.

BASICS

- Scarring alopecia, also known as **cicatricial alopecia,** comprises a large group of heterogenous disorders. Based on the pathogenic mechanism, they can be divided into inflammatory and noninflammatory categories. The inflammatory alopecias can be further subdivided into either infectious (see Chapter 7, "Superficial Fungal Infections: Tinea Capitis") or noninfectious groupings.
- This section will focus on the scarring alopecias that are caused by an inflammatory noninfectious process. Such scarring alopecias affect all ethnic groups and races; however, certain types of scarring alopecias are more prevalent in African-American and Afro-Caribbean women.
- Because many African-American and Afro-Caribbean women use grooming techniques to straighten the natural kinkiness of their hair, a traumatic alopecia can be a consequence of these practices. Alopecia may result from the use of hair reshaping products (e.g., relaxers, straighteners, hot combs, foam rollers, and permanent wave products) or hair braiding methods (e.g., cornrows) that are popular in the black community.
- It is a common misconception that these techniques are used solely to make hair more becoming and stylish; in fact, they are used as much to make hair more manageable. Traction alopecia, chemical alopecia, and hot-comb alopecia (also known as follicular degeneration syndrome) may be caused by the use of any of these methods, either alone or in combination, and may ultimately result in permanent alopecia.

Pathogenesis

- There are many hypotheses regarding the pathogenesis of some of the scarring alopecias, including autoimmune phenomena, superantigen response of cytokines, infection, and altered host response.
- Also, certain hairstyling practices can result in damage and permanent destruction of the hair follicles (see discussion of the variant central centrifugal cicatricial alopecia).

CLINICAL MANIFESTATIONS AND COURSE

- The initial symptoms of scarring alopecia are caused by inflammation of the scalp. The patient may complain of an itching or burning sensation. In its early stages, there is no

obvious hair loss or scarring noted. The diagnosis is often missed in this initial presentation, and the patient may be told by the clinician that he or she has "excessive dandruff" or "seborrheic dermatitis." The patient may then be advised to shampoo more often with an antidandruff shampoo; this often results in exacerbation of symptoms.
- As the disease progresses, the hair loss becomes more apparent. The loss of follicular orifices (ostia or pores) is a key feature of scarring alopecia, differentiating it from AA (see earlier discussion), a nonscarring inflammatory alopecia in which the follicular orifices remain intact and indicate that scarring has not taken place.
- The process can further evolve into patches of alopecia that can coalesce into larger areas. The skin within the areas of hair loss may have a thin, shiny, atrophic appearance and may spread centrifugally, with an area of central scarring surrounded by an expanding periphery of erythema (inflammation).

Chronic Cutaneous Lupus Erythematosus

See also Chapter 25, "Cutaneous Manifestations of Systemic Disease."

BASICS

- Chronic cutaneous lupus erythematosus (CCLE) accounts for about one third of cases of cicatricial alopecia. It occurs more frequently in African-American women. Evidence of SLE or other cutaneous signs of lupus may or may not be present.
- Discoid lupus erythematosus—so-named for its discoid, or disk-shaped, lesions—is by far the most common form of CCLE.
- SLE, unlike CCLE, may lead to telogen effluvium, which typically presents as a diffuse nonscarring type of hair loss (see earlier discussion). Occasionally, the scarring alopecia of CCLE can be seen in a patient with SLE.

CLINICAL MANIFESTATIONS

- Typically, the patient with CCLE presents with patches of alopecia on the scalp that are red, atrophic, and mottled (representing areas of hypo- and hyperpigmentation) (FIG. 10.13).
- Lesions may be quite pruritic.
- Other similar lesions may be observed on the conchae of the external ears or elsewhere on the body.

DIAGNOSIS

- A scalp biopsy for regular hematoxylin/eosin (H/E) staining demonstrates a lymphocytic infiltrate, and direct immunofluorescence may be helpful in making the diagnosis.
- Serologic studies can be helpful; however, the vast majority of CCLE cases do not demonstrate the presence of antinuclear antibodies.

> **SOME COMMON CAUSES OF SCARRING ALOPECIA**

- Chronic cutaneous lupus erythematosus
- Lichen planopilaris
- Central centrifugal cicatricial alopecia
- Traction alopecia
- Sarcoidosis
- Folliculitis decalvans
- Pseudofolliculitis barbae (see later in this chapter)
- Acne keloidalis (see later in this chapter)

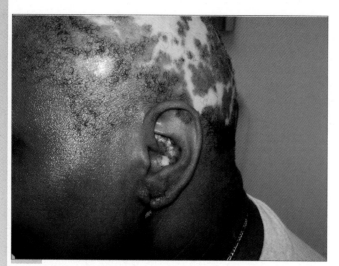

10.13 *Chronic cutaneous lupus erythematosus.* Extensive scarring alopecia, as well as typical discoid lesions, are seen in this patient.

 MANAGEMENT

- Topical **superpotent corticosteroids** or **intralesional corticosteroid injections** are the first-line therapy for CCLE. **Hydroxychloroquine** (200 to 400 mg/day) is often effective, but glucose-6-phosphate dehydrogenase (G6PD) deficiency screening is required prior to treatment because patients with G6PD deficiency are more prone to the hematologic side effects of this drug. Patients taking hydroxychloroquine need to be monitored for anemia and require retinal examination prior and during treatment because of the potential retinopathy.
- Other therapies that have been used include **dapsone**, **isotretinoin,** and **thalidomide.** The goal of treatment is to alleviate the scalp pruritus or discomfort, decrease inflammation, and prevent further destruction of the hair follicles.

 HELPFUL HINT

- When faced with a scarring alopecia in a woman of color, it is very important to rule out fungal infection of the scalp (tinea capitis), which can lead to a scarring alopecia.

Lichen Planopilaris

BASICS

- Lichen planopilaris (LPP) accounts for approximately another third of cases of scarring alopecia. Lichen planus (LP) is an idiopathic eruption with characteristic papules on the skin, nails, and mucous membranes (see Chapter 4, "Inflammatory Eruptions of Unknown Cause"); however, sometimes the scalp may be involved.
- The inflammation may result in a scarring alopecia, which is then referred to as LPP to highlight the hair follicle involvement (*pilaris* refers to hair).
- In most cases of LPP, the inflammation is limited to the scalp, and typical LP lesions are not seen elsewhere on the skin.

Etiology

- LPP and LP are considered to result from a cell-mediated immune response of unknown origin.

CLINICAL MANIFESTATIONS

- Patients who have LPP initially present with erythema and burning of the scalp; the condition progresses to the development of patchy alopecia, most commonly on the vertex of the scalp. Typically, there is perifollicular erythema and scale (FIG. 10.14).
- Hair casts, which are white, sleevelike structures that encircle the hair shaft, can sometimes be noted in LPP.
- Tufting or polytrichia, which are clumped hairs caused by surrounding scarring, are often seen. The condition tends to be progressive but "burns out" after several years.

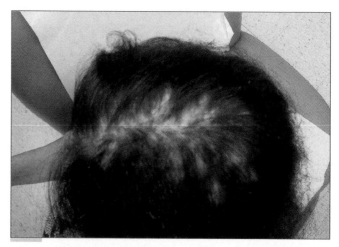

10.14 *Lichen planopilaris.* This woman has patchy areas of cicatricial alopecia. The affected skin is smooth, white, and devoid of erythema or pores, causing the so-called "footprints in the snow" appearance.

- There is great variability in the severity of LPP. **Frontal fibrosing alopecia** (which affects the frontal area of the scalp) has recently been described and is believed to be a subtype of LPP.

DIAGNOSIS

- A scalp biopsy for regular H/E staining, demonstrating a lymphocytic infiltrate, may be helpful in making the diagnosis.
- Serologic studies to help exclude connective tissue disease are recommended. Hepatitis C as well as certain medications (gold, atabrine, and quinacrine) have been associated with LPP. Fungal cultures and or periodic acid–Schiff (PAS) staining should be performed to rule out tinea capitis.

 MANAGEMENT

- **Topical superpotent topical** or **intralesional corticosteroid injections** are the first line of therapy for LPP.
- **Doxycycline** or **minocycline** (100 to 200 mg/day) is often effective in mild cases of LPP.
- Other therapies that have been used include **cyclosporine**, **hydroxychloroquine, dapsone,** and **oral isotretinoin.**

Central Centrifugal Cicatricial Alopecia

BASICS

- Central centrifugal cicatricial alopecia (CCCA) is the current terminology used to describe a type of scarring alopecia mostly seen in African-American women; it is believed to be caused by the use of various chemicals and/or heat to relax the hair. Previously, the traditional terms *hot-comb alopecia* and *follicular degeneration syndrome* were coined to describe this condition.
- Chemicals such as thioglycolates, which are found in commercial styling products, create curls by destroying the disulfide bonds of keratin. These chemicals may also have irritant effects on the scalp that can result in hair shaft damage as well as inflammation of the scalp and loss of hair roots.
- Hot-comb alopecia results from the excessive use of pomades with a hot comb or iron. (Hot combs or pomades alone do not cause permanent alopecia.) On contact with the hot comb or hot iron (i.e., marcelling iron), the pomade liquefies and drips down the hair shaft into the follicle; this results in a chronic inflammatory folliculitis that, in time, can lead to scarring alopecia and permanent hair loss.

CLINICAL MANIFESTATIONS

- Early hair loss is usually asymptomatic and gradual. Later, particularly if chemical relaxers and hot combs are used, scaling, pustules, and itching may occur and result in scarring alopecia.
- Hypopigmentation and hyperpigmentation can be observed in affected scalp areas.
- Tufting or polytrichia can also be noted. Patients often complain of burning or stinging in affected areas.
- As the name CCCA implies, patches of scarring alopecia initially present on the central vertex of the scalp, and the alopecia progressively extends outward in a centrifugal pattern (FIG. 10.15).

DIAGNOSIS

Diagnosis is based on the following:

- Clinical appearance
- History of hair reshaping techniques
- Scalp biopsy, if necessary

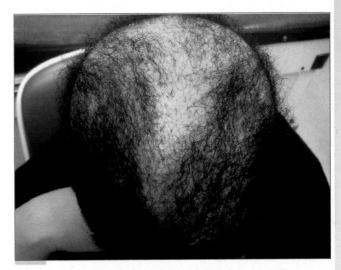

10.15 *Central centrifugal cicatricial alopecia.* The continuous use of chemical relaxers resulted in permanent hair loss at the vertex of this woman's scalp.

 DIFFERENTIAL DIAGNOSIS

- CCCA is not uncommon in black women.
- However, it is important to rule out other causes of scarring alopecias, such as CCLE, LPP, tinea capitis, sarcoidosis, and traction alopecia, which are described in this chapter.

MANAGEMENT

- Treatment of CCCA consists of removing changing or eliminating the damaging hairstyle practices as well as reducing the inflammation. Encouraging the patient to change hairstyle practices requires sensitivity as well as a good understanding of the different hairstyles and practices of black women.
- Natural hairstyles that do not place traction on the hair shaft are recommended.
- Use of mild, lye-free chemical relaxants once every 2 months is suggested, and the use of heat-relaxing devices such as hot combs and hood dryers should be discouraged.
- Anti-inflammatory therapy with an oral tetracycline such as minocycline or doxycycline as well as **topical** or **intralesional corticosteroids** are helpful in the initial phases.
- Once the inflammation is completely resolved, hair transplantation into scarred areas can be used to improve cosmesis.

 POINTS TO REMEMBER

- Although a great majority of black women are using or have used chemical and thermal relaxers, a diagnosis of CCCA should not be made presumptively. A scalp biopsy for H/E staining and direct immunofluorescence, a negative PAS stain, as well as negative or nonreactive connective tissue serologies, helps rule out other causes of scarring alopecias.
- The importance of early diagnosis and initiation of treatment of a scarring alopecia is of the utmost importance, because it can result in the complete destruction of the hair follicle. Once the follicle is replaced by scar tissue, the hair loss is irreversible.

Traction Alopecia

BASICS

- Traction alopecia is seen almost exclusively in African-American and African-Caribbean women of all ages, who are more likely to braid their hair.
  - The condition results from the prolonged trauma to the hair follicle by such hairstyles such as cornrows and braiding.
  - The persistent physical stress of traction injury caused by tight rollers and tight braiding or ponytails causes hair loss.
- In addition, the use of hair dryers (with resultant overheating of hair shafts) and the practices of vigorous combing or brushing as well as bleaching can also contribute to hair breakage.

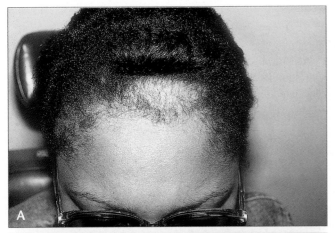

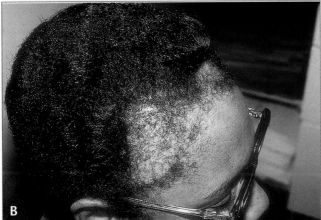

10.16 A and B *Traction alopecia.* A: This woman's alopecia is the result of the use of tight curlers. Note the symmetric loss of hair in a frontotemporal distribution and the "relaxed" curl that was chemically straightened. **B:** Note the fringe of residual hairs at the distal margin of alopecia. These hairs were too short to be "grabbed" by the hair curlers.

CLINICAL MANIFESTATIONS

- Traction alopecia is manifested by a symmetric pattern of hair loss, with broken hairs.
- A characteristic border of residual hairs is often at the distal margin of the hair loss.
- Follicular papules and pustules may be present and can result in permanent scarring alopecia.

DISTRIBUTION OF LESIONS

- Traction pattern: alopecia is evident at the temples and along the frontal hairline (FIGS. 10.16 A and B). Hair loss later extends to the vertex and occipital areas.
- Chemical or hot-comb pattern: hair loss is more irregular (less symmetric) and reflects the areas where the chemicals or hot comb were applied.

- A combination of these patterns may be seen if both traction and hot combs or chemicals are used.

DIAGNOSIS

- The clinical presentation and history are usually sufficient to make the diagnosis.

 MANAGEMENT

- Early intervention and discontinuation of the damaging hairstyles are the mainstays of therapy, because delay may result in irreversible hair loss.

Sarcoidosis

- Hair loss may closely resemble that of traumatic alopecia. However, other signs and symptoms of sarcoidosis are usually apparent. A scalp biopsy of lesional skin may be necessary to distinguish sarcoidosis from traumatic alopecia.
- Sarcoidosis of the scalp is seen most commonly in African-American women. It is usually seen in patients who have other cutaneous or noncutaneous involvement, such as pulmonary sarcoidosis.
- This contrasts with CCLE and LPP, where the scarring alopecia is less likely to be seen in conjunction with other cutaneous or systemic features of these diseases. Clinically, in sarcoidosis, atrophic patches of alopecia that mimic CCLE may be seen.

DIAGNOSIS

- Indications that may be helpful:
  - Scalp biopsy for regular H/E staining demonstrating non-caseating granulomas
  - Evidence of cutaneous sarcoidosis elsewhere on the body or systemic involvement
- Serologic studies to exclude connective tissue diseases are recommended.

 MANAGEMENT

- Potent topical, **intralesional,** or **oral corticosteroids** may be used to control sarcoidosis of the scalp.
- Antimalarial agents such as **hydroxychloroquine** may be used in refractory cases.

Folliculitis Decalvans

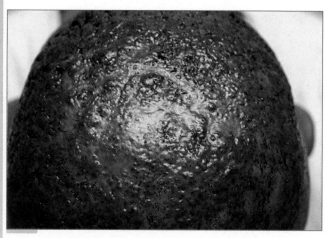

10.17 *Folliculitis decalvans.* Extensive inflammation, pustules, and scarring are present.

BASICS

- Folliculitis decalvans presents as a scarring patch surrounded with follicular pustules.
- Successive crops of peripheral pustules result in an expanding patch or patches of scarring alopecia (FIG. 10.17).

DIAGNOSIS

Bacterial cultures from the follicular pustules often grow *Staphylococcus aureus*. This condition does not merely represent a bacterial folliculitis; rather, an abnormal immune response to possible staphylococcal antigens may be involved.

- A scalp biopsy for H/E staining demonstrates a scarring alopecia with a neutrophilic infiltrate.
- It is important to rule out tinea capitis, which can also present as a pustular scarring alopecia.

Rx MANAGEMENT

- Prolonged antistaphylococcal treatment is recommended, either **monotherapy (erythromycin, tetracycline, cephalexin)** or **combination therapy (rifampin plus clindamycin or cephalexin)**.
- **Topical antibiotic agents** and topical corticosteroids may be used in conjunction with systemic therapy.
- **Zinc sulfate** (30 to 60 mg, three times daily) has been reported to be helpful in some cases.

Pseudofolliculitis Barbae and Acne Keloidalis

BASICS

Hair follicle problems are very common in men and women of African-American, African-Caribbean, and Hispanic origin who have tightly curled hair. Postadolescent African-American men, in particular, experience "shaving bumps" (pseudofolliculitis barbae) and a characteristic acnelike, scarring condition located on the occiput referred to as acne keloidalis.

Pseudofolliculitis Barbae

- Tightly coiled hairs emerge from curved hair follicles (ILL. 10.1)
  - When shaved, the hair becomes a sharp tip that curves downward as it grows and reenters the epidermis, or the sharpened hair may grow parallel to the skin and penetrate it.
  - Furthermore, newly erupting hairs from below may pierce and aggravate areas that are already inflamed.
- Thus, growing hairs act as traumatic vehicles that produce an inflammatory foreign body–like reaction.

DESCRIPTION OF LESIONS

- On close inspection, tight, curly hairs that have been sharpened by shaving and penetrate the skin are noted.
- Inflammatory papules and pustules ensue (FIG. 10.18).
- Ultimately, persistent flesh-colored papules that represent hypertrophic scars and postinflammatory pigmented lesions become prominent clinical features.

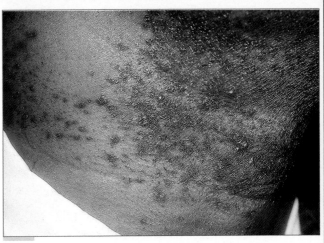

10.18 *Pseudofolliculitis barbae.* Tight, curly hairs that have been sharpened by shaving penetrate the skin. Inflammatory papules and pustules that resemble acne are evident.

DISTRIBUTION OF LESIONS

- Lesions are seen on the beard, particularly on the neck and the submental areas.

 DIFFERENTIAL DIAGNOSIS

- Acne vulgaris
- Bacterial folliculitis

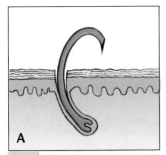 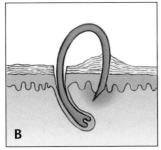 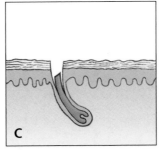 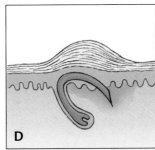

I10.1 Pseudofolliculitis barbae, or "razor bumps," showing extrafollicular and transfollicular penetration. **A:** A curly hair grows from a sharply curved hair root. When shaved, the hair is left with a sharp point. As this hair grows, the sharp tip curves back and pierces the skin. **B:** The sharpened hair penetrates the skin. **C and D:** When hairs are cut too closely, they can penetrate the side of the hair root. Both types of follicular reentry cause a foreign body–like reaction (papule). (Modified from Crutchfield CE III. The causes and treatment of pseudofolliculitis barbae. *CUTIS* 1998;61:351–356, with permission.)

MANAGEMENT

Preventive Measures

- Discontinuance of shaving is only partially helpful; however, this is generally not a choice desired by most patients.
- Patients may avoid close shaving by using a guarded razor (e.g., PFB Bump Fighter). This razor is covered with a plastic coating that prevents the razor from contacting the skin directly. The use of an electric razor is another method that reduces the closeness of the shave.
- Hairs may be lifted with a fine needle or a toothpick before they penetrate the skin (Fig. 10.19).
- Patients should be advised not to pluck hairs because new hairs will again grow from below and penetrate a site that is already inflamed.

Treatment

- Treatment is difficult.
- **Nonfluorinated, class 5 or 6 topical steroids** are used for inflammation and itching.
- Used once daily, topical antibiotics such as erythromycin 2% (**Akne-mycin**) ointment or **BenzaClin** or **Duac gel** (these combine clindamycin and benzoyl peroxide) often reduce inflammation.
- Systemic antibiotics such as **minocycline** are helpful when marked inflammation and pustulation are present.
- Chemical depilatories such as **Magic Shave** and **Royal Crown powders** are effective in removing and softening

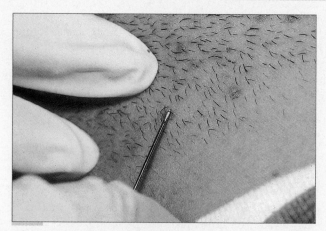

10.19 *Pseudofolliculitis barbae.* A curled hair is lifted with a fine needle after it had penetrated the skin.

hairs; the main disadvantages are that they are irritating and they have an unpleasant odor.
- Hair destruction using an **extended-pulse width laser** has been shown to be effective.
- Eflornithine hydrochloride 13.9% (**Vaniqa**) is an enzyme inhibitor that slows hair growth (see Chapter 11, "Hirsutism").
- **Electrolysis** is difficult to use on inflammatory foci, but it can be partially effective as an adjunctive treatment method.

Acne Keloidalis (Folliculitis Keloidalis)

BASICS

- The name **acne keloidalis** is actually a misnomer. It has nothing to do with acne but is actually a type of folliculitis.
- The pathogenesis of acne keloidalis is similar to that of pseudofolliculitis barbae (see previous section), in which coiled hairs produce a reentry phenomenon that results in characteristic features.

DESCRIPTION OF LESIONS

- Initially, inflammatory papules and pustules are noted.
- Ultimately, hypertrophic scarring occurs, characterized by flesh-colored papules (FIG. 10.20) and possibly keloid formation.

DISTRIBUTION OF LESIONS

- This condition is characteristically seen in the lower occipital area, but it can extend to the adjacent or the entire scalp and thus may be indistinguishable from folliculitis decalvans (FIG. 10.21; see FIG. 10.17).

 MANAGEMENT

- **Potent topical or intralesional steroids** (5 to 10 mg/mL) help decrease itching and inflammation.
- **Topical antibiotics** are used when papules and pustules are present.
- A systemic antibiotic such as **minocycline** seems to be helpful because of its anti-inflammatory effect.
- Surgical treatment is not without risk. It is reserved for extreme cases and may result in worse scarring.

 SEE PATIENT HANDOUT "Pseudofolliculitis Barbae (Razor Bumps)" ON THE SOLUTION SITE

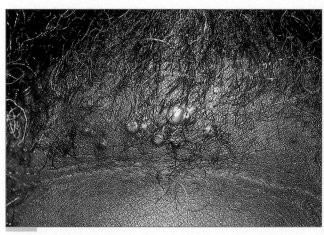

10.20 *Acne keloidalis.* Hypertrophic scarring and flesh-colored papules are seen in this patient.

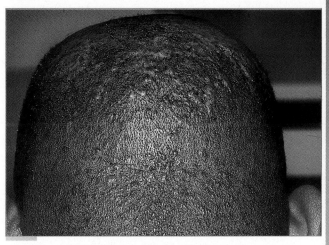

10.21 *Acne keloidalis and scalp folliculitis.* Here the problem extends to the adjacent scalp.

 POINTS TO REMEMBER

- When bacterial folliculitis is present, it is usually the result of secondary, not primary, pathogens.
- Prevention of these disorders also depends on avoidance of close "clipper" shaves and haircuts.

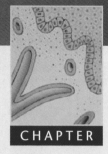

Hirsutism

11

OVERVIEW

Hirsutism is defined as the excessive growth of thick, dark hair in locations where hair growth in women is normally minimal or absent. Such male-pattern growth of terminal body hair usually occurs in androgen-stimulated locations, such as the face, chest, and areolae.

Although the terms *hirsutism* and *hypertrichosis* are often used interchangeably, hypertrichosis actually refers to excess hair (terminal or vellus) in areas that are not predominantly androgen dependent. Whether a given patient is hirsute is often difficult to judge because hair growth varies among individual women and across ethnic groups. What is considered hirsutism in one culture may be considered normal in another. For example, women from the Mediterranean region and Indian subcontinent have more facial and body hair than do women from Asia, sub-Saharan Africa, and Northern Europe. Dark-haired, darkly pigmented individuals of either sex tend to be more hirsute than blond or fair-skinned persons. In women, hirsutism exceeding culturally normal levels can be as distressing an emotional problem as the loss of scalp hair.

BASICS

- Hirsutism, by itself, is a benign condition primarily of cosmetic concern.
- However, when hirsutism in women is accompanied by masculinizing signs or symptoms, particularly when these arise well after puberty, it may be a manifestation of a more serious underlying disorder, such as an ovarian or adrenal neoplasm. Fortunately, such disorders are rare.

Pathogenesis

- Hirsutism can be caused by abnormally high androgen levels or by hair follicles that are more sensitive to normal androgen levels. Therefore, increased hair growth is often seen in patients with endocrine disorders characterized by hyperandrogenism, which may be caused by abnormalities of either the ovaries or the adrenal glands.

- The physiologic mechanism proposed for androgenic activity consists of three stages: (a) production of androgens by the adrenals and ovaries, (b) androgen transport in the blood on carrier proteins (principally sex hormone–binding globulin [SHBG]), and (c) intracellular modification and binding to the androgen receptor.
- In short, central overproduction of androgen, increased peripheral conversion of androgen, decreased metabolism, and enhanced receptor binding are each potential causes of hirsutism. For circulating testosterone to exert its stimulatory effects on the hair follicle, it first must be converted into its more potent follicle-active metabolite, dihydrotestosterone. The enzyme 5-α-reductase, which is found in the hair follicle, performs this conversion.
- The severity of hirsutism does not correlate with the level of increased circulating androgens because of individual differences in androgen sensitivity of the hair follicles.
- Testosterone stimulates growth, thereby increasing size and intensifying the pigmentation of hair. Estrogens act in an opposite manner by slowing growth and producing finer, lighter hairs. Progesterone has minimal effect on hair growth.

Cycles of Hair Growth

Hair grows in long cycles over many months: an anagen (active) phase (ILL. 11.1) is followed by a catagen (degenerative) phase, then a telogen (resting) phase, with different hairs alternating phases. The anagen and telogen phases are hormonally regulated. During the telogen phase, the hair shaft eventually separates from the follicle and falls out.

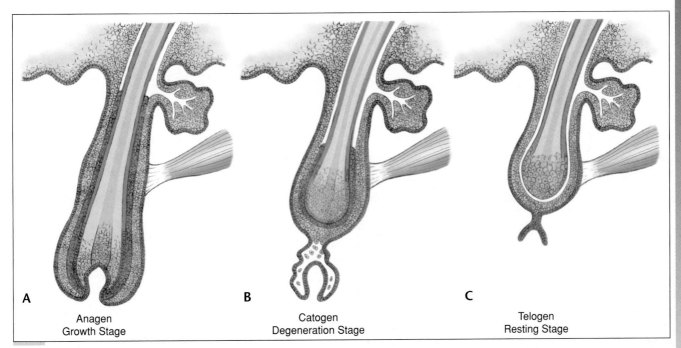

A   Anagen Growth Stage

B   Catogen Degeneration Stage

C   Telogen Resting Stage

I11.1   *Cycles of hair growth.* (Modified from Structure and function of the skin. Sams WM Jr, Lynch PJ, eds. In: *Principles and Practice of Dermatology.* New York: Churchill Livingstone, 1990:8, with permission.)

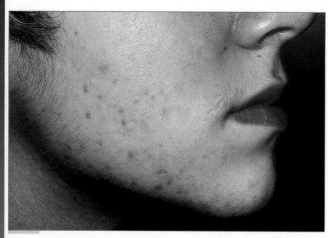

11.1 *Hirsutism.* This patient has PCOS. This is the most common cause of androgen excess and hirsutism. Note the lesions of acne.

The amount of free testosterone—the biologically active androgen that, after conversion to dihydrotestosterone, causes hair growth—is regulated by SHBG. Lower levels of SHBG increase the availability of free testosterone. SHBG decreases in response to the following:

- Exogenous androgens
- Certain disorders that affect androgen levels, such as polycystic ovary syndrome
- Congenital or delayed-onset adrenal hyperplasia
- Cushing's syndrome
- Obesity
- Hyperinsulinemia
- Hyperprolactinemia
- Excess growth hormone
- Hypothyroidism

Conversely, SHBG increases with higher estrogen levels, such as those that occur during oral contraceptive therapy. The resulting increased SHBG levels lower the activity of circulating testosterone.

Disorders Associated with Hirsutism

Polycystic Ovary Syndrome
- The most common cause of androgen excess and hirsutism is polycystic ovary syndrome (PCOS).
  - Virilization is minimal, and hirsutism is often prominent.
  - Characteristic features include menstrual irregularities, dysmenorrhea, occasional glucose intolerance and hyperinsulinemia, and, often, obesity.
  - The hyperinsulinemia is believed to hyperstimulate the ovaries into producing excess androgens.
- Women with PCOS may show other cutaneous manifestations of androgen excess in addition to hirsutism, such as recalcitrant acne (FIG. 11.1), acanthosis nigricans, and alopecia on the crown area of the scalp (a pattern that contrasts with the bitemporal and vertex androgenic alopecia seen in men) (see FIG. 10.2).
- Hirsutism may also be seen in the following ovarian conditions, most of which are associated with virilization:
  - Luteoma of pregnancy
  - Arrhenoblastomas
  - Leydig cell tumors
  - Hilar cell tumors
  - Thecal cell tumors

Familial Hirsutism
- This type of hirsutism is not associated with androgen excess. Familial hirsutism is both typical and natural in certain populations, such as in some women of Mediterranean or Middle Eastern ancestry (FIG. 11.2).

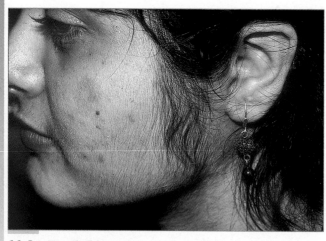

11.2 *Familial hirsutism.* As seen in this Pakistani woman, familial hirsutism is both typical and natural in certain populations.

Drug-Induced Hirsutism

- Drugs that can induce hirsutism by their inherent androgenic effects include dehydroepiandrosterone sulfate (DHEA-S), testosterone, danazol, and anabolic steroids.
- The current low-dose oral contraceptives are less likely to cause hirsutism than were previous formulations.

Adrenal Causes

- Children with **congenital adrenal hyperplasia (CAH)**, the classic form of adrenal hyperplasia, may exhibit hirsutism. Such children may be born with ambiguous genitalia and symptoms of salt wasting and failure to thrive, and they may develop masculine features.
- **Late-onset CAH** affects about 1% to 5% of hyperandrogenic women. Although these patients have clinical features that resemble PCOS, they manifest no salt-wasting symptoms and may not develop signs of virilization and menstrual irregularities until puberty or adulthood (Fig. 11.3).
- **Cushing's syndrome** is a noncongenital form of adrenal hyperplasia. It is characterized by an excess of adrenal cortisol production.
- **Androgen-producing adrenal tumors** are extremely rare.

Other Associated Disorders

- Other less common but potentially serious disorders associated with hirsutism include anorexia nervosa, acromegaly, hypothyroidism, porphyria, and cancer.

Idiopathic Hirsutism

- The few hirsute women who do not have a familial form of hirsutism or any detectable hormonal abnormality are usually given a diagnosis of idiopathic, or end-organ, hirsutism.
  - Such patients have normal menses, normal-sized ovaries, no evidence of adrenal or ovarian tumors or dysfunction, and no significant elevations of plasma testosterone or androstenedione.
- Antiandrogen therapy may improve hirsutism in some idiopathic cases.
  - This suggests that this form of hirsutism may be androgen induced.
  - It is believed that many of these women may have mild or early PCOS and androgen levels in the upper range of normal.

CLINICAL MANIFESTATIONS

The onset of hirsutism can take one of the following forms:

- For example, in women with familial hirsutism, it often appears during puberty.
- Excess growth of facial hair is seen in elderly postmenopausal women and may be caused by unopposed androgen.
- It appears rather abruptly when an androgen-secreting tumor arises.

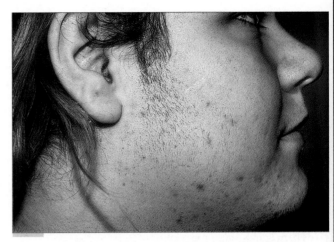

11.3 *Hirsutism in late-onset congenital adrenal hyperplasia.* An 18-year-old woman with clinical features that are similar to those of PCOS: acne, hirsutism, menstrual irregularities, and obesity.

DESCRIPTION OF LESIONS AND OTHER PHYSICAL FINDINGS

- Excess terminal hair grows in a masculine pattern.
- Other accompanying signs and symptoms to look for may include the following:
  - Acanthosis nigricans
  - Obesity
  - Pelvic mass
  - Signs or symptoms of virility
  - Signs or symptoms of Cushing's syndrome
  - Acne
  - Alopecia

DISTRIBUTION OF LESIONS

A woman with hirsutism has excess terminal hair in a masculine pattern in key anatomic sites, including the following:

- Face, particularly the moustache, beard, and temple areas
- Chest, areolae, linea alba, upper back, lower back, buttocks, inner thighs, and external genitalia

DIAGNOSIS

- After familial and drug-induced causes for hirsutism have been excluded, hirsutism resulting from androgen excess should be considered.
- Initial screening for total or free testosterone and DHEA-S often determines whether further testing is necessary. Testosterone and DHEA-S levels may provide clues to the source of excessive androgen production.

Serum Testosterone

- Whether total testosterone is a better screening test than free testosterone is controversial.
  - The evaluation of total testosterone is less expensive and probably easier to interpret.
  - However, free testosterone may be a more sensitive indicator of hormonal level abnormality.
- Testosterone levels vary during the different phases of the menstrual cycle by approximately 25%.
- Early morning measurement of testosterone levels is advised. The upper limit of the reference range for total plasma testosterone levels is 70 to 90 ng/dL.
- No direct correlation exists between the levels of testosterone and the degree of hirsutism, because hirsutism is caused by the action of dihydrotestosterone, which is the more potent testosterone metabolite.
  - Elevated free serum testosterone levels (>80 ng/dL) are found in most women with anovulation and hirsutism.

- In most patients in whom the total testosterone level is greater than 200 ng/dL (>100 ng/dL in postmenopausal women), a tumor workup is indicated. This workup includes a pelvic examination and ultrasound, which usually are adequate to diagnose PCOS. If the test results are negative, an adrenal computed tomography scan is performed.

Serum DHEA-S

- In some patients who are hirsute, DHEA-S is elevated. Moderate elevations suggest an adrenal origin of the hirsutism.
- Normal levels of DHEA-S accompanied by high levels of testosterone indicate that the ovaries, and not the adrenals, are producing the excess androgen.
- A tumor workup is indicated in most patients in whom the DHEA-S level is greater than 700 μg/dL (400 μg/dL in postmenopausal women). An increase of this magnitude usually results from adrenal hyperplasia rather than the extremely rare adrenal carcinomas.

Other Tests

If a woman shows severe or rapidly progressive hirsutism or signs or symptoms of virilism (e.g., infrequent or absent menses, acne, deepening of the voice, male-pattern balding, increased muscle mass, increased libido, clitoral hypertrophy), it may be necessary to perform additional tests.

Serum Androstenedione

- Androstenedione can originate in the adrenal glands or in the ovaries and often is elevated in patients with hyperandrogenism.
- A serum androstenedione level above 100 ng/dL suggests an ovarian or adrenal neoplasm.

Luteinizing Hormone and Follicle-Stimulating Hormone

- Often, in women with PCOS, luteinizing hormone (LH) levels are elevated and follicle-stimulating hormone (FSH) levels are depressed, which results in elevated LH/FSH ratios (>2 is common).
- The evaluation of late-onset CAH and other types of adrenal abnormalities is beyond the scope of this chapter. If Cushing's syndrome is suspected, a 24-hour urinary cortisol or an overnight dexamethasone suppression test should be performed.

DIFFERENTIAL DIAGNOSIS

- **Drug-induced hypertrichosis** should be distinguished from drug-induced hirsutism. In drug-induced hypertrichosis there is a uniform growth of fine hairs that appear over extensive areas of the trunk, hands, and face. This growth is not androgen dependent.
- **Precipitating drugs** include phenytoin, minoxidil (Fig. 11.4), diazoxide, cyclosporine, penicillamine, high-dose corticosteroids, phenothiazines, acetazolamide, and hexachlorobenzene. The exact mode of action is not known, but presumably these agents also exert their effects independent of androgens.

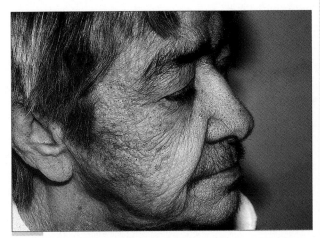

11.4 *Drug-induced hypertrichosis.* Oral minoxidil was the cause of hypertrichosis in this patient.

 ## MANAGEMENT

Overview

- Treatment of hirsutism is unnecessary if no abnormal origin can be diagnosed and if the patient does not find the hirsutism cosmetically objectionable. Treatment should be offered, however, if an underlying disorder is identified or if the patient is troubled by the hair growth.
- Management depends on the underlying cause. For example, non–androgen-dependent excess hair, such as hypertrichosis, is treated primarily with physical hair removal methods. In contrast, those patients who have androgen-dependent hirsutism may require a combination of physical hair removal and medical antiandrogen therapy.
- As an alternative to hair removal, simple bleaching of hair is an inexpensive method that works well when hirsutism is not too excessive. Bleaches lighten the color of the hair so that it is less noticeable.

Hair Removal

Depilation

Depilatories remove hair from the surface of the skin. Depilatory methods include ordinary shaving and the use of chemicals, such as thioglycolic acid.

- **Shaving** removes all hairs, but it is immediately followed by growth of hairs that were previously in anagen; as these hairs grow in, they produce rough stubble. There is no evidence that shaving increases the growth or coarseness of subsequent hair growth. However, most women prefer not to shave their facial hair.
- **Chemical depilation** may be best suited for treatment of large hairy areas in patients who are unable to afford more expensive treatments, such as electrolysis and laser epilation. Chemical depilatories separate the hair from its follicle by reducing the sulfide bonds that are found in abundance in hairs. Irritant reactions and folliculitis may result.

Temporary Epilation

- **Epilation** involves the removal of the intact hair with its root. **Plucking** or **tweezing** is widely performed. This method may result in irritation, damage to the hair follicle, folliculitis, hyperpigmentation, and scarring.
- **Waxing** entails the melting of waxes that are then applied to the skin. When the wax cools and sets, it is abruptly peeled off the skin, and embedded hair is removed with it. This method is painful and sometimes results in folliculitis. Repetitive waxing may produce miniaturization of hairs, and, over the long run, it may permanently reduce the number of hairs.
- Certain **natural sugars,** long used in parts of the Middle East, are becoming popular in place of waxes. They appear to epilate as effectively as, but less traumatically than, waxing.
- **Threading,** a method used in some Arab countries, is a technique in which cotton threads are used to pull out hairs by their roots. Home epilating devices that remove hair by a rotary or frictional method are also available. Both methods may produce traumatic folliculitis.
- **Radiation therapy** was a popular method of hair removal in the past. However, it has fallen out of favor and is no longer acceptable.

continued on page 242

MANAGEMENT *Continued*

Permanent Epilation
Electrolysis and Thermolysis
- Hair destruction by electrolysis, thermolysis, or a combination of both is performed with a fine, flexible electrical wire that produces an electrical current after it is introduced into the hair shaft. Thermolysis (diathermy) uses a high-frequency alternating current and is much faster than the traditional electrolysis method, which uses a direct galvanic current.
- Electrolysis and thermolysis are slow processes that can be used on all skin and hair colors, but multiple treatments are required.
- Electrolysis and thermolysis can be uncomfortable and may produce folliculitis, pseudofolliculitis, and postinflammatory pigmentary changes in the skin.

Laser Epilation
- Lasers can treat larger areas and can do so faster than electrolysis and thermolysis. They have skin-cooling mechanisms that minimize epidermal destruction during the procedure.
- Skin and hair color often determine whether a laser should be used. Lasers are most effective on dark hairs on fair-skinned people. In such patients, lighter skin does not compete with darker hairs for the laser, which selectively targets the pigment (melanin). In dark-skinned people, a newer approach that delivers more energy to the hairs over a longer period may prove safe and effective.
- As with electrolysis and thermolysis, multiple treatments are necessary for long-term hair destruction.
- Folliculitis, pseudofolliculitis, discomfort, and pigmentary changes may result from laser therapy.

- It remains to be proven whether lasers are more effective in permanent hair removal than the more traditional methods. They are certainly more costly.

Pharmacologic Treatment
- In general, pharmacologic treatments for hirsutism are selected based on the underlying cause.
- Medications (**antiandrogens**) are often administered while cosmetic hair removal techniques are being used. All these drugs must be given continuously, because when they are stopped, androgens will revert to their former levels.
- The following medications are all absolutely contraindicated for use during pregnancy because of the risk of feminization of a male fetus:
  - Ovarian suppression (**oral contraceptives**)
  - Androgen receptor blockade and inhibition (spironolactone, flutamide, and cyproterone acetate)
  - Adrenal suppression (**oral corticosteroids**)
  - 5-α-reductase inhibition (**finasteride**)
- These agents can be used singly or in combination.

New Treatments
- **Eflornithine hydrochloride** cream 13.9% (Vaniqa) is a prescription topical cream that acts as a growth inhibitor, not a depilatory. The agent inhibits ornithine decarboxylase, an enzyme required for hair growth. It is indicated for the reduction of unwanted facial hair in women. Twice-daily use for at least 4 to 8 weeks is necessary before effectiveness is noted.
- **Metformin (Glucophage)** reduces insulin levels, and this change in turn reduces the ovarian testosterone levels by competitive inhibition of the ovarian insulin receptors. This drug is effective in treating hirsutism in women with PCOS.

 POINTS TO REMEMBER

- Androgen-stimulated hirsutism may be a marker for androgen excess and may occasionally signal a potentially serious underlying metabolic disorder or potentially fatal neoplasm.
- Expensive hormonal laboratory tests for a woman with simple hirsutism are usually not cost-effective. However, if a woman shows a constellation of virilizing signs or symptoms, such as infrequent or absent menses, acne, deepening of the voice, male-pattern balding, increased muscle mass, increased libido, and clitoral hypertrophy, she should be referred to an endocrinologist.

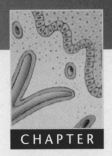

Disorders of the Mouth, Lips, and Tongue

OVERVIEW

Oral mucous membrane lesions are often clues to the presence of systemic illnesses, such as acquired immunodeficiency syndrome (AIDS), syphilis, and systemic lupus erythematosus. They may also be helpful in diagnosing dermatologic conditions, including lichen planus and pemphigus. Lesions such as "canker sores" are often seen as isolated phenomena but may also be an accompaniment or a precursor to a symptom complex, such as that seen in Behçet's syndrome or ulcerative colitis.

It is often difficult to make a clinical diagnosis in the oral cavity. Lesions may resemble normal variants, or they may look like each other.

Inflammatory oral lesions—particularly those that are vesicobullous—rarely remain intact and unruptured. Instead, such lesions usually become erosions and ulcers by the time clinicians see them, adding to the difficulty of diagnosis.

> ➤ **COMMON MANIFESTATIONS INCLUDE:**
>
> - Erosions, blisters, fissures, and ulcers
> - Erosions and ulcers of the tongue
> - Whitish plaques
> - Pigmentary changes
> - Neoplasms
> - Cystic lesions
> - Normal variants

Aphthous Stomatitis

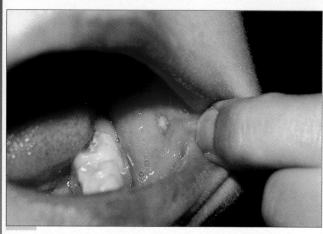

12.1 *Aphthous stomatitis.* A small punched-out erosion has a bright red margin surrounding a gray-white or yellowish center.

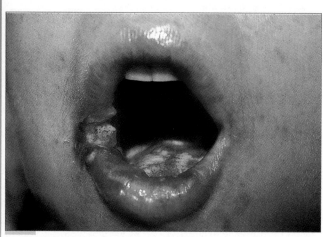

12.2 *Aphthous stomatitis in Behçet's syndrome.* Large, painful erosions and extensive aphthae are evident on the lips and tongue of this woman.

DIFFERENTIAL DIAGNOSIS

The presence of persistent or large painful aphthae broadens the differential diagnosis to include:

- Primary HSV infection
- Autoimmune bullous diseases such as pemphigus vulgaris and bullous pemphigoid
- Recurrent erythema multiforme
- Systemic lupus erythematosus
- Cyclic neutropenia
- Erosive oral lichen planus
- Ulcerative colitis
- Behçet's disease

BASICS

- Commonly known as "canker sores," aphthous stomatitis lesions (aphthous ulcers) are a common, recurrent problem consisting of shallow erosions of the mucous membranes.
- They are seen in children and adults and appear to be more common in women than men.
- Aphthous stomatitis has no known cause, but an immune mechanism is considered the most likely contributory factor.
  - Patients often ascribe recurrences to psychologic stress or local trauma.
  - Women may correlate them with their menstrual cycle.
- Most cases heal spontaneously, only to recur unexpectedly.
- Oral erosions that are indistinguishable from aphthous stomatitis are sometimes seen in primary herpes simplex virus (HSV) infections.

DESCRIPTION OF LESIONS

- The lesions of aphthous stomatitis are small (2 to 5 mm), shallow, well-demarcated, punched-out erosions.
- Lesions typically have a ring of erythema, with a gray or yellowish center (FIG. 12.1).

DISTRIBUTION OF LESIONS

- Lesions may be seen on the buccal, labial, and gingival mucosa, as well as on the tongue (see FIG. 6.27).

CLINICAL MANIFESTATIONS

- The lesions are usually painful.
- They tend to heal in 4 to 14 days, a duration similar to that of HSV lesions.
- Patients with human immunodeficiency virus (HIV) or Behçet's disease may develop aphthous stomatitis lesions that are larger and more persistent, painful, and extensive than those seen in other patients (FIG. 12.2).

DIAGNOSIS

- The diagnosis is made clinically.
- Most intraoral ulcers in immunocompetent patients are canker sores, not HSV lesions.

MANAGEMENT

Therapeutic options for aphthous stomatitis lesions include:

- Symptomatic therapy with topical anesthetic viscous lidocaine (**Xylocaine**) may help.
- **Vanceril** (beclomethasone dipropionate) aerosol can be sprayed directly on lesions.
- Superpotent topical steroids are applied directly to lesions and held there by pressure with a finger.
- **Tetracycline suspension** (250 mg/tsp); patients should "swish and swallow."
- Diphenhydramine (**Benadryl**) suspension; patients are to "gargle and spit."
- Tacrolimus ointment (**Protopic**) 0.1% and (**Elidel**) pimecrolimus cream 1% applied at bedtime may accelerate healing.

- **Silver nitrate,** applied directly to lesions, also can promote healing.
- **Intralesional corticosteroid injections** or a brief course of **systemic corticosteroids** are effective in reducing pain and healing lesions in patients with large, persistent, painful ulcers.
- Recently, **thalidomide** has been used with some success in healing large, painful, persistent aphthae in persons with HIV infection.
  - However, even a single dose of thalidomide has been known to cause fetal malformation.
  - Consequently, women of childbearing potential should use thalidomide only if they receive counseling and use effective contraception.

 POINT TO REMEMBER

- Most intraoral ulcers in immunocompetent patients are canker sores, not HSV lesions; recurrent HSV infection rarely occurs inside the mouth.

HELPFUL HINT

- A single, nonhealing ulcer (lasting more than 2 months) should undergo biopsy to rule out squamous cell carcinoma (FIG. 12.3).

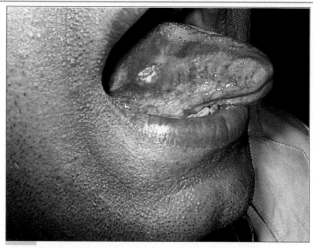

12.3 *Squamous cell carcinoma.* This persistent, non-healing ulceration proved to be a squamous cell carcinoma. (Image courtesy of Ashit Marwah, M.D.)

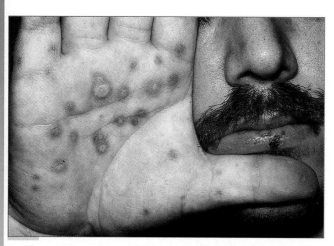

12.4 *Erythema multiforme caused by herpes simplex virus.* This patient has a recurrent HSV infection. Note the drying crust of the herpetic "cold sore" on his lower lip and the targetlike lesions on his palm.

Erythema Multiforme

See also Chapter 18, "Diseases of Vasculature."

Erythema Multiforme Minor

- Erythema multiforme minor is a self-limited eruption characterized by symmetrically distributed erythematous macules or papules, which develop into the characteristic target-like lesions consisting of concentric color changes with a dusky central zone that may become bullous. This is not a disease but a syndrome with multiple underlying causes and associations such as drug reactions, poison ivy contact dermatitis, and, most often, recurrent herpes virus infection.
- A crusted lesion of recurrent HSV may be present on the vermilion border of the lip during an outbreak of erythema multiforme (FIG. 12.4).

Erythema Multiforme Major (Stevens-Johnson Syndrome)

- This is the more serious variant of erythema multiforme. It has extensive mucous membrane involvement, systemic symptoms, and widespread lesions.
- Erythema multiforme major is often accompanied by fever, malaise, myalgias, and severe, painful mucous membrane involvement.
- Hemorrhagic crusts on lips and other mucous membranes are seen in addition to the extensive targetoid lesions elsewhere (Fig. 12.5).

Systemic Lupus Erythematosus

- Erosions or ulcerations can be seen on the oral mucosa.
- See also Chapter 25, "Cutaneous Manifestations of Systemic Disease."

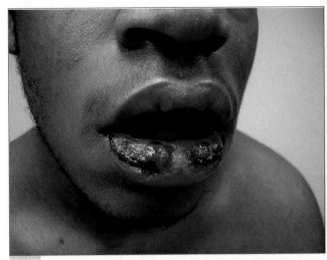

12.5 *Erythema multiforme major (Stevens-Johnson Syndrome).* Bullae and hemorrhagic crusts are noted on the lips of this patient. He has targetoid lesions elsewhere on his body.

Perlèche

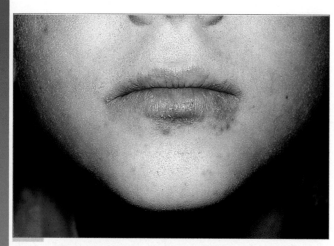

12.6 *Perlèche (angular cheilitis) and atopic cheilitis.* This child has scaling, fissuring, and crusting at the corners of her mouth, as well as eczema of her lips. She also has eczema on other areas of her skin.

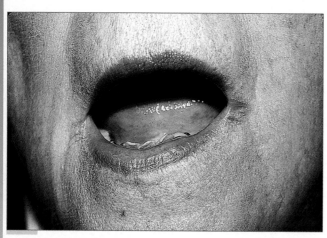

12.7 *Perlèche (angular cheilitis).* This patient's problem was believed to be caused by a problem with her dentures.

- Perlèche (derived from the French word meaning "to lick") is an erythematous eruption that occurs at the corners of the mouth. It is also known as angular cheilitis.
- It is sometimes seen in young patients who have atopic dermatitis, specifically atopic cheilitis (FIG. 12.6).
- It also appears in the elderly and may be caused by aging and atrophy of the muscles of facial expression that surround the mouth, which results in "pocketing" at the corners of the mouth (FIG. 12.7). These pockets become macerated and serve as nidi for the retention of saliva, resulting in the secondary overgrowth of microorganisms such as yeasts and/or bacteria.
- In many instances, perlèche is often simply a form of intertrigo, a common inflammatory condition of skin folds that occurs when opposing moist skin surfaces are in constant contact with each other (see Chapter 3, "Psoriasis").
- Other factors such as poor-fitting dentures, malocclusion, anodontia, and bone resorption may lead to drooling or vertical shortening of the face, thus accentuating the melolabial crease.
  - Lip licking in children, mouth breathing, and orthodontic devices are also risk factors.
  - Vitamin deficiency is often blamed but rarely proved as a cause of perlèche.

CLINICAL MANIFESTATIONS

- Redness, scaling, fissuring, and crusting occur at the corners of the mouth.
- Patients may also have evidence of atopic cheilitis and/or atopic dermatitis elsewhere on the body.

 MANAGEMENT

- A mild topical steroid such as desonide (**DesOwen**) 0.05% ointment, **Elocon** ointment, or over-the-counter **hydrocortisone 1%** cream or ointment often helps resolve the inflammation.
- Petrolatum or other ointments are used to protect and moisturize the area.
- Topical anticandidal (**ketoconazole, clotrimazole, nystatin**) and antibacterial agents (**mupirocin**), either alone or in combination with a class 6 **topical hydrocortisone ointment,** are often effective.
- Topical immunomodulators such as **Protopic ointment 0.1%** or **Elidel 1%** cream may also be tried.
- If necessary, a dental referral is suggested to correct potential causative factors mentioned earlier.
- Injection of **collagen** into the responsible overlapping skin folds has been beneficial in some selected patients.

Mucous Patches of Secondary Syphilis

- The lesions of secondary syphilis on the tongue are known as mucous patches (FIG. 12.8). (For a full discussion of this condition, see Chapter 19, "Sexually Transmitted Diseases," and FIG. 19.18.)
- This condition is characterized by asymptomatic, round or oval, eroded lesions or papules that are devoid of epithelium. The lesions teem with spirochetes.
- A Venereal Disease Research Laboratory test is reactive.

Geographic Tongue

- Geographic tongue, or benign migratory glossitis, is a common idiopathic finding (FIG. 12.9).
- The lesions are areas that are shiny, red, and devoid of papillae and resemble mucous patches. These lesions seem to move about on the surface of the tongue and change configurations from one day to the next, thus accounting for the bizarre, shifting patterns.
- Reports have suggested an association of geographic tongue with psoriasis; however, its 2% incidence in patients with psoriasis is no greater than would be expected in the otherwise healthy population.
- No treatment is necessary.

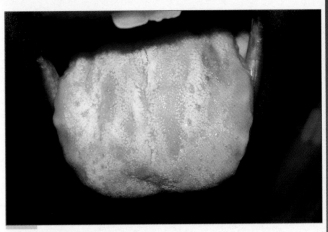

12.8 *Mucous patches of secondary syphilis.* These mucous patches result from eroded epithelium of the tongue.

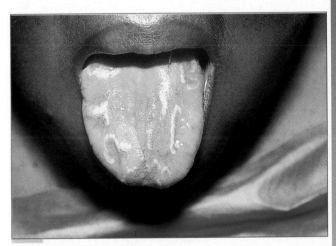

12.9 *Geographic tongue.* Shiny, red patches are devoid of papillae (note the resemblance to the mucous patches shown in FIG. 12.8).

Whitish Plaques

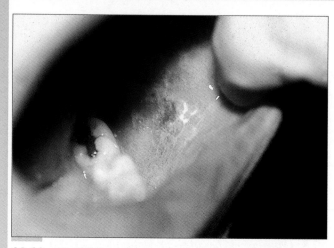

12.10 *Oral lichen planus.* A white, lacy network of lesions and erosions is present on the buccal mucosa. Note the erosions.

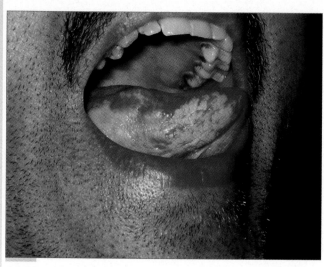

12.11 *Leukoplakia.* (Image courtesy of Ashit Marwah, M.D.)

Lichen Planus

- For a full discussion of this condition, see Chapter 4, "Inflammatory Eruptions of Unknown Cause."

DESCRIPTION OF LESIONS

- A white, lacy network of lesions is present on the buccal mucosa (Fig. 12.10), tongue, or gums.
- The lesions may be erosive, ulcerative, and painful.
- Typical lesions of lichen planus may or may not be present elsewhere on the body.

 DIFFERENTIAL DIAGNOSIS

- White oral lichen planus lesions are often confused with oral candidiasis, oral leukoplakia, and a normal bite line (see Fig. 4.23).

Oral Leukoplakia

- This white macular or plaquelike lesion is considered a precursor to squamous cell carcinoma of the mucous membranes.
- Smoking, chewing tobacco, and ethanol abuse are all contributing factors.
- White adherent plaques are present.
- Lesions occur on the tongue (Fig. 12.11), buccal mucosa, hard palate, and gums.
- Oral leukoplakia may resemble oral lichen planus, oral hairy leukoplakia (see Fig. 12.12), or white plaques caused by trauma.
- Less than 5% of lesions have been reported to develop into squamous cell carcinoma.

Oral Hairy Leukoplakia

- Oral hairy leukoplakia is associated with the Epstein-Barr virus (FIG. 12.12).
- It is seen in patients with HIV infection (see Chapter 24, "Cutaneous Manifestations of HIV Infection") and in transplant recipients.
- Filiform papules that resemble white hairs are seen on the sides of the tongue.
- Lesions are usually asymptomatic.

Candidiasis ("Thrush")

- Oral candidiasis is seen in immunocompromised patients (see Chapter 24, "Cutaneous Manifestations of HIV Infection") and in neonates.
- Curdlike or erosive lesions are easily removed with gauze.
- Lesions may involve the tongue, the oropharynx, and the angles of mouth (angular cheilitis).
- A potassium hydroxide examination or fungal culture is positive.

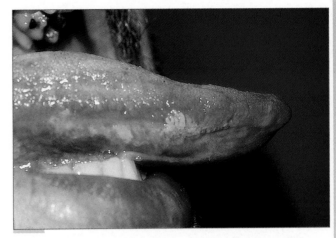

12.12 *Oral hairy leukoplakia.* This patient has AIDS. Note the papules on the sides of the tongue that resemble white hairs.

Pigmentary Changes

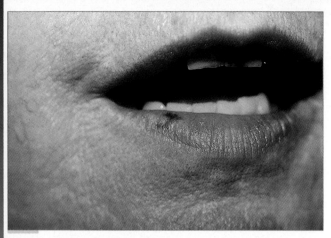

12.13 *Labial melanotic macule.* This is a common, benign, pigmented macule on the lower lip of adults. It is probably caused by sun exposure.

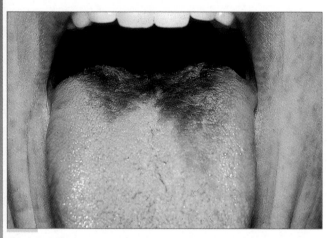

12.14 *Black hairy tongue.* A velvety, hairlike thickening of the tongue's surface is noted. The color can range from a yellowish-brown or -green to jet black.

Labial Melanotic Macule

- This is a common, benign, pigmented macule on the lower lip of adults.
- It is probably caused by sun exposure (FIG. 12.13).

Black Hairy Tongue

- Black hairy tongue is more than just a pigmentary change. Actually, it represents benign, asymptomatic hyperplasia (an accumulation of keratin) or hypertrophy of the filiform papillae of the tongue. The pigmentation results from the normal pigment-producing bacterial flora that colonize the keratin.
- It has been debatably associated with smoking, excessive coffee or tea drinking, and the prolonged use of oral antibiotics, and it is considered by some clinicians as a possible marker for AIDS.

CLINICAL MANIFESTATIONS

- A velvety, hairlike thickening of the tongue's surface is apparent (FIG. 12.14).
- The color can range from a yellowish brown or green to jet black.

 MANAGEMENT

- Brushing with a dilute hydrogen peroxide solution may bleach the pigmented tissue.
- A toothbrush can be used to scrape off the excess keratin.
- Tretinoin 0.05% gel or lotion has also been used.

Pigmentation from Drugs

- A black discoloration of the tongue should be distinguished from black hairy tongue (described earlier). In these cases, there is no hyperkeratosis or hypertrophy of papillae. Oral mucous membrane pigmentation has been noted to result from the following agents:
- Antimalarials (FIG. 12.15), bismuth (FIG. 12.16), chlorhexidine mouth rinses, doxorubicin, fluoxetine, inhalation of heroin smoke, ketoconazole, lomefloxacin, propranolol, risperidone, sulfonamides, terbinafine, tobacco, zidovudine, and all tetracyclines have been associated with pigmentation.
- Artifactual pigmentation has been noted to result from amalgam tattoos and dental fillings.

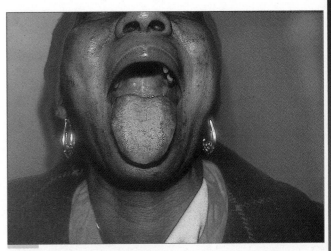

12.15 *Antimalarial hyperpigmentation.* Pigmentation of this patient's tongue is secondary to antimalarial therapy with hydroxychloroquine (Plaquenil).

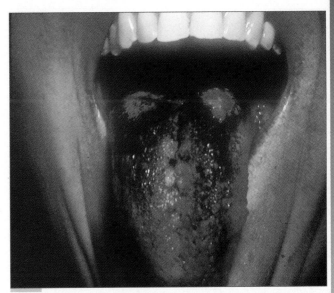

12.16 *Pigment artifact.* The black pigmentation on this patient's tongue was caused by the deposition of bismuth, the active ingredient in Pepto-Bismol. It was easily removed.

Neoplasms

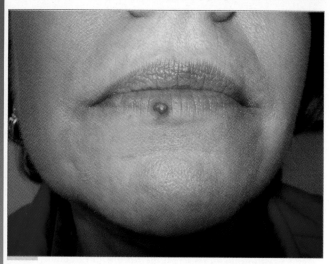

12.17 *Pyogenic granuloma.* This angiomatous-appearing lesion proved to be a pyogenic granuloma after it was biopsied.

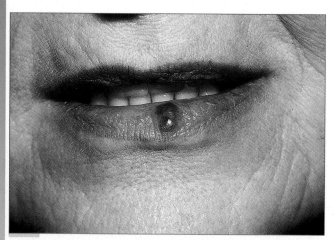

12.18 *Venous lake.* These soft, compressible blebs are common findings on the lips of the elderly.

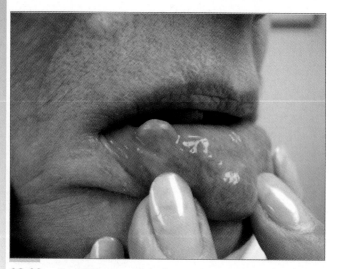

12.19 *Oral fibroma.* This firm nodule may appear on the lip, tongue, or buccal mucosa.

Pyogenic Granuloma

- Pyogenic granuloma is a benign neoplasm (FIG. 12.17) seen on the lips and gums, particularly in pregnant women (see Chapter 21, "Benign Skin Neoplasms").

Venous Lake

- A venous lake (venous varix) is another common benign vascular neoplasm; it usually occurs in patients older than 60 years of age.
- This neoplasm is generally characterized by dark blue to purple macules or papules that may be seen on the lower lip (FIG. 12.18), face, ears, and eyelids.

Oral Fibroma

- Most often observed in adults, oral fibromas are the most common oral neoplasm. Most represent reactive fibrous hyperplasia caused by trauma or local irritation.
- They are seen most often on the buccal mucosa along the plane of occlusion of the maxillary and mandibular teeth. Oral fibromas present as asymptomatic, smooth-surfaced, firm, solitary papules. The diameter may vary from 1 mm to 2 cm. Ulceration caused by repeated trauma may occur (FIG. 12.19).

- The clinical differential diagnosis of a fibroma includes giant cell fibroma, neurofibroma, peripheral giant cell granuloma, mucocele, benign and malignant salivary gland tumors, as well as squamous cell carcinoma (FIG. 12.20).

Solar Keratosis

- For a full discussion, see Chapter 22, "Premalignant and Malignant Skin Neoplasms."
- These lesions are most often seen in elderly men with fair complexions.
- Generally, the lesion is a slow-growing, firm papule or ulcer.
- Initially, it may appear as a nonhealing erosion.
- Solar keratoses are seen most often on the lower lip, where there is maximal sun exposure (FIG. 12.21).

SEE PATIENT HANDOUT "Solar Keratosis (Actinic Keratosis)" ON THE SOLUTION SITE

Squamous Cell Carcinoma

- A squamous cell carcinoma may evolve from a solar keratosis in this area (FIG. 12.22), or it may arise de novo inside the oral cavity.

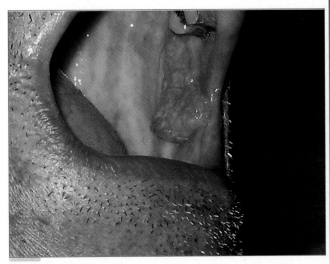

12.20 *Squamous cell carcinoma.* This patient has a nodular squamous cell carcinoma on the buccal mucosa. (Image courtesy of Ashit Marwah, M.D.)

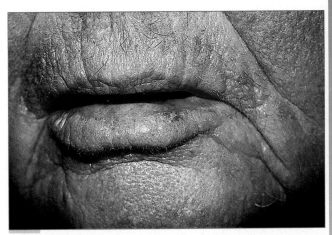

12.21 *Solar keratosis.* Note the erosions and crusting on the lower lip of this elderly patient.

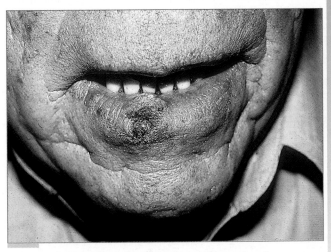

12.22 *Squamous cell carcinoma.* This patient has a squamous cell carcinoma of the lower lip.

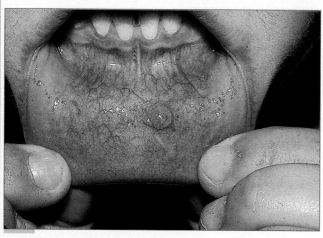

12.23 **Mucocele.** Cystic lesion on the lingual mucosa.

Mucous Cyst

- A mucous cyst (mucocele) (FIG. 12.23) is a common, mucus-filled, blisterlike lesion of the minor salivary glands in the oral cavity. Some authors prefer the term *mucocele* since most of these lesions are not true cysts because of the absence of an epithelial lining. The lesions are considered to be caused by trauma to the openings of salivary glands.
- This condition is seen most commonly in infants, young children, and young adults.

CLINICAL MANIFESTATIONS

- A bluish or clear papule contains mucoid material.
- It is easily ruptured and sometimes recurrent.
- Eventually, the surface of the lesion turns irregular and whitish because of multiple cycles of rupture and healing caused by trauma or puncture.
- The most frequent locations are in the lower lip, floor of the mouth, cheek, palate, retromolar fossa, and dorsal surface of the tongue. These lesions spare the upper lip.
- They may spontaneously disappear, particularly in infants.

 MANAGEMENT

- Patients with a superficial mucous cyst require reassurance only.
- **Cryosurgery** with liquid nitrogen spray may be performed. After 4 to 7 days, a necrotic surface is observed in the treated area. The treated area separates from the surrounding mucosa in 1 to 2 weeks to expose a new epithelialized surface.
  - The advantages of the procedure include simple application, minor discomfort during the procedure, and low incidence of complications (e.g., secondary infection, hemorrhage).
  - However, the possibility of recurrence exists.
- Another therapeutic strategy is **argon laser treatment.**
- **Partial or total electrodesiccation** is also performed.
- **Intralesional injections of triamcinolone acetonide** also have been reported as treatments for mucous cysts; however, these are not used routinely.
- Oral surgery is the treatment of choice for deeper, recalcitrant lesions. **Surgical excision** should include the immediate adjacent glandular tissue.

Odontogenic Sinus
(Cutaneous Dental Sinus Tract)

- Most often, these lesions appear on the chin or lower jaw. The lesion often has a small indentation that results from scarring (FIG. 12.24).
- The pathologic process evolves from an intraoral abscess that forms a sinus tract that dissects subcutaneously and exits through the face or neck. The patient is usually unaware of the underlying dental etiology.
- Often diagnosed incorrectly, this lesion of dental origin often resembles a furuncle, a cyst, a pyogenic granuloma, or an ulceration.

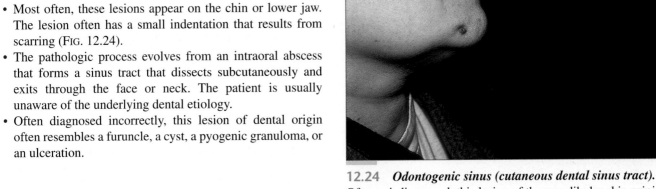

12.24 *Odontogenic sinus (cutaneous dental sinus tract).* Often misdiagnosed, this lesion of the mandibular skin originated in a subjacent dental abscess.

 MANAGEMENT

- Panoramic or apical radiographic examinations help make the diagnosis.
- Treatment may require oral antibiotics, tooth extraction, and/or root canal therapy.

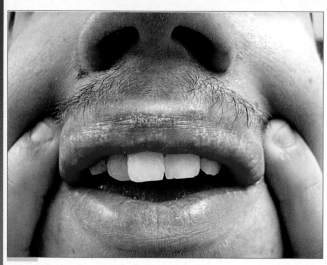

12.25 *Fordyce spots.* Yellow papules on the labial mucosa. These papules are normal variants.

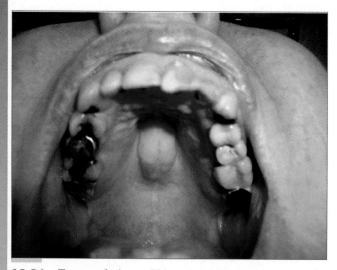

12.26 *Torus palatinus.* This woman has an asymptomatic bony hard swelling located on the midline of her hard palate. The location, clinical appearance, and texture of tori and exostoses are so characteristic that the diagnosis can be made without resorting to biopsy.

Fordyce Spots

- Fordyce spots (FIG. 12.25) are normal findings that represent ectopic mucous glands. They are brought to medical attention when they are noted by the patient.
- The yellow papules occur on the lips or buccal mucosa.
- The lesions are more obvious when the skin is stretched.
- They are incidental findings that require no treatment.

Torus

- Tori are developmental abnormalities that result in overgrowth of mature bone (FIG. 12.26); they differ only by their location.
- These findings have been known to occur more commonly in certain ethnic groups (e.g., Native Americans, Inuit, African Americans, and certain Asian populations). In these groups, the conditions show an autosomal dominant inheritance pattern.
- Treatment is not necessary.

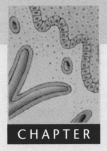

Diseases and Abnormalities of Nails

Herbert P. Goodheart and Hendrick Uyttendaele

OVERVIEW

Mammals use their nails as weapons, as primitive tools, for grooming purposes, for scratching, and for the removal of infestations. Similarly, humans use their fingernails to help pick up small objects and to scratch itchy areas. Fingernails protect vulnerable fingertips; toenails protect toes from the impact of footwear and external trauma. Nails also are important contributors to the aesthetic appearance of the hands and feet.

For the health care provider, nail abnormalities may be the first signal that a systemic disease is present.

➤ **COMMON NAIL PROBLEMS**

- Longitudinal ridging (onychorrhexis)
- Brittle nails (onychoschizia)
- Onycholysis
- Green nail syndrome

➤ **TRAUMATIC LESIONS**

- Subungual hematoma
- Median nail dystrophy

➤ **INFLAMMATORY DISORDERS**

- Psoriasis

➤ **INFECTIONS OF THE NAIL AND SURROUNDING TISSUES**

- Acute paronychia
- Chronic paronychia
- Onychomycosis
- Digital mucous (myxoid) cyst

➤ **NAIL PROBLEMS: MISCELLANEOUS DISORDERS**

- Leukonychia striata
- Yellow nail syndrome
- Koilonychia
- Dermatomyositis
- Subungual verruca
- Junctional nevus
- Terry's nails
- Half-and-half nails
- Dystrophy from preformed artificial nails

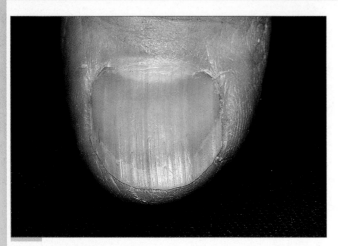

13.1 ***Longitudinal ridging.*** Parallel elevated ridges are characteristic of this normal variant. The ridges may have a beaded appearance.

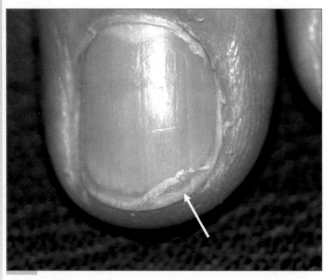

13.2 ***Onychoschizia.*** The distal nail splits into layers parallel to the nail's surface.

Longitudinal Ridging (Onychorrhexis)

Longitudinal ridging is a very common and normal variant in elderly persons. It consists of parallel ridges that run lengthwise along the nail plates (FIG. 13.1). Such ridges are more commonly observed in fingernails than in toenails. Occasionally, longitudinal ridging is seen in younger persons. The etiology is unknown and the condition is not indicative of any trauma, infection, or nutritional deficiency.

 MANAGEMENT

- There is no treatment available to decrease longitudinal ridging, except for filing and buffing the ridges down with a soft file.

Brittle Nails (Onychoschizia)

Brittle and split (onychoschizia) nails are common in adults (FIG. 13.2). In some people, nails become fragile and easily break off at the free edge. This has traditionally been considered a sign of nail plate dehydration; however, a recent study has indicated that the water content of brittle nails is not significantly different from that of normal nails.

Brittle nails are a common complaint in adult and elderly women and can also be observed in people with iron deficiency and thyroid disease. Elderly men are less apt to present with this problem. The increased incidence in women may be a result of their higher cosmetic awareness, their frequent use of nail products, menopausal status, or frequent exposure to harmful extrinsic factors (e.g., detergents or water).

 MANAGEMENT

Traditionally, distal nail splitting has been compared to scaly, dry skin elsewhere on the body. Thus, many treatment recommendations are similar to those for dry skin:

- Avoid excessive contact with water soaps, and other detergents. Wear gloves when washing dishes.
- Gloves should be worn in cold weather.
- Apply moisturizing creams or ointments (e.g., **lactic acid creams** in 5% to 12% concentrations) at bedtime or after bathing or washing.
- Keep the nails short; trim them when they are well hydrated and less likely to be frayed and use a soft file to keep the distal nail edge smooth.
- Consider taking the B_2-complex vitamin supplement **biotin** (2.5 mg/day). Some observers claim to have had some success in increasing nail integrity and thickness with this regimen.

Onycholysis

This finding represents a separation of the nail plate from its underlying attachment to the pink nail bed (FIG. 13.3). The separated portion is white and opaque, in contrast to the pink translucence of the attached portion. Normal physiologic onycholysis is seen at the distal free margin of healthy nails as they grow. It usually starts distally and progresses proximally, causing an uplifting of the distal nail plate. When separation is more proximal, the onycholysis becomes more obvious and becomes cosmetically objectionable. In some patients, the nail takes on a green or yellow tinge (see the discussion of green nail syndrome later in the next section).

Onycholysis is most frequently seen in women, particularly in those with long fingernails. It may become painful and may interfere with routine function of the nails (e.g., picking up small objects, such as coins and paper clips).

Pathogenesis

Whereas onycholysis may sometimes result from onychomycosis (tinea unguium), fungal nail infection is only one cause of onycholysis. The causes of this disorder can be divided into two main types, external and internal.

External Causes

- Irritants such as nail polish, nail wraps, nail hardeners, and artificial nails can cause the problem. Onycholysis may also be seen in persons who frequently come into contact with water, such as bartenders, hairdressers, manicurists, citrus fruit handlers, and domestic workers.
- Trauma, especially habitual finger sucking, athletic injuries to the toes, wearing of tight shoes, and the use of fingernails as a tool, can all cause the disorder.
- Traumatic onycholysis of the toenails can be caused by a lack of appropriate nail care. It is often difficult for elderly patients to trim toenails frequently. This may be a result of arthritis, decreases in fine motor control, or a decline in flexibility. Such difficulties may result in long nails that interfere with shoes fitting properly.
- Fungal infections (e.g., chronic paronychia or onychomycosis) are another cause.
- Some drugs can act as phototoxic agents to induce fingernail onycholysis. Photo-onycholysis usually occurs abruptly on multiple nails at the same time (rather than slowly progressing). Such drugs include diuretics, sulfa drugs, tetracycline, doxycycline, and, particularly, demethylchlortetracycline.

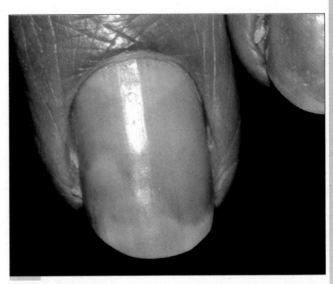

13.3 *Onycholysis.* The separated portion of the nail is white and opaque; the attached portion is pink and translucent.

Internal Causes

- Psoriasis is the most common cause. Patients generally have evidence of psoriasis elsewhere on the body, or there may be other psoriatic nail findings, such as pitting.
- Inflammatory skin diseases of the nail matrix (root), such as eczematous dermatitis or lichen planus, can cause onycholysis.
- Neoplasms and subungual warts are possible causes, especially if only one nail is involved (See FIG. 13.20).
- Other possible internal causes include thyroid disease, pregnancy, and anemia.

 MANAGEMENT

The goal of management is to keep the newly growing nail attached by:

- Keeping nails dry and cut closely; proper trimming (along the contour) on a regular basis can protect the nails from injury
- Using nail polish sparingly
- Avoiding unnecessary manipulation of nails
- Treating or avoiding the underlying cause of the problem, if known

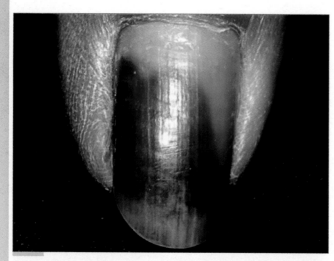

Green Nail Syndrome

This is a consequence of onycholysis. Green nail syndrome is a painless discoloration under the nail and should not be confused with a subungual fungal infection (FIG. 13.4).

Pathogenesis
- The "dead space" under the onycholytic nail serves as an excellent breeding ground for microbes.
- Often, *Pseudomonas* species are present; their presence usually accounts for the green or green-black nail color.

13.4 *Green nail syndrome.* The "dead space" under the nail often harbors *Pseudomonas* species. The green color is virtually pathognomonic for *Pseudomonas*.

 MANAGEMENT

- Soak the affected nail twice daily in a mixture either of one part **chlorine bleach** and four parts **water** or of equal parts **acetic acid (vinegar)** and **water**. This generally eliminates the discoloration.
- If possible, avoid or minimize the underlying cause (i.e., the factor that led to onycholysis, as described in the previous section).

BASICS

- Injuries to the nail root (the matrix that directly underlies the proximal nail fold) may be caused by direct trauma, microbes (e.g., fungi, bacteria), inflammatory conditions (e.g., eczema), or a digital myxoid cyst.
- These disorders sometimes result in characteristic deformities; for example, nail pitting, "oil spots," and onycholysis may be seen in patients with psoriasis.
- At other times, deformities result from eczema in the proximal nail fold.

Traumatic Lesions

Trauma is the most common cause of nail disorders.

Subungual Hematoma

This condition results from trauma to the nail matrix or nail bed, such as repeated minor injuries (e.g., tight shoes, sports injuries) or substantial impact (as from a hammer).

- An acute subungual hematoma that results from rapid accumulation of blood under the nail plate can be very painful (FIG. 13.5), whereas small lesions may be painless and may go unnoticed for some time.
- Chronic, painless subungual hematomas that are clearly not the result of trauma may appear similar to a neoplasm, such as an acral lentiginous melanoma (which is very rare). Because the coagulated bloodstains remain until the nail grows out (for 6 to 12 months), the diagnosis may be in doubt for some time.

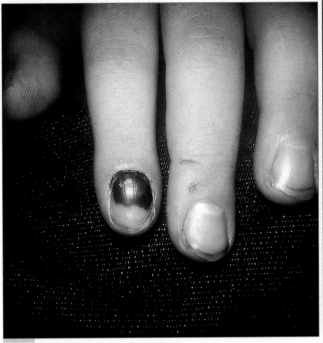

13.5 *Acute subungual hematoma.* This results from the rapid accumulation of blood.

 DIFFERENTIAL DIAGNOSIS

- Junctional nevus is a possibility (see FIG. 13.21; see FIG. 22.51).
- Acral lentiginous melanoma should be considered (see FIG. 22.52).

 MANAGEMENT

- An acute, painful, swollen subungual hematoma may be incised and drained by placing the red-hot end of a heated paper clip on the area elevated by the hematoma. The small hole created with this procedure allows the blood to drain and thus quickly relieves the pain. (Note: This technique is best left to a health professional. Patients with hematomas should not be encouraged to try it themselves.)
- Twirling a 27-gauge needle to create a similar hole is an alternative method for draining the blood.

 POINT TO REMEMBER

- If there is a strong suspicion of melanoma, the nail bed should undergo biopsy.

 HELPFUL HINT

- A rapid method to substantiate the presence of a hematoma is to pare the nail plate gently with a no. 15 scalpel blade or to file it down until the coagulated blood can be visualized.

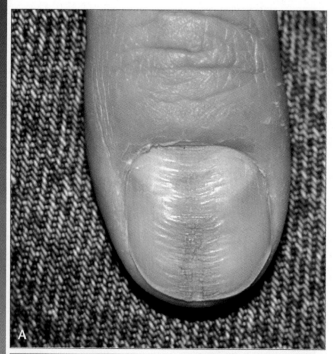

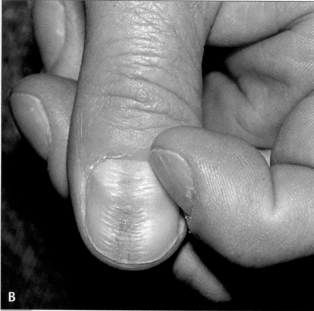

13.6 A and B *Median nail dystrophy.* **A:** Note the vertical ridging ("washboard" appearance) in the nails caused by a habitual tic. After repeated trauma to the proximal nail fold, median nail dystrophy can result. **B:** Most often, the patient habitually presses the nail of the adjacent finger against the proximal nail fold.

Median Nail Dystrophy

- This condition results from a compulsive habit—repeated trauma to the proximal nail fold of the thumb, usually inflicted by the nail of the adjacent index finger (FIG. 13.6). Some patients may do this with both hands, and this causes bilateral damage.
- The resultant nail deformity is analogous to an injury to the root of a tree that deforms the growing tree trunk.

Diagnosis

- The patient can sometimes be observed performing the repeated action without being aware of it. (This is particularly true in children.)

 MANAGEMENT

- Treatment of any habit is difficult; the habit and resultant nail deformity are usually chronic by the time medical attention is sought.
- It can be suggested to patients that breaking this habit may be aided by an alternative activity, such as knitting or needlepoint. Parents may be advised to have children keep tape or another dressing on the affected nails.

Inflammatory Disorders

Inflammatory disorders that involve the nail matrix, such as psoriasis, can result in distinctive deformities of the nails, whereas other conditions, such as eczema of the proximal nail fold, result in nonspecific deformities.

Psoriasis
- The typical nail changes are pitting (FIG. 13.7), onycholysis, thickening (subungual hyperkeratosis), and "oil spots."
- For a more comprehensive discussion, see Chapter 3, "Psoriasis."

Eczematous Dermatitis with Secondary Nail Dystrophy
- Nail deformity secondary to eczematous dermatitis is a problem that is often overlooked in patients with severe atopic dermatitis (FIG. 13.8).
- It results when eczematous dermatitis involves the distal extensor surface of the fingers, and the associated inflammation also involves the matrix, or "root," of the nail. The inflamed matrix, which underlies the proximal nail fold, consequently gives rise to a dystrophic nail plate.

DESCRIPTION OF LESIONS

- Eczematous dermatitis that involves the nail plate is located on the dorsum of the distal part of the finger (the proximal nail fold).
- The nails generally have a ripplelike deformity that corresponds to the time of activity of the inflammation.

 MANAGEMENT

- Improvement of the appearance of the nail plate follows control of inflammation of the proximal nail fold skin with the use of topical steroids.

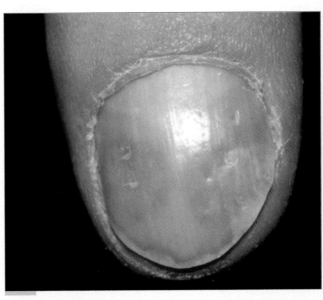

13.7 _Psoriasis._ Pitting, onycholysis, and "oil spots" are evident in this nail.

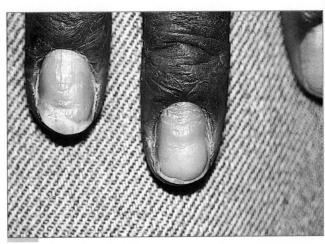

13.8 _Eczematous dermatitis._ The eczema of the proximal skin also affects the matrix (root) of the nail; this results in nail dystrophy.

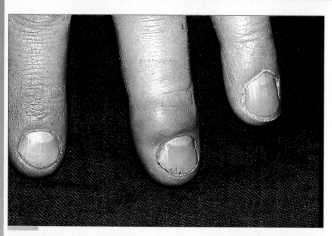

13.9 *Acute paronychia.* Acutely red, tender, unilateral involvement of the proximal nail fold. Often, pus is visible through the proximal or lateral nail fold.

The term *paronychia* refers to inflammation of the nail folds surrounding the nail plate. The condition can be either acute or chronic.

Acute Paronychia

Pathogenesis

- Acute paronychia usually results from an infection caused by *Staphylococcus aureus;* less commonly, it may be caused by streptococci or *Pseudomonas* species.
- Generally, only one nail is involved.
- The condition may occur spontaneously, or it may follow trauma or manipulation, such as nail biting, a manicure, or removal of a hangnail.

CLINICAL MANIFESTATIONS

- Acute paronychia is heralded by the rapid onset of bright red swelling of the proximal or lateral nail fold behind the cuticle.
- A throbbing, tender, and intensely painful lesion often results (FIG. 13.9).

 DIAGNOSIS AND DIFFERENTIAL DIAGNOSIS

- Acute bacterial paronychia can be confused with herpetic whitlow.
- A Tzanck preparation (see FIG. 6.26), bacterial culture, or both must be performed when the diagnosis is in doubt.

 MANAGEMENT

- Mild cases may require only warm saline or aluminum acetate (**Domeboro 1:40**) soaks for 10 to 15 minutes two to four times daily.
- In more severe cases, simple **incision and drainage** (with a no. 11 surgical blade) usually afford rapid relief of pain.
- Occasionally, systemic therapy with antistaphylococcal antibiotics, such as **dicloxacillin,** or a **cephalosporin**, may be needed.

Chronic Paronychia

This condition primarily results from a combination of chronic moisture, irritation, and trauma to the cuticle and proximal nail fold (FIG. 13.10). It occurs much more often in women than in men, and it is particularly common in persons whose hands are frequently exposed to a wet environment, such as housewives, domestic workers, bartenders, janitors, bakers, dishwashers, dentists, dental hygienists, and children who habitually suck their thumbs. It is also seen more often in patients with diabetes and in persons who manicure their cuticles.

The predisposing factor is usually trauma or maceration that produces a break in the barrier (cuticle) between the nail fold and nail plate. This allows moisture to accumulate and microbial colonization to follow.

Pathogenesis
- Although *Candida* is frequently isolated from the proximal nail fold of patients with chronic paronychia, a primary pathogenesis for this organism has never been proven.
  - In fact, evidence indicates that this condition is not a fungal infection at all but is actually an eczematous process.
  - Instances in which *Candida* may play a primary pathogenic role include patients who are diabetic and those with primary mucocutaneous candidiasis.
- For this reason, topical steroids are often a more effective therapy than topical or even systemic antifungal agents.

CLINICAL MANIFESTATIONS
- Chronic paronychia usually develops slowly and asymptomatically.
- Secondary nail plate changes often occur, including onycholysis (see earlier discussion). A greenish or brown discoloration along the lateral borders and transverse ridging of the nails may appear.
- One or more fingers can be involved.

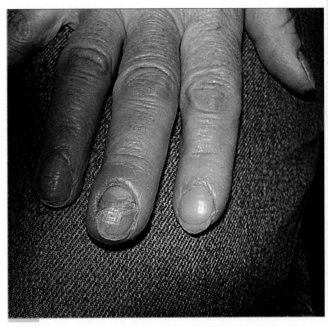

13.10 *Chronic paronychia.* In addition to erythema and edema of the proximal nail fold, nail dystrophy and the absence of a cuticle is noted here.

  DIFFERENTIAL DIAGNOSIS

- The diagnosis can generally be established based on the typical clinical appearance of the fingers and the patient's history. The presence of a candidal infection can be confirmed with a potassium hydroxide preparation or fungal culture, if necessary.
- Various pathogens and contaminants—including *Candida* species, gram-positive or gram-negative organisms, or mixed flora—may be cultured from the pus obtained from under the proximal nail fold. Bacterial culture often grows a mixed flora.

MANAGEMENT

- Avoid prolonged exposure to moisture and trauma, especially frequent hand washing and manicures.
- Wear gloves (the cotton-under-vinyl variety is best) when performing tasks such as washing dishes.

In addition, one or more of the following treatments should be considered:

- A superpotent topical steroid such as **clobetasol cream** 0.05% can be applied once or twice daily to the proximal nail fold. Alternatively, **Cordran tape** may be applied nightly to this area.

- One to two drops daily of **3% thymol in 70% ethanol** (compounded by a pharmacist) can be placed under the proximal nail fold.
- A topical broad-spectrum antifungal agent, such as **clotrimazole**, **ketoconazole**, **econazole**, or **miconazole,** is often combined with a potent topical corticosteroid (see earlier discussion) to provide antifungal as well as anti-inflammatory effects.
- If topical therapy is ineffective, oral broad-spectrum antiyeast therapy such as itraconazole (**Sporanox**) or ketoconazole (**Nizoral**) may be prescribed if clinically indicated and there are no contraindications to their use.

 POINTS TO REMEMBER

- Chronic paronychia is frequently misdiagnosed—and treated—as an acute staphylococcal paronychia.
- Chronic paronychia is distinct from onychomycosis, which is a fungal infection of the nail itself.

Onychomycosis

For a complete discussion, see Chapter 7, "Superficial Fungal Infections."

 SEE PATIENT HANDOUT "Fungal Nails (Onychomycosis)" ON THE SOLUTION SITE

Digital Mucous (Myxoid) Cyst

This is not a true cyst, because it lacks an epidermal lining. It is actually a focal collection of clear, gelatinous, viscous mucin (focal mucinosis) that occurs over the distal interphalangeal joint or, more commonly, at the base of the nail.

DESCRIPTION OF LESIONS

- Pressure from the lesion on the nail matrix (root) often results in a characteristic longitudinal groove in the nail plate (FIG. 13.11).
- When the lesion occurs more proximally, such as over the distal interphalangeal joint, there is no longitudinal groove (FIG. 13.12).
- This dome-shaped, rubbery lesion occurs exclusively in adults, particularly in women older than 50 years of age. Some myxoid cysts are believed to be a consequence of osteoarthritis, rather than trauma.

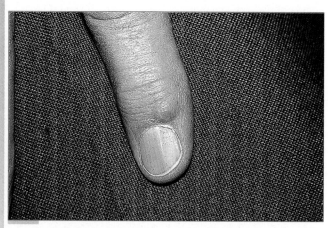

13.11 *Digital mucous (myxoid) cyst.* Note the longitudinal groove in the nail plate.

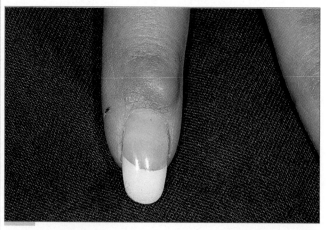

13.12 *Digital mucous (myxoid) cyst over the distal interphalangeal joint.* Notice the absence of the longitudinal groove.

MANAGEMENT

This benign lesion may be treated as follows:

- It may be ignored, particularly if it is asymptomatic.
- Lesions have reportedly resolved after several weeks of daily firm compression.
- Incision and drainage (Fig. 13.13), cryosurgery with liquid nitrogen, and intralesional triamcinolone injections may be performed, with varying results.
- Surgical excision is reserved for the occasional painful or otherwise troublesome lesion.

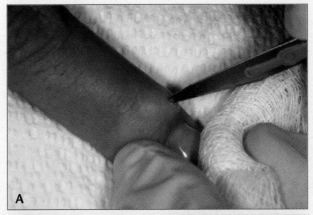

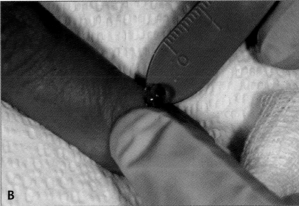

13.13 A and B *Digital mucous (myxoid) cyst.* Incision and drainage. Blood-tinged, viscous, jellylike mucoid material is expressed.

Miscellaneous Nail Disorders

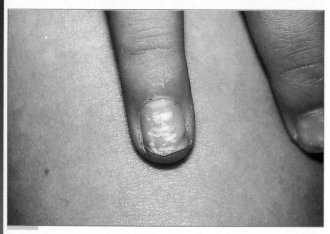

13.14 *Leukonychia striata.* These white spots caused by trauma are extremely common.

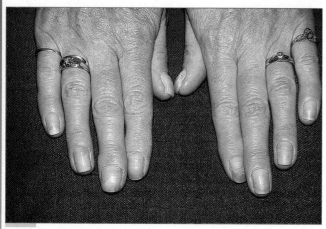

13.15 *Yellow nail syndrome.* These are thickened, slow-growing nails.

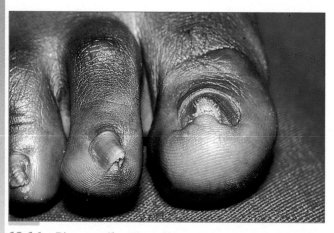

13.16 *Pincer nails.* The nails curve inward and pinch the nail bed.

- In addition to the disorders already described, various other conditions can affect the nails.
- Some of these disorders produce characteristic nail findings that may serve as clues to unrecognized systemic disease.

Leukonychia Striata
FIGURE 13.14.

- Leukonychia striata, which is also called transverse striate leukonychia, is often mistaken for a fungal nail infection.
- These white lines result from an injury to the nail matrix that occurred about 2 to 3 months earlier. The underlying injury is often an antecedent illness or the repeated trauma of manicuring; occasionally, it develops after liquid nitrogen therapy for warts.

Yellow Nail Syndrome
FIGURE 13.15.

- The nails are yellow, curved, and grow slowly. Yellow nail discoloration also has been reported in patients with acquired immunodeficiency syndrome.
- This syndrome is associated with certain respiratory disorders (e.g., bronchiectasis, chronic respiratory infections, lymphedema, pleural effusion, ascites).

Increased Transverse Nail Curvature (Pincer Nails)
FIGURE 13.16.

- Increased transverse curvature is often manifested as a pincer nail deformity.
- In this deformity, the nails' normal transverse curvature increases along the longitudinal axis and becomes more pronounced at the distal edge, which results in "pinching" of the underlying skin. This condition can become quite painful and may predispose the patient to infections and ingrown nails.
- Pincer nails are often congenital and may be seen in persons with the yellow nail syndrome or as a normal variant. They are also seen in women who wear ill-fitted shoes as well as those who also have inflammatory osteoarthritis.

Half-and-Half Nails
FIGURE 13.23.

- The proximal half of the nail is white and the distal portion retains the normal pink color.
- These characteristic color changes may be seen in chronic renal failure.

Dystrophy from Preformed Artificial Nails
FIGURE 13.24.

- Acrylic sculptured nails and the less expensive preformed plastic artificial nails are used for nail elongation. They are attached directly to the natural nail plate, which they cover entirely. The artificial nails are glued to the natural nail plate with an acrylate-based adhesive.
- Minor upward pressure on the distal tip of the artificial nail can result in significant distal onycholysis; complete nail avulsion can even result. Any space between the natural nail plate and the artificial nail may become infected (bacterial or fungal) or deformed, and this will often not be noticed until removal of the artificial nail.

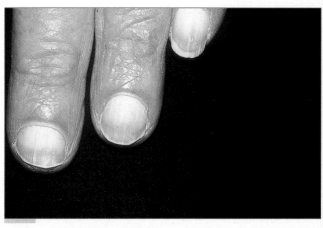

13.23 *Half-and-half nails.* Note that the proximal half is white and the distal half is pink. This patient had renal failure.

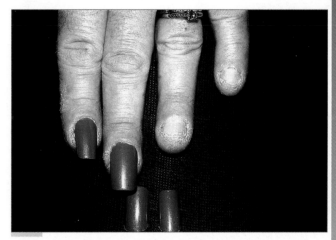

13.24 *Nail dystrophy from artificial nails.* The nail deformity in this woman was noticed when her artificial nails were removed.

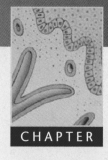

Pigmentary Disorders

> **DISORDERS OF HYPOPIGMENTATION**

- Vitiligo vulgaris
- Other forms of hypopigmentation
- Postinflammatory hypopigmentation
- Idiopathic guttate hypomelanosis
- Other types of hypomelanosis

> **DISORDERS OF HYPERPIGMENTATION**

- Melasma
- Postinflammatory hyperpigmentation
- Phyto-photodermatitis and berloque dermatitis
- Poikiloderma of Civatte
- Confluent and reticulated papillomatosis (Gougerot-Carteaud disease)
- Acanthosis nigricans
- Carotinemia

OVERVIEW

Skin color is mainly due to melanin. The amount of melanin is determined primarily by hereditary factors and by the result of exposure to ultraviolet radiation (tanning).

Melanogenesis

Melanocytes in the basal layer of the epidermis produce melanin. The melanin pigment is manufactured on melanosomes (intracytoplasmic organelles). Once made, the melanosomes are carried along dendrites and delivered to neighboring keratinocytes of the epidermis.

Darkly pigmented skin has melanosomes that contain more melanin and are larger in diameter than in light skinned individuals, and when those melanosomes are transferred to keratinocytes, they are singly dispersed and degrade more slowly.

Increase in melanin (hyperpigmentation or hypermelanosis) can be due to an increased number melanocytes or from increased production of melanin. Reduction in melanin production or a loss of melanocytes results in pale patches (hypopigmentation or hypomelanosis) or white patches (leukoderma). Vitiligo is a specific type of leukoderma characterized by depigmentation of the epidermis due to a partial or complete loss of melanocytes.

Vitiligo Vulgaris

BASICS

- An acquired disorder of skin depigmentation, vitiligo vulgaris (common vitiligo) affects 1% to 2% of the world's population.
- Thirty percent of patients with vitiligo report a positive family history of the disorder.
- A distinct form of vitiligo occurs in children, and this form is often segmental or dermatomal in its distribution. Some children may develop halo nevi, which are melanocytic nevi encircled by a white halo of depigmentation (see Chapter 21, "Benign Skin Neoplasms").

Pathogenesis

- Although the cause of vitiligo vulgaris is still unknown, the condition is thought to result from an autoimmune process that prompts the loss of melanocytes. Vitiligo may develop in patients with other diseases that are believed to have an autoimmune basis (e.g., thyroid dysfunction, Addison's disease, alopecia areata, diabetes mellitus, and pernicious anemia), and this finding supports the hypothesis that an immune mechanism may be involved in its pathogenesis.
- Another theory proposes that vitiligo is caused by an abnormality of nerve endings adjacent to skin pigment cells.

DESCRIPTION OF LESIONS

- Physical examination of a patient with vitiligo reveals hypopigmented (FIG. 14.1) or depigmented, chalk-white macules.
- Occasionally, the lesions may have various shades of color and may include islands of repigmentation (FIG. 14.2).
- In dark-skinned people, pigmentary loss may be observed at any time of year, whereas in light-skinned people, the lesions may be most obvious in the summer, because the tanning effects of the summer sun can accentuate the contrast between the light and dark skin.

DISTRIBUTION OF LESIONS

- Vitiliginous lesions tend to have a bilateral, symmetric distribution.
- They frequently occur on acral areas (e.g., the hands and feet), body folds, bony prominences, and external genitals.
- Lesions characteristically appear around orifices (e.g., the mouth, eyes, nose, and anus), but they may also involve the eyebrows, eyelashes, and scalp hair, resulting in white hairs (**leukotrichia**).
- In severe cases, vitiligo may be more widespread (FIG. 14.3) or even total (**vitiligo universalis**).

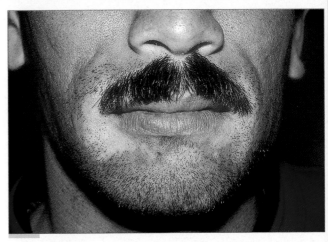

14.1 *Vitiligo.* Depigmented macules are characteristic of vitiligo vulgaris. Note the characteristic periorificial distribution in this patient.

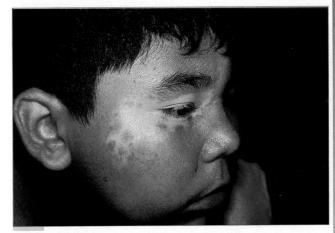

14.2 *Vitiligo.* Various shades of hypopigmentation, depigmentation, and islands of spontaneous repigmentation can be seen in this patient. Note the white eyelashes.

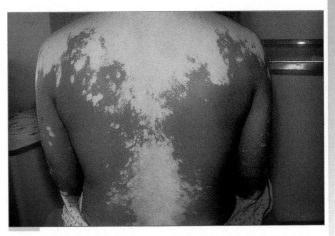

14.3 *Vitiligo.* Extensive depigmentation is evident in this patient.

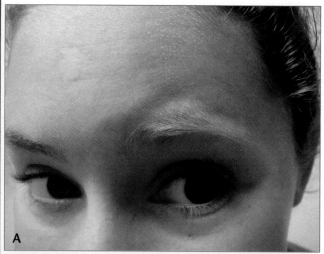

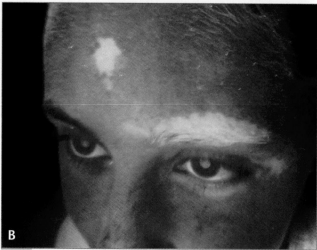

14.4 A and B *Vitiligo.* Wood's lamp examination reveals a "milk-white" fluorescence in areas depigmented by vitiligo. Note the depigmented eyebrows and eyelashes.

CLINICAL MANIFESTATIONS

- Clinical manifestations often develop cyclically. A rapid loss of pigment is followed by a stable period (during which some repigmentation may occur), and then generally by recurrence.
- Some patients spontaneously experience partial repigmentation; total repigmentation is unusual.
- Patients with severe vitiligo may experience embarrassment and lowered self-esteem.

DIAGNOSIS

- A clinical diagnosis of vitiligo is usually based on the characteristic appearance of the skin lesions.
- The diagnosis can be aided by Wood's lamp examination; this should reveal a milk-white fluorescence. Wood's lamp is a handheld black light that makes hypopigmented areas appear lighter and depigmented areas (e.g., those produced by vitiligo) appear as a pure white or bluish white fluorescence (FIG. 14.4).

DIFFERENTIAL DIAGNOSIS

Postinflammatory Hypopigmentation

See also later discussion.

- Because the lesions of this disorder are not totally depigmented, they are generally off-white in color.
- Often, patients who have postinflammatory hypopigmentation reveal a history of preexisting inflammatory dermatitis, such as eczema or tinea versicolor.

Hypopigmented Tinea Versicolor

- This disorder is frequently mistaken for vitiligo vulgaris. Patients with active, untreated tinea versicolor have a whitish scale.
- In addition, under Wood's lamp examination, the lesions may appear as a yellow-orange fluorescence, and skin scrapings tested with potassium hydroxide are positive for the hyphae and spores of the responsible yeast. Inactive, or postinflammatory, spots of tinea versicolor lack scale and are hypopigmented (see Chapter 7, "Superficial Fungal Infections").

Chemical Leukoderma

- This develops on the hands of persons who work with germicidal detergents or with certain rubber-containing compounds that destroy melanocytes.
- The diagnosis is established based on the location of the lesions (e.g., only on the hands) and a history of exposure (FIG. 14.5).

Leprosy

- Cutaneous leprosy often manifests with areas of hypopigmentation. The lesions may appear as hypopigmented macules, plaques, or nodules that become insensitive to touch.
- Leprosy is extremely rare in the United States, but it may be seen occasionally in patients who emigrate from endemic areas, such as India or parts of South and Central America.

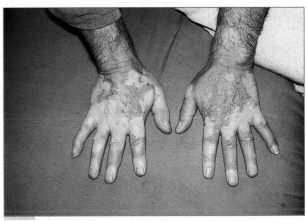

14.5 ***Chemical leukoderma.*** Chemically induced depigmentation is limited to this patient's hands. Exposure to a cleaning product containing phenol caused the areas of depigmentation in this patient, who routinely used the product at work.

 MANAGEMENT

- Treatment options for vitiligo include repigmentation therapies for the macules and depigmentation of the remaining healthy skin in patients with extensive disease.
- If administered early to patients with limited disease, **potent** (class 2) and **superpotent** (class 1) **topical corticosteroids** are occasionally helpful in promoting repigmentation.
  - The hands and feet respond poorly to this treatment as well as other therapies mentioned in this section.
  - Less potent topical steroids such as 1% hydrocortisone should be used on eyelid skin.
- Reports of repigmentation have been noted in some patients who applied tacrolimus (**Protopic**) 0.1% ointment or picrolimus (**Elidel**) 1% cream twice daily for 2 to 3 months.

- **Photochemotherapy** (see Chapter 3, "Psoriasis"), using psoralens and natural sunlight or psoralens and ultraviolet A light (PUVA) in a phototherapy light box, is sometimes tried. However, this treatment is time-consuming and often ineffective. It should generally not be used for children younger than 9 years.
  - The treatments are 50% to 70% successful in restoring some color on the face, trunk, and upper arms and legs.
  - Again, the hands and feet respond poorly to this method.
  - **Narrow-band UVB** and **excimer laser** therapy are expensive and not readily available.
- **Surgical transplants** may be attempted. The following methods may be tried for small, stable areas of vitiligo.
  - **Punch grafts:** Punch biopsy specimens from a pigmented donor site are transplanted into depigmented

continued on page 278

sites, however, a residual, pebbled pigmentary pattern may result.

- **Minigrafting:** Small donor grafts are inserted into incisional recipient areas of vitiligo and held in place with pressure dressings. As with punch grafting, this procedure does not result in total return of normal pigment, and a mottled pigmentation may result.
- Special cosmetic makeup that is formulated to match the patient's normal skin color (e.g., **Dermablend** or **Covermark**) or self-tanning compounds that contain dihydroxyacetone may effectively hide the white patches.
- Sunscreens can be used to avoid exacerbating the contrast between normal skin and lesions and to protect the lesions, which are sensitive to the sun.
- If attempts at repigmentation do not produce satisfactory results, depigmentation may be attempted in selected patients. Those with extensive vitiligo (more than 50% loss of pigment) may elect to have the remaining skin "bleached" with **Benoquin** (20% monobenzyl ether of hydroquinone). The results are permanent (FIG. 14.6).

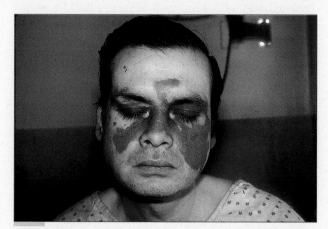

14.6 *Vitiligo.* Extensive depigmentation. The residual normal pigmentation was treated with Benoquin.

 POINTS TO REMEMBER

- Health care professionals should resist the tendency to trivialize vitiligo by referring to it as simply a cosmetic disorder.
- Patients should be urged to use sunscreens whenever they are exposed to the sun. By minimizing tanning, sunscreens lessen the contrast between healthy skin and lesions; they also protect the vitiliginous skin, which is sensitive to the sun.
- If indicated by positive findings in the patient's history or physical examination, screening of vitiligo patients for autoimmune diseases should be done; however, the frequency of these associations is not sufficiently high to warrant routine blood tests.
- Response rates to treatments for vitiligo often are disappointing, and lesions on the backs of the hands and feet are very resistant to therapy.

 HELPFUL HINTS

- Clinicians should be sensitive to patients who have emigrated from countries in which leprosy is endemic—and generally dreaded. Such patients may feel particularly embarrassed and stigmatized by focal areas of lightened skin color, regardless of the cause of the hypopigmentation.
- For children who have light skin tones, sunscreens and observation may be the best course.

SEE PATIENT HANDOUT "Vitiligo" ON THE SOLUTION SITE

Other Forms of Hypopigmentation

BASICS

- Although hypopigmentation and depigmentation are more obvious in dark-skinned persons, they can cause problems even in light-skinned persons, particularly those who tan.
  - Persons with dark complexions appear to be at an increased risk of developing these pigmentary changes.
  - Postinflammatory reactions are the most common cause of hypopigmentation. Localized alterations in skin color are not uncommon after many cutaneous inflammatory conditions. In addition, neonates and toddlers may exhibit congenital areas of hypopigmentation.
- Occasionally, a combination of light and dark patches may develop.
- Often, the pigmentary changes are self-limited; they require only time for resolution. Nevertheless, they can be a source of embarrassment for many patients. Providing reassurance and practical advice on how best to conceal the areas of altered skin color can help patients cope better with these disorders.

Postinflammatory Hypopigmentation

- Lightening of the skin may follow nearly any inflammatory cutaneous eruption (e.g., **eczema** or **psoriasis; FIG. 14.7**).
- In **pityriasis alba**, hypopigmented round spots are commonly seen on the face and other areas of the skin in children with atopic dermatitis. Occasionally, the slightly scaly patches that precede the hypopigmentation may be seen (FIG. 14.8).
- Postinflammatory hypopigmentation may also develop after an injury to the skin, such as a burn or surgical scar. The areas of hypopigmentation roughly correspond to the location and shape of the antecedent eruption ("footprints").

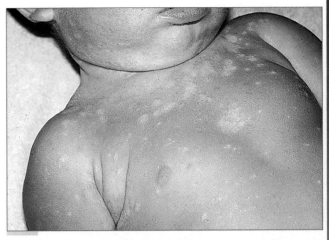

14.7 *Atopic dermatitis.* Postinflammatory hypopigmented macules can be seen in this infant who has atopic dermatitis. Note active areas of inflammation on the neck and axillary areas.

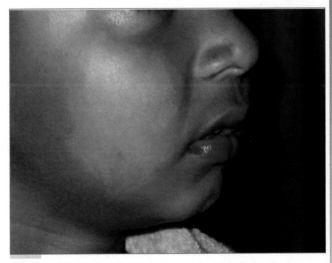

14.8 *Pityriasis alba.* Hypopigmented round spots are commonly seen on the faces in children who have atopic dermatitis.

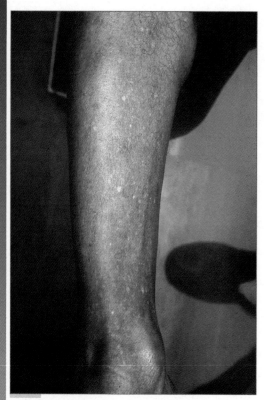

14.9 *Idiopathic guttate hypomelanosis.* Note the white spots on this elderly woman's shin.

 MANAGEMENT

- In general, the pigmentary changes that follow mild inflammatory dermatoses slowly revert to normal over several months. However, those that follow more severe inflammation or injury may be permanent.
- For facial lesions, if there is any scale or erythema, treatment with a mild class 6 topical steroid such as over-the-counter **1% hydrocortisone** cream twice daily may be helpful.
- The passage of time often improves the cosmetic abnormality.
  - In the interim, makeup products such as **Covermark** and **Dermablend** can be used to conceal the areas of hypopigmentation.
- Artificial tanning lotions can also be useful.

Idiopathic Guttate Hypomelanosis

Idiopathic guttate hypomelanosis (IGH) is the formal name for the idiopathic white spots that often appear on the arms and lower legs of middle-aged and elderly people. This condition occurs in all races, but as with vitiligo, it is more apparent in persons with darker skin. Typically, IGH develops first on the legs of women in early adult life (Fig. 14.9). Later, it may spread to other sun-exposed areas, such as the arms and the upper part of the back.

- The characteristic discrete, angular, or circular macules are 1 to 3 mm in diameter. However, lesions may measure up to 10 mm in diameter.
- These spots tend to develop more commonly in areas of chronic sun damage, particularly on the anterior lower legs and forearms. Inexplicably, the face is not involved.
- They produce no symptoms other than skin discoloration.
- There is no effective treatment.

Other Types of Hypomelanosis

Numerous systemic and congenital conditions may cause hypopigmentation. They include the following:

- Endocrine diseases, such as Addison's disease and hypothyroidism, may cause hypopigmentation.
- Genetic conditions, such as congenital vitiligo, tuberous sclerosis, and albinism, may also cause this condition.
- Congenital areas of hypopigmentation (FIG. 14.10).
- Infectious diseases, such as leprosy, pinta, and yaws, may be causes.
- In addition, hypomelanosis may result from the use of topical therapeutic agents, such as corticosteroids, hydroquinone, and retinoids. Nutritional deficiencies (especially vitamin B_{12} deficiency and kwashiorkor) may also cause a loss of pigmentation. These disorders should be considered in the appropriate clinical or environmental context.

 POINT TO REMEMBER

- The likelihood that normal pigmentation will return depends on the degree and type of injury.

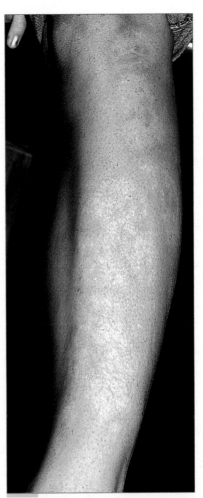

14.10 *Nevus depigmentosus.* This off-white linear hypomelanosis has been present since birth. It has enlarged commensurate with the patient's growth.

Disorders of Hyperpigmentation

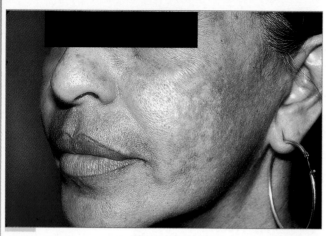

14.11 *Melasma of cheeks.* Melasma may result from pregnancy, oral contraceptive use, or menopause, or it may arise de novo for no apparent reason.

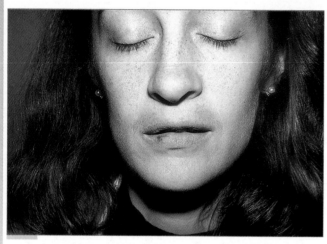

14.12 *Melasma of the "moustache" area.* Note the darkening above the patient's upper lip.

Melasma

BASICS

- Formerly known as chloasma, melasma, or the "mask of pregnancy," is an acquired form of hyperpigmentation that is seen most commonly on the face.
  - It may result from pregnancy, oral contraceptive use, or menopause, or it may arise de novo for no apparent reason. It is exacerbated by exposure to sunlight. Melasma is rare before puberty and most commonly occurs in women during their reproductive years.
  - When men are affected, the clinical and histologic picture is identical; however, the explanation for this condition is unknown.
- Melasma is seen most frequently in young women of childbearing age, particularly those who have darker complexions and live in sunny climates. It is seen in Asia, the Middle East, South America, Africa, and the Indian subcontinent. In North America, melasma is most prevalent among Hispanics, African-Americans, and immigrants from countries in which it is common.

CLINICAL MANIFESTATIONS AND DESCRIPTION OF LESIONS

- Clinically, melasma is primarily a cosmetic problem.
- It consists of asymptomatic, blotchy darkening of the facial skin.
- Lesions are tan to brown, hyperpigmented macules that may coalesce into symmetric, well-demarcated patches (FIG. 14.11).
- During pregnancy, the darkening of the skin often occurs in the second and third trimesters and spontaneously fades after termination of pregnancy.
- Melasma also tends to fade on discontinuance of oral contraceptives or avoidance of sunlight; however, it may persist indefinitely.

DISTRIBUTION OF LESIONS

- Lesions are found mainly on the cheeks, angles of the jaw, forehead, nose, chin, and above the upper lip (FIG. 14.12).

DIFFERENTIAL DIAGNOSIS

Postinflammatory Hyperpigmentation

See also the discussion in the subsequent section.

- This may often be explained by a previous inflammatory eruption or injury. In general, lesions roughly correspond to the location of inflammation or injury, and they have less clearly defined margins than are seen in melasma.

Solar Lentigines ("Liver Spots")

- These lesions (referred to in the singular as *lentigo*) have uniform coloration and are acquired during middle age on sun-exposed areas, such as the face and backs of the hands (see also Chapter 21, "Benign Skin Neoplasms").

MANAGEMENT

- Treatment of melasma involves a combination approach using one or more bleaching agents and cosmetic camouflage. In addition, sun avoidance and the use of sunblocks are essential.
- Bleaching creams that contain the tyrosinase inhibitor hydroquinone are readily available. Over-the-counter preparations such as **Ambi** and **Esoterica** contain 2% hydroquinone.
- Preparations of 3% hydroquinone (**Melanex**) and 4% hydroquinone (**Eldoquin Forte**) are available by prescription only. Some products such as **Eldopaque** contain a sunblock; **Lustra,** a 4% hydroquinone agent, also contains vitamins C and E and glycolic acid.
- Hydroquinone preparations are applied twice daily to areas of darkening only.

- Other lightening agents include the tyrosinase inhibitor azelaic acid (**Azelex** 20% cream), which may be used in addition to hydroquinone.
- Topical **tretinoin** can also be used in combination with both hydroquinone and a topical steroid (**Tri-Luma cream**).
- **Alpha-hydroxy acid** products, such as mild **glycolic acid** peels, may also be used to hasten the effect of other topical lightening agents. They should be used cautiously in darkly pigmented Hispanics, Asians, and blacks because of the risk for postinflammatory pigmentary hyperpigmentation (see next section).
- **Kojic acid,** a tyrosinase inhibitor, is used in Japan and the Middle East, and it seems to have an efficacy similar to that of hydroquinone.

POINTS TO REMEMBER

- Treatment requires patience during the many months in which lightening agents must be applied.
- Without the strict avoidance of sunlight, potentially successful treatments for melasma are doomed to failure.

HELPFUL HINTS

- Patients receiving treatment should be cautioned to expect slow but gradual lightening.
- Destructive modalities (e.g., cryotherapy, medium-depth chemical peels, lasers) yield unpredictable results and are associated with numerous potential adverse effects.
- Sunscreens that contain opaque physical blockers such as titanium dioxide and zinc oxide are preferred over chemical sunscreens because of their broader protection.

SEE PATIENT HANDOUT "Melasma" ON THE SOLUTION SITE

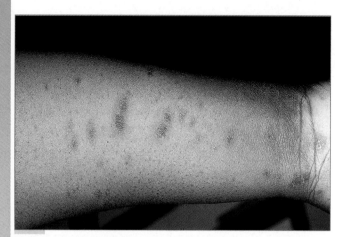

14.13 *Lichen planus, postinflammatory hyperpigmentation.* Hyperpigmentation is quite characteristic of healing lesions of lichen planus.

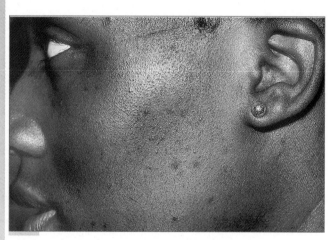

14.14 *Postinflammatory hyperpigmentation.* In this patient, healing acne lesions resulted in hyperpigmentation.

Rx MANAGEMENT

- Often, the passage of time, coupled with sun protection, affords a gradual lightening of darkened areas.
- Avoidance of the inciting event may prevent future lesions. Treatment of acne, for example, prevents the formation of new inflammatory lesions and allows old pigmented lesions to fade.
- When lesions persist, many of the measures used to treat melasma (see earlier discussion) may be tried. However, persistent postinflammatory hyperpigmentation tends to be much more recalcitrant than is melasma to therapeutic measures, and cosmetic cover-ups may be used.

Postinflammatory Hyperpigmentation

BASICS

- Darkening of the skin may occur after nearly any inflammatory eruption, including eczema, lichen planus (FIG. 14.13), or acne (FIG. 14.14), or after an injury such as a burn. Elective skin treatments (e.g., chemical peels, laser resurfacing, or dermabrasion) may also precipitate it.
- The hyperpigmentation stems from the melanocytes' exaggerated response to cutaneous insult, which results in an increased or abnormal distribution of the pigment melanin.
- Like melasma, postinflammatory hyperpigmentation tends to develop more often in people with dark complexions.

DESCRIPTION AND DISTRIBUTION OF LESIONS

- Lesions tend to conform in location and shape to the preceding eruption or injury.
- On occasion, lesions may mimic the exact shape of the inciting insult (FIG. 14.15).

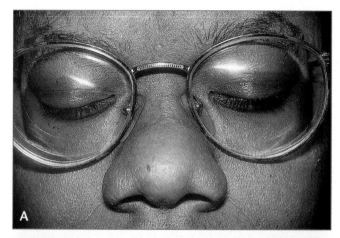

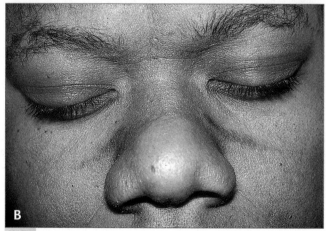

14.15 A and B *Postinflammatory hyperpigmentation.* In this patient, the cause was contact dermatitis from his eyeglasses. Note how the lesions conform to the shape of the frames.

Phytophotodermatitis and Berloque Dermatitis

BASICS

- A botanical cause for dermatitis is suspected when the pattern of the eruption is linear or streaky, such as that noted in the contact dermatitis caused by poison ivy (see Chapter 2, "Eczema"). The pattern is nearly always asymmetric. Some plants cause an eruption only after the skin is exposed to the sun; this is referred to as *photocontact dermatitis* or *phytophotodermatitis*.
- When the phytophotodermatitis is caused by perfume or other agents such as oil from the bergamot lime (*Citrus bergamia*), an ingredient in perfumes and fragrances, it is referred to as *berloque dermatitis*. Bergapten is also a naturally occurring component of the following:
  - Various other fruits, such as lemon oil
  - Plants such as false Queen Anne's lace (*Ammi majus*) and the giant Russian hogweed (*Heracleum mantegazzianum*)
- The initial skin response on exposed parts that have been in contact with the plant or perfume and then exposed to the sun resembles an exaggerated sunburn with (FIG. 14.16A) or without blistering.
  - Ultimately, postinflammatory hyperpigmentation that may last several weeks (FIG. 14.16B) or months occurs.
  - The reaction is a chemically induced, nonimmunologic, acute skin irritation requiring light (usually within the UVA spectrum; i.e., 320 to 400 nm) on bergapten, or 5-methoxypsoralens, a furocoumarin, the photoactive component of bergamot oil.

Poikiloderma of Civatte

BASICS

- This common condition occurs primarily in middle-aged, fair-skinned women.
- It is primarily of cosmetic concern to patients. Hormonal changes related to menopause or low estrogen levels may be a causal factor.
- Lesions consist of erythema associated with a mottled pigmentation located on the sides of the neck and other sun-exposed areas.
- The distribution of skin changes—the sparing of the shaded submental and submandibular areas—supports chronic sunlight exposure as the apparent cause of this condition (FIG. 14.17).

 MANAGEMENT

- There is no very effective medical treatment; however, the patient should be advised about avoidance of sun exposure and the proper use of sunscreens to prevent further skin involvement.
- The pulsed-dye laser has been noted to decrease the redness of this condition.

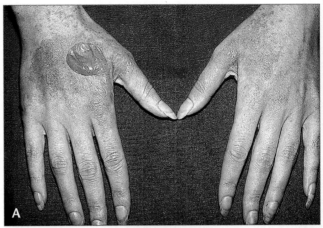
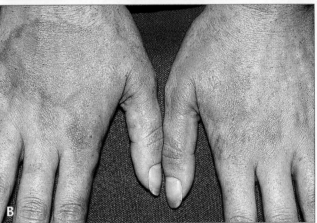

14.16 A and B *Berloque dermatitis.* **A:** This woman was squeezing limes for an outdoor barbecue 2 days before this blistering, hyperpigmented eruption began. **B:** This is the same patient 2 weeks later. Note the postinflammatory hyperpigmentation.

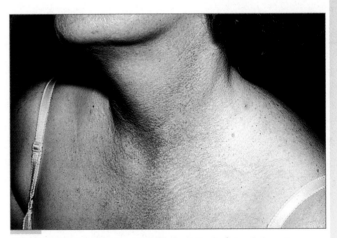

14.17 *Poikiloderma of Civatte.* The persistent erythema in this patient is characteristic. Note the sparing of the shaded areas under the chin and jawline.

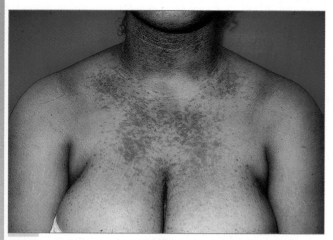

14.18 *Confluent and reticulated papillomatosis.* The darkly pigmented, coalescing papules are shown here in a typical distribution. Note that this patient also has evidence of acanthosis nigricans on her neck and axillae.

 DIFFERENTIAL DIAGNOSIS

- **Acanthosis nigricans** (see following section), which CRP resembles histopathologically, and darkly pigmented **tinea versicolor** are the most common conditions that may be confused with CRP.

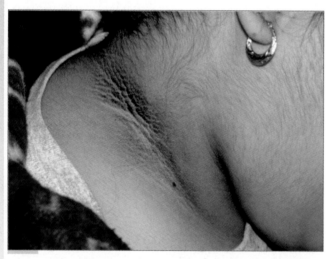

14.19 *Acanthosis nigricans.* This patient has diabetes. Note the marked hyperpigmentation.

Confluent and Reticulated Papillomatosis (Gougerot-Carteaud Disease)

BASICS

- Confluent and reticulated papillomatosis (CRP) is an uncommon condition of unknown etiology. Causal theories include an endocrine disruption, a disorder of keratinization, and an abnormal host reaction to *Pityrosporum* organisms or bacteria.
- It usually has its onset shortly after puberty.
- CRP is characterized by hyperkeratotic papules, usually located on the trunk. The lesions coalesce to form hyperpigmented, confluent plaques centrally and a reticular pattern peripherally (FIG. 14.18).

 MANAGEMENT

- CRP responds to oral tetracycline, such as minocycline 100 mg twice a day.

Acanthosis Nigricans

BASICS

- A characteristic hyperpigmented skin pattern, acanthosis nigricans occurs primarily in flexural folds. The skin is thought to darken and thicken in reaction to circulating growth factors.
- Most cases of acanthosis nigricans, including idiopathic cases and those associated with obesity, are referred to as *benign acanthosis nigricans*. Other benign forms of acanthosis nigricans are associated with endocrine disorders, such as insulin-resistant diabetes, polycystic ovary syndrome, Cushing's disease, Addison's disease, pituitary tumors, pinealomas, and hyperandrogenic syndromes with insulin resistance (FIG. 14.19). Acanthosis nigricans is sometimes related to drug use, most commonly secondary

to glucocorticoids, nicotinic acid, diethylstilbestrol, or growth hormone therapy. Acanthosis nigricans may also be inherited without any disease associations.

- The rare, so-called *malignant acanthosis nigricans* is associated with an internal malignant disease, usually an intra-abdominal adenocarcinoma. Affected patients generally have a poor prognosis. The skin condition is sometimes seen before the cancer is recognized; it can also be associated with recurrences and metastases.

DESCRIPTION OF LESIONS

- Acanthosis nigricans generally presents with a gradual evolution of symmetric, asymptomatic, tan or brown to black, leathery or velvety plaques. The plaques are sometimes "warty" (papillomatous) and studded with skin tags. They have linear, alternating, dark and light pigmentation that becomes more apparent when the skin is stretched (FIG. 14.20).

DISTRIBUTION OF LESIONS

- The most common sites of involvement are the axillae, the base of the neck, the inframammary folds, the inguinal areas, and the antecubital fossae.
- The dorsa of the hands (especially the knuckles), the elbows, and the knees are also common locations.
- Less commonly, mucous membranes, the vermilion border of the lips, and the eyelids are involved.

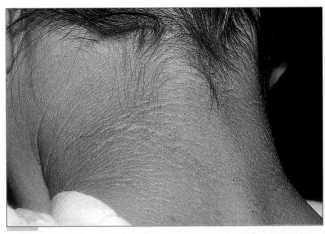

14.20 *Acanthosis nigricans.* Linear, alternating dark and light pigmentation becomes more apparent when the skin is stretched.

 POINTS TO REMEMBER

- Malignant acanthosis nigricans generally has a sudden onset, but otherwise it clinically resembles the benign form of the disorder.
- Concern is greatest when acanthosis nigricans suddenly arises in a nonobese adult who has no family history of the condition.

 MANAGEMENT

- Acanthosis nigricans is primarily a cosmetic concern.
- Treatment is generally not effective

Carotenemia

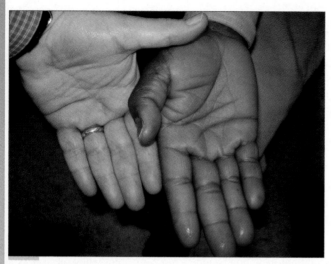

14.21 *Carotenemia.* The yellow-orange palms in this patient from West Africa were attributed to his diet, which consisted of an abundance of yams.

BASICS

- Carotenemia is characterized by yellow pigmentation of the skin caused by an increased level of beta-carotene in the blood. Most cases result from prolonged and excessive consumption of carotene-rich foods, such as carrots, squash, and yams (sweet potatoes).
- Less commonly, carotenemia has been associated with diabetes mellitus and hypothyroidism.

DESCRIPTION OF LESIONS

- The yellow-orange pigmentation often appears on the palms and soles (FIG. 14.21).
- The tip of the nose, the nasolabial folds, the palate, and other areas of the skin may become involved.
- The sclerae are spared, which distinguishes carotenemia from jaundice.

Rx MANAGEMENT

- Diet-induced carotenemia is a benign condition. The yellow pigmentation generally resolves with dietary changes.

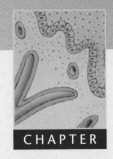

Pruritus: The "Itchy" Patient

OVERVIEW

Pruritus, the most common symptom of all skin diseases, can be simply defined as an unpleasant sensation that elicits the urge to scratch.

Pruritus may result from the following:

- Common primary skin disorders such as eczema, lichen simplex chronicus, xerosis, psoriasis, lichen planus, or, rarely, dermatitis herpetiformis
- Exogenous causes such as drugs, contact dermatitis (e.g., poison ivy), scabies, lice, fiberglass, and aquagenic pruritus
- Internal disorders such as chronic renal failure, acquired immunodeficiency syndrome, polycythemia vera, cholestasis, pregnancy-related disorders, primary biliary cirrhosis, diabetes mellitus, thyroid disease, and carcinoid syndrome
- Psychogenic causes such as delusions of parasitosis, neurotic excoriations, pruritus ani, and obsessive-compulsive disorder
- Associated malignant diseases such as Hodgkin's disease, leukemia, and multiple myeloma

> ➤ **PRURITUS OF UNKNOWN ORIGIN (PUO)**
>
> - Neurotic excoriations (factitia)
> - Pruritus of chronic renal disease
> - Pruritus caused by liver disease
> - Pruritus resulting from hypothyroidism
> - Pruritus resulting from hyperthyroidism
> - Pruritus resulting from Hodgkin's disease
>
> ➤ **CLINICAL VARIANTS**
>
> - Aquagenic pruritus
> - Notalgia paraesthetica
> - Brachioradial pruritus

Pruritis of Unknown Origin

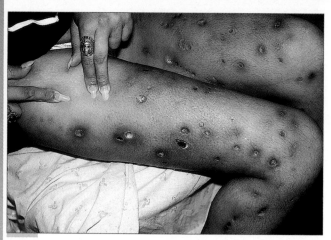

15.1 *Neurotic excoriations (factitia).* These self-induced ulcers convinced the patient that she was infested with lice.

BASICS

Pruritus of unknown origin (PUO) is itching for more than 2 to 6 weeks with no determined cause.

DESCRIPTION OF LESIONS

- Linear excoriations, crusts, lichenified plaques, and wheals may be present.
- Pruritus with no lesions is also quite common.
- When lesions have bizarre appearances, **facticia** or **"neurotic excoriations"** should be suspected. (FIG. 15.1) (see also Chapter 2, "Eczema").

DISTRIBUTION OF LESIONS

- Symptoms or clinical lesions may be localized (FIG. 15.2) or widespread.

DIAGNOSIS

- A search for the cause of the pruritus is based on the following:
  - A careful history
  - Physical evidence (linear excoriations, crusts)
- The workup for PUO includes the following:
  - Rectal and pelvic examinations, if indicated
  - Complete blood count
  - Stool examination for parasites and occult blood
  - Chest radiograph
  - Thyroid, renal, and liver function tests
  - Follow-up of the patient for as long as necessary to make a diagnosis

MANAGEMENT

- Whenever possible, treatment of the underlying systemic disease that causes the pruritus may bring relief.
- **Antihistamines** are of more benefit in the treatment of allergic conditions, urticaria, and drug reactions than they are for the treatment of itching and may be no more effective than placebo. Despite this finding, the powerful effect of antihistamines as placebos should not be overlooked.
- Topical therapy that can be soothing and helpful in some patients includes the following:
  - Menthol, phenol, camphor, and calamine lotions (e.g., **Sarna, Prax, PrameGel**) may be used.
  - Topical steroids are generally not very helpful when no lesions are apparent.
  - **Cold applications** of frozen vegetable packets may be useful.

For Pruritus of Chronic Renal Disease
- Renal pruritus occurs most often in those receiving hemodialysis.
- **Ultraviolet B (UVB) therapy** is often effective. **Narrow-band UVB** is particularly effective.
- Oral ingestion of **activated charcoal** may be helpful. It is inexpensive and generally well tolerated; therefore, it is considered a reasonable treatment when UV therapy has failed.

- Successful **kidney transplantation** is the only definitive treatment for chronic renal pruritus.

For Pruritus Caused by Liver Disease
- Cholestyramine (**Questran**), a bile acid sequestrant, can be used to treat the pruritus that often occurs during liver failure because of the liver's inability to eliminate bile. Cholestyramine binds bile in the gastrointestinal tract to prevent its reabsorption.
- Pruritus associated with obstructive malignancy of the biliary tract (e.g., primary sclerosing cholangitis) may be relieved by placing a stent to relieve the obstruction.

For Pruritus Resulting from Hypothyroidism
- The pruritus of hypothyroidism is primarily secondary to xerosis and should be treated with emollients and thyroid hormone replacement.

For Pruritus Resulting from Hyperthyroidism
- Pruritus secondary to hyperthyroidism generally improves with correction of thyroid function.

For Pruritus Resulting from Hodgkin's Disease
- Pruritus caused by lymphoma may precede the diagnosis.
- Systemic corticosteroids with palliative chemotherapy in late-stage Hodgkin's disease often provide relief.

 POINTS TO REMEMBER

- Antihistamines often exert their antipruritic action by inducing sleep (soporific effect).
- Topical emollients are an essential component of the therapy of pruritus when xerosis is present.

 HELPFUL HINTS

- The dosage of antihistamines should be titrated gradually upward using nonsedating agents during the daytime and sedating agents at bedtime.
- Scabies should be considered if more than one family member itches.
- Hodgkin's disease may present with pruritus that precedes the diagnosis by up to 5 years.

Clinical Variants

- A patient may complain of itching caused by reasons that seem totally inexplicable or bizarre. Many histories have various twists and turns, such as the following.

AQUAGENIC PRURITUS

- The person with aquagenic pruritus experiences intense itching *only* after exposure to water.

NOTALGIA PARESTHETICA

- This not uncommon condition is seen most often in middle-aged and elderly patients. Notalgia paresthetica is thought to represent a sensory neuropathy that is caused by nerve impingement for spinal arthritis.
- It most often consists of a localized, very focal, often unilateral area of recurrent itching that characteristically occurs on the lower or mid-scapula. The postinflammatory hyperpigmentation that sometimes results from the chronic rubbing and scratching reveals the diagnosis (see Fig. 15.2).
- Treatment is often futile. Capsaicin (**Zostrix**) cream, which depletes nerve endings of their chemical transmitters, may be tried.

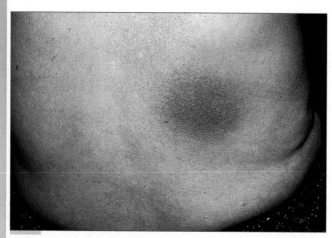

15.2 *Notalgia paraesthetica.* Note the typical location on the lower scapula. The postinflammatory hyperpigmentation resulted from the chronic rubbing and scratching of this itchy area.

BRACHIORADIAL PRURITUS

- Brachioradial pruritus (BRP) is an intense itching sensation of the arm, usually between the shoulder and elbow of either or both arms.
- There is ongoing debate regarding whether BRP is caused by a nerve entrapment in the cervical spine or a prolonged exposure to sunlight, because the outer, sun-exposed aspects of the arms are most often affected.
- Measures to treat BRP include the following:
  - **Sun protection;** wearing clothing with long sleeves is more effective than use of sunscreens alone
  - Capsaicin (**Zostrix**) cream
  - Ice packs
  - **Amitriptyline** tablets at night
  - Anticonvulsant agents, including **gabapentin** 300 mg three times daily
  - Electrical cutaneous nerve field stimulation

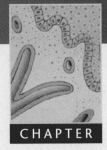

Xerosis: The "Dry" Patient

OVERVIEW

Xerosis, or dry skin, is a common occurrence in winter climates, particularly in conditions of cold air, low relative humidity, and indoor heating. Xerosis can affect anyone, but it tends to be more severe in certain persons, especially those with a hereditary predisposition.

Modern lifestyles are also contributing factors. In Western societies, people tend to overbathe, and they often live and work in overheated spaces.

The word "dry" is sometimes misapplied. Skin that appears to be dry (i.e., that shows a buildup of scale) may not always be suffering from a lack of water but rather from an overadherence or hyperproliferation of scale. Overadherence of scale may occur in patients with ichthyosis (see Chapter 2, "Eczema"). Hyperproliferation of scale is noted in atopic dermatitis, psoriasis, seborrheic dermatitis, and common dandruff.

- ➤ **XEROSIS**
- ➤ **ASTEATOTIC ECZEMA**
- ➤ **ATOPIC DERMATITIS**

XEROSIS

- Xerosis, or dry skin, tends to be most apparent on the hands and lower legs.
- It becomes especially common in persons who are older than 65 years of age (FIG. 16.1).

Pathogenesis

- The reasons why the skin becomes—or appears to become—dry are not well understood. It has been proposed that xerosis may be secondary to diminished production of sebum (asteatosis), as well as to reduced eccrine gland activity. However, other biochemical factors related to aging skin have also been implicated.
- Popular folklore and the lay literature often blame xerosis on inadequate water ingestion, but there is no scientific basis for this claim.

Asteatotic Eczema
See also FIGURE 2.52.

- Asteatotic eczema (**winter eczema**) is caused by a relative loss of water from the skin through evaporation, a lack of normal desquamation, and, possibly, a decline in the production of sebum (the skin's natural lubricant and sealant).
- Most often seen on the shins, with seasonal recurrences during the winter months, this form of eczema is a common, sometimes pruritic, low-grade dermatitis. Early on, the affected skin feels and looks dry (FIG. 16.2); later, an inflammatory dermatitis may evolve.

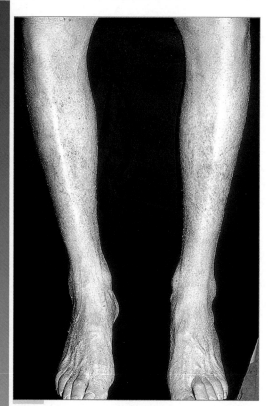

16.1   *Xerosis.* Dry skin tends to be most apparent on the hands and lower legs. This elderly patient's legs are dry and scaly.

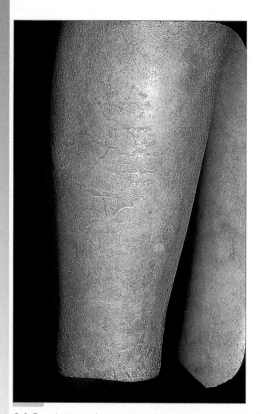

16.2   *Asteatotic eczema.* Xerosis and subtle changes consisting of exaggerated skin markings are seen in this patient.

- Occurring exclusively in adults, lesions most commonly appear on the shins, arms, hands, and trunk (see Chapter 2, "Eczema"). Because the eruption often resembles the surface of a cracked porcelain vase, it is often referred to as *erythema craquelé*. It is also likened to the appearance of a dry riverbed (FIG. 16.3).
- A clinical variant consists of small, square, scaly plaques that are often mistaken for tinea corporis (ringworm) or psoriasis and treated as such (FIG. 16.4).

Atopic Dermatitis

- Dry, xerotic, exquisitely sensitive, itchy skin is the major feature of atopic dermatitis (eczema) (see Chapter 2, "Eczema," for management of this condition). Atopic skin is often characterized by decreased water content, increased water loss, and reduced water-binding capacity, as well as epidermal hyperproliferation, resulting in lichenification (an exaggeration of normal skin markings) and buildup of scale.
- Patients usually have a personal or family history of allergies, asthma, or hay fever. In addition to scaly eczematous plaques, such patients may develop painful linear cracks or fissures from xerosis, particularly on the palms, soles, and fingertips (FIG. 16.5).

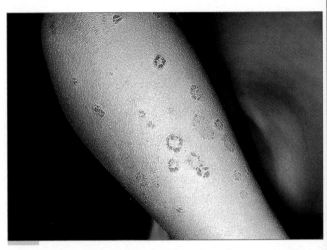

16.4 *Asteatotic eczema.* In this patient there are small, squarish plaques that resemble ringworm.

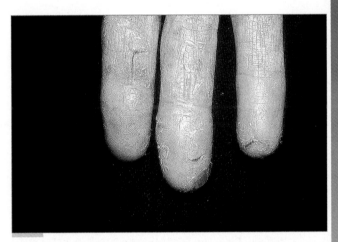

16.5 *Atopic dermatitis, hand eczema.* Dry, sensitive, itchy, lichenified skin is characteristic of this condition. This patient has painful fissures of the distal fingers.

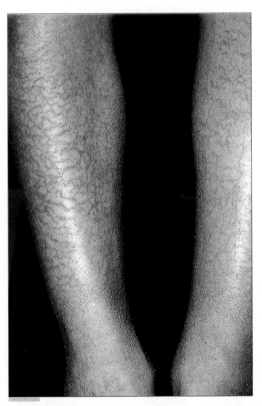

16.3 *Asteatotic eczema.* Here the skin resembles a cracked porcelain vase (erythema craquelé).

DIFFERENTIAL DIAGNOSIS

Ichthyosis Vulgaris

See FIGURE 2.21.

- Ichthyosis vulgaris (the most commonly seen variant of ichthyosis) resembles dry skin; however, it is actually caused by overadherence of scale.
- It is frequently associated with atopy.
- Skin with ichthyosis vulgaris resembles fine fish scales and tends to be most clinically obvious on the shins.
- Ichthyosis vulgaris is inherited in an autosomal dominant fashion and tends to improve with age.

Dry Skin That's Not "Dry"

- Many patients complain of "dry skin" from the use of topical retinoids such as Retin-A for the treatment of acne. Actually, the "dryness" is scaling that results from the exfoliative effect of the topical retinoid.
- Another common complaint is that of scaling and "dryness" from seborrheic dermatitis of the face and scalp. In such cases, the skin is not dry and deprived of moisture; rather, it scales and flakes from the inflammatory process.

 MANAGEMENT

Moisturizers

- Moisturizers do not add water to the skin, but they help retain or "lock in" water that is absorbed while bathing. Therefore, moisturizers should be applied while the skin is still damp.
- There are numerous over-the-counter moisture preparations in ointment bases, cream bases, and lotions. Some moisturizers contain alpha-hydroxy acids. The choice of product is based on personal preference, ease of application, cost, and effectiveness.
- Ammonium lactate 12% (**Lac-Hydrin**) lotion or cream is a prescription alpha-hydroxy acid preparation that may be applied after bathing. It is very effective and is used for more severe cases of xerosis. The 12% ammonium lactate preparation may be purchased over the counter as **AmLactin**.
- A 40% urea lotion (**Carmol 40**) is useful for moderate to severe dryness.

Other Strategies

- For the dermatitis, itching, and erythema of atopic dermatitis or asteatotic eczema, low- to medium-potency (class 4 to 6) **topical corticosteroids** are valuable. In severe cases, more potent topical corticosteroids (class 1 to 3) may be applied for brief periods when necessary.
- Showers and baths that are less frequent and shorter may be helpful. Only tepid water should be used.
- Soap avoidance (on affected areas) or mild soaps (e.g., **Dove, Basis**) or a soap substitute (e.g., **Cetaphil lotion**) may be tried. However, excessive use of any soap or substitute should be avoided, especially on affected areas.
- Adhesive dressings (**Band-Aids**) are effective in promoting healing of fissures.
- Lined gloves, worn while washing dishes, can keep hands dry.
- Scarves, gloves, and other apparel can help to provide adequate protection from exposure to outdoor cold.
- The use of room humidifiers and the ingestion of copious amounts of water are of questionable value.

 POINTS TO REMEMBER

- Dry skin and persistent pruritus—especially in elderly patients—may be evidence of a systemic condition (e.g., hypothyroidism or hypoparathyroidism), renal disease, or an underlying malignant disease.
- Dry or scaly skin may be associated with the use of cholesterol-lowering agents, in particular nicotinic acid.
- A genetically determined ichthyosis should be distinguished from simple xerosis, although the management of both conditions is similar.

HELPFUL HINTS

- Cocoa butter, petroleum jelly, or even vegetable shortening (e.g., **Crisco**) can be used as inexpensive moisturizers when cost is a consideration. These are very effective and do not contain many additives that may be sensitizing.
- For fissures, **Krazy Glue**, a cyanoacrylate glue that is carefully applied to "seal the cracks," is a nontoxic dressing that is reported to promote healing.

 SEE PATIENT HANDOUT "Dry Skin (Xerosis)" ON THE SOLUTION SITE

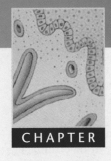

Drug Eruptions

OVERVIEW

An adverse drug reaction is any nontherapeutic deleterious effect of a prescribed or over-the-counter medication. Drug eruptions can mimic almost any dermatosis. Drug reactions may be allergic (immunologic) or nonallergic (toxic). Allergic-type drug reactions are not dose dependent. They are classified as the four following types of immunologic reactions:

- Type I: classic immediate hypersensitivity (urticaria, angioedema, anaphylaxis)
- Type II: cytotoxic (hemolysis, purpura)
- Type III: immune complex (vasculitis, serum sickness, urticaria, angioedema)
- Type IV: delayed hypersensitivity (contact dermatitis, exanthematous reactions, photoallergic reactions)

Nonallergic drug eruptions are more common than allergic-type eruptions; they may be dose related or idiosyncratic. Vertigo caused by high-dose minocycline, demethylchlortetracycline-related photosensitivity reactions, and irritant reactions from topical retinoids are examples.

BASICS

- Most drug eruptions are exanthematous (red rashes) and usually fade in a few days.
- More serious reactions include erythema multiforme major (Stevens-Johnson syndrome), toxic epidermal necrolysis, and serum sickness.

The presence of urticaria, mucosal involvement, extensive or palpable purpura, or blisters almost always requires discontinuation of the responsible drug. Certain classes of systemic medications, such as antimicrobial agents, nonsteroidal anti-inflammatory drugs (NSAIDs), cytokines, chemotherapeutic agents, and psychotropic agents, are associated with a high rate of cutaneous reactions. Risk factors include the following:

- Age: Drug eruptions are more commonly seen in elderly persons because they often take more drugs than younger people and they often take more than one drug at a time; consequently, they are more likely to have been previously sensitized.

- ➤ EXANTHEMATOUS DRUG ERUPTION
- ➤ URTICARIAL DRUG ERUPTION
- ➤ DRUG PHOTOSENSITIVE OR PHOTOTOXIC ERUPTION
- ➤ FIXED DRUG ERUPTION
- ➤ ERYTHRODERMA
- ➤ HYPERSENSITIVITY SYNDROME
- ➤ LEUKOCYTOCLASTIC VASCULITIS
- ➤ ERYTHEMA MULTIFORME MAJOR
- ➤ TOXIC EPIDERMAL NECROLYSIS
- ➤ LICHENOID DRUG ERUPTION
- ➤ LUPUS-LIKE DRUG ERUPTION
- ➤ ACNEIFORM DRUG ERUPTION

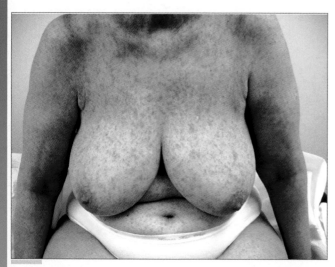

17.1 *Drug eruption.* Exanthematous reaction to a sulfa drug.

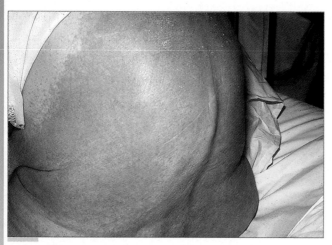

17.2 *Drug eruption.* Note the "drug red" color of this confluent eruption caused by a penicillin derivative.

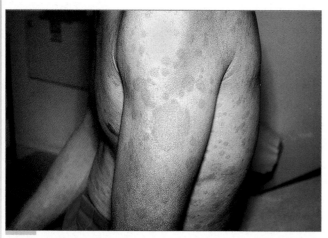

17.3 *Urticarial drug eruption.* Note the bizarre shapes of the urticarial plaques.

- A history of previous drug reactions is a risk factor.
- A family history of drug eruptions is another factor.
- Prolonged use of a drug can predispose patients to drug eruptions.
- Paradoxically, although human immunodeficiency virus (HIV) infection causes profound anergy to other immune stimuli, the frequency of drug hypersensitivity reactions is increased markedly compared with both immunocompetent and HIV-negative immunocompromised populations.

Characteristic Skin Reactions Produced by Drugs

Adverse cutaneous drug reactions can mimic many common non-drug-related skin eruptions, and certain drugs are more likely to cause characteristic reactions in the skin, as follows:

- **Exanthems and urticarial reactions:** sulfonamides, penicillins, hydantoins, allopurinol, quinidine, angiotensin-converting enzyme inhibitors, barbiturates, carbamazepine, isoniazid, NSAIDs, and phenothiazine, as well as thiazide diuretics, aspirin, blood products, cephalosporins, dextran, opiates, radiocontrast dye, ranitidine, and vaccines
- **Acneiform eruptions:** systemic steroids, topical steroids, lithium, oral contraceptives, and androgenic hormones
- **Photo-induced:** tetracyclines, particularly demethylchlortetracycline and doxycycline; griseofulvin; certain diuretics; sulfonylurea agents used to treat diabetes; NSAIDs; and phenothiazines
- **Erythema nodosum:** iodides, oral contraceptives, penicillin, gold, amiodarone, sulfonamides, and opiates
- **Bullous eruptions:** penicillin, sulfonamides, captopril, iodides, gold, and furosemide
- **Purpura:** anticoagulants and thiazides
- **Vasculitic eruptions:** allopurinol, aspirin or other NSAIDs, cimetidine, gold, hydralazine, penicillin, phenytoin, propylthiouracil, quinolones, sulfonamide, tetracycline, and thiazides
- **Erythema multiforme major (Stevens-Johnson syndrome)** and **erythema multiforme minor:** sulfonamides, penicillins, tetracyclines, hydantoins, and barbiturates
- **Fixed drug eruptions:** tetracyclines, sulfonamides, griseofulvin, barbiturates, phenolphthalein, and NSAIDs
- **Contact dermatitis:** neomycin and preservatives in topical medications

DESCRIPTION OF LESIONS

- The morphology of a drug eruption can often provide clues to the most likely responsible agent.

Exanthematous Drug Eruption

- Lesions are morbilliform (resembling measles) (FIG. 17.1).
- There may be areas of confluence.
- Lesions are pink, "drug red," or purple (FIG. 17.2).

Urticarial Drug Eruption

- Urticarial drug eruptions usually occur as wheals that may coalesce or take cyclic or gyrate forms (FIG. 17.3).

- Lesions usually appear shortly after the start of drug therapy and resolve rapidly when the drug is withdrawn (see also Chapter 18, "Diseases of Vasculature").

Drug Photosensitivity or Phototoxic Eruption
- This may appear as erythematous (an exaggerated sunburn; Fig. 17.4), eczematous, or lichenoid (resembling lichen planus).
- Lesions generally occur on sun-exposed areas such as the "V" of the neck, extensor forearms, and the face (Fig. 17.5).

Fixed Drug Eruption
- This is a reaction of circular red plaques or blisters that recurs at the same cutaneous site each time the drug is ingested. In other words, a rechallenge of the drug results in an identical eruption at the same site or sites.
- Lesions may be round or oval, single (Fig. 17.6), or multiple (Fig. 17.7).

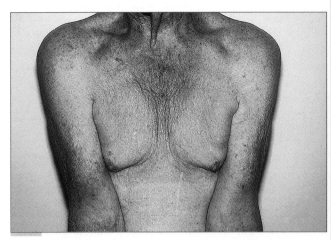

17.5 *Phototoxic drug eruption.* This is a phototoxic eruption caused by hydrochlorothiazide. The eruption appears in a photo distribution—the "V" of the neck and the extensor forearms.

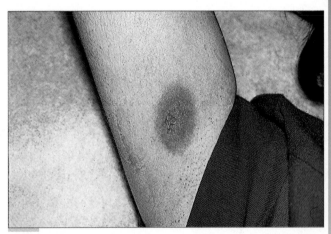

17.6 *Fixed drug eruption.* An oval lesion occurred at the identical site where it had occurred previously. In both episodes, the rash emerged after this patient ingested a sulfonamide antibiotic. Note the eroded blister in the center of the lesion.

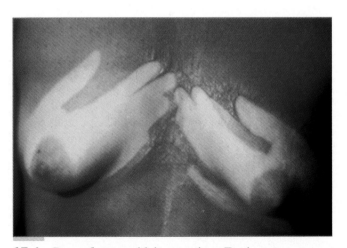

17.4 *Drug photosensitivity eruption.* Erythematous (exaggerated sunburn) reaction in a person who was taking demeclocycline (Declomycin) and fell asleep on the beach. (Courtesy of the Albert Einstein College of Medicine, Division of Dermatology, Bronx, New York.)

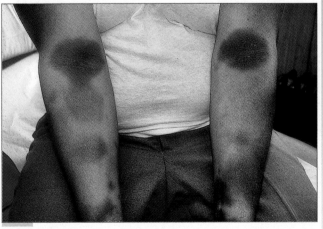

17.7 *Fixed drug eruption, multiple lesions.* These lesions are postinflammatory and were caused by phenytoin (Dilantin).

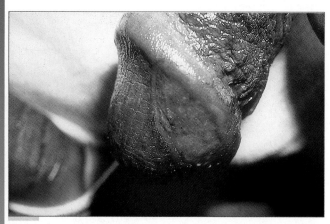

17.8 *Fixed drug eruption.* An oval erosion on the glans penis occurred in this patient who was taking minocycline. According to the patient, an identical lesion—in the same location—appeared when he was given minocycline previously.

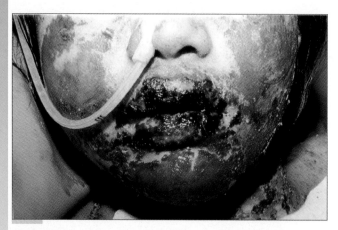

17.9 *Toxic epidermal necrolysis.* A child with a severe, generalized eruption with epidermal necrosis and denuded erosive areas. (Image courtesy of Ashit Marwah, M.D.)

- A lesion on the glans penis is not unusual (FIG. 17.8).
- Lesions initially are erythematous; later they become violaceous.
- Lesions often blister and erode.
- The eruption often heals with characteristic postinflammatory hyperpigmentation.

Erythroderma (Exfoliative Dermatitis)
- This is widespread inflammation of the skin (see Chapter 25, "Cutaneous Manifestations of Systemic Disease"), and it may result from an underlying skin condition, drug eruption, internal malignancy, or immunodeficiency syndrome.
- Lymphadenopathy is often noted, and hepatosplenomegaly, leukocytosis, eosinophilia, and anemia may be present.

Hypersensitivity Syndrome
- This is a potentially life-threatening complex of symptoms often caused by anticonvulsants. It usually begins within 1 to 3 weeks after a new drug is started, but it may develop 3 months or later into therapy.
- Patients have fever, sore throat, rash, lymphadenopathy, hepatitis, nephritis, and leukocytosis with eosinophilia.
- Aromatic anticonvulsant drugs cross-react (i.e., phenytoin, phenobarbital, carbamazepine); valproic acid is a safe alternative.

Leukocytoclastic Vasculitis
- This is a common drug eruption.
- It is characterized by palpable purpura. Fever, myalgias, arthritis, and abdominal pain may be present.
- A laboratory evaluation to exclude internal involvement is mandatory (see Chapter 18, "Diseases of Vasculature").

Erythema Multiforme Major
- Stevens-Johnson syndrome can be caused by drugs and infections (see Chapter 18, "Diseases of Vasculature").
- It is characterized by widespread skin involvement, large and atypical targetoid lesions, significant mucous membrane involvement, constitutional symptoms, and sloughing of the skin (see Chapter 18, "Diseases of Vasculature").

Toxic Epidermal Necrolysis
- This is a severe skin reaction that involves a prodrome of painful skin, followed by rapid, widespread, skin sloughing (FIG. 17.9).
- Most cases are the result of drugs (see also Chapter 24, "Cutaneous Manifestations of HIV Infection").
- Secondary infection and sepsis are major concerns.

Erythema Nodosum
- This is characterized by tender, red, subcutaneous nodules that typically appear on the anterior aspect of the legs.
- Erythema nodosum is a reactive process often secondary to infection, but it may be caused by medications, especially oral contraceptives and sulfonamides (see Chapter 18, "Diseases of Vasculature").

Lichenoid Drug Eruption

- This reaction appears similar to lichen planus (see Chapter 4, "Inflammatory Eruptions of Unknown Cause").

Lupuslike Drug Eruption

- Symptoms are identical to those of systemic lupus erythematosus, but skin findings are uncommon.
- Lesions are also identical to drug-induced subacute cutaneous lupus erythematosus, which is characterized by annular, psoriasiform, nonscarring lesions in a photodistributed pattern (see Chapter 25, "Cutaneous Manifestations of Systemic Disease").

Acneiform Drug Eruptions

- The usual responsible agents are systemic steroids.
- Lesions generally appear on the trunk as monomorphic papules and pustules (FIG. 17.10).

DISTRIBUTION OF LESIONS

Drug eruptions have specific regional predilections. For example:

- Exanthems tend to be symmetric and occasionally generalized in distribution; they are noted particularly on the trunk, thighs, upper arms, and face.
- The distribution of a contact dermatitis most often corresponds the area of initial insult to the skin (FIG. 17.11).
- A fixed drug eruption may present as a solitary isolated lesion occurring most often on the hands, feet, and genitalia; multiple lesions may occur on the trunk and extremities.
- A photo-induced drug eruption occurs on the face, dorsal forearms, and "V" of the neck and upper sternum.
- Erythema nodosum occurs characteristically in the pretibial area.
- Purpura and vasculitic drug eruptions also tend to occur on the lower extremities.
- Topical steroid-induced rosacea occurs on the face.
- Steroid atrophy most often occurs in body folds (axillae and inguinal creases).
- Urticaria can be seen anywhere on the body.
- Angioedema occurs in a periorbital, labial, and perioral distribution.
- Erythema multiforme lesions commonly manifest on mucous membranes as well as on the palms and soles; they can also be widespread (see Chapter 18, "Diseases of Vasculature").

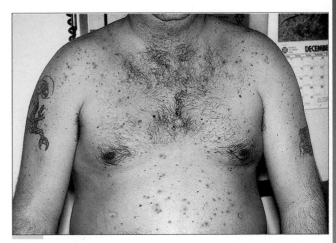

17.10 *Acneiform eruption caused by oral steroids.* This patient developed multiple papules and pustules in a characteristic distribution.

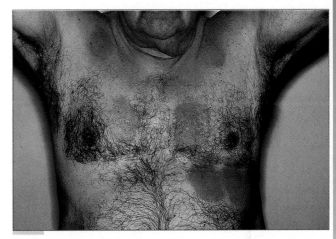

17.11 *Contact dermatitis.* The geometric, erythematous lesions in this patient were caused by a reaction to leads used for a cardiac stress test.

MANAGEMENT

- The drug should be discontinued, *if feasible*. However, the decision to discontinue a potentially vital drug presents a dilemma.
- Oral antihistamines, such as diphenhydramine (**Benadryl**), hydroxyzine (**Atarax**), or the nonsedating agents cetirizine (**Zyrtec**) and loratadine (**Claritin**), may be helpful.
- **Systemic steroids** are given only in severe cases in which an infectious cause has been excluded.

 POINTS TO REMEMBER

- Prompt recognition and withdrawal of an offending drug are important, particularly in patients with severe reactions.
- If it is necessary to continue the drug (i.e., there is no alternative medication) and the adverse reaction is mild or tolerable, the difficulty may be minimized by decreasing the dosage or treating the adverse reaction.
- Persons who are immunocompromised have a greater risk of developing a drug eruption than the general population.

 HELPFUL HINTS

- Drug reactions can occur even after years of continuous therapy with the same drug.
- Drug reactions can occur days after a drug has been discontinued.
- A drug eruption may easily be confused with a feature of the condition that it is intended to treat (e.g., a viral exanthem treated with an antibiotic).
- Patients with infectious mononucleosis are likely to develop a morbilliform rash when they are given ampicillin.
- Exanthematous eruptions in adults are mostly the result of medications; in children, however, they are more likely to be a result of a viral infection.

CLINICAL MANIFESTATIONS

- Pruritus is a common complaint; however, adverse drug reactions also can cause pruritus unaccompanied by a rash.
- Acute urticarial lesions usually appear shortly after the onset of drug therapy and resolve rapidly when the drug is withdrawn.
- Mucous membrane lesions are often painful (e.g., erosions, ulcers).
- Drug eruptions may be associated with systemic anaphylaxis or with extensive mucocutaneous exfoliation and multisystemic involvement; however, most drug eruptions are mild and self-limited, resolving after the offending agent is discontinued.
- In drug eruptions with vasculitis, fever, myalgias, arthritis, and abdominal pain may be present. Vasculitis typically begins 7 to 21 days after the onset of drug therapy. The vasculitic process also may include other organ systems.

DIAGNOSIS

- Obtaining a detailed, careful history from the patient or family is paramount.
- A handy reference to drug eruptions and interactions should always be available.
- Patients occasionally have eosinophilia.
- Skin biopsy of an exanthem showing perivascular lymphocytes and eosinophils may be helpful, but it is not diagnostic. Characteristic histopathologic changes may occur in some cases, such as leukocytoclastic vasculitis in palpable purpura and panniculitis in erythema nodosum; however, these findings are not necessarily diagnostic of a drug-related origin.
- Rechallenging with a suspected drug as a diagnostic tool is generally discouraged, unless:
  - Alternative agents are not available and the drug is indispensable to the patient.
  - The reaction is minor.

 DIFFERENTIAL DIAGNOSIS

- **Viral or bacterial exanthems** generally occur with fever and other symptoms; however, they are often indistinguishable from a drug eruption.
- **Pityriasis rosea** should be considered.
- **Acute urticaria (not drug-induced)** is another possible diagnosis.
- **Chronic urticaria (not drug-induced)** should be considered.

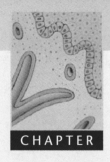

Diseases of Vasculature

OVERVIEW

Cutaneous manifestations of vascular disorders range from a mild rash, urticaria, or angioedema to severe, life threatening vasculitis or anaphylaxis. Diseases featuring inflammation of the wall of blood vessels due to leukocyte migration and resultant damage can affect various organ systems. Large, medium, and/or small vessels may be involved.

> **URTICARIA AND ANGIOEDEMA**

- Acute urticaria
- Chronic urticaria
- Dermatographism
- Cold urticaria
- Light-induced (solar) urticaria
- Cholinergic urticaria
- Other physical urticarias

> **ERYTHEMA MULTIFORME**

> **NON-PALPABLE PURPURA AND BENIGN SMALL VESSEL VASCULITIS**

- Actinic (senile purpura)
- Schamberg's purpura
- Majocchi's purpura (purpura annularis telangiectodes).

HYPERSENSITIVITY VASCULITIS

- Palpable purpura

Urticaria and Angioedema

BASICS

- Urticaria, commonly known as hives, is a reaction of cutaneous blood vessels that produces a transient dermal edema consisting of papules or plaques of different shapes and sizes.
- *Angioedema* refers to edema that is deeper than urticaria and involves the dermis and subcutaneous tissue.
- By definition, an individual urticarial lesion lasts less than 24 hours.
- A total of 10% to 20% of the population has at least one episode of urticaria or angioedema at some point in his or her lifetime.

Pathophysiology

- Release of histamine and other compounds by mast cells and basophils causes the appearance of urticaria. Mast cell activation causes degranulation of intracellular vesicles that contain histamine, leukotriene C_4, prostaglandin D_2, and other chemotactic mediators that recruit eosinophils and neutrophils into the dermis. Histamine and chemokine release lead to extravasation of fluid into the dermis (edema). Histamine effects account for many of the clinical and histologic findings of urticaria.
- As with drug reactions, urticaria may be immune mediated or nonimmune mediated (see Chapter 17, "Drug Eruptions"). Causes of urticaria and angioedema include the following:
  - Immunologic causes, mediated by immunoglobulin E (IgE), include food, drugs, and parasites.
  - Complement-mediated causes include serum sickness and whole blood transfusions.
  - Physical stimuli that are non–IgE-mediated include cold, sunlight, and pressure (e.g., dermatographism).
  - Occult infections include sinusitis, dental abscesses, and tinea pedis. However, such problems are rarely associated with chronic urticaria.
- In 85% to 90% of patients with chronic urticaria, the origin is unknown (i.e., chronic idiopathic urticaria).

CLASSIFICATION

- Urticaria may be classified as acute or chronic urticaria, physical urticaria, urticarial vasculitis, and hereditary angioedema (rare).

Acute Urticaria

Acute urticaria, by definition, lasts less than 6 weeks.

- Outbreaks are often IgE-mediated.
- Many patients have an atopic history.
- There may be an obvious precipitant such as an acute upper respiratory infection, drug, parasitic infection, or bee sting.
- The most common drugs that may cause acute hives are antibiotics (especially penicillin and sulfonamides), pain medications such as aspirin, nonsteroidal anti-inflammatory drugs (NSAIDs), narcotics, radiocontrast dyes, diuretics, and opiates such as codeine.
- The most common foods associated with acute urticaria are milk, wheat, eggs, chocolate, shellfish, nuts, fish, and strawberries. Food additives and preservatives such as salicylates and benzoates may also be responsible.
- Systemic diseases such as lymphomas and collagen vascular diseases may have an associated urticaria.
- Acute urticaria also may be caused by physical stimuli such as pressure, cold, sunlight, or exercise. Such hives are called physical urticarias (see later discussion).
- Anaphylaxis or an anaphylactoid reaction can occur.

Chronic Urticaria

Chronic urticaria is, by definition, urticaria that lasts longer than 6 weeks, although the cutoff point is an arbitrary one.

- Chronic urticaria occurs in a 2:1 female-to-male ratio.
- It is seen predominantly in adults.
- The cause is usually unknown; however, chronic urticaria may, very infrequently, be a sign of one of the following systemic diseases: systemic lupus erythematosus (SLE), serum hepatitis, lymphoma, polycythemia, macroglobulinemia, or thyroid disease.

DESCRIPTION OF LESIONS

- Papules and plaques are of varying sizes.
- Wheals are the color of the patient's skin or pale red; a white halo may be noted at the periphery of the lesions (FIG. 18.1).
- Lesions have various shapes; they can be annular, linear, arciform, or polycyclic, and frequently they are multiple, with bizarre shapes (FIGS. 18.2 and 18.3).
- Individual lesions disappear within 24 hours (evanescent wheals).
- Lesions may be accompanied by a deep swelling (angioedema) around the eyes, lips, and tongue that often looks frightening. Fortunately, angioedema usually lasts less than 24 hours.

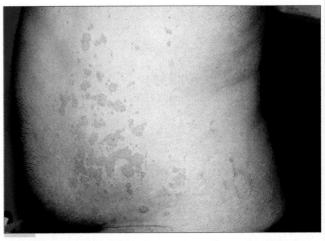

18.2 *Urticaria.* Multiple lesions have various shapes and sizes.

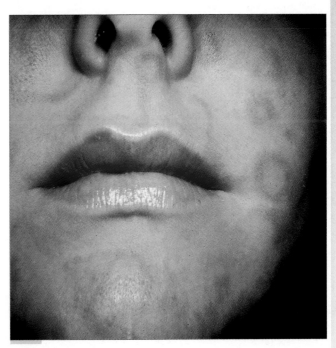

18.3 *Acute urticaria.* Lesions are annular, arciform, and polycyclic, with bizarre shapes.

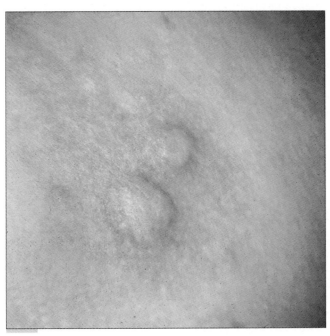

18.1 *Urticaria.* Skin-colored wheals are present.

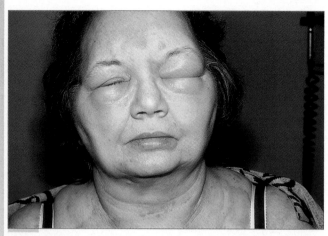

18.4 *Urticaria.* Marked angioedema is noted.

DISTRIBUTION OF LESIONS

- Angioedema is noted primarily in the periorbital area (FIG. 18.4), lips, and tongue.
- Urticarial lesions may occur anywhere on the body and may be localized or generalized.

CLINICAL MANIFESTATIONS

- Lesions generally itch.
- Arthralgia, fever, malaise, and other symptoms may accompany urticaria when it is the result of hepatitis or serum sickness, for example.
- Scratching and rubbing of lesions generally do not produce scabs or crusts similar to those seen in atopic dermatitis.
- Episodes of acute urticaria lasts for hours to days (generally less than 30 days).
- Approximately 50% of patients with chronic urticaria are free of lesions in 1 year; in other patients, lesions may recur for many years.
- Emotional stress may trigger recurrences.

DIAGNOSIS OF CHRONIC URTICARIA

The diagnosis of acute and chronic urticarias is usually made on clinical observation and history. If a complete review of systems is normal, and a physical urticaria is ruled out, it is often futile to perform multiple laboratory tests to determine a cause for chronic urticaria. Nonetheless, a positive symptom-directed search for underlying illness (e.g., SLE, thyroid disease, lymphoma, and necrotizing vasculitis) may warrant evaluations such as:

- Complete blood count
- Erythrocyte sedimentation rate
- Fluorescent antinuclear antibody test
- Thyroid function studies
- Hepatitis-associated antigen test
- Assessment of the complement system
- Radioallergosorbent test for IgE antibodies
- In the presence of eosinophilia, stool examination for ova and parasites
- CD203c assay, a new in vitro diagnostic test that is used to detect autoimmune urticaria and identifies antibodies that are responsible for many cases of chronic idiopathic urticaria

Clinical Variants

Physical Urticarias

Physical factors are the most commonly identified causes of chronic urticaria. Physical urticarias are diagnosed by challenge testing.

Dermatographism ("Skin Writing")

FIGURE 18.5.

- Dermatographism affects more than 4% of the general population, in whom it is physiologic and asymptomatic.
- Linear erythematous wheals occur 3 to 4 minutes after firmly stroking the skin with the wooden handle of a cotton swab; they fade within 30 minutes. A delayed form also exists.
- Lesions are seen under constrictive garments, such as belts and bras, or after a person scratches.
- In some persons, itching is the primary symptom.
- Episodes of dermatographism may persist for years.

Cold Urticaria

FIGURES 18.6 A and B.

- Cold urticaria occurs mainly in young adults and children.

> **SOME PHYSICAL URTICARIAS AND THEIR CAUSES**
>
> - Dermatographism results from firm stroking or scratching.
> - Cold urticaria is caused by exposure to cold.
> - Aquagenic urticaria results from contact with water.
> - Cholinergic urticaria is caused by heat or exercise.
> - Solar urticaria results from sun exposure.

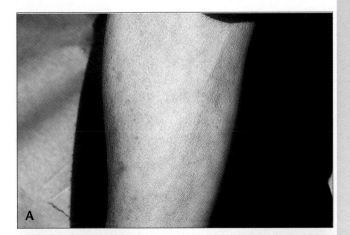

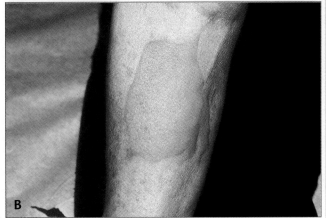

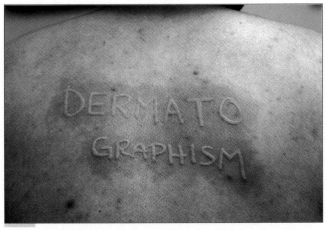

18.5 *Dermatographism ("skin writing").* These lesions occurred 3 minutes after stroking with the wooden tip of a cotton swab.

18.6 and B *Cold urticaria.* The "ice cube test." Before **(A)** and 5 minutes after **(B)** application of an ice cube. A large wheal and surrounding erythema have appeared.

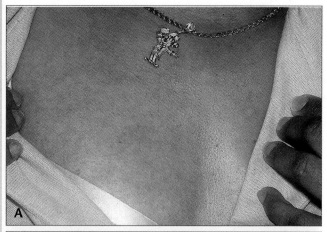

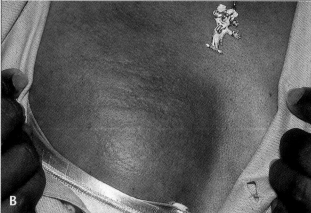

18.7 A and B *Solar urticaria induced by ultraviolet A light.* Before sun exposure (**A**) and after 15 minutes of sun exposure through a glass window (**B**). The glass window filters out ultraviolet B light.

- Itchy hives occur at sites of cold exposure, such as areas exposed to cold winds or immersion in cold water.
- In the "ice cube test," a wheal arises on the skin after application of an ice cube.

Light-Induced (Solar) Urticaria
FIGURES 18.7 A and B.

- Solar urticaria occurs in sun-exposed areas of the skin and is triggered by different wavelengths of light.

Cholinergic Urticaria
- This type of urticaria is induced by exercise or a hot shower.
- The patient exercises to the point of sweating, which provokes lesions and establishes the diagnosis.
- Typical lesions are multiple, small, monomorphic wheals.

Other Physical Urticarias
- These include those induced by pressure, heat, vibration, and water (aquagenic urticaria).

DIFFERENTIAL DIAGNOSIS

Insect Bite Reactions

These reactions are also known as papular urticaria. For a full discussion of insect bite reactions, see Chapter 20, "Bites, Stings, and Infestations."

- Reactions to insect bites may be indistinguishable from ordinary hives.
- Bites are generally seen on exposed areas.
- They may have a central punctum and crust; they also may blister.
- Individual lesions may last more than 24 hours.

Erythema Multiforme Minor

See also subsequent detailed discussion.

- Lesions are targetoid.
- Lesions last more than 24 hours.
- Lesions are generally nonpruritic.

Erythema Migrans (Acute Lyme Disease)

For a full discussion of this condition, see Chapter 20, "Bites, Stings, and Infestations."

- Erythema migrans may be indistinguishable from urticaria.

- Lesions are usually solitary, annular, and targetlike.
- Lesions may last more than 24 hours.
- Lesions are generally nonpruritic.

Urticarial Vasculitis

This condition is rare and is probably related to circulating immune complexes.

- Persistent hivelike lesions last more than 24 hours.
- Lesions may be tender rather than itchy.
- Residual purpura or hyperpigmentation often ensues on resolution of lesions.
- Evidence of vasculitis (e.g., purpura) is occasionally seen in the lesions.
- The diagnosis is confirmed by skin biopsy.
- Patients may have hypocomplementemia and an elevated erythrocyte sedimentation rate.
- Urticarial vasculitis may be associated with collagen vascular diseases.

 MANAGEMENT

- If possible, the cause of the hives should be eliminated, and tight clothing and hot baths and showers should be avoided, particularly in people who have physical urticaria.
- Salicylates, NSAIDs, and narcotics, which are all histamine-releasing agents, may aggravate both acute and chronic urticaria and should be avoided.
- Histamine H_1 blockers include hydroxyzine (**Atarax**), diphenhydramine (**Benadryl**), and cyproheptadine (**Periactin**); H_1 and H_2 blockers may be used in combination, such as cimetidine (**Tagamet**) plus hydroxyzine. These first-generation antihistamines compete with histamine at the tissue receptor level. Patients with chronic urticaria often require much higher than the usual doses of antihistamines.
- Nonsedating antihistamines, such as loratadine (**Claritin**) 10 mg, desloratadine (**Clarinex**) 5 mg, fexofenadine (**Allegra**) 60/180 mg, and cetirizine (**Zyrtec**)

10 mg, may be used during the day, and a more sedating H1 blocker or a tricyclic antidepressant drug, such as doxepin (**Sinequan**), may be tried at bedtime. Doxepin can be given at much lower dosages than when it is used as an antidepressant (e.g., from 5 mg two times daily to 50 mg three times daily).

- *For the pediatric age group*:
  - Fexofenadine (**Allegra**) is approved for use in children as young as 6 months of age in a liquid form dosed at 15 mg twice a day and 30 mg twice a day for children aged 2 to 11 years.
  - A sedating antihistamine such as diphenhydramine or hydroxyzine may be added at bedtime.
- **Systemic steroids** are sometimes used for short periods to break the cycle of chronic urticaria; however, they are not indicated for long-term use in the treatment of chronic idiopathic urticaria.
- If all else fails, a diary of daily foods eaten may be kept, with subsequent food elimination. However, this approach is rarely successful.

POINTS TO REMEMBER

- Except for the physical urticarias and urticaria that is obviously associated with drugs and systemic disease, determining the cause of chronic urticaria is generally a fruitless task.
- Most often, routine blood tests are of little or no value in determining the cause of acute or chronic urticaria.
- Antihistamines remain the mainstay for treating chronic urticaria; a combination of these agents may be necessary for control.
- Allergies are almost never the cause of chronic urticaria. Allergy testing is expensive and often tests that are positive for allergies have no relation to the patient's urticaria.
- When individual wheals persist for more than 24 hours, the process is unlikely to be urticaria.

 HELPFUL HINTS

- **Epinephrine,** which is often administered by intramuscular or subcutaneous injection for acute urticaria, **should not** be used for routine cases of hives. It should be reserved for cases of acute anaphylaxis.
- Patients with documented cold urticaria should be advised not to immerse themselves abruptly in cold water.
- Patients with severe reactions should consider wearing a **medical alert bracelet** that describes their problem.
- Montelukast (**Singulair**), a leukotriene receptor antagonist used to treat asthma, has been found to be effective in some cases of chronic idiopathic urticaria that are refractory to antihistamines.
- Immunotherapies using prednisone, plasmapheresis, intravenous immunoglobulin, low-dose methotrexate, oral psoralens plus ultraviolet A treatment, oral tacrolimus, azathioprine, and cyclosporine have been used in severe, recalcitrant cases.
- Children with chronic urticaria occasionally have an underlying autoimmune disease; thyroid antibodies are the most common positive finding.

 SEE PATIENT HANDOUT "Hives (Urticaria)" ON THE SOLUTION SITE

BASICS

- Erythema multiforme (EM) is a confusing condition for many health care providers. The classic description of EM made by Ferdinand von Hebra in the late 19th century was very specific and is still currently used. He described "a self-limited eruption characterized by symmetrically distributed erythematous papules, which develop into characteristic targetlike lesions consisting of concentric color changes with a dusky central zone that may become bullous" (FIG. 18.8). This classic form of EM is currently defined as EM minor.
- The more serious variant, with extensive mucous membrane involvement, systemic symptoms, and more widespread lesions, is called EM major (Stevens-Johnson syndrome).
- EM is a reaction pattern of dermal blood vessels with secondary changes noted in the epidermis that results clinically in curious targetlike shapes.
- EM is most commonly seen in late adolescence and in young adulthood. Affected persons are generally in good health.

Causes

The list of causes of EM is long and is, in many, a duplication of the list of causes of urticaria (see previous section). Most instances of both EM major and minor are idiopathic; however, the following are the most well-documented associations.

- The most common precipitating cause of EM minor is recurrent labial herpes simplex virus infection (FIG. 18.9); recurrences of herpes progenitalis also have been reported to precede or sometimes occur simultaneously with episodes of recurrent EM minor. EM minor is unlikely related to drugs.
- Precipitating factors in EM major are drugs (sulfonamides, penicillin, hydantoins, barbiturates, allopurinol, NSAIDs); *Mycoplasma* infection; pregnancy; *Streptococcus* infection; hepatitis A and B; coccidioidomycosis; and Epstein-Barr virus infection.
- Poison ivy (rhus dermatitis) has also been reported to be associated with erythema multiforme.

DESCRIPTION OF LESIONS

- Lesions begin as round, erythematous macules.
- Some lesions evolve to form targetoid plaques (iris lesions) with a dark center that may become vesicobullous.
- Lesions persist (are "fixed") for at least 1 week.
- Erosions and crusts form.

DISTRIBUTION OF LESIONS

- Lesions are bilateral and symmetric.
- The palms and soles, dorsa of hands and feet, extensor forearms and legs, face, and genitalia are affected.
- Mucous membrane lesions are limited to the mouth in EM minor.
- Extensive mucous membrane lesions in EM major may be located in multiple sites, including the mouth, pharynx, eyes, and genitalia (FIG. 18.10).

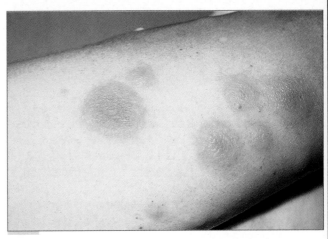

18.8 *Erythema multiforme.* Characteristic targetlike lesions are noted here.

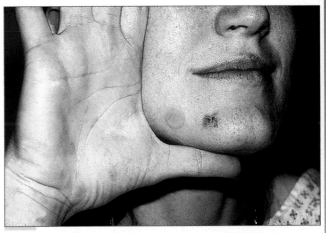

18.9 *Erythema multiforme minor.* This patient has a recurrent herpes simplex virus infection. Note the drying crust of the herpetic "cold sore" on her upper lip and the targetlike lesions on her palm (see also FIG. 12.4).

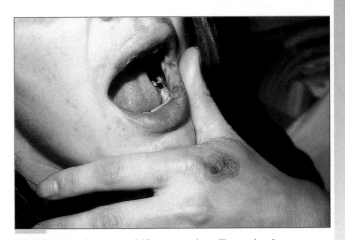

18.10 *Erythema multiforme major.* Extensive hemorrhagic crusting on mucous membranes is noted in a patient with fever and extensive erythematous lesions (see also FIG. 12.5).

MANAGEMENT

- If known, the precipitating cause should be eliminated or treated.
- Suspected etiologic drugs should be discontinued.
- Empiric treatment with oral acyclovir, famciclovir (**Famvir**), or valacyclovir (**Valtrex**) may prevent or mitigate recurrences if EM is a result of herpes simplex virus infection (see Chapter 6, "Superficial Viral Infections," for dosages).
- Wet dressings (e.g., **Burow's solution**) and topical steroids may be applied to oozing lesions.
- In life-threatening situations, such as may occur in EM major, hospitalization is often essential. The use of systemic steroids in such severe cases is controversial, and their effectiveness has not been established.
- The use of intravenous gamma globulin and cyclosporine is also controversial, and the effectiveness of these treatments has not been confirmed by double-blind studies.

 POINTS TO REMEMBER

- EM is not a disease but a syndrome, a reaction to underlying stimuli, with multiple causes and various degrees of severity.
- Even in the clinical absence of herpes simplex virus infection, recurrent EM may be suppressed with oral acyclovir, famciclovir, or valacyclovir.

CLINICAL MANIFESTATIONS

Erythema Multiforme Minor
- The eruption is acute, self-limited, and often recurrent.
- Evidence of herpes labialis may be present.
- Little or no mucous membrane involvement is noted.

Erythema Multiforme Major
- EM major is often accompanied by symptoms of fever, malaise, and myalgias.
- Severe, painful mucous membrane involvement occurs.
- Possible complications include keratitis, corneal ulcers, upper airway damage, and pneumonia.

DIAGNOSIS
- Typical target lesions are present.
- Skin biopsy is performed, if necessary.

DIFFERENTIAL DIAGNOSIS

Urticaria
- Lesions are transient, not "fixed."
- Lesions are pruritic.
- The center of annular lesions is not dusky in color.

Primary Herpes Gingivostomatitis and Primary Bullous Diseases of the Oral Cavity
- In the absence of nonmucous membrane skin lesions, other diseases of the mucous membranes may be clinically indistinguishable from those of EM.
- Mucous membrane biopsy may be necessary to distinguish oral bullous EM from primary bullous diseases such as pemphigus vulgaris or bullous pemphigoid (see also Chapter 12, "Disorders of the Mouth, Lips, and Tongue").

BASICS

Purpura is defined as a hemorrhage of blood into the skin or mucous membranes (FIG. 18.11). It is most commonly seen on dependent areas (i.e., the lower legs and ankles). Purpuric skin is purple, violaceous, or dark red in color and is nonblanchable because blood is present *outside* of vessel walls. In contrast, erythema is red in color and blanches on compression because blood remains *within* the vessels. Nonpalpable purpuric lesions that are smaller than 3 mm in size are referred to as *petechiae*; those larger than 3 mm are called *ecchymoses*. Purpura is further subdivided into *nonpalpable* (macular) and *palpable* (papular) categories.

The lower legs are the most common location for purpuras as well as the primary site of peripheral venous disease such as stasis dermatitis (see Chapter 2, "Eczema"). Purpuric lesions can be a sign or symptom of other vascular disorders such as coagulopathies or vasculitis and may serve as clues to systemic diseases such as SLE. Of lesser concern are the so-called "benign" variants—the benign pigmented purpuras (BPPs) that are caused by capillaritis, which allows blood to exit small vessels (extravasation) and create petechiae. As their name implies, BPPs are not associated with any systemic disease.

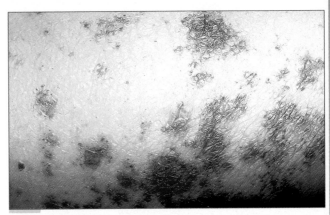

18.11 *Purpura.* Petechiae and ecchymoses combine and form areas of nonblanching purpura.

Nonpalpable Purpura and Small Vessel Vasculitis

BASICS

- Nonpalpable purpura may be seen after the following:
  - Minor trauma to the skin. This may precipitate purpura, particularly when a patient is taking drugs such as aspirin, clopidogrel (Plavix), NSAIDs, and warfarin (Coumadin), all of which increase clotting time.
  - Long-term application of potent topical steroids on the skin of elderly patients.
- It also may be seen in association with:
  - BPP (see subsequent discussion).
  - Blood dyscrasias and coagulopathies, such as thrombocytopenia, leukemia, and disseminated intravascular coagulopathy. Lesions are more commonly on dependent areas (i.e., lower legs and ankles; buttocks in bedridden patients).
  - **Actinic purpura** (formerly known as senile purpura), which is a prevalent finding on the dorsal forearms in elderly persons. Such ecchymoses are believed to result from minor trauma to an area of chronic sun exposure. Thinning of skin and "fragile capillaries" are considered the cause (FIG. 18.12).
  - Chronic venous insufficiency of the lower extremities.

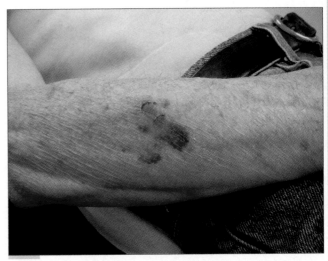

18.12 *Senile, or actinic, purpura.* Ecchymoses are present on the dorsal forearms in an elderly person.

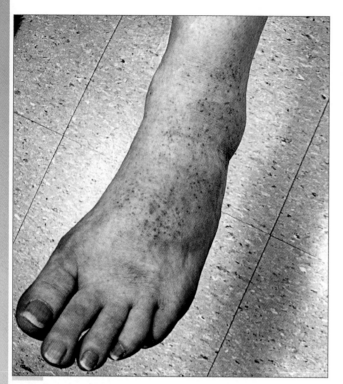

18.13 *Schamberg's purpura.* "Cayenne pepper" petechiae are seen on the lower extremities.

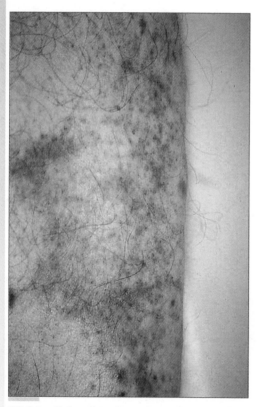

18.14 *Schamberg's purpura.* In this patient, the lesions are more extensive. Coalescence of petechiae has created large areas of nonpalpable purpura. Note the hyperpigmented macules indicating the presence of hemosiderin in the skin. (Image courtesy of Art Huntley, M.D.)

DESCRIPTION OF LESIONS

- Lesions begin as nonblanching, red, pinpoint-size macules (petechiae) or bruises (ecchymoses) that may coalesce.
- Older lesions become purple, then brown as hemosiderin forms.

CLINICAL MANIFESTATIONS

- Lesions are generally asymptomatic, but they may be mildly pruritic.
- BPP may be of cosmetic concern to patients; other patients wish to be reassured that purpura is not a sign of a serious disease.
- Lesions may persist for months to years or indefinitely.

Variants of Benign Pigmented Purpura

Schamberg's Purpura

- This is most commonly seen on the lower extremities.
- It is the most common of the BPPs and occurs primarily in adults, especially in the elderly. It is characterized by so-called "cayenne pepper" purpura (FIGS. 18.13 and 18.14).

Majocchi's Purpura (Purpura Annularis Telangiectodes)

- Also a capillaritis, these asymptomatic annular lesions may be seen especially in adolescents and young adults and may appear at any site.
- Lesions consist of pigmentation that is annular in configuration, often with a central clearing. The purple, yellow, or brown patches consist of telangiectases and hemosiderin deposition (Fig. 18.15).

DIAGNOSIS

- The diagnosis is made on clinical presentation.
- Lesions are not palpable and are nonblanching on diascopy (direct pressure).

 DIFFERENTIAL DIAGNOSIS

- Biopsy may be necessary at times to distinguish benign purpura from leukocytoclastic vasculitis, the histopathologic finding in palpable purpura (see next section).

 MANAGEMENT

- BPP generally requires no workup; however, if a blood dyscrasia or coagulopathy is suspected, appropriate laboratory tests should be ordered.
- Possible offending drugs should be evaluated regarding their risk-to-benefit ratio.
- A coagulopathy or blood dyscrasia should be ruled out, if it is clinically suspected.

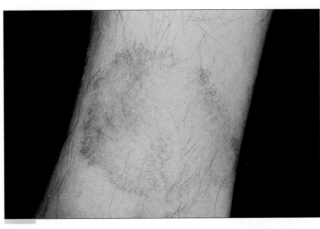

18.15 Majocchi's purpura (purpura annularis telangiectodes). This is the characteristic ring-shaped nonblanching purpuric lesion that has become hyperpigmented because of the presence of hemosiderin. (Image courtesy of Art Huntley, M.D.)

BASICS

- Palpable purpura (PP) is a vasculitis of the skin. It involves a group of conditions that affect the vessels that lie within the middle to upper dermis. When the vasculitis is more extensive and affects internal organs—most commonly the gastrointestinal tract, kidneys, central nervous system, and joints—it may then be referred to as *hypersensitivity vasculitis* (HV).
- The prognosis is good when no internal involvement is present. PP and HV may be acute or chronic. Common to all forms of vasculitis are the inflammation and destruction of blood vessel walls by inflammatory cells. Palpability of lesions is caused by the accumulation of inflammatory cells and the leakage of blood from the vessels.

Pathophysiology

- It is believed that the deposition of circulating immune complexes in the postcapillary venules is the cause of vasculitis. The circulating immune complexes may also deposit in organs, causing a vasculitis with resultant gastrointestinal bleeding, hematuria, and arthralgias.
- **Leukocytoclastic vasculitis** is the characteristic histopathologic finding of PP and HV. Biopsy of lesions shows characteristic leukocytoclastic vasculitis ("nuclear dust").
- The cutaneous vasculitis may be associated with a hypersensitivity to antigens from drugs (most often antibiotics), NSAIDs, allopurinol, thiazide diuretics, and hydantoins. Conditions that may be associated with HV include malignancies; infectious diseases; cryoglobulinemias; other underlying diseases such as SLE, Sjögren's syndrome, rheumatoid arthritis, and inflammatory bowel diseases; paraproteinemia; ingestants and infections such as beta-hemolytic streptococcal infection; viral hepatitis, particularly hepatitis C; and human immunodeficiency virus infection.
- More than 50% of cases are idiopathic and may occur in the absence of any systemic disease.

DESCRIPTION OF LESIONS

- Lesions tend to appear in crops; they are red to violaceous to purple in color and are nonblanching (FIG. 18.16).
- Infrequently, hemorrhagic vesicles or bullae may occur and develop into painful ulcerations (FIG. 18.17).
- Healing takes place within 1 to 2 weeks and may result in postinflammatory hyperpigmentation and/or scarring.

DISTRIBUTION OF LESIONS

- The lesions are characteristically symmetric in distribution. They are most often seen in dependent areas such as the lower legs and ankles and on the buttocks in bedridden patients, but any area of the skin can be involved.
- In severe forms, lesions can become generalized.

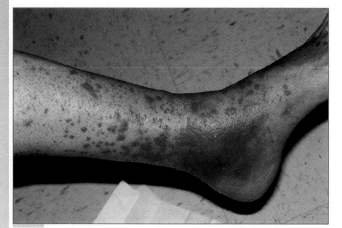

18.16 *Palpable purpura.* Nonblanching papules suggest vasculitis. Hemorrhagic blisters and coalescence of lesions arise from purpuric areas and are indicative of more severe vessel involvement.

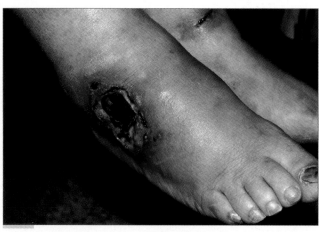

18.17 *Vasculitis.* This patient has cryoglobulinemic vasculitis. Hemorrhagic blisters are forming a large ulceration on her ankle.

CLINICAL MANIFESTATIONS

- Lesions may be asymptomatic, mildly pruritic, slightly painful, or very painful (ulcers) and may occur in the absence of any systemic disease.
- Lesions can be recurrent; however, the majority of patients (90%) have only a single episode.
- There may be associated malaise and possible fever.
- In systemic vasculitis, symptoms are referable to the organ involved.

DIAGNOSIS

- Laboratory investigations that are useful for identifying any underlying disease include complete blood count, a blood chemistry panel, erythrocyte sedimentation rate, urinalysis, and stool examination for occult blood. Further studies (e.g., serum complement, antinuclear antibodies) should be directed by the patient's symptoms. Other testing may include serum protein electrophoresis, cryoglobulins, and hepatitis C antibody for patients who have no identifiable disease.
- Biopsy of fresh lesions shows characteristic leukocytoclastic vasculitis ("nuclear dust"). A biopsy performed too early or too late in its evolution may not reveal these findings.

 DIFFERENTIAL DIAGNOSIS

Henoch-Schönlein Purpura

- Henoch-Schönlein purpura (HSP) is a term that should be reserved for disease that follows an upper respiratory infection, generally in children. It is a type of HV caused by group A streptococci.
- HSP generally occurs in persons 20 or younger but may also be seen in adults.
- Clinical and histopathologic findings are similar to those of HV. Abdominal pain, arthralgia, hematuria, and proteinuria may be present.
- Patients with HSP caused by group A streptococci have a perivascular IgA immunofluorescent deposition in the skin and kidneys. In children and in some adults, serologic testing for a possible streptococcal infection should be considered (streptozyme or antistreptolysin O titer).

Arthropod Bite Reactions

- When these appear on the lower extremities, they can mimic PP.
- The history of exposure to bites is often obtainable (FIG. 18.18).

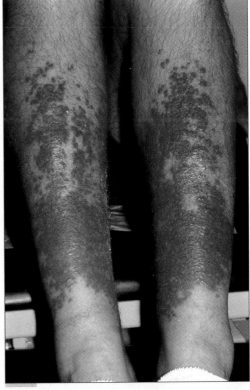

18.18 *Arthropod bite reaction.* These intensely pruritic discrete and confluent nonblanching purpuric lesions occurred several days after this patient walked in tall grass, where he was bitten by chigger mites.

continued on page 318

Septic Vasculitis

- Palpable and nonpalpable purpura may also be seen in septic vasculitis, in which lesions are more often acral (i.e., distal on toes or fingertips) and tend to be few in number (e.g., gonococcemia) (Fig. 18.19).
- Lesions also tend to lack the characteristic symmetry of HV.
- Patients who have septic vasculitis may also be febrile and show other signs and symptoms of their underlying infection.

Other Vasculitides

- It should be kept in mind that cutaneous vasculitis, and thus PP, may be seen in patients with rare diseases such as Wegener's granulomatosis, polyarteritis nodosa, cryoglobulinemic vasculitis, antiphospholipid syndrome, microscopic polyangiitis, and Churg-Strauss syndrome (allergic granulomatosis).
- Many of these conditions involve larger vessels than are typically involved in HV.

Atrophie Blanche (Livedoid Vasculopathy)

- Patients present with small, porcelain-white, stellate (star-shaped) scars with surrounding telangiectasias (Fig. 18.20). The initial lesions are typically painful purpuric macules or papules on the malleoli and the adjacent dorsa of the feet that often appear in clusters and form irregular patterns of superficial punched-out ulcers.
- The white scars result from the healing of such ulcerations and represent an end-stage feature of chronic venous insufficiency.
- Livedoid vasculopathy has become the more dynamic, more inclusive term because it better explains the pathogenic process that leads to the condition.
- In addition to chronic venous hypertension, atrophie blanche has been associated with conditions that have a vascular occlusive component to them, such as deficiencies in a variety of blood factors, a history of increased plasma homocysteine levels, the presence of antiphospholipid antibodies, and abnormalities in fibrinolysis and platelet function. There is also a primary or idiopathic type of atrophie blanche that is a distinct condition and is not usually the result of other diseases. As with secondary atrophie blanche, women are affected more often than men.

Pyoderma Gangrenosum

- Ulcerative lesions that evolve from PP may resemble the chronic ulcers of this disease.

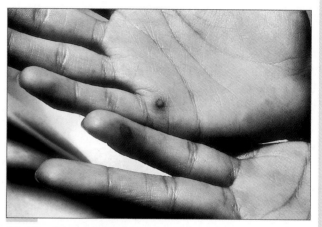

18.19 ***Disseminated gonococcemia.*** This is an example of septic vasculitis. Note the two palpable purpuric hemorrhagic vesicles.

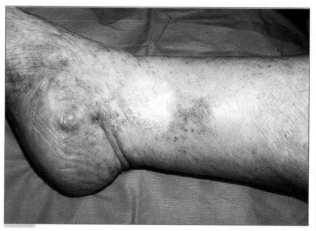

18.20 ***Atrophie blanche (livedoid vasculopathy).*** White, stellate scars are present. The proximal erythema and the superficial varicosities that surround the affected area (corona phlebectasia) suggest that stasis dermatitis is the cause of her vasculitis.

POINTS TO REMEMBER

- PP may be a sign of systemic vasculitis, sepsis, drug allergy, underlying disease, or an idiopathic benign reaction pattern.
- Patients with PP that primarily affects the skin, and not the internal organs, have a good prognosis.
- When evaluating purpura (both palpable and nonpalpable, septic and nonseptic) of the lower extremities, other, often rare, entities must also be considered as diagnostic possibilities in the proper clinical context.
- The diagnosis of BPP is generally made on clinical grounds, and the patient should be reassured about the benign nature of these lesions.

 HELPFUL HINT

- Vasculitis in patients with Wegener's granulomatosis, polyarteritis nodosa, or Churg-Strauss syndrome can be considered a potentially fatal disease. Treatment with systemic corticosteroids and/or immunosuppressive/cytotoxic agents is necessary.

MANAGEMENT

- If known, the precipitating cause (e.g., drug) should be eliminated or the responsible underlying disease (e.g., SLE) should be treated.
- Elevation of the legs (above the level of the heart) and/or compression stockings may be useful because the disease often affects dependent areas.
- In general, no treatment is necessary for mild, self-limited episodes.
- For painful cutaneous lesions or arthralgias, **NSAIDs** may be used (e.g., ibuprofen, indomethacin, or naproxen).
- For severe, extensive or recalcitrant cases, **oral corticosteroids** are indicated. The dose is slowly reduced over the course of several weeks.
- For recurrent or persistent lesions, **dapsone** and **colchicine** have also been reported to be effective.
- In cases of rapid progression or systemic involvement, immunosuppressants such as cyclophosphamide (**Cytoxan**), azathioprine (**Imuran**), methotrexate (**Rheumatrex**), and mycophenolate mofetil (**CellCept**) have been used in conjunction with systemic steroids as steroid-sparing agents.
- Recently the use of rituximab (**Rituxan**) has been reported to be helpful in some cases of vasculitis.

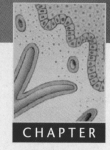

19

Sexually Transmitted Diseases

Mary Ruth Buchness and Herbert P. Goodheart

OVERVIEW

• Until the 1990s, sexually transmitted diseases (STDs) were commonly known as venereal diseases. *Veneris* is the Latin form of the name Venus, the Roman goddess of love.

• **Syphilis** is common worldwide, and since the late 1990s infectious early syphilis has re-emerged as an important disease in western Europe and the United States and is an important facilitator of human immunodeficiency virus (HIV) transmission.

• An estimated 1% of the population of the United States has clinically evident lesions of the **human papilloma virus (HPV),** and 15% have latent HPV infection. HPV is thought to be one of the main causes of cervical cancer, and it has also been linked with other types of cancers of the female and male reproductive system.

• **Herpes simplex virus (HSV)** infection is another STD that presently has no cure. The incidence of HSV-2 infection is also one of the most rapidly increasing among STDs in the United States.

• **Chancroid** is rare in the United States and Western Europe. In the United States, it is associated with the use of crack cocaine.

• **Lymphogranuloma venereum** and **granuloma inguinale** are also reported rarely in the United States and Western Europe and are more frequently seen in tropical and subtropical regions.

BASICS

- Anogenital warts, for the most part, are sexually transmitted viral warts caused by infection with specific types of HPV. Despite the generally benign nature of the proliferations, certain types of HPV can place patients at a high risk for anogenital cancers.
- Treatment of genital warts can be difficult and lengthy. Patients should be counseled about their risk of infectivity to others. They also should be advised of their increased risk of having other STDs.
- The incubation period is variable, ranging from 3 weeks to 8 months, with a reported average, in one study, of 2.8 months.
- HPV has been identified in the skin of infected persons at a distance of up to 1 cm from the actual lesion; this feature may explain the high recurrence rate. HPV types 16, 18, 31 to 35, 39, 42, 48, and 51 to 54 have been identified in cervical and anogenital cancers.
- The median duration of infection is 8 months. In a study of college women, only 9% had persistence of infection after 2 years, even among those infected with oncogenic subtypes.
- Lesions tend to be more extensive and recalcitrant to treatment in immunocompromised persons; they also tend to grow larger and more numerous during pregnancy.
- Women with HPV infection who are pregnant or who are considering pregnancy pose specific challenges. In addition to the potential for rapid proliferation of external genital warts during pregnancy, the presence of HPV infection raises concerns regarding the risk of laryngeal papillomatosis or genital HPV infections in the newborn; however, cesarean section does not eliminate the risk of transmission.
- More than half of children with anogenital warts have a manifestation of viral inoculation at birth or incidental spread of cutaneous warts. Such cases often are caused by nongenital HPV infections.

Risk Factors

- Transmission of anogenital HPV infection occurs largely by sexual intercourse.
- Other risk factors for infection include cigarette smoking, participating in sexual activity at an early age, having a high number of sexual partners, having another STD, immunosuppression, and having an abnormal Pap smear result.

DESCRIPTION OF LESIONS

There are five morphologic types of anogenital warts, and a patient may manifest more than one type. The appearance of warts depends on its location; for example, the condyloma acuminatum type tends to occur on moist surfaces.

- Condyloma acuminatum may resemble small cauliflowers (FIG. 19.1).
- Warts may appear as smooth, dome-shaped, papular lesions (FIG. 19.2).

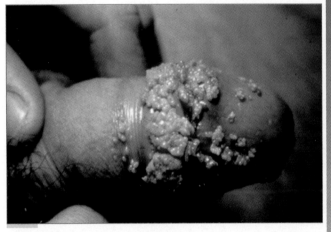

19.1 *Condyloma acuminatum.* Lesions resemble small cauliflowers.

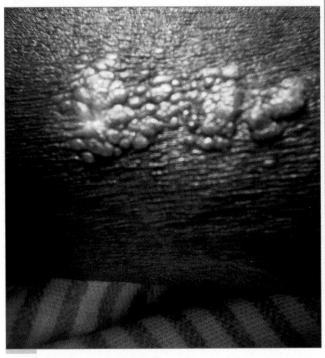

19.2 *Condyloma acuminatum.* Smooth, dome-shaped papular lesions are present.

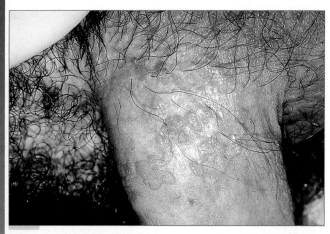

19.3 *Condyloma acuminatum.* These papules have the appearance of common warts.

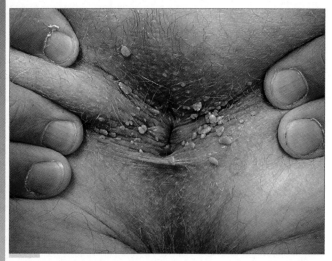

19.4 *Condyloma acuminatum.* Perianal warts are seen in this patient.

- They can look like typical verrucous papules or plaques that resemble common warts (FIG. 19.3).
- Occasionally, they present as flat papules that may be hyperpigmented.

DISTRIBUTION OF LESIONS

Anogenital Lesions

- In men, lesions occur on the penis, scrotum, mons pubis, inguinal crease, and perianal area (FIG. 19.4).
- In women, the vagina, labia (FIG. 19.5), mons pubis, perianal area, and uterine cervix are the most common locations.
- Intra-anal warts are seen predominantly in patients who have engaged in receptive anal intercourse.
- Warts may also be found in the peri- and intraurethral areas in men.

Outside the Genital Area

- HPV has been associated with conjunctival, nasal, oral, and laryngeal warts.

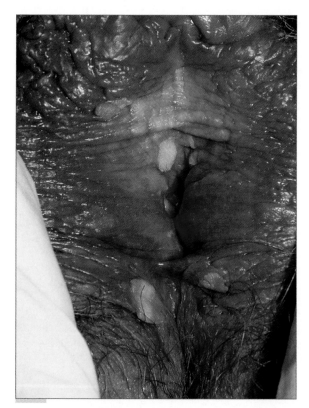

19.5 *Condyloma acuminatum.* Note the labial warts in this patient. Compare to FIGURE 19.7.

CLINICAL MANIFESTATIONS

- Genital warts are usually asymptomatic.
- Lesions may become pruritic, particularly perianal and inguinal lesions.
- They may be painful or bleed if traumatized.
- Genital warts may resolve spontaneously or, rarely, progress to invasive squamous cell carcinoma.

DIAGNOSIS

- The diagnosis of anogenital warts is generally straightforward when the patient presents with the typical cauliflower-like lesions of condyloma acuminatum or with characteristic verrucous or filiform warts.
- However, when lesions are papular (flat-topped), pigmented, moist, or erosive, the diagnosis may not be as clinically obvious.

Acetowhite Test on Mucous Membranes

- In women, colposcopy is performed using 35% acetic acid, which produces an acetowhitening of subclinical lesions on the vaginal and cervical mucosa (Fig. 19.6).
- Atypia or koilocytosis found on Pap smears represents early changes resulting from HPV infection.

Acetowhite Test on Non-Mucous Membrane Areas

- Application of a 5% concentration of acetic acid for 15 to 20 minutes makes subclinical lesions turn white.
- Any lesion with epidermal hyperkeratosis appears white. Thus, this method often produces false-positive results and is no longer recommended for routine screening for genital warts.

Biopsy

A biopsy may be needed to identify confusing anogenital lesions.

- After local anesthesia with lidocaine, curved iris scissors are used to obtain a small specimen (snip biopsy) from the labia minora or perianal area. A punch biopsy or, more simply, a shave biopsy may be obtained from non-mucous membrane skin (see Chapter 26, "Diagnostic and Therapeutic Procedures"). If an ulcer or an indurated nodule is present—particularly if carcinoma is suspected—a punch or excisional biopsy should be performed.
- A biopsy is used to rule out anogenital bowenoid papulosis or frank squamous cell carcinoma in atypical or recalcitrant lesions.

(text continued on page 327)

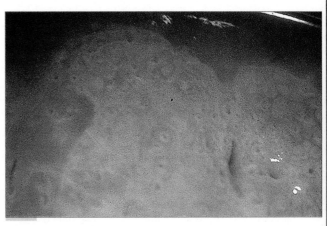

19.6 *Cervical warts.* Acetowhitening of subclinical lesions on the cervical mucosa is shown here.

DIFFERENTIAL DIAGNOSIS

Normal Anatomic Structures

- In women, **vestibular papillae** are normal anatomic structures. Unlike warts, vestibular papillae (vulvar papillomatosis) occur near the vaginal vestibule in symmetric clusters or in a linear pattern. They often appear as monotonous, small, smooth projections that resemble cobblestones (Fig. 19.7).
- In men, **pearly penile papules** are frequently mistaken for warts. They are small, skin-colored to shiny, pearly papules that are located around the rim of the corona of the glans penis (Figs. 19.8 and 19.9).
- **Fordyce spots** are angiokeratomas. They occur on the medial labia minora in many women (see Fig. 21.47).

Benign Lesions

- Common benign skin lesions, such as **skin tags, seborrheic keratoses,** and **melanocytic nevi,** may also be easily mistaken for warts.
- Skin tags are smooth and may be pigmented or skin-colored. Seborrheic keratoses and melanocytic nevi often have a verrucous (keratotic) appearance and may be pigmented.

Other Conditions

- **Hemorrhoids.** Not infrequently, anal hemorrhoids are mistaken for warts. Hemorrhoids are smooth and compressible.
- **Molluscum contagiosum.** This pox virus infection can easily be confused with, and may coexist with, genital warts. It is seen most often in young children and in patients with HIV infection and in sexually active young

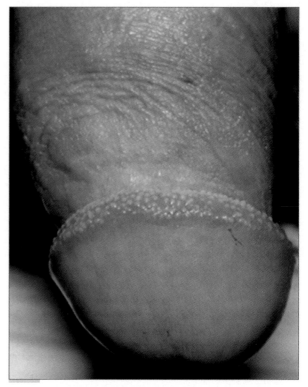

19.8 *Pearly penile papules.* These normal anatomic structures occur as shiny papules that are present around the corona of the glans penis and the frenum of the penis.

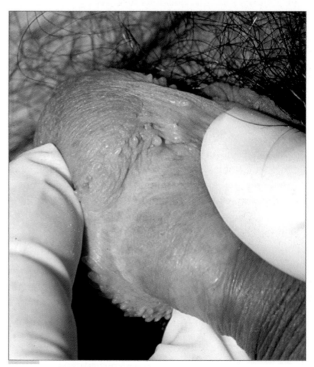

19.9 *Pearly penile papules.* These hairlike papules are sometimes referred to as "hirsutoid papules." They are also frequently misdiagnosed and treated as warts.

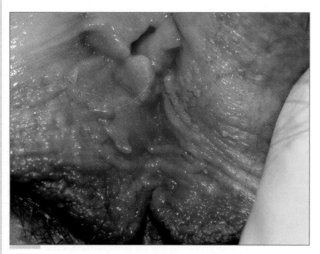

19.7 *Vestibular papillae (vulvar papillomatosis).* These normal anatomic structures occur near the vaginal vestibule in symmetric clusters or in a linear pattern. They are frequently mistaken for warts.

continued on page 325

adults (see Chapter 6, "Superficial Viral Infections," and Chapter 24, "Cutaneous Manifestations of HIV Infection"). The lesions are dome-shaped, waxy or pearly white papules with a central white core, which is often revealed by inspection with a handheld magnifier.

- **Condyloma latum of secondary syphilis.** Lesions are moist, smooth-surfaced, and, usually, whitish and flat-topped. Serologic tests for syphilis are positive (see FIG. 19.20).

Malignant Neoplasms

When any of the following conditions are suspected, a biopsy should be performed.

- **Bowenoid papulosis.** These lesions are clinically similar to, and often indistinguishable from, flat or dome-shaped genital warts. They are associated with HPV type 16 or 18. Histologically, bowenoid papulosis demonstrates squamous cell carcinoma in situ; however, it follows a largely benign clinical course.
- **Giant condyloma acuminatum.** Also known as a Buschke-Löwenstein tumor, this lesion is a low-grade, locally invasive squamous cell carcinoma that can arise from and appear as a fungating condyloma (FIG. 19.10). It is associated with HPV types 6 and 11 and should be considered in the differential of lesions measuring greater than 1 cm in diameter. Only radical surgical extirpation is considered appropriate treatment.
- **Squamous cell carcinoma.** These lesions are rapidly growing nodules or tumors, and they may be erosive or ulcerative.

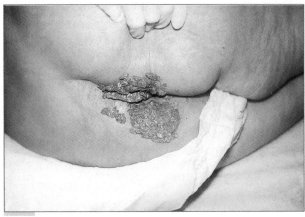

19.10 *Giant condyloma acuminatum.* This low-grade, locally invasive malignant tumor can arise from and appear as a fungating condyloma.

 MANAGEMENT

Counseling

- Patients should be advised about the long latency period of HPV; thus, a patient may not have contracted condyloma from his or her current partner.
- Male patients should use condoms at least 1 year after clinical infection is treated; however, condoms are not perfect protection because warts can occur on genital areas other than the penis or vagina.
- In affected women, there is a risk of malignant degeneration to cervical intraepithelial neoplasia or squamous cell carcinoma. If cervical warts are found during examination or if vulvar neoplasia is confirmed by biopsy, referral for colposcopic evaluation is indicated.
- It is recommended that anogenital warts be treated in pregnant women during the second and third trimesters and that vaginal delivery be performed if possible.
- In affected men with perianal warts, there is a risk of malignant degeneration to anal intraepithelial neoplasia or anal carcinoma. Atypical lesions should be biopsied.
- The U.S. Centers for Disease Control and Prevention (CDC) recommends cesarean section only when the vaginal outlet is obstructed by extensive condylomata or if vaginal delivery would cause excessive bleeding.

- Patients who have internal anal or rectal warts tend to have continual recurrences of external warts and should be referred to a rectal surgeon.
- Diagnosis of genital warts in a child requires that the clinician report suspected abuse to begin an evaluation process that may or may not confirm sexual abuse (FIG. 19.11).

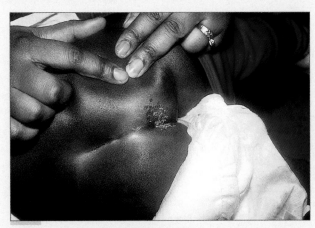

19.11 *Perianal warts in an infant.* The possibility of child abuse should always be considered in these cases.

continued on page 326

Surgical Therapy

- **Cryosurgery with liquid nitrogen.** Cryosurgery is very effective for treating multiple, small warts (e.g., lesions on the shaft of the penis and vulva). Cryotherapy is also safe for the mother and fetus when used during the second and third trimesters of pregnancy.
- **Electrodesiccation and curettage.** This is quite effective for a limited number of lesions on the shaft of the penis.
- **Carbon dioxide laser treatment.** This is more expensive and includes a danger of the operator developing laryngeal lesions from virus in the laser plume.
- **Surgical excision** (useful for debulking large "cauliflower" lesions). Large, unresponsive lesions around the rectum or vulva can be treated with scissor excision of the bulk of the mass followed by electrocautery of the remaining tissue down to the skin surface.

Intralesional Therapy

- **Interferon-α2b** (11.5 units three times weekly for 3 weeks). This is not recommended by the CDC because of high expense and a lack of increased efficacy over other treatments. It may also cause flulike symptoms.

Topical Therapy

See Table 19.1.

Vaccine

- Quadrivalent vaccine (**Gardasil**) protects against HPV subtypes 6, 11, 16, and 18.
- A bivalent vaccine protects against subtypes 16 and 18. Approval is pending.

- The Advisory Committee on Immunization Practices of the CDC recommends routine immunization of girls at 11 and 12 years of age, with the vaccine being made available to girls as young as 9 and women as old as 26. Efficacy has not been studied in women older than 26 or in males.
- Women younger than 26 years of age with abnormal or equivocal Pap smears, known HPV infection, or genital warts can be vaccinated. However, the vaccine does not protect against HPV subtypes that the vaccine recipient already has.
- Gardasil can be used in women younger than 26 years of age who are breastfeeding or are immunocompromised; however, those women who are immunodeficient may not produce an adequate number of antibodies in response to the vaccine.
- Pregnant women should not be vaccinated.
- The goal is to reduce the incidence of anogenital cancers by immunizing against the most common oncogenic subtypes.
  - Postmarket research has shown the quadrivalent vaccine to be almost 100% effective in preventing infection with HPV 16 and 18. It is also effective, to a lesser extent, in preventing infection with an additional 10 subtypes of HPV, including oncogenic subtypes responsible for 20% of cervical cancers.
  - Refer to the CDC Web site (www.cdc.gov/std/) for the most current updates.

Treatment for Pregnant Women

- In the ambulatory setting, appropriate treatment choices include trichloroacetic or bichloracetic acid and ablative procedures, such as cryosurgery.

 POINTS TO REMEMBER

- Immunosuppressed patients, such as those with acquired immunodeficiency syndrome (AIDS) and those taking immunosuppressive therapy (e.g., renal transplant recipients), are more likely than others to develop persistent HPV infection and subsequent dysplasia and malignant disease.
- Malignant degeneration may be indicated by increases in size, pain, or bleeding.
- Pearly penile papules, vestibular papillae, and other normal anatomic structures are often mistaken for condyloma acuminatum.

 SEE PATIENT HANDOUT "Genital Warts" ON THE SOLUTION SITE

 HELPFUL HINTS

- Although skin warts are common in the general pediatric population, genital warts are uncommon in children. Consequently, the diagnosis of genital warts in children should alert the health care provider to the possibility of sexual abuse.
- Confusing condyloma lata for genital warts misses the diagnosis of highly infectious secondary syphilis and leads to inappropriate therapy and potentially disastrous sequelae for the patient.
- Confusing pearly penile papules, vestibular papillae, or Fordyce spots with genital warts results in unnecessary treatment and unwarranted psychosocial stress.
- Cesarean delivery should not be performed solely to prevent transmission of HPV infection to the newborn; however, it is advisable to remove visible lesions during pregnancy.

Table 19.1 TOPICAL THERAPIES FOR ANOGENITAL WARTS

TREATMENT	APPLICATION
Patient-applied therapies	
Imiquimod 5% (**Aldara**) cream	It is used three times weekly at bedtime for up to 16 weeks.
	It enhances a patient's immunity to HPV by increasing local production of interferon.
	Efficacy in immunocompromised patients is unknown.
	Safety for use in pregnancy is not known.
Podofilox (**Condylox**) 0.5% solution or gel	It is used twice daily (morning and evening) for 3 days, then followed by 4 days without therapy. This 1-week cycle of treatment may be repeated up to four times until no wart remains.
	Safety for use in pregnancy is not known.
Provider-applied therapies	
Podophyllin resin 10% to 25% in tincture of benzoin	It is carefully applied to the wart surface. The patient is instructed to wash the area in 4 to 6 hours, and the interval is increased for subsequent treatments.
	It is most effective on warts on moist surfaces (perianal, labial, under the prepuce).
	Podophyllin is an antimitotic agent that causes local tissue destruction. It should not be used in pregnant women or on extensive mucosal surfaces.
Trichloroacetic or **bichloracetic acid** 80% to 90%	First, the surrounding normal epithelium is coated with a protective substance, such as 2% lidocaine jelly or Vaseline petroleum jelly, and then a small, cotton-tipped applicator is used to apply the medication carefully to the wart surface.
	These agents can cause intense burning of mucosal surfaces. They are most effective on small warts and on nonmucosal surfaces.
	They may be followed by the use of podophyllin on nonmucosal surfaces.

Herpes Simplex Genitalis

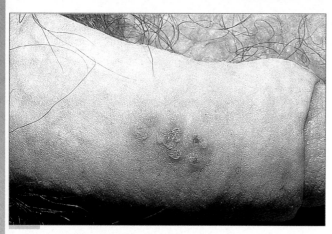

19.12 *Herpes simplex genitalis.* Grouped vesicles on an erythematous base are evident in this patient.

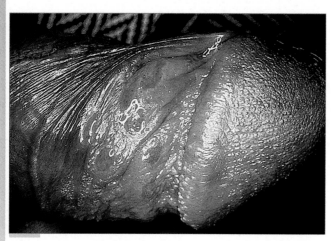

19.13 *Herpes simplex genitalis.* Vesicles have become grouped erosions in this patient.

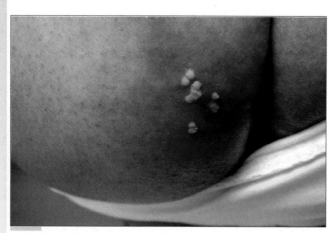

19.14 *Herpes simplex.* This is a common site of HSV-2 in women.

BASICS

- Herpes simplex genitalis is a genital disease caused most commonly by HSV-2, although HSV-1 can also infect genital skin. It is most commonly, but not invariably, sexually transmitted.
- HSV is the most common cause of ulcerative genital lesions. The disease is highly contagious during the prodrome and while the lesions are active.
- HSV establishes latency in the dorsal root ganglia and reappears after different triggers in individual patients. Triggers include psychologic or physiologic stress, physical trauma such as from sexual intercourse, menses, and immunosuppression.
- Affected patients may have recurrences that are infrequent or as common as once monthly. Patients who have six or more episodes per year are candidates for long-term suppressive therapy.

Risk Factors

- Women have higher acquisition rates and more recurrences than do men.
- People between 15 and 35 years of age have a greater chance to contract HSV-2.
- For those individuals who are infected with HPV (see earlier discussion) and HSV, those who have a greater number of sexual partners are also more likely to develop HSV.

DESCRIPTION OF LESIONS

- Initially, lesions appear as grouped vesicles on an erythematous base (FIG. 19.12).
- Lesions may then become pustular, crusted, and eroded (FIG. 19.13).
- Crusting of the lesions occurs over 15 to 20 days, before reepithelialization begins.
- Chronic ulcerations or crusted or verrucous papules may develop in immunocompromised patients (see FIGS. 24.3 and 24.4).

DISTRIBUTION OF LESIONS

- In women, the vulvae, perineum, inner thighs, buttocks, and sacral area (FIG. 19.14) are the most common sites of involvement.
- In men, the penis, scrotum, thigh, and buttocks are the typical locations.

CLINICAL MANIFESTATIONS

Primary Herpes Simplex

- As with HSV-1, this may be more severe than recurrent infections (see Chapter 6, "Superficial Viral Infections").
- The duration is generally from 10 to 14 days.
- Regional adenopathy may be present.
- Fever, dysuria, urinary retention, and constipation may also occur.
- Alternatively, the initial outbreak may be mild or asymptomatic, so that the patient sheds virus intermittently without realizing that he or she is infected.

Recurrent Herpes Simplex

- There is often a prodrome of itching, burning, numbness, tingling, or pain 1 to 2 days before a clinical outbreak.
- Lesions are localized and recur at the same site or in close proximity each time.
- Regional adenopathy may be present.
- Vulvar involvement may cause dysuria.
- The duration is generally from 3 to 5 days.
- Chronic ulcerative lesions are indicative of immunosuppression.
- The risk of neonatal transmission is less than 3% and is greatest in patients with primary HSV at the time of delivery.

COMPLICATIONS

- Genital ulcer disease puts the patient at an increased risk of HIV infection.

- The risk of neonatal transmission depends on when the maternal infection is acquired. The risk to the neonate is less than 1% if the maternal infection is recurrent or is acquired at the beginning of pregnancy and is 30% to 50% if the maternal infection is acquired near term.
- If maternal HSV is acquired near the time of delivery, cesarean section is usually advised.
- Patients with certain skin diseases, such as atopic dermatitis, are in danger of developing dissemination of herpes simplex, also known as Kaposi's varicelliform eruption (see FIG. 6.29).

DIAGNOSIS

- Most often, the diagnosis is based on the clinical appearance.
- The Tzanck preparation (see Chapter 6, "Superficial Viral Infections") may be helpful, but it lacks sensitivity.
- Viral culture is the current standard of diagnosis, but the sensitivity declines rapidly as the lesions begin to heal.
- Diagnosis in tissue culture using monoclonal antibodies or polymerase chain reaction is sensitive; however, it is very expensive and has not been approved by the U.S. Food and Drug Administration for the diagnosis of genital lesions.
- Serologic testing may be useful, according to CDC guidelines, for those with (a) recurrent genital signs and symptoms and negative cultures, (b) a clinical diagnosis of genital herpes without laboratory confirmation, and (c) a partner with genital herpes. It is not recommended for screening of the general population.

DIFFERENTIAL DIAGNOSIS

Herpes Zoster
See Chapter 6, "Superficial Viral Infections."

- Herpes simplex may be dermatomal and may appear clinically identical to herpes zoster.
- A history of recurrences suggests HSV.

Primary Syphilis (Chancre)
See Figs. 19.15 and 19.16.

- Classically, the lesion has been described as being "painless"; however, secondarily infected lesions may be painful.
- The border is indurated.

Chancroid
- There are multiple painful ulcers (see Figs. 19.22 and 19.23).

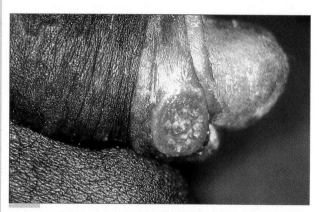

19.15 *Chancre of primary syphilis.* This ulcer has a rolled, indurated border (chancre) and a "clean" base.

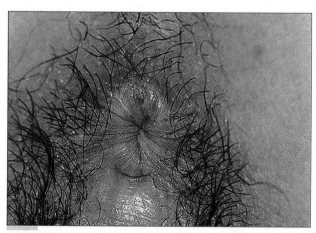

19.16 *Chancre of primary syphilis.* Note the lesion on the anus.

 MANAGEMENT

Patient Education
- The patient should be given written educational materials and clear instructions regarding safe sexual practices.
- The use of **condoms** should be encouraged.
- The patient should be advised about asymptomatic viral shedding.
- The risk of neonatal infection should be emphasized to both female *and* male patients.

Topical Therapy
- **Topical antivirals** are of limited effectiveness and are not recommended.
- Symptomatic relief may be achieved with cold compresses, viscous lidocaine (**Xylocaine**), **EMLA** (eutectic mixture of lidocaine and prilocaine), or **oral analgesics**.

Systemic Antiviral Therapy
Primary Herpes Simplex
- **Acyclovir** (200 mg five times daily or 400 mg three times daily for 10 days) *or*
- Famciclovir (**Famvir**) (250 mg three times daily for 10 days) *or*
- Valacyclovir (**Valtrex**) (1 g twice daily for 7 to 10 days)

Recurrent Herpes Simplex: Episodic Therapy
Treat at the first sign of the prodrome.

- Acyclovir (400 mg three times daily for 5 days, 800 mg twice daily for 5 days, or 800 mg three times daily for 3 days) *or*
- Famciclovir (125 mg twice daily for 5 days or 1,000 mg twice daily for 1 day *or*
- Valacyclovir (500 mg twice daily for 3 days or 1,000 mg daily for 5 days

continued on page 331

Recurrent Herpes Simplex with More than Six Recurrences per Year or Chronic Recurrent Erythema Multiforme (Daily Suppressive Therapy)

- Treat as for recurrent HSV for 5 days, then continue therapy with acyclovir (400 mg twice daily) *or*
- Famciclovir (250 mg twice daily) *or*
- Valacyclovir (500 mg once daily or 1,000 mg once daily)
- After 1 year of treatment with these agents, the medication should be discontinued to determine the recurrence, and the dosage can be adjusted as needed.
- The safety of daily acyclovir has been established for a period of 6 years and for famciclovir and valacyclovir for 1 year.

Acyclovir-Resistant Herpes Simplex

- This is seen in patients with AIDS.
- Coresistance to famciclovir and valacyclovir has been reported.
- **Foscarnet** can be given (40 mg/kg IV two to three times daily for 14 to 21 days).

- Recurrent HSV after foscarnet treatment is often acyclovir sensitive.

Herpes Simplex in Pregnant Women

- The safety and efficacy of oral antiviral therapy during pregnancy have not been established.
- Although acyclovir readily crosses the placenta, several studies did not reveal any increased risk to the developing fetus.
- Antiviral therapy is recommended for pregnant women who are experiencing a primary HSV infection.
- If vaginal delivery occurs through an infected birth canal, the neonate should be observed, and any suspicious lesions should be cultured.
- If no symptoms or signs are present during labor, vaginal delivery is recommended.
- Although the risk of neonatal infection is lower in women with recurrent HSV than it is in women with primary infection, the presence of active herpetic lesions or symptoms of vulvar pain or burning may call for cesarean delivery, regardless of the type of maternal herpetic infection.

 POINTS TO REMEMBER

- Oral antiviral treatment should be initiated, if possible, during the prodromal phase.
- Asymptomatic infections are common and contribute significantly to HSV transmission because of subclinical viral shedding.
- Condoms are clearly not foolproof, because the virus spreads by contact with herpes sores and condoms may not cover all sores.

 HELPFUL HINTS

- A recent study found that 500 mg Valtrex, taken once daily by people with HSV-2, decreased by 50% the risk of transmitting the infection to uninfected partners. This suggests that Valtrex can be prescribed in so-called discordant couples—those in which one partner is infected and the other is not.
- Maternal acquisition of HSV-1 or HSV-2 during pregnancy accounts for most neonatal HSV infections, which often result in infant deaths.

Syphilis

BASICS

- Syphilis is a systemic STD caused by the spirochetal bacterium *Treponema pallidum.* It is divided into primary, secondary, early latent, late latent, and tertiary stages.
- Tertiary syphilis is exceedingly rare in the modern era, presumably because most infected patients have had exposure to multiple courses of antibiotics during the course of their lives, and this treatment prevents the infection from progressing.

Primary Syphilis

DESCRIPTION OF LESIONS

- A painless ulceration is seen, with a rolled, indurated border (chancre) (see FIG. 19.15).
- Lesions are usually single, but they may be multiple.
- The base of the ulcer is "clean" unless it is superinfected.
- There are no vesicles.

DISTRIBUTION OF LESIONS

- The primary chancre most often presents on or near the glans penis in men; it appears less commonly on the shaft of the penis.

- The chancre may occur at the base of the penis in condom wearers.
- A visible chancre is less common in women.
- In women, lesions may occur on the labia majora or minora, the clitoris, or the posterior commissure.
- Anal lesions may occur after receptive anal intercourse (see FIG. 19.16).
- Less frequently, extragenital chancres can occur.

CLINICAL MANIFESTATIONS

- The primary chancre is usually asymptomatic.
- Regional adenopathy may be present.
- An untreated chancre heals within 3 months.

DIAGNOSIS

The following diagnostic methods are used:

- Darkfield examination of the ulceration
- Skin biopsy
- Nontreponemal serologic tests such as Venereal Disease Research Laboratory, rapid plasma reagin, and the automated reagin test; these become positive at a rate of 25% of patients per week of infection

 DIFFERENTIAL DIAGNOSIS

Herpes Simplex
- Lesions are generally painful.
- Vesicles precede the ulceration.

Chancroid
- Chancroid is unusual in the United States.
- In Africa, chancroid is often present as a coinfection.
- Lesions are painful.

MANAGEMENT

- Test for HIV infection and retest 3 months later if negative.

Non–Penicillin-Allergic Patients
- **Benzathine penicillin G** (2.4 million units IM in a single dose)

Penicillin-Allergic Nonpregnant Patients
- **Doxycycline** (100 mg PO twice daily for 2 weeks) *or*
- **Tetracycline** (500 mg four times daily for 2 weeks)

Penicillin-Allergic Pregnant Patients
- Desensitization to penicillin
- Subsequent treatment with benzathine penicillin G (2.4 million units IM, with a second dose 1 week later)

HIV-Infected Patients
- **Benzathine penicillin G** (2.4 million units IM in one dose)
- Some experts recommend repeated treatment

 POINTS TO REMEMBER

- Patients should be evaluated at 3 and 6 months after treatment. Nontreponemal tests should be negative or have decreased fourfold in titer.
- If the antibody titer does not drop fourfold, suspect treatment failure, reinfection, or HIV infection.

Secondary Syphilis

DESCRIPTION OF LESIONS

- Scaly, erythematous, oval, papulosquamous papules appear (Fig. 19.17) and are usually asymptomatic.

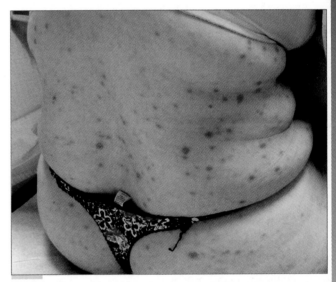

19.17 *Secondary syphilis.* Scaly, erythematous oval patches and papules are noted. (Image courtesy of Ed Zabawski, D.O.)

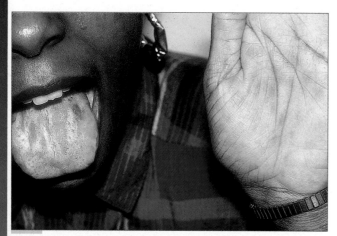

19.18 *Secondary syphilis.* Mucous patches are present, and characteristic copper-colored palmar lesions are seen.

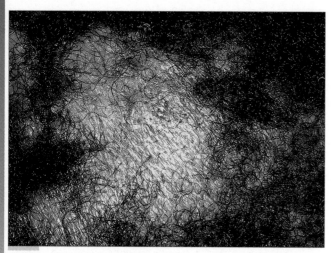

19.19 *Secondary syphilis.* Note the "moth-eaten" appearance of alopecia in this patient.

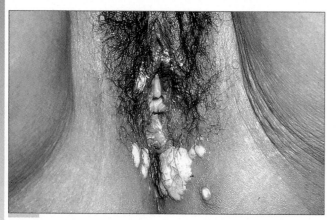

19.20 *Secondary syphilis.* Condyloma latum is noted. These moist, wartlike papules are highly infectious.

- Mucous patches may be noted (FIG. 19.18).
- "Moth-eaten" alopecia (FIG. 19.19) and condyloma latum (FIG. 19.20) are also seen in secondary syphilis.

DISTRIBUTION OF LESIONS

- Lesions are widespread and include the palms (FIG. 19.21), soles, scalp, and mucous membranes.

CLINICAL MANIFESTATIONS

- Generalized adenopathy and mild systemic symptoms are often present.

DIAGNOSIS

- The diagnosis is often suggested by the clinical presentation.
- If available, a darkfield examination of serum expressed from lesions can confirm the diagnosis, *or*
- Positive treponemal (fluorescein treponemal antibody) and nontreponemal serologic tests (100% of non-HIV-infected patients, usually at a titer greater than 1:16 for the nontreponemal test) confirm the diagnosis, *or*
- A skin biopsy with silver or immunoperoxidase stain may confirm the diagnosis.
- Serologic titers may be negative in HIV-infected persons.

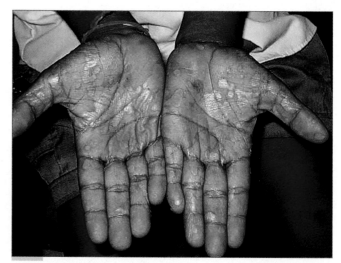

19.21 *Secondary syphilis.* Characteristic copper- or "ham"-colored, papulosquamous lesions are seen on this patient's palms. (Image courtesy of Ashit Marwah, M.D.)

Latent Syphilis

- Latent syphilis is manifested by positive serologic tests for nontreponemal and treponemal antibodies in the absence of clinical manifestations. It is divided into early latent syphilis and late latent syphilis.
- Early latent syphilis is syphilis documented to be of less than 1 year in duration and is treated with the same regimen as primary and secondary infections.
- The duration of late latent syphilis is more than 1 year or is unknown. The recommended treatment is benzathine penicillin 2.4 million units intramuscularly weekly for 3 weeks. HIV-infected patients with latent syphilis of any duration should have a cerebrospinal fluid examination to rule out neurosyphilis before treatment.

Tertiary Syphilis

- Tertiary syphilis occurs about 20 years after the onset of untreated syphilis, and it is rare in the antibiotic era.
- Treatment is the same as for late latent syphilis.

Congenital Syphilis

- Congenital syphilis can affect infants born to mothers with untreated syphilis, with syphilis treated during pregnancy with erythromycin, with syphilis treated less than 1 month before delivery, and with syphilis treated with penicillin without a fourfold decrease in serologic titer.
- The CDC recommends that all pregnant women be tested for syphilis at least once during pregnancy and at the time of delivery in at-risk populations.

 DIFFERENTIAL DIAGNOSIS

Pityriasis Rosea
See FIGURES 4.1 to 4.4.

- Usually, pityriasis rosea is confined to the skin above the knees, and it spares the face, palms, and soles. It is prudent to check syphilis serologic tests in patients with pityriasis rosea.

Other Diagnoses
- Other papulosquamous eruptions such as psoriasis, lichen planus, and drug eruptions should be considered.

 MANAGEMENT

- This is the same as for primary syphilis.
- The serologic titer should fall fourfold in 6 months. If it does not, the patient should have a cerebrospinal fluid examination. If it is negative, some experts advise retreatment with benzathine penicillin (2.4 million units weekly for 3 weeks).

Chancroid

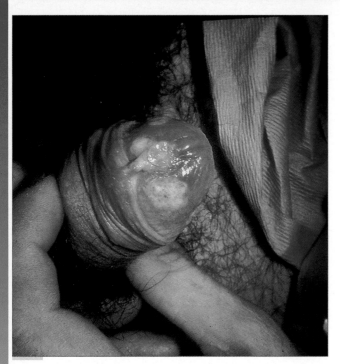

19.22 *Chancroid.* This patient has multiple painful ulcers on the glans penis.

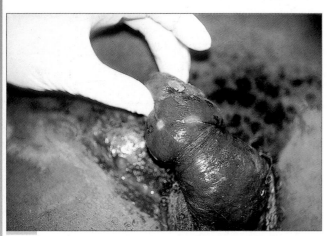

19.23 *Chancroid.* Multiple painful ulcers and a bubo are present.

BASICS

- Chancroid is an ulcerative STD that is most common in developing countries and is rare in the United States and Western Europe. In the United States, it is associated with the use of crack cocaine.
- The causative organism, *Haemophilus ducreyi,* a gram-negative rod, is fastidious and requires specific conditions for culture.
- Chancroid occurs as a mixed infection with syphilis or herpes simplex in 10% of cases.
- Clinical infection is more common in men than in women.

DESCRIPTION OF LESIONS

- The earliest manifestation is a papule, which becomes a pustule and ulcerates.
- Fully developed lesions are painful, with undermined borders and peripheral erythema (FIGS. 19.22 and 19.23).
- Borders are not indurated.
- There may be satellite ulcers.

DISTRIBUTION OF LESIONS

- The location of lesions depends on the site(s) of inoculation.
- In **men,** the prepuce, balanopreputial fold, and the shaft of the penis are the typical sites.
- In **women,** lesions are noted on the labia majora, posterior commissure, or perianal area.
- Extragenital lesions have been described.

CLINICAL MANIFESTATIONS

- The incubation period is 25 days.
- Tenderness and pain are common.
- Unilateral or bilateral inguinal adenopathy (buboes) may be present.

DIAGNOSIS

- The diagnosis is often made based on the clinical appearance.
- A negative darkfield examination, syphilis serologic testing, and HSV cultures help to exclude other diagnoses.
- Obtaining a culture is difficult.
- A Gram stain shows characteristic "schools of fish" or "Chinese characters."
- Polymerase chain reaction may help in making a diagnosis.

MANAGEMENT

- **Drug Therapy**
  - **Azithromycin** (1 g PO in a single dose) *or*
  - **Ceftriaxone** (250 mg IM in a single dose) *or*
  - **Erythromycin** (500 mg PO four times daily for 7 days) *or*
  - **Ciprofloxacin** (500 mg PO twice daily for 3 days)
- Pregnant women and HIV-infected patients should be treated with erythromycin.
- Symptomatic improvement usually occurs in 3 days; objective improvement is seen in 7 days.
- Complete healing may take more than 2 weeks.
- HIV testing should be performed on all patients and repeated 3 months later if negative.

POINTS TO REMEMBER

- Chancroid is rare in the United States, but epidemics have been described in crack cocaine users.
- Chancroid predisposes to HIV infection because of recruitment of CD4 cells into the ulcer.
- Always test for coinfection with HIV, syphilis, and HSV.

DIFFERENTIAL DIAGNOSIS

Herpes Simplex
- **Herpes simplex** is preceded by blisters, and the borders are not undermined.

Chronic HSV
- **Chronic HSV** in patients with AIDS may resemble chancroid.

Primary Syphilis
- In **primary syphilis,** the borders are indurated, not undermined, and the lesion is generally painless.

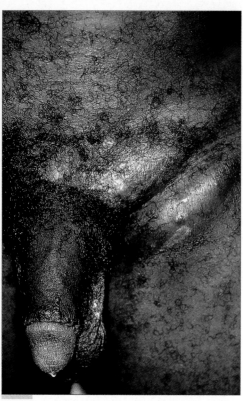

19.24 *Lymphogranuloma venereum.* Regional lymphadenitis ("the groove sign") is present.

BASICS

- Lymphogranuloma venereum (LGV) is caused by *Chlamydia trachomatis* types L1, L2, and L3. It is most often sexually transmitted.
- LGV is most common in Southeast Asia, Africa, Central America, and the Caribbean. LGV accounts for 2% to 10% of genital ulcer disease in India and Africa.
- An inconspicuous cutaneous ulceration occurs at the site of inoculation, and it often heals without being noticed.

DESCRIPTION OF LESIONS

- Evanescent papulopustule or ulceration occurs.
- Regional lymphadenitis is characteristic. The groin fold divides lymph nodes into upper and lower groups ("the groove sign") (FIG. 19.24). Sometimes, the adenopathy is bilateral.
- Fluctuance and sinus tracts may develop.

DISTRIBUTION OF LESIONS

- The primary lesion, if present, is found on the penis, vaginal wall, cervix, or perirectally. It is rarely seen in women.

CLINICAL MANIFESTATIONS

- LGV may be associated with malaise and joint stiffness.
- Scarring may result in genital lymphedema.
- Erythema nodosum occurs in 10% of women with LGV.
- Rectal exposure can lead to proctocolitis, which if not treated promptly leads to chronic colorectal strictures and fistulas.

DIAGNOSIS

- The diagnosis of LGV depends mainly on the exclusion of other causes of suppurative adenopathy and serologic testing: a complement fixation test, and two immunofluorescent tests.
- Culture of the organism is also available.

 MANAGEMENT

- **Doxycycline** (100 mg PO twice daily for 3 weeks minimum) *or*
- Alternative regimen (and in pregnant women): **erythromycin** (500 mg PO four times daily for 3 weeks minimum)
- Buboes may need to be aspirated or incised and drained.

 POINTS TO REMEMBER

- Infection is rare in the United States.
- Cutaneous manifestations are usually inapparent.

DDx **DIFFERENTIAL DIAGNOSIS**

Catscratch Disease
- Usually, there is a history of traumatic contact with cats at a site proximal to involved lymph nodes.

Pyogenic Adenitis
- A positive Gram stain and bacterial cultures may be found.

Tuberculous Adenitis
- A positive acid-fast bacillus stain and cultures and a positive purified protein derivative test are obtained.

Granuloma Inguinale (Donovanosis)

BASICS

- Granuloma inguinale is a chronic granulomatous ulcerative disease of the genitalia caused by the gram-negative bacillus *Calymmatobacterium granulomatis*. It is thought to be sexually transmitted, with low infectivity.
- It is rare in the United States and is widespread in the tropics and subtropics. The frequency of the disease in homosexuals suggests that the causative organism may reside in the gastrointestinal tract.

DESCRIPTION OF LESIONS

- The initial lesion is a papule or a nodule that ulcerates.
- The ulcer is painless and has an undermined border.
- There is no regional adenitis.

DISTRIBUTION OF LESIONS

- Granuloma inguinale appears in the genital, pubic, perineal, groin, or perianal areas.
- Extragenital lesions occur in 3% to 6% of cases.

CLINICAL MANIFESTATIONS

- The presence of pain or adenitis suggests superinfection.

DIAGNOSIS

- Smears from the edge of the lesion may show characteristic Donovan bodies (organisms within macrophages).
- The biopsy specimen should be taken from the edge of the lesion.

 DIFFERENTIAL DIAGNOSIS

Syphilis
- Syphilis must be excluded by darkfield and serologic examinations.
- The borders of the ulcers are indurated, not undermined.

 MANAGEMENT

- The treatment of choice is doxycycline (100 mg twice daily for 3 weeks minimum or until the ulcers have healed).
- Alternative regimens:
  - **Azithromycin** (1,000 mg once weekly for at least 3 weeks or until the ulcers have healed) *or*
  - **Ciprofloxacin** (750 mg twice daily for at least 3 weeks or until the ulcers have healed) *or*
  - **Erythromycin** (500 mg four times daily for at least 3 weeks or until the ulcers have healed) *or*
  - **Trimethoprim-sulfamethoxazole** (one double-strength tablet twice daily for at least 3 weeks or until the ulcers have healed)

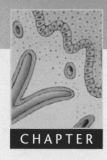

Bites, Stings, and Infestations

- ➤ **INSECTS, TICKS, MITES**

  - Insect bite reactions
  - Lyme disease (lyme borreliosis)
  - Scabies: mite infestation

- ➤ **LICE INFESTATIONS (PEDICULOSIS)**

  - Head lice (pediculosis capitis)
  - Body lice (pediculosis corporis)
  - Pubic lice

- ➤ **WATERBORNE STINGS AND SEASHORE INFESTATIONS**

  - Jellyfish stings
  - Seabather's eruption ("sea lice")
  - Cutaneous larva migrans ("creeping eruption")

OVERVIEW

In much of the world, insect bites commonly serve as vectors that transport diseases such as malaria, leishmaniasis, filariasis, and rickettsial diseases. In modern industrial societies, insect bites are more of a nuisance than a potential carrier of a life-threatening illness. On the East Coast and in the Midwest of the United States, mosquitoes and biting flies as well as ticks account for most bites. In arid areas, including much of the Southwest and parts of California, flying insects are less common, and crawling arthropods are the primary cause of bites and stings.

West Nile virus, of much concern in the United States, is a mosquito-borne infection that can cause encephalitis. It was originally seen in New York State in 1999 and is now being reported throughout the country.

BASICS

- Insects that bite include mosquitoes, fleas, flies, ticks, chiggers, and lice. Mosquito and fly bites occur most often from outdoor exposures, particularly in the summer. Flea bites are most often acquired indoors from pets.
- Insects that sting include bees, wasps, hornets, and fire ants.
- There is individual variability in the attraction of insects, possibly related to pheromones. Furthermore, reactions to bites and stings are probably related to individual hypersensitivity.
- The physical insult of an insect bite or sting causes little injury; instead, lesions occur as a result of the body's immune response to injected foreign chemicals and proteins introduced by the bite or sting. The time it takes for reactions to develop reflects the immune mechanism involved.

Pathogenesis

- Immediate hivelike skin lesions reflect hypersensitivity to the bite or sting. They are mediated by immunoglobulin E (FIG. 20.1).
- Delayed pruritic papules, nodules, and vesicles usually become symptomatic within 48 hours after the insult. They are manifestations of delayed hypersensitivity (type IV cell-mediated immunity).

DESCRIPTION OF LESIONS

- Bite reactions typically present as intensely pruritic erythematous papules that commonly are excoriated.
- Bite reactions may be indistinguishable from ordinary hives.
- Grouping of lesions often occurs, particularly after flea bites ("breakfast, lunch, and dinner"; FIG. 20.2).

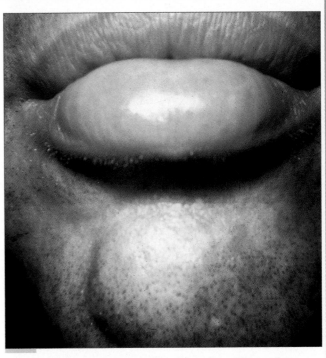

20.1 *Angioedema caused by a bee sting.* This patient developed an immediate hypersensitivity reaction after being bitten on the lip.

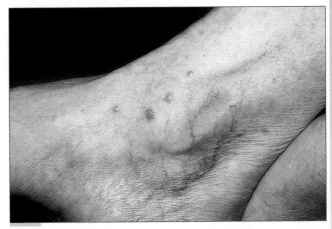

20.2 *Flea bites.* Note the arrangement of lesions in groups of three ("breakfast, lunch, and dinner"); the fourth lesion probably represents a "midnight snack."

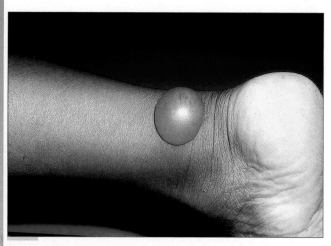

20.3 *Bullous arthropod bite reaction.* Note the tense bulla that resulted from a chigger bite.

- Lesions may have a central punctum and crust and also may become vesicobullous (FIG. 20.3).
- Insect bite reactions are also known as papular urticaria when lesions persist for longer than 48 hours.

DISTRIBUTION OF LESIONS

- Lesions are found on exposed areas, more often on non-clothed body parts such as distal lower extremities, forearms, and hands.
- The papules of flea bites are typically asymmetric in distribution.
- Lesions are also commonly seen on the lower legs, forearms, lower trunk, and waist; the axillary and anogenital areas are usually spared. Flying insects tend to bite on the upper trunk or extremities, whereas crawling insects tend to bite or sting on the lower trunk or extremities. Although this is not always true, it often helps narrow down the cause.

CLINICAL MANIFESTATIONS

- Insect bites may be a chronic, recurrent problem or simply a nuisance.
- The purpose of bites is usually to obtain a blood meal, which means that they often occur in multiples. The purpose of stings is usually self-defense, which means that they occur singly; the glaring exception is fire ants, which sting as much as they can.
- Itching may be intense and may persist for weeks.
- Secondary bacterial infection may occur.
- Stings generally cause immediate pain and are therefore usually remembered.
- Bites often go unnoticed, and the lesions that arise from them may not appear for days after the bite because of what is often a delayed immune-mediated hypersensitivity reaction. Consequently, a patient may seek medical advice for unexplained itchy bumps or blisters. Presumably, bites go unnoticed because it is to the arthropod's advantage to obtain its blood meal without being detected, which serves to increase its survival value.

DIAGNOSIS

- The diagnosis is usually made on clinical appearance and history.
- Inquiry about household pets currently and formerly residing in the house may be a clue to the diagnosis. If the residence was formerly host to a dog or cat infested with fleas, the fleas left behind may have found new human hosts.
- A skin biopsy is not diagnostic, but it may show suggestive findings consisting of a dense lymphocytic infiltrate (resembling lymphoma) with many eosinophils. The responsible agent is rarely found in a biopsy specimen.

DIFFERENTIAL DIAGNOSIS

Urticaria Unrelated to Insect Bites

See also Chapter 17, "Drug Eruptions."

- This type of urticaria lacks a central punctum.
- It is often indistinguishable from insect bites.

Fiberglass Dermatitis

- Nonspecific itching is noted.
- The patient has a history of exposure (e.g., works with roofing materials).

Scabies

- See the discussion later in this chapter.

 POINTS TO REMEMBER

- A careful history and knowledge of the patient's environment and possible exposures should be sought.
- Symptoms may persist for weeks after the original bites.
- Other causes should be diligently sought if symptoms persist for more than 4 to 6 weeks.

 HELPFUL HINTS

- Patients who seek medical help generally do not consider "mundane" insect bites to be the cause of their dermatosis or itching; rather, they seek attention because they assume that other factors cause their problem.
- Poisons normally used by exterminators do not kill fleas.

 MANAGEMENT

- **Insect repellents** that contain N,N-diethyl-m-toluamide (**DEET**) help prevent bites and stings.
- Acute reactions to stings are treated symptomatically with **topical** or **intralesional steroids** and **oral antihistamines**; people with severe reactions from stings may profit from desensitization therapy.
- Anaphylactic reactions require epinephrine, **systemic steroids,** and antihistamines.
- If flea infestation is suspected, pets should be evaluated by a veterinarian. If fleas are present in the home, thorough vacuuming and shampooing of flea-infested areas and sometimes even **fumigation** may be necessary.

Lyme Disease (Lyme Borreliosis)

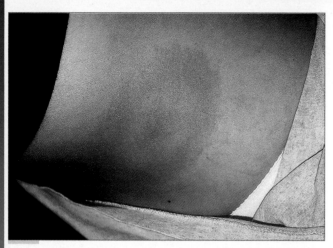

20.4 ***Lyme disease, erythema migrans.*** A solitary, annular, targetlike, erythematous plaque of erythema migrans is seen.

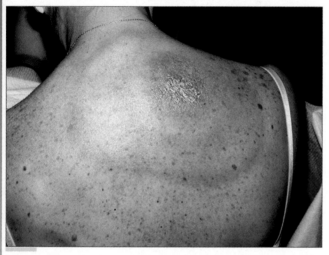

20.5 ***Lyme disease.*** In this patient, erythema migrans is manifested by concentric rings with resolving central vesicles.

BASICS

- Lyme disease, or Lyme borreliosis (LB), is a systemic infection caused by the spirochete *Borrelia burgdorferi*. Bacteria are introduced into the skin via a bite from an infected *Ixodes* tick.
- The tick has to be attached for 24 hours for the organism to be transmitted.
- Once in the skin, the spirochete may stay localized at the site of inoculation, or it may disseminate via the blood and lymphatics. Hematogenous dissemination can occur within days or weeks of the initial infection. The organism can travel to other parts of the skin, the heart, the joints, the central nervous system, and other parts of the body.
- The tick vector of LB, *I. dammini,* is found in the northeastern and midwestern United States, where most cases are reported. *I. scapularis* in the southeastern United States, *I. pacificus* on the Pacific coast, and *I. ricinus,* the sheep tick, in Europe are also vectors. Because the disease depends on deer, mice, ticks, and bacteria, it is limited geographically to the areas where all these organisms are present.
- LB can occur in any season, although it is most prevalent during the warmer months from May through September during the nymphal stage of the tick. The ticks cling to vegetation (not trees) in grassland, marshland, and woodland habitats. They transfer to animals and humans brushing against the vegetation.

DESCRIPTION OF LESIONS

- Initially, the LB lesion is a red macule or papule at the site of a tick bite. The bite itself usually goes unnoticed (only 15% of patients report a tick bite). Approximately 2 to 30 days after infection, the rash appears.
- The lesion expands to form an annular erythematous lesion, erythema migrans (EM), which is the classic lesion of LB (FIG. 20.4). The lesion measures from 4 to 70 cm in diameter, generally with central clearing.
- The center of the lesion, which corresponds to the putative site of the tick bite, may become darker, vesicular, hemorrhagic, or necrotic (FIG. 20.5).

- Lesions may be confluent (not annular), and concentric rings may form.
- Multiple lesions occur in approximately 20% of patients, likely a result of bacteremia (FIGS. 20.6 and 20.7). These secondary lesions tend to be more uniform in morphology than the primary lesion.

DISTRIBUTION OF LESIONS

- Common sites are the thigh, groin, trunk, and axillae.
- Because secondary lesions spread hematogenously, they are less restricted than primary lesions in terms of location.

CLINICAL MANIFESTATIONS

Early Lyme Disease

- At the early stage of disease, flulike symptoms, such as malaise, arthralgias, headaches, and a low-grade fever and chills, may occur. Other symptoms include stiffness of the neck and difficulty in concentrating.
- The EM rash itself is usually asymptomatic.

Intermediate, Chronic, and Late Lyme Disease

- Some of the signs and symptoms of LB may not appear for weeks, months, or even years after the initial tick bite and are believed to be caused by immunopathogenic mechanisms. The signs and symptoms of intermediate, chronic, and late Lyme disease include:
  - **Arthritis** in one or more large joints; nervous system problems that may include pain, paresthesias, Bell's palsy, headaches, and memory loss; and cardiac dysrhythmias.
  - Rarely, a lesion of lymphocytoma cutis may develop, usually occurring on the earlobe or nipple. These lesions are bluish red nodules.
  - **Acrodermatitis chronica atrophicans (ACA)** is a manifestation of chronic LB that begins as an inflammatory phase marked by edema and erythema, usually on the distal extremities. Later, atrophy occurs, and thin "cigarette-paper" skin is seen. Because of the loss of subcutaneous fat, underlying venous structures are more visible, and the skin becomes thin, atrophic, and dry.
  - Both **lymphocytoma cutis** and ACA are very rare findings in the United States and are seen primarily in Europe. The clinical differences probably result from the different antigenic strains of *Borrelia*.
- **Late Lyme disease** refers to symptoms, primarily rheumatologic and neurologic, that occur months to years after initial infection. It is not unusual for patients to first present with late extracutaneous symptoms without ever having had an initial EM lesion or other overt symptoms of early Lyme disease. This may occur because the patient was asymptomatic or because early disease was not recognized by the patient or correctly diagnosed by the health care provider.

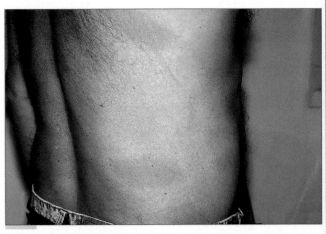

20.6 *Lyme disease.* Multiple confluent lesions of erythema migrans are noted.

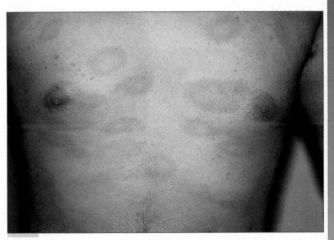

20.7 *Lyme disease.* Multiple annular lesions of erythema migrans are seen here.

DIAGNOSIS

- The diagnosis of LB is often difficult because the disease mimics many other conditions.
  - Viral infections, such as influenza and mononucleosis, also may manifest with rash, aches, fever, and fatigue.
  - Drug eruptions and insect bite reactions other than those caused by the *Ixodes* tick closely match the rash of early LB.

Early Diagnosis

To diagnose early LB, the following are important:

- There is a history of tick exposure or bite in an area endemic for LB.
- The specific tick is identified as a potential vector of LB.
- The various presentations of EM are recognized.

Laboratory Testing

- Serologic testing, using enzyme-linked immunosorbent assay (ELISA) and Western blot analyses for *B. burgdorferi,* is notoriously unreliable.
  - At the early presenting stage of LB, serologic testing has been reported to be positive in only 25% of infected patients. After 4 to 6 weeks, approximately 75% of these patients test positive, even after antibiotic therapy.
- Patients with past LB and those who have been vaccinated may be persistently seropositive.
- The poor reputation of serologic testing is derived somewhat from the many false-negative test results of patients treated very early in the course of the disease and from the many misdiagnosed cases of supposed LB.
- The U.S. Centers for Disease Control and Prevention currently recommends a two-step testing procedure consisting of a screening ELISA or immunofluorescent assay followed by a confirmatory Western immunoblot test on any samples with positive or equivocal results on ELISA.
- Infrequently, spirochetes may be identified using silver or antibody-labeled stains.
- Other diagnostic measures, such as polymerase chain reaction and cultures for *B. burgdorferi* have met with some success; however, these techniques are time-consuming and expensive. The *Borrelia* organism is fastidious, and culture of skin biopsy specimens is not readily available.

(text continued on page 350)

DIFFERENTIAL DIAGNOSIS

Tinea Corporis

- See Chapter 7, "Superficial Fungal Infections."
- There may be a history of exposure to fungus.
- Lesions are also annular (ringlike) and clear in the center; however, tinea corporis has an "active" scaly border (epidermal involvement).
- Lesions are potassium hydroxide positive (FIG. 20.8), or the fungal culture grows dermatophytes.
- Tinea corporis generally itches.

Acute Urticaria

- See Chapter 18, "Diseases of Vasculature."
- At times, this may be indistinguishable from LB.
- Lesions may have eccentric shapes (FIG. 20.9).
- Individual lesions disappear within 24 hours.
- It generally itches.

Granuloma Annulare

- For a full discussion of this condition, see Chapter 4, "Inflammatory Eruptions of Unknown Cause."

Erythema Multiforme

- For a full discussion of this condition, see Chapter 25, "Cutaneous Manifestations of Systemic Disease."

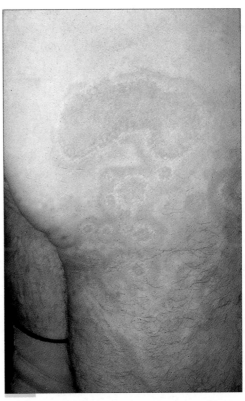

20.9 *Acute urticaria.* Lesions have bizarre, eccentric shapes in this patient.

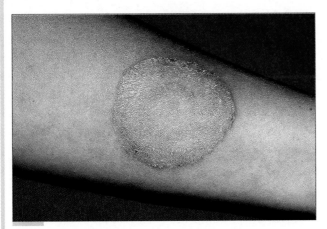

20.8 *Tinea corporis.* The scaly border is potassium hydroxide–positive.

Tick Recognition

- *Ixodes* ticks are much smaller than dog ticks. In their larval and nymphal stages, they are no bigger than a pinhead; unengaged adult ticks are the size of the head of a match (FIG. 20.10).

Tick Removal

- An attached tick should be removed carefully by using a pair of tweezers. The tick should be grasped by the head (not the body), as close as possible to the skin, to avoid force that may crush it. It is then gently pulled straight out of the patient's skin (FIG. 20.11).

Treatment of Erythema Migrans (Early Lyme Borreliosis)

- **Doxycycline** (100 mg twice per day for 21 days [do not use in children younger than 10 years or in pregnant women]) *or*
- **Amoxicillin** (500 mg three times per day for 21 days) *or*
- **Ceftriaxone** or **cefuroxime** (500 mg twice per day for 21 days [expensive; use only if patient is unable to tolerate the other antibiotics])
- **Azithromycin** (Zithromax) and erythromycin: second-line drugs that should be considered in pregnant patients who are allergic to beta-lactam antibiotics

Prevention

- People who are outdoors in endemic areas in the summer should wear long pants and socks, use insect repellents, and frequently look for ticks on themselves and their clothing.

Lyme Disease Vaccine (LYMErix)

- A vaccine directed against the outer surface protein A of *B. burgdorferi* was removed from the United States market in 2002.

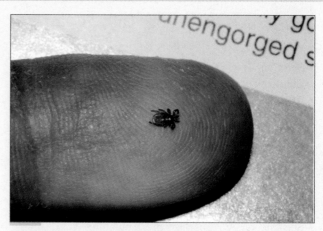

20.10 *Ixodes tick.* An adult tick is the size of the head of a match.

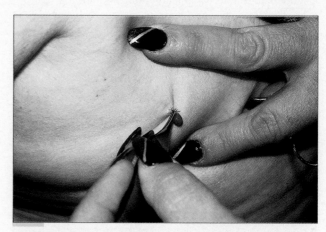

20.11 *Dog tick.* An intact engorged adult dog tick being removed by the head.

HELPFUL HINTS

- Patients can be reinfected. There is no lasting immunity to LB.
- Most patients at the EM stage are seronegative.
- An additional tick-borne coinfection by *Ehrlichia* species and *Babesia microti* has been reported with increasing frequency. Such coinfection is suggested by a very high fever or toxicity.
- Antibiotic prophylaxis after tick bites is controversial. Clearly, prevention of bites is a better means of avoiding disease.
- Health care providers must understand the limitations of serologic tests.
- Wearing clothing with white colors improves the odds of seeing ticks on clothing before they attach.
- Regular tick inspections and removal of ticks before they have been attached for 24 hours is another important way to reduce the risk of contracting Lyme disease.

POINTS TO REMEMBER

- Serologic testing is usually negative early in the course of infection.
- Serologic testing should not be used to make a diagnosis, only to help confirm it.

SEE PATIENT HANDOUT "Lyme Disease" AND "Lyme Disease: Prevention" ON THE SOLUTION SITE

Scabies: Mite Infestation

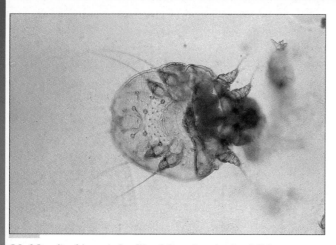

20.12 *Scabies.* A fertilized female mite is visible.

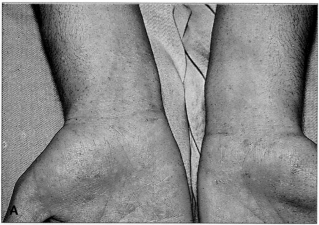

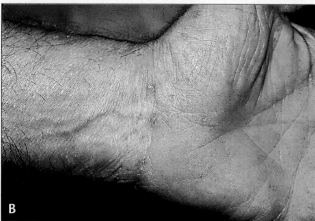

20.13 A and B *Scabies.* Lesions are present on the flexor wrists. Note linear burrows.

BASICS

- Scabies is a skin infestation caused by the mite *Sarcoptes scabiei* var. *hominis.* It is usually spread by skin-to-skin contact, most frequently among family members and by sexual contact in young adults. Occasionally, epidemics occur in nursing homes and similar extended-care institutions, where scabies is spread by person-to-person contact and possibly by mite-infested clothing and bed linen. The diagnosis can be easily overlooked, and treatment is often delayed for long periods.
- The diagnosis of scabies should be considered when an individual complains of intractable, persistent pruritus, especially when other family members, consorts, or fellow inhabitants of an institution, such as a nursing home or school, have similar symptoms.
- Although scabies is found more commonly in poor, crowded living conditions, it occurs worldwide and is not limited to the impoverished or those who practice poor personal hygiene. African-American and Afro-Caribbean individuals infrequently acquire scabies; the reason is unknown.

Pathogenesis

- A fertilized female mite (FIG. 20.12) excavates a burrow in the stratum corneum, lays her eggs, and deposits fecal pellets (scybala) behind her as she advances.
- The egg laying, scybala, or other secretions act as irritants or allergens, which may account for the itching and the subsequent delayed type IV hypersensitivity reaction that occurs approximately 30 days after infestation.

DESCRIPTION OF LESIONS

- The initial lesions of scabies include tiny pinpoint vesicles and erythematous papules, some of which evolve into burrows, the classic telltale lesions of scabies (FIGS. 20.13 and 20.14).

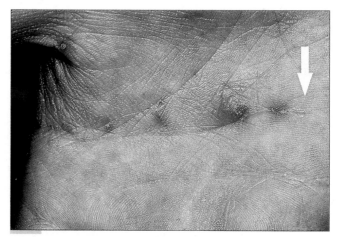

20.14 *Scabies.* This close-up view shows a burrow (*arrow*) on the palm.

- The burrow is a linear or S-shaped excavation that is pinkish-white and slightly scaly and ends in the pinpoint vesicle or papule. This is where the mites may be found.
- Burrows are easiest to find on the hands, particularly in the finger webs and wrists in adults and on the palms and soles in infants.
- Sometimes burrows can be highlighted by applying black ink with a felt-tipped pen to the suspected areas.

DISTRIBUTION OF LESIONS

- Lesions are most often located on the interdigital finger webs (FIG. 20.15), sides of the hands and feet, flexor wrists, umbilicus, waistband area, axillae, ankles, buttocks, and groin.
- Children and adults rarely have lesions above the neck; this is an important diagnostic sign.
- Infants tend to have more widespread involvement, including the face and scalp and especially the palms and soles.
- Immunocompromised patients also tend to have a widespread distribution of lesions.

CLINICAL MANIFESTATIONS

- Because the incubation period from initial infestation to the onset of pruritus is approximately 1 month, it is not uncommon for contacts to be asymptomatic, especially if they have been recently infested.
- Itching (nocturnal pruritus) has traditionally been considered a symptom that is characteristic of scabies; however, it should be kept in mind that pruritus that occurs in many other skin conditions also tends to be more severe during the nighttime hours, when people are inclined to be less distracted by their daytime routines.

Course and Secondary Lesions
- Initially, itching is rather mild and focal, but when lesions begin spreading rapidly, usually after 4 to 6 weeks, it can sometimes become intolerable.
- A generalized distribution of lesions is probably the result of a hypersensitivity reaction. In this case, a more pleomorphic array of lesions, such as "juicy" papules and nodules, may be seen.
- Hemorrhagic crusts and ulcerations may replace the primary lesions.
- In men, itchy papules and nodules, particularly on the penis and scrotum, are virtually pathognomonic for scabies (FIG. 20.16).

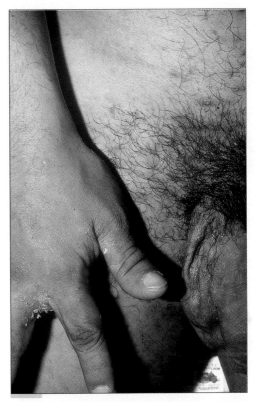

20.15   *Scabies.* Finger web and groin lesions are noted.

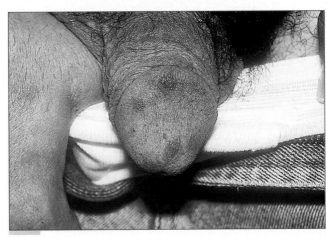

20.16   *Scabies.* Characteristic pruritic papules are present on this patient's penis.

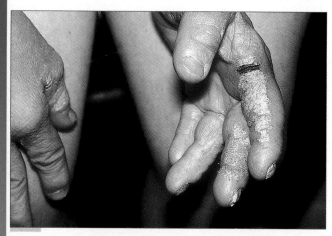

20.17 *Norwegian scabies.* This child with Down's syndrome has verrucous plaques on his hands and thickened dystrophic nails. The lesions are teeming with scabies mites.

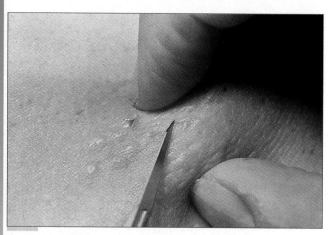

20.18 *Scabies.* Scraping for scabies is performed.

 DIFFERENTIAL DIAGNOSIS

- Insect bites, such as fleas, generally spare areas that are covered (e.g., the groin and axillae).
- Pruritus associated with systemic diseases, such as renal disease, hepatic disease, lymphomas, AIDS, leukemias, and Hodgkin's disease, should be excluded.

Other Diagnoses
- Atopic dermatitis or dyshidrotic eczema should be considered.
- Drug eruptions and other itchy rashes, including urticaria, tinea, xerosis, and contact dermatitis, should also be kept in mind.

Clinical Variants

Scabies in Infants
- Frequently, intact vesicles are seen on the palms and soles. A typical clinical picture of an infant with scabies is one who doggedly pinches his or her skin.

Scabies in the Elderly
- Patients, particularly in an institutional setting, can have intense pruritus and few papular lesions, excoriations, or simply have dry, scaly skin.

Norwegian or Crusted Scabies
- Norwegian, or crusted, scabies (FIG. 20.17) occurs in people with varying degrees of immune deficiency such as that seen in Down's syndrome, leukemia, nutritional disorders, and acquired immunodeficiency syndrome (AIDS) (see also Chapter 24, "Cutaneous Manifestations of HIV Infection," and FIG. 24.14).
- The lesions tend to involve large areas of the body.
- The hands and feet may be scaly and crusted with a thick keratotic material that can also be seen under the nails.
- There may be wartlike vegetations on the skin; these are hosts to thousands of mites and their eggs.

DIAGNOSIS

A conclusive diagnosis is made by finding scabies mites, eggs, or feces.

- A drop of mineral oil is applied to the most likely lesion (usually a vesicle on the finger web or wrist is chosen). The site is then scraped with a surgical blade (FIG. 20.18), the scrapings are placed on a slide, and a cover slip is then applied (see also FIGS. 24.15 and 24.16).
- Adults, who are more efficient scratchers than children, tend to remove the definitive evidence of scabies (i.e., mite) with their fingernails. Because mites are few and are particularly difficult to find in adults, the time and effort spent searching for the mite may be better used by taking a thorough history and counseling the patient and his or her contacts. Thus, if scabies is strongly suspected on clinical grounds, scabicidal treatment should be initiated.

MANAGEMENT

- Treatment is directed at killing the mites with a scabicide. It is also aimed at affording rapid symptomatic relief using appropriate oral antihistamines and topical corticosteroids, if necessary.
- **Management of institutional scabies:**
  - Treatment must be conducted in an organized, cooperative fashion.
  - A scabicide and/or oral ivermectin (see below) is administered to all patients, staff, family members, and frequent visitors.
  - Laundering of all bed linen and clothes is necessary shortly after treatment.

Permethrin (Elimite and Acticin)

- The prescription drugs Elimite and Acticin both contain permethrin cream 5%. They are safe and effective scabicides that are currently considered the treatment of choice for scabies.
- They have not been proven to be safe in infants younger than 2 months or in pregnant and nursing women.
- These instructions for use should be followed:
  - After a warm bath, the cream is applied to all skin surfaces "from head to toe" (including the palms, soles, and scalp in small children) and is left on for 8 to 12 hours, usually overnight. It is washed off the next morning.
  - If indicated, other family members and contacts should be treated simultaneously. All bed linen and intimate undergarments should be washed in hot water after treatment is completed.
  - Generally, only one treatment is necessary; however, a second treatment is often recommended in 4 to 5 days, especially in long-standing cases and for infants with scabies of the palms and soles.
  - Patients should be advised that it is normal to continue itching for days or weeks after treatment, albeit less intensely. The medication should *not* be applied repeatedly. Systemic antihistamines and a potent class 3 or 4 topical corticosteroid can be used for these symptoms.

Lindane (Kwell Lotion, Scabene)

- This is the generic name for gamma benzene hexachloride. This agent is available as a 1% lotion or cream. Lindane stimulates the nervous system of the parasite, causing seizures and death. Until recently, it was the mainstay of scabies treatment; now it is recommended as an alternative agent, to be used only if other agents fail or are not tolerated.
- It also requires a prescription.
- It is also safe and effective, but controversy has arisen about its safety after several reports of neurotoxicity in infants. Ultimately, it was concluded that the drug was overused in these cases and led to systemic absorption. California has banned the use of lindane for treatment of lice and scabies.

- Lindane is to be avoided in infants, in pregnant or nursing women, or in people with a history of seizure disorders.
- There have been reports of resistance to this agent.
- These instructions for use should be followed:
  - Used as an overnight treatment, it is applied from the neck to toes, and the patient is instructed to wash it off in 8 to 12 hours.
  - Treatment may be repeated in 4 to 5 days if there is little symptomatic improvement.

Precipitated Sulfur Ointment (6%)

- This is used in pregnant or lactating women and in infants younger than 2 months. It is applied nightly for 3 nights.
- Although it is messy and malodorous, it is effective and safe.

Ivermectin

- Ivermectin (**Stromectol**) is an antihelmintic that can be administered (off-label) in a single oral dose. This agent is not currently approved by the U.S. Food and Drug Administration for the treatment of scabies in humans, and no studies have been done to establish its safety for use in pregnancy or in children.
- It may be used when topical therapy is difficult or impractical (e.g., widespread infestations in nursing homes).
- It has been used safely and effectively in patients who are seropositive for human immunodeficiency virus and in some patients with Norwegian scabies.
- This agent may be administered adjunctively with a topical scabicide.
- It is available in 3- and 6-mg tablets.
- **Dosage:** 0.2 mg/kg in a single oral dose that is repeated in 10 days. For 6-mg tablets, the dosages are given in TABLE 20.1.

Crotamiton (Eurax Lotion and Cream)

- This preparation, a 10% cream or lotion, has an unknown mechanism of action.
- It is not very effective against scabies.

Table 20.1 IVERMECTIN DOSAGE FOR TREATMENT OF SCABIES WITH 6-MG TABLETS

WEIGHT (KG)	NO. OF TABLETS
15–24	0.5
25–35	1
36–50	1.5
51–65	2
66–79	2.5
> 80	3–4

HELPFUL HINTS

Think scabies when you see:

- An infant with palmar or plantar vesicles or pustules
- More than one family member, roommate, or sexual partner who is itching
- Pruritic scrotal or penile nodules
- Vesicles in the finger webs

SEE PATIENT HANDOUT "Scabies" ON THE SOLUTION SITE

POINTS TO REMEMBER

- Scabies mimics other skin diseases.
- Scabies rarely occurs above the neck in immunocompetent adults.
- Contacts should be treated simultaneously to avoid "ping-ponging" (reinfection).
- Treatment failure may result from noncompliance (i.e., treating lesions only) or reinfection.
- Symptoms may persist after appropriate treatment.
- Lesions that resemble insect bites, an eczematous dermatitis, and so-called neurotic excoriations may confuse an unsuspecting diagnostician.
- Because the scabies mite can survive away from the skin for 2 to 5 days on inanimate objects such as clothing of an affected person, it is believed that indirect contact with such personal items can transmit the organism. This is most applicable in immunocompromised and institutionalized elderly patients.

BASICS

- There are two species of sucking lice: *Pediculosis humanus* and *Phthirus pubis* (pubic lice, sometimes called "crabs").
- *P. humanus* is further divided into two subspecies: *P. humanus capitis* (the head louse) and *P. humanus corporis* (the body louse).

Head Lice (Pediculosis Capitis)

- Head lice spread from human to human; epidemics of head lice are most commonly seen in schoolchildren.
- Head lice occur more often in girls and women than in boys and men; they are unusual in African-Americans, but not in African blacks.

Body Lice (Pediculosis Corporis)

- Body lice are most often found in situations of poor personal hygiene, such as in homeless people.
- They are historically prevalent in war conditions.

Pubic Lice

- Pubic lice are generally transmitted by sexual contact.

DESCRIPTION OF LESIONS

Head Lice

- There are no primary lesions; however, secondary crusts and eczematous dermatitis resulting from scratching may be present.
- Nits (louse eggs) are cemented to the hairs (FIG. 20.19).
- It is difficult to find living lice.

Body Lice

- Lesions begin as small papules.
- Later, secondary lesions develop from scratching and may produce crusted papules, infected papules, and ulcerations.

Pubic Lice

- Small living brown lice may be seen at the base of hairs (FIG. 20.20).
- Blue macules (maculae ceruleae) may occur on nearby skin.

DISTRIBUTION OF LESIONS

Head Lice

- Only the scalp is involved.

Body Lice

- Covered areas (under infested clothing) of the body may be affected.

Pubic Lice

- Pubic hair, eyebrows, eyelashes, and axillary hair may be infested.

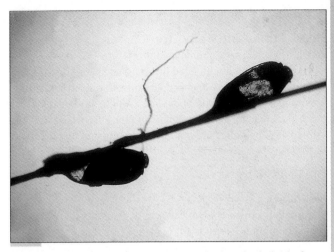

20.19 *Head lice.* The nits are attached to the hair shaft.

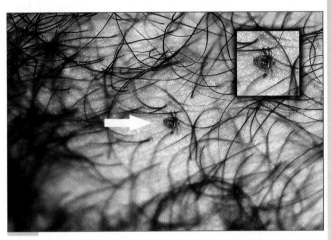

20.20 *Pubic lice.* A small brown living crab louse is seen at the base of hairs *(arrow)*.

CLINICAL MANIFESTATIONS

Head, Pubic, and Body Lice
- Itching is the predominant symptom.
- Affected children with head lice may be asymptomatic.
- There is a possibility of secondary infection from scratching.
- With the exception of body lice, which have historically been known to carry epidemic typhus, trench fever, and relapsing fever, lice are not known to transmit any disease.

DIAGNOSIS

Head Lice
- Knowledge of an epidemic at school generally alerts parents or school nurses to look for evidence of lice.
- White nits may be very obvious on a background of darker hair.

- A hair may be plucked and examined for nits using the low power of a microscope.
- A nit is attached to the base of a hair shaft when the egg is first laid and remains cemented to the growing hair.

Body Lice
- The diagnosis is made not from examining the patient but closely inspecting the seams of his or her clothing, where the lice are found.

Pubic Lice
- Lice may be present.
- Pruritus is noted.
- Blue macules may be seen.
- Often, a sexual partner has "crabs."

 DIFFERENTIAL DIAGNOSIS

Head Lice
- Atopic dermatitis of the scalp should be considered.

Body Lice and Pubic Lice
- Atopic dermatitis or another type of eczematous dermatitis should be considered.
- Scabies should be excluded.

MANAGEMENT

Head Lice

- Remove nits with a fine-tooth comb after soaking the hair in a vinegar solution; this helps soften the cementing substance that attaches the nit to the hair.

First-Line Treatment
Nix **Creme Rinse, RID**, and **Acticin** (over-the-counter)

- These products all contain low concentrations of permethrin; they are very effective in killing adult lice and nymphs but not as effective in killing nits (eggs).
- There has been a growing resistance of head lice to these agents.
- How to use these products:
  - The hair is washed with a nonmedicated shampoo and is towel dried; the agent is applied as a cream rinse, allowed to remain in place for 10 minutes, and then rinsed off thoroughly.
  - Because these agents do not destroy nits effectively, a second application (using the same technique) often is recommended 7 to 10 days after the initial therapy.
- The latest treatment resembles a powerful blow-dryer, which delivers a blast of heated air to dry out lice and their eggs in one half-hour treatment. The practicality and efficacy of this device remain to be proven.

Strategies for Resistant Cases
Ovide (Malathion Lotion 0.5%)

- This agent is considered the most effective treatment for head lice.
- It is both a pediculicide and an ovicide.
- Caution: Ovide Lotion is flammable. Treated areas that are wet with this product should be kept away from open flames and electric heat sources such as hair dryers.
- How to use Ovide:
  - The lotion is applied to **dry** hair in a quantity sufficient to wet hair and scalp.

- It is then massaged into the scalp and is left on for 8 to 12 hours. Heat (e.g., hairdryers, hot curlers) should **not** be used to dry the lotion.
- The hair is then rinsed, and the nits are removed with a fine-tooth (nit) comb.
- Treatment should be repeated in 7 to 10 days if lice are still present (using the same technique).

Elimite Cream (5% Permethrin Cream)

- This is available by prescription.
- It is left on overnight under an occlusive shower cap.
- The application is repeated in 1 week to destroy any remaining eggs.

Other Treatment Options

- **Oral ivermectin** has not yet been approved for the treatment of head lice. The dosage is 0.2 mg/kg in a single dose. A second treatment may be required.
- Petrolatum such as **Vaseline Petroleum Jelly** is quite messy and difficult to remove, but it is an inexpensive and sometimes effective method that asphyxiates the lice and nits. It is applied to the entire scalp and is left on under a shower cap overnight.

Pubic Lice

- **Kwell (Lindane) shampoo** USP 1% is an ectoparasiticide and ovicide effective against *Sarcoptes scabiei*. It is lathered and is left on for 10 minutes.
- **RID** and **Nix** lotions are also effective.
- Treatment should include contacts of infested patients, especially sexual partners.

Body Lice

- A shower and clean clothing generally cure body lice.
- Clothing should be washed at hot temperatures to kill the lice.

 HELPFUL HINTS

- Shaving of pubic, scalp, or body hair is not necessary to treat lice.
- In resistant cases, particularly after repeated treatment failures, delusions of parasitosis should be considered in the differential diagnosis in adult patients.

 SEE PATIENT HANDOUT "Head Lice" ON THE SOLUTION SITE

Visiting the beach and swimming in saltwater or freshwater expose people to a variety of creatures. Encounters with jellyfish (e.g., sea nettle, Portuguese man-of-war, thimble jellyfish) can cause skin reactions.

Jellyfish Stings

BASICS

- Two types of stinging jellyfish are seen floating in the coastal waters off North America: the smaller sea nettle and the rarer, more dangerous Portuguese man-of-war, whose poison can be fatal.
- The tentacles of jellyfish have many stinging nematocysts, which contain a hollow poisonous tip and hooks. The hooks hold the jellyfish onto the victim while the nematocysts discharge the toxic venom.

DESCRIPTION OF LESIONS

- The shape of the lesions, which resemble linear welts that develop at the site of contact, often give the victim the appearance of having been whipped (FIG. 20.21).
- Lesions may fade or may blister and become necrotic, depending on the amount of injected venom and the victim's sensitivity.

DISTRIBUTION OF LESIONS

- The distribution is asymmetric and unilateral.

CLINICAL MANIFESTATIONS

- Victims usually describe a stinging or burning sensation.
- The sting of the Portuguese man-of-war is more painful than a common jellyfish sting. It has been described as feeling like being struck by a lightning bolt, and some victims dread it more than a shark bite (FIG. 20.22).
- There have been reported cases of anaphylactic reactions and fatalities from both sea nettle and Portuguese man-of-war stings.

DIAGNOSIS

- The diagnosis is based on the reported sting occurring in an endemic area and its characteristic eruption.

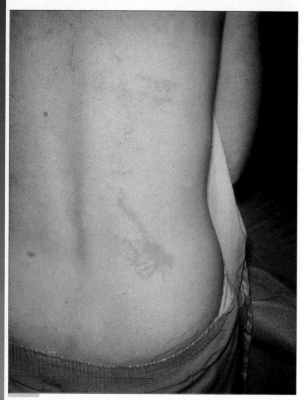

20.21 *Jellyfish sting.* Note the curvilinear, whiplike shape of the lesions.

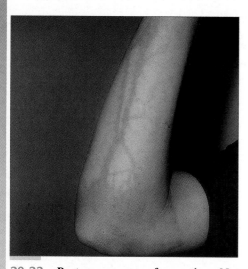

20.22 *Portuguese man-of-war sting.* Note the linear shape of the lesions. The sting of the Portuguese man-of-war is more painful than a common jellyfish sting.

POINT TO REMEMBER

- Severe stings that result in systemic reactions may require life-support measures such as on-site resuscitation.

 DIFFERENTIAL DIAGNOSIS

- Other bites or stings should be considered.

Seabather's Eruption ("Sea Lice")

 MANAGEMENT

- Mild stings may be treated symptomatically with cool soaks and **topical steroids.**
- For more severe reactions, the affected area should be washed with **seawater, alcohol,** or **vinegar** to remove nematocysts and to inactivate any toxins that remain.

BASICS

- This intensely pruritic eruption develops *under* swimwear, presumably because the responsible larvae become trapped under the garments.
- It occurs several minutes to 12 hours after exposure to the larvae of the thimble jellyfish (*Linuche unguiculata*) in the saltwater off the coast of Florida and in the Caribbean.
- This condition has also been contracted off the coast of Long Island, New York, where it has been reputedly caused by the larvae of a sea anemone.

DISTRIBUTION AND DESCRIPTION OF LESIONS

- Erythematous macules and papules occur *under* swimwear (Figs. 20.23 A and B).

CLINICAL MANIFESTATIONS

- The pruritus is worse at night and tends to prevent the patient from sleeping.
- Fever and malaise, the next most common symptoms, are experienced more often by children than by adults.
- Lesions last for 2 to 14 days and resolve spontaneously.

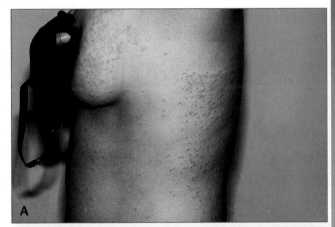

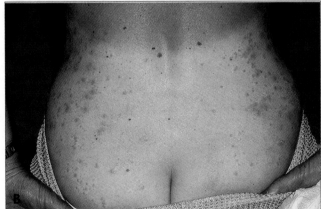

20.23 A and B *Seabather's eruption.* This patient has just returned from bathing off the coast of Florida. The lesions are confined to the area covered by her bathing suit.

MANAGEMENT

- Treatment for both seabather's eruption and swimmer's itch is symptomatic.
- After bathing, immediate removal of the swimwear for washing, or rinsing of the swimwear while it is still being worn, may help prevent seabather's eruption.
- Immediate towel drying after swimming in freshwater may prevent swimmer's itch.

DIAGNOSIS

- The diagnosis can be made when the patient has bathed in an endemic area and displays inflammatory papules on the area covered by the bathing suit.

 DIFFERENTIAL DIAGNOSIS

- **Swimmer's itch** (cercarial dermatitis) occurs on *exposed* sites after freshwater swimming.
  - It is caused by *Schistosoma* organisms that invade the skin. These organisms are the microscopic larvae of the parasitic flatworm.
  - After being released from host snails, the larvae swim in water until they penetrate the skin of a warm-blooded host, such as a duck or a human.

BASICS

- As the name suggests, cutaneous larva migrans is a cutaneous eruption that creeps or migrates in the skin. It results from the invasion and movement of various hookworm larvae that have penetrated the skin through the feet, lower legs, or buttocks.
- *Ancylostoma braziliense, A. caninum, A. ceylanicum, Uncinaria stenocephala* (dog hookworm), *Bunostomum phlebotomum* (cattle hookworm), *A. duodenale,* and *Necator americanus* are the primary hookworms that cause cutaneous larvae migrans in the United States.
- The adult hookworm (nematode) resides in the intestines of dogs, cats, cattle, and monkeys. The feces of these animals contain hookworm eggs that are deposited on sand or soil, hatch into larvae if conditions are favorable, and then penetrate human skin, which serves as a "dead-end" host.
- At greatest risk are gardeners, farm workers, and people who sunbathe or walk on sandy beaches by the seashore.
- Larva currens, a distinct variant of cutaneous larva migrans, is caused by *Strongyloides stercoralis* and may produce visceral disease. Visceral larva migrans is caused by another species of hookworm.

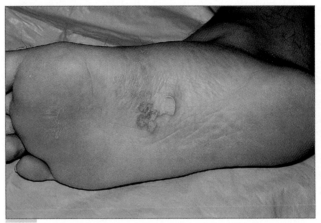

20.24 *Cutaneous larva migrans.* Note the serpiginous, erythematous, raised, tunnellike lesions in typical locations.

DESCRIPTION OF LESIONS

- Lesions have a characteristic curvilinear, serpentine shape (FIG. 20.24).

DISTRIBUTION OF LESIONS

- Areas that come into contact with sand or contaminated soil, most commonly the feet (farmers) or buttocks (sunbathers on nude beaches), are affected.

CLINICAL MANIFESTATIONS

- This benign eruption is usually pruritic and self-limited because the larvae usually die within 4 to 6 weeks.

DIAGNOSIS

- The diagnosis is based on the characteristic clinical appearance.
- If the patient has been vacationing on the beach in an area endemic for cutaneous larva migrans, consider the condition when diagnosing a local itchy eruption on one foot.

MANAGEMENT

- **Class 1 superpotent topical steroids** (e.g., clobetasol cream) for itching
- **Topical thiabendazole** suspension (500 mg/5 mL under occlusion three times per day for 1 week)
- **Oral thiabendazole** (Mintezol; 50 mg/kg/day in two daily doses for 2 to 5 days) *or*
- **Albendazole** (400 mg daily for 3 days [this drug has fewer side effects than thiabendazole])
- **Liquid nitrogen,** applied to the active, advancing end of the lesion

DIFFERENTIAL DIAGNOSIS

Granuloma Annulare
- Lesions are annular.
- It lacks scale and vesicles and does not itch.

Tinea Pedis
- Potassium hydroxide examination is positive.

Other Diagnoses
- Other bites or stings (e.g., jellyfish) should be considered.

HELPFUL HINT

- If the patient has been vacationing on the beach in an endemic area, consider cutaneous larva migrans as a cause of a local itchy eruption on one foot.

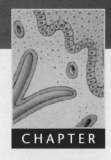

Benign Skin Neoplasms

OVERVIEW

- Benign lesions such as melanocytic nevi, skin tags, seborrheic keratoses, cherry angiomas, and epidermoid cysts are expected consequences of the skin's normal, age-appropriate, often hereditary, maturation process.
- As with most skin lesions, familiarity breeds recognition. This chapter, along with Chapter 22, presents the various common benign and malignant neoplasms in their diverse clinical guises.
- Skin lesions—particularly pigmented skin lesions—often present a difficult and puzzling conundrum for the nondermatologist health care provider. Questions such as "Am I missing a melanoma?" "Is this mole suspicious?" and "Is this a skin cancer?" may arise. In reality, the answer is not always apparent. In fact, the decision of whether a lesion is benign or malignant is often a challenge for many dermatologists as well. Distinguishing between a benign pigmented lesion such as melanocytic nevus or a seborrheic keratosis and a potentially fatal skin cancer such as melanoma creates the most concern among health care providers.

➤ **MELANOCYTIC NEVI**

- Junctional melanocytic nevus
- Compound melanocytic nevus
- Dermal melanocytic nevus
- Blue nevus
- Halo nevus
- Spitz nevus
- Congenital melanocytic nevus
- Atypical nevus (dysplastic nevus, Clark's nevus)

➤ **SEBORRHEIC KERATOSIS**

- Stucco keratosis
- Dermatosis papulosa nigra
- Sign of Leser-Trélat

➤ **SKIN TAGS**

➤ **SEBACEOUS HYPERPLASIA**

➤ **CYSTS**

- Epidermoid
- Pilar
- Milium

➤ **LIPOMA**

➤ **CHONDRODERMATITIS NODULARIS CHRONICA HELICIS**

➤ **DERMATOFIBROMA**

➤ **FIBROUS PAPULE**

➤ **HYPERTROPHIC SCAR**

➤ **KELOID**

➤ **COMMON ANGIOMAS**

- Cherry angioma
- Venous lake
- Angiokeratomas
- Spider angioma
- Pyogenic granuloma

Melanocytic Nevi

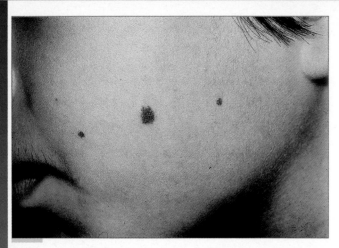

21.1 *Junctional melanocytic nevi.* These small, flat, lesions are uniform in color.

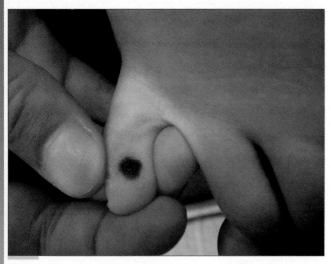

21.2 *Junctional melanocytic nevus (congenital).* This small lesion is extremely unlikely to become malignant.

BASICS

- Melanocytic nevi (MN), commonly called moles or "beauty marks," are, most often, benign proliferations of normal skin components. They are composed of nevus cells that are derived from melanocytes, the pigment-producing cells that colonize the epidermis.
- The acquisition of MN is greatest in childhood and adolescence. In addition to an hereditary predisposition, it has been suggested that their onset is a response to sun exposure.
- During adulthood, the development of new lesions tapers off, and many existing lesions gradually lose their capacity to form melanin and become skin-colored or disappear completely.
- MN may be congenital or acquired, and they are much more often seen in patients with light or fair skin than in blacks or Asians.
- Acquired MN are sometimes associated with melanoma; however, the frequency of transformation into a melanoma is not known. Congenital nevi, on the other hand, especially when very large, hold the greater risk of malignant transformation (see later discussion).

Junctional Melanocytic Nevi

- These small, macular (flat), frecklelike lesions are uniform in color. Individual lesions may be brown to dark brown to black (FIG. 21.1).
- Histologic examination reveals melanocytic nevus cells located at the dermoepidermal junction.
- Whether acquired or congenital, junctional MN are most prevalent on the face, arms, legs, trunk, genitalia, palms, and soles (FIG. 21.2).

The most important lesions in the differential diagnosis of junctional MN include:

- Dysplastic nevus (atypical mole; see later discussion)
- Lentigo maligna (see FIG. 22.47)
- Melanoma (see Chapter 22)

Freckles (Ephelides)
- These small, tan macules appear on the sun-exposed skin of fair-skinned people (FIG. 21.3).
- They darken after sun exposure and lighten when they are no longer exposed to the sun.

Lentigo (Plural: Lentigines) or "Liver Spot"
These small, acquired tan macules occur on sun-exposed areas during middle and elderly age. They are uniform in color (FIG. 21.4). Most often, they appear on the face, dorsal hands (FIG. 21.5), extensor forearms, and anterior legs.

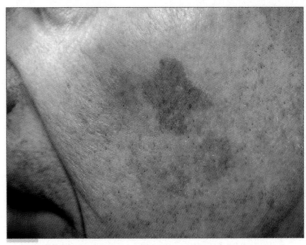

21.4 *Solar lentigines.* Note the uniformity in color (compare with FIGS. 22.47 and 22.48).

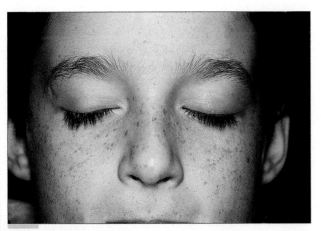

21.3 *Freckles (ephelides).* Freckles come and go with sun exposure. They are most often seen in people who have fair skin.

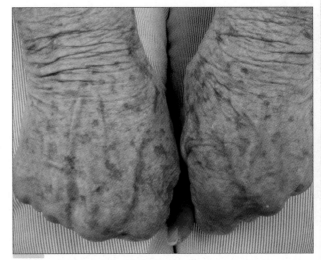

21.5 *Solar lentigines.* These extremely common tan macules arise on sun-exposed areas during middle age.

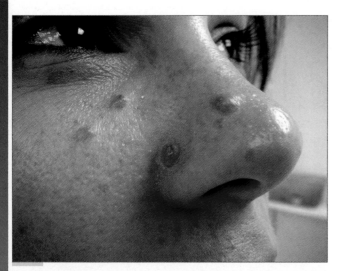

21.6 *Compound melanocytic nevi.* Elevated, dome-shaped papules that are most often seen on the face, arms, legs, and trunk. These lesions tend to lose pigmentation as the patient ages.

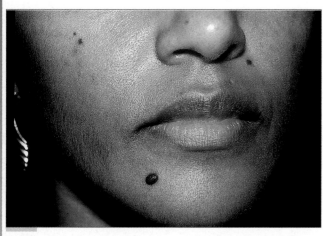

21.7 *Compound melanocytic nevi.* In individuals with dark skin, such lesions tend to be more intensely pigmented.

 DIFFERENTIAL DIAGNOSIS OF DERMAL NEVI AND COMPOUND NEVI

Dermal nevi and compound nevi often resemble one another as well as the following:

- Atypical nevus
- Neurofibromas
- Skin tags (acrochordons)
- Basal cell carcinomas
- Seborrheic keratoses
- Angiofibroma (fibrous papules)
- Nodular melanoma

Compound Melanocytic Nevi

- Compound MN are elevated, dome-shaped papules or papillomatous nodules.
- Uniformly brown to dark brown, they may contain hairs and are seen most often on the face, arms, legs, and trunk (FIGS. 21.6 and 21.7).
- Their histologic structure combines features of junctional and dermal nevi (see next section).

Dermal Melanocytic Nevi

- Dermal MN may be elevated and dome-shaped, wartlike, or pedunculated.
- Most often skin-colored, they may be tan or brown, or they may be dappled with pigmentation. Lesions tend to lose pigmentation with age and become skin-colored (FIG. 21.8).
- They are most often seen on the face and neck.
- Microscopy reveals that dermal MN cells are located in the dermis.

CLINICAL MANIFESTATIONS OF DERMAL NEVI AND COMPOUND NEVI

- Dermal nevi and compound nevi are asymptomatic unless they are irritated or inflamed.
- Very rarely do they transform to malignant melanoma.

DIAGNOSIS

- The diagnosis is based on clinical appearance or, if necessary, a histopathologic evaluation after removal.

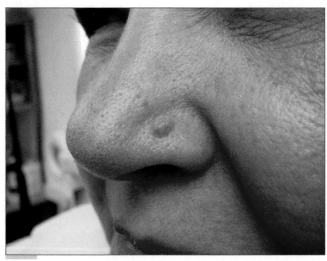

21.8 *Dermal melanocytic nevus.* This lesion was pigmented when the patient was in her teens and twenties.

Clinical Variants

Blue Nevi

- These lesions are a benign variant of dermal MN that are heavily pigmented. They occur as blue-gray or blue-black macules, papules, or nodules (FIG. 21.9) and are rarely malignant. The dark brown pigment that creates a bluish color to these lesions is caused by the Tyndall phenomenon.
- Like the more common dermal and compound MN, blue nevi usually begin to appear in adolescence or early adulthood.

Halo Nevi

- Halo nevi are MN that are encircled by a white halo of depigmentation. The halo represents a regression of a preexisting nevus caused by a lymphocytic infiltrate. Frequently, the entire nevus disappears, and the area regains normal pigmentation.
- Most often, halo nevi are initially seen on preadolescents; they usually appear on the trunk (FIG. 21.10).
- If a halo nevus is seen on an adult, two very rare possibilities should be considered: the lesion may be malignant, or a melanoma may be present elsewhere on the body. Biopsy and removal are indicated in this situation. Also bear in mind that in a patient of any age, a biopsy should be performed if the nevus has an atypical clinical appearance.

Spitz Nevi

- These nevi are a distinctive variant of MN. In the past, they were referred to as "juvenile melanomas," but now they are recognized as benign. In children, the lesions may appear as pink papules; sometimes they are heavily pigmented and are jet black in color.
- A heavily pigmented, small, spindle-cell variant of Spitz nevus may be seen on the legs of women.
- It is prudent to completely excise these lesions to minimize the risk of recurrence and possible confusion with a malignant lesion.

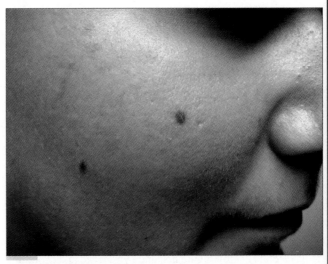

21.9 ***Blue nevus.*** This is a variant of melanocytic nevus. Note the blue-gray color caused by the Tyndall effect. Compare to the tan-colored nevus on this boy's face.

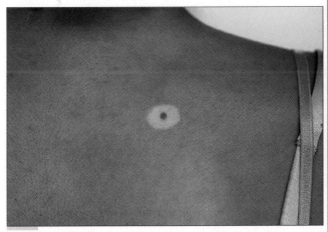

21.10 ***Halo nevus.*** An inflamed compound nevus has lost some of its original tan pigmentation. It is encircled by a white halo of depigmentation. Ultimately, the nevus may disappear, and the area will regain normal pigmentation.

Congenital Melanocytic Nevi

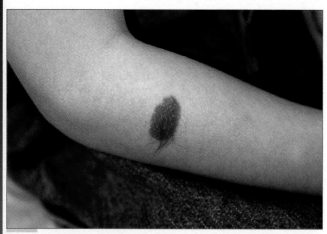

21.11 Small to medium-sized congenital hairy nevus. This lesion is evenly pigmented and symmetric and probably has little, if any, malignant potential.

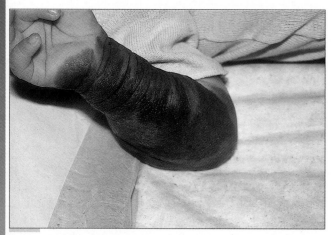

21.12 *Giant pigmented hairy nevus.* A patient with this lesion may have a greater than 6% lifetime risk of melanoma.

- Often generating great concern in both patents and pediatricians, congenital melanocytic nevi (CMN) are MN that are present at birth or arise during the first year of life.
  - By definition, CMN are present at birth or soon thereafter, although some small CMN are clearly so-called "tardive" and may appear as late as up to 2 years of age.
  - CMN occur in about 1% of children.
- On histopathology, in contrast to acquired MN described above, the nevus cells of CMN tend to be deeper in the dermis and subcutaneous fat and are often present in the skin appendages such as nerves and hair follicles.
- CMN vary considerably in size and are commonly classified as small (under 1.5 cm), intermediate (1.5 to 19.9 cm) (Fig. 21.11), or large/giant (20 cm). (These figures are based on the predicted final adult size of lesions.)
- Physical findings include the following:
  - CMN are generally relatively evenly pigmented and tan or brown, especially those that are thin.
  - Some lesions can have an array of colors.
- The malignant potential of small or medium-sized CMN is controversial. However, many experts believe that a small nevus does not significantly increase the lifetime risk of developing melanoma.
- CMN are of the greatest concern when they are 20 cm or larger in diameter. These nevi, which are often called giant pigmented hairy nevi, "garment nevi," or "bathing trunk nevi," may develop into melanoma—the lifetime risk is estimated to be between 3.3 and 6.0% (Fig. 21.12).

MANAGEMENT OF MELANOCYTIC NEVI

- All MN should be carefully examined and biopsy should be considered, particularly if there is any suggestion of clinical atypia.
- However, for most MN, biopsy is not indicated. Persons with numerous MN, particularly atypical nevi (see later discussion), are at greater risk for developing malignant melanoma.

Indications for Removal
- Atypical appearance
- Cosmetic reasons
- Repeated irritation by clothing, such as a bra strap
- Persistent discomfort (a lesion that itches, hurts, or bleeds)

Methods of Removal
Lesions can be removed by shave excision (which is often followed by electrodesiccation) or by elliptic excision (see Chapter 26, "Diagnostic and Therapeutic Procedures").

- *Shave (tangential) excision*: This method is fast and economical, and it generally provides satisfactory cosmetic results. Its disadvantage is that it often results in only partial removal of the lesions, which infrequently necessitates a second excisional procedure.
- *Elliptic excision*: This technique is performed with the intent of removing lesions completely. Surgical margins can be identified. However, elliptic excision is slower than shave excision. It also requires suturing and suture removal, and it results in linear scars that may not be as cosmetically pleasing as scars that result from shave excisions.

 POINTS TO REMEMBER

- Any pigmented lesion that changes rapidly in size or color or that has an atypical appearance should be removed for biopsy.
- A primary care physician should have a low threshold for referral to a dermatologist if there is any concern regarding the diagnosis and management of a pigmented lesion.
- All MN that are removed should be submitted for microscopic evaluation.
- Large CMN have a low but real risk of malignant transformation and the development of melanoma.

Atypical Nevus (Dysplastic Nevus, Clark's Nevus)

BASICS

- The atypical nevus, which is also called dysplastic nevus, an atypical mole, or Clark's nevus, is a controversial and confusing lesion. Even among dermatopathologists, there is no consensus regarding the histopathologic criteria for its diagnosis.
- Some individuals have only a few atypical nevi, and their risk of melanoma may not be much higher than those individuals without such nevi.
- This much is agreed: When a patient has numerous atypical nevi and there is a positive family history of melanoma, the potential for melanoma in that patient and in his or her family is extremely high. Such dysplastic nevi may be inherited as an autosomal dominant trait (see discussion of familial atypical mole syndrome).
- Atypical nevi are rarely seen in black, Asian, or Middle Eastern populations.

DESCRIPTION OF LESIONS

Atypical nevi have some or all of the following features:

- They are usually larger than common moles and frequently measure 5 to 15 mm in diameter.
- Their borders are usually irregular, notched, and ill-defined.
- They have a macular appearance, but the centers may be raised (for this reason, they are sometimes called "sunny-side-up egg lesions") (FIG. 21.13).
- Their coloration (tan, brown, black, pink, or red) is irregular.

DISTRIBUTION OF LESIONS

- Atypical nevi are most often found on the trunk, legs, and arms; generally, the face is spared.

CLINICAL MANIFESTATIONS

- The exact risk of an individual atypical nevus developing into a melanoma is uncertain.
- Unlike dermal and compound nevi, these lesions often continue to appear into adulthood.
- Differentiating them clinically from melanoma is often difficult.

Clinical Variants

Sporadic Atypical Nevi

- A patient with an isolated atypical nevus and no family history of multiple atypical nevi or melanoma probably carries little risk of developing melanoma and should not necessarily be identified as prone to melanoma.

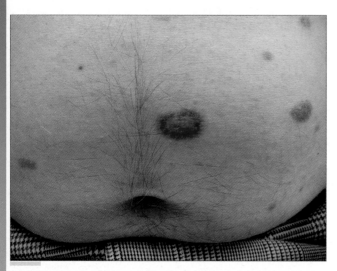

21.13 *Atypical nevus (dysplastic nevus).* Note the raised center and indistinct border; such a nevus is sometimes called a "sunny-side-up egg lesion." It is generally larger than a common mole.

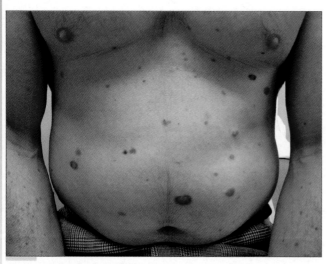

21.14 *Multiple dysplastic nevi.* Note the characteristic distribution on the trunk.

Multiple Atypical Nevi

- The exact risk of an individual nevus developing into a melanoma is uncertain (Fig. 21.14).
- In certain situations, atypical nevi are considered possible precursors to, as well as potential markers for, the development of melanoma that may occur de novo without evolving from a precursor dysplastic nevus.

Familial Atypical Mole Syndrome

- Those persons who meet the following criteria are considered to have an extremely high potential for developing malignant melanoma:
  1. Patients with a first-degree (e.g., parent, sibling, or child) or second-degree (e.g., grandparent, grandchild, aunt, uncle) relative who has a history of malignant melanoma have heightened risk.

2. Many nevi—often more than 50—are present, and some of them are atypical moles.
3. Moles show certain dysplastic features when examined under the microscope.

 DIFFERENTIAL DIAGNOSIS

- Other MN (see earlier discussion)
- Malignant melanoma
- Pigmented basal cell carcinoma

 MANAGEMENT

- The method chosen for removing suspected atypical nevi depends on the purpose of treatment.
  - If melanoma is suspected, complete excision should be performed.
  - If melanoma is not suspected, the lesion can be removed and prepared for biopsy with a shave or punch biopsy technique.

Prevention

- Patients with many atypical nevi should avoid excessive sun exposure and should routinely use a sunscreen with a sun protective factor of 15 or greater.

- Patients who meet the criteria for familial atypical mole syndrome should examine their own skin every 2 to 3 months, in addition to having a full body examination and regular screening visits performed by a dermatologist.
- High-risk patients and their families should be taught self-examination to detect changes in existing moles and should be given printed material with photographs to help them recognize the features of malignant melanoma.

 POINTS TO REMEMBER

- The risk of melanoma is greatly increased in patients with multiple atypical nevi and a personal or family history of melanoma.
- Once a diagnosis of multiple atypical nevi is established, other family members should be examined.
- A person with an isolated atypical nevus probably carries little risk of developing melanoma and should not be identified as melanoma prone.
- Melanoma risk is greater in those persons who have one relative with melanoma than in those with no affected relative. The lifetime risk of melanoma may approach 100% in persons with atypical nevi who are from melanoma-prone families (i.e., individuals having two or more first-degree relatives with melanoma).
- Patients with the familial atypical multiple mole and melanoma syndrome (also known as the dysplastic nevus syndrome) should be monitored vigilantly.

 HELPFUL HINT

- Despite the fact that patients with many dysplastic nevi are at a very high risk of developing a melanoma, the notion of removing *all* of their dysplastic nevi to reduce their risk of melanoma is generally believed to be ill advised. To consider these nevi to be precursors of melanomas creates undo anxiety for patients but does not appear to decrease their potential for developing melanomas.

 SEE PATIENT HANDOUT "Atypical Nevus (Mole)" ON THE SOLUTION SITE

Seborrheic Keratosis

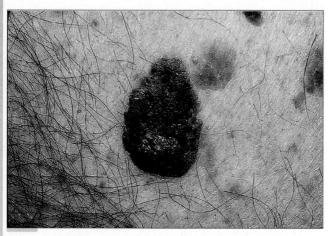

21.15 *Seborrheic keratoses.* The largest, darkest, lesion has a warty, rough-surfaced, tortoise shell-like, "stuck-on" appearance. The lesions in the background are also SKs; these lesions are unusual before 30 years of age. (Compare with images of melanoma in Chapter 22: Figs. 22.35–22.43.)

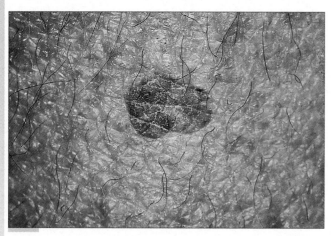

21.16 *Seborrheic keratoses.* This lesion is almost flat. Lesions are found on the arms and legs.

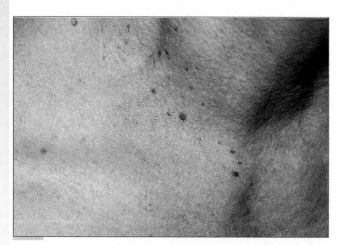

21.17 *Seborrheic keratoses.* Multiple pigmented papules, some of which are clinically indistinguishable from skin tags, are evident. (See Fig. 21.22.)

BASICS

- A seborrheic keratosis (SK) is an extremely common benign skin growth that becomes apparent in people older than 40 years of age. These lesions are the most common neoplasms in the elderly, and they have virtually no malignant potential.
- Patients often report a positive family history of SKs, and men and women are equally frequently affected.
- SKs have been whimsically described as "barnacles in the sea of life" and "maturity spots"; these metaphors are intended to allay patients' anxieties.

DESCRIPTION OF LESIONS

- The typical SK has a warty, "stuck-on" appearance that ranges from tan to dark brown to black. The "dry," crumbly, keratotic surface of some lesions is sometimes rubbed or picked off, only to recur later.
- The use of the word "seborrheic," a misnomer, stems from the occasional "greasy" or shiny appearance of the lesions; SKs are actually epidermal in origin, with no sebaceous derivation.
- The appearance of individual lesions tends to vary considerably, even on the same patient. Lesions may be warty and tortoiseshell-like (Fig. 21.15); scaly, flat, or almost flat (Fig. 21.16); or small pigmented papules similar to skin tags (discussed later) (Fig. 21.17).
- The color, shape, and surface characteristics of SKs can change with the age and location of individual lesions. Lesions are often smooth and symmetric, uniformly pigmented, and small. To the untrained eye, however, these lesions may resemble melanomas (i.e., they may be asymmetric, have irregular or notched borders, and vary in color).

DISTRIBUTION OF LESIONS

- SKs most often are located on the back, chest, and face, particularly along the frontal hairline (FIG. 21.18) and scalp. They are also frequently found on the arms, legs, and abdomen (FIG. 21.19).
- Smaller lesions similar to skin tags can be seen around the neck, under the breast, or in the axillae.
- In women, lesions are often seen under and between the breasts.
- When many lesions are present, the distribution is usually bilateral and symmetric.

DIAGNOSIS

- With experience, SKs are easily recognized.
- If necessary, a shave biopsy (using a no. 15 scalpel blade) or curettage (see Chapter 26, "Diagnostic and Therapeutic Procedures") may be performed for histologic confirmation.

 DIFFERENTIAL DIAGNOSIS

- Malignant melanoma
- Pigmented basal cell carcinoma
- Verruca vulgaris
- Solar lentigo (especially early flat SKs)
- Pigmented solar keratosis (actinic keratosis)
- MN
- Dysplastic nevus

Clinical Variants

Stucco Keratoses
- These are a nonpigmented variant of SK; they are seen most often in the elderly.

Description of Lesions
- Stucco keratoses are skin-colored or whitish papules that become whiter and scalier when they are scratched. They typify the "dry, stuck-on" type of seborrheic keratosis.

Distribution of Lesions
- They are commonly found on the distal lower leg, particularly around the ankles (FIG. 21.20), and they may also be seen on the dorsal forearms.

Dermatosis Papulosa Nigra
- This common manifestation is diagnosed primarily in African-American, Afro-Caribbean, and sub-Saharan African blacks; however, it is also seen in darker-skinned persons of other races. Lesions start appearing in adolescence and increase in number as persons age.

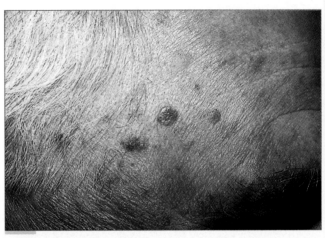

21.18 *Seborrheic keratoses.* The frontal hairline and temples are common locations.

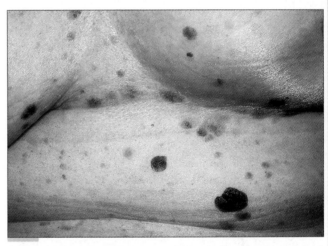

21.19 *Seborrheic keratoses.* These lesions are in a typical location. Note the different colors, sizes, and shapes of the various lesions in this patient.

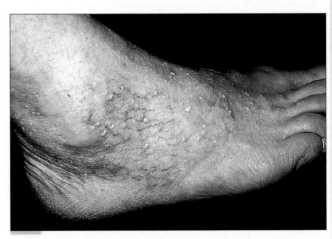

21.20 *Stucco keratoses.* These lesions have a whitish, "stuck-on" appearance. They occur especially on the dorsum of the foot and around the Achilles tendon area.

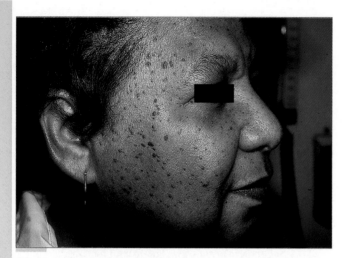

21.21 ***Dermatosis papulosa nigra.*** The lesions of this common inherited condition appear as small, pigmented papules on the face that resemble SKs and are histologically indistinguishable from them.

- Dermatosis papulosa nigra (DPN) lesions are histopathologically identical to SKs and are considered to be of autosomal dominant inheritance.

Description of Lesions
- Lesions are darkly pigmented and, in contrast to typical SKs, they have minimal, if any, scale.

Distribution of Lesions
- DPNs are generally seen on the face, especially the upper cheeks and lateral orbital areas (FIG. 21.21).

Sign of Leser-Trélat
- This condition refers to the sudden appearance of multiple SKs in a short period or a rapid increase in their size.
- It is a rare phenomenon and is presumed by some observers to be a cutaneous sign of leukemia or internal malignant disease, especially of the gastrointestinal tract, prostate, breast, ovary, uterus, liver, or lung. However, in light of the frequency of malignant disease in the elderly, and the ubiquitous presence of SKs in this age group, the relationship is believed by some observers to be fortuitous.

 MANAGEMENT

- Patients with SKs are often referred to dermatologists with a presumptive diagnosis of warts or moles or to have these lesions evaluated for cancer, particularly melanoma.
- Learning to recognize SKs should obviate the need for many of these referrals. When a patient is referred, a biopsy (generally a shave biopsy) is performed if necessary to confirm the diagnosis or to distinguish SK from a pigmented basal cell carcinoma, MN, wart, or melanoma.
- Because some patients have numerous lesions, it is an impractical expenditure of time and money to perform multiple biopsies of lesions, as long as the clinical appearance is typical.
- An excisional biopsy should always be performed whenever malignant melanoma is suspected.

Treatment
- Cryosurgery is performed with liquid nitrogen spray, cotton swab application, or light electrocautery and curettage (treating the base of the lesion helps to prevent recurrence) (see Chapter 26, "Diagnostic and Therapeutic Procedures"); *or*
- Excisional surgery, which results in scar formation, is unnecessary, unless a biopsy of a completely removed lesion is required to rule out malignant disease.

 HELPFUL HINT

- SKs present in many shapes, colors, and sizes. It is a good idea to become familiar with these lesions by consistently examining the skin of all adult patients.

 POINTS TO REMEMBER

- SKs are mainly a cosmetic concern, except when they are inflamed or irritated and can be an annoyance. The challenge for primary care clinicians is to distinguish these lesions from skin cancer, particularly malignant melanoma.
- Lesions may be quite numerous on some persons. Because SKs may, at times, be confused with melanoma, careful visual examination of all lesions should be performed.

BASICS

- These benign skin lesions are extremely common. They are sometimes referred to as *acrochordons, fibroepithelial polyps,* or, if large, *soft fibromas* or *pedunculated lipofibromas.* They are often seen in the body folds of obese persons.
- Skins tags were formerly suspected by several investigators to be markers for intestinal polyps or, possibly, internal malignant diseases, but current evidence suggests that this association is not justifiable.

DESCRIPTION OF LESIONS

- Skin tags are generally 1- to 10-mm fleshy papules.
- They may be skin-toned, tan, or darker than the patient's skin. They are sessile or pedunculated in shape.
- They are most often found on the neck (FIG. 21.22), the axillae, the inframammary area, the groin (especially the inguinal creases), the upper thighs, and the eyelids (FIG. 21.23).

CLINICAL MANIFESTATIONS

- Skin tags are primarily of cosmetic concern; however, they may become a nuisance from the irritation of necklaces and underarm shaving, for example.
- In women, they tend to grow larger and more numerous over the course of a pregnancy.
- They are often seen in association with acanthosis nigricans (See Chapter 14, "Disorders of Pigmentation").

DIAGNOSIS

- Skin tags are easy to recognize; a skin biopsy is rarely necessary.

 DIFFERENTIAL DIAGNOSIS

- Pedunculated SKs
- Compound or dermal nevi
- Neurofibromas

 MANAGEMENT

- Small skin tags are easily removed by snipping them off at their base using iris scissors, with or without prior local anesthesia (see Chapter 26, "Diagnostic and Therapeutic Procedures"). The crushing action of the scissors results in little bleeding or pain.
- Skin tags, if disregarded, occasionally may spontaneously self-destruct. After torsion, they become necrotic and autoamputate.

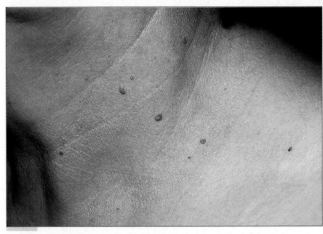

21.22 *Skin tags (acrochordons).* Pigmented papules are present around this patient's neck.

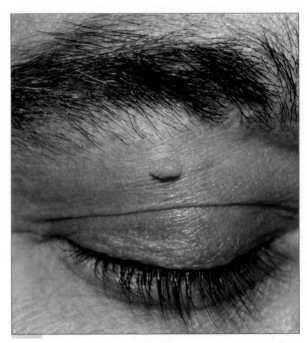

21.23 *Skin tag (acrochordon).* A solitary, skin-colored skin tag is present on the eyelid.

- A rapid and painless treatment for small skin tags is to dip a needle holder or nontoothed forceps into liquid nitrogen for 15 seconds and then gently grasp each skin tag for about 10 seconds. There is little or no collateral damage, just a narrow rim of erythema. Multiple lesions can be treated using this method. The frozen skin tag will be shed in approximately 10 days. This is a good approach for skin tags hanging on the eyelids (FIGS. 21.24 and 21.25).

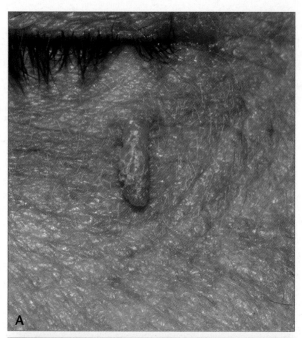

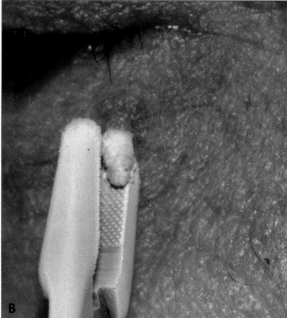

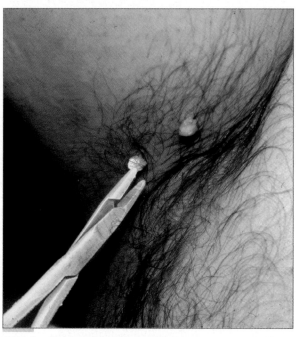

21.25 *Skin tags (acrochordons).* Axillary lesions treated with liquid nitrogen.

21.24 A and B *Pedunculated fibroepithelioma (skin tag).* **A:** Skin tag on eyelid. **B:** Treatment is performed with liquid nitrogen. Frost appears at the tip of the needle holder and on the skin tag. The frozen skin tag will be shed in 7 to 10 days.

BASICS

- Sebaceous hyperplasia refers to small, benign papules on the face of adults representing hypertrophy of the sebaceous glands.
- These fairly common lesions are often confused with basal cell carcinomas.

DESCRIPTION OF LESIONS

- The yellow or cream-colored papules are often doughnut-shaped with a dell (umbilication) in the center (FIGS. 21.26 A and B).
- They are small in diameter (1 to 3 mm).
- Telangiectasias are present on the raised borders.

DISTRIBUTION OF LESIONS

- Lesions occur on the forehead and cheeks.

CLINICAL MANIFESTATIONS

- Lesions are asymptomatic.
- They may be of cosmetic concern.

DIAGNOSIS

- The diagnosis is made by the lesion's typical clinical appearance ("little bagels").
- Biopsy is indicated if basal cell carcinoma is suspected.

 DIFFERENTIAL DIAGNOSIS

- Basal cell carcinoma (see Chapter 22, "Premalignant and Malignant Skin Neoplasms")

 MANAGEMENT

- The patient should be reassured about the benign nature of this condition.
- Light electrocautery, shave biopsy, or laser ablation may be performed to remove lesions, if desired, although these lesions tend to recur.

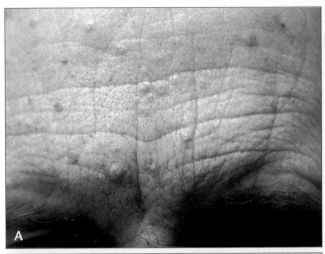

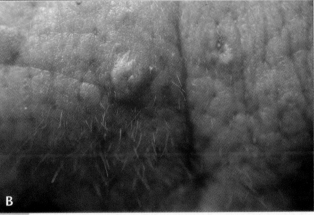

21.26 A and B *Sebaceous hyperplasia.* **A:** Multiple yellowish papules are present. Note the central dell and telangiectasias. **B:** Close-up view.

Cysts

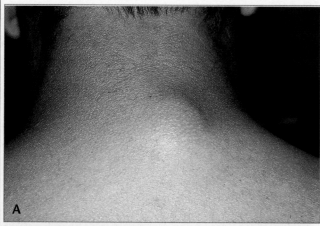

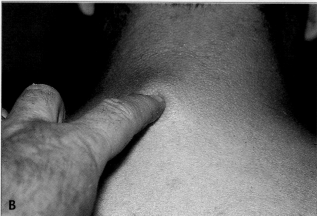

21.27 A and B *Epidermoid cyst.* These lesions often occur on the back. They appear as smooth, discrete, freely movable, dome-shaped ballotable masses. **A:** Cyst. **B:** Compression of the lesion, which has the same consistency as an eyeball or a fully inflated balloon.

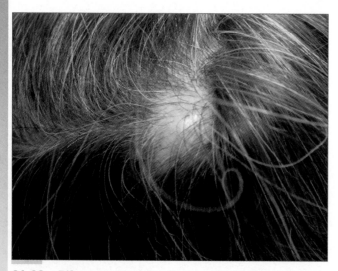

21.28 *Pilar cyst.* Note the absence of hair. The pressure from the enlarging cyst has destroyed the hair follicles. These lesions are freely movable.

BASICS

- A cyst is a sac containing semisolid or liquid material. The sac contains keratin and lipid-rich debris. A cyst has an epithelial lining that produces keratin.
- Cysts tend to be hereditary, arise in adulthood, and may occur as multiple lesions.
- **Epidermoid cysts,** the most common type, are derived from the epithelium of the hair follicle and connect to the surface of the skin with a keratin-filled central pore that looks like a blackhead (FIGS. 21.27 A and B).
- **Pilar cysts,** the second most common type, have a thicker wall that develops from a stratified epithelium. Pilar cysts lack a central pore (FIG. 21.28).

DESCRIPTION OF LESIONS

- Lesions appear as smooth, discrete, freely movable, dome-shaped nodules.
- Cysts that have previously been infected, ruptured, drained, or scarred may be firmer and less freely movable.
- Lesions range from 0.5 to 5.0 cm in diameter.
- Often, there is a central pore (seen in epidermoid cysts), from which cheesy-white, malodorous keratin material can be expressed.

DISTRIBUTION OF LESIONS

- Epidermoid cysts occur most often on the face, behind the ears, and on the neck, trunk, scrotum, and labia.
- Pilar cysts are most often located on the scalp.

CLINICAL MANIFESTATIONS

- Cysts are usually asymptomatic, unless they are inflamed or infected.
- Scrotal and pilar cysts may calcify.
- Pilar cysts are generally devoid of overlying scalp hair.

Clinical Variants

Milia
Basics
- Milia (singular, milium) are extremely common epidermal cysts that contain keratin.
- They can occur in people of any age. They may arise in traumatic scars or in association with certain scarring skin conditions, such as porphyria cutanea tarda.

Description of Lesions
- They are 1.0 to 2.0 mm in diameter and are white to yellow (FIG. 21.29).
- They are often mistaken for the closed comedones of acne ("whiteheads") (FIG. 21.30; see FIG. 1.4).

Distribution of Lesions
- Milia are most often noted on the face, especially around the eyes and on the cheeks and forehead.

DIAGNOSIS

- On palpation, an intact epidermoid or pilar cyst feels smooth; when compressed, it feels like an eyeball or a fully expanded balloon (see FIGS. 21.27 A and B).
- If necessary, a biopsy or an incision and drainage can be performed to confirm the diagnosis.

DIFFERENTIAL DIAGNOSIS

- Lipoma should be considered when cystlike lesions are found on the trunk, the back of the neck, and extremities. However, the consistency of a lipoma is rubbery and somewhat softer than that of a cyst (see FIGS. 21.27 A and B). Lipomas are also irregular in shape.

MANAGEMENT

Epidermoid and Pilar Cysts
- The entire cyst wall does not have to be completely removed to prevent recurrence. However, a large epidermoid or pilar cyst can be removed through a small hole created by a punch biopsy tool (see Chapter 26, "Diagnostic and Therapeutic Procedures").
- For incision and drainage, a fluctuant, infected cyst may be incised with a no. 11 blade, drained, and then packed with iodoform gauze.
- The contents of inflamed or so-called "infected" cysts are most often sterile or contain normal skin flora; thus pre- or postoperative antibiotics are probably unnecessary.

Milia
- In contrast to closed comedones (which they resemble), milia must first be incised (usually with a no. 11 blade) before their contents can be expressed.
- Alternatively, they can be destroyed with light electrodesiccation.

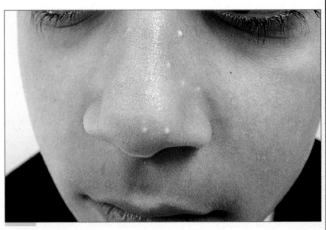

21.29 *Milia.* These epidermal cysts contain keratin. They are 1.0 to 2.0 mm in diameter and are white to yellow.

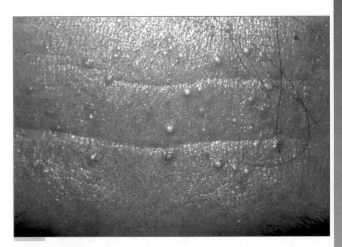

21.30 *Milia.* These lesions are often mistaken for the closed comedones of acne ("whiteheads").

HELPFUL HINT

- Erythematous, tender, or draining epidermal and pilar cysts are often misdiagnosed as being infected rather than inflamed, and patients are accordingly treated unnecessarily with oral antibiotics.

Lipoma

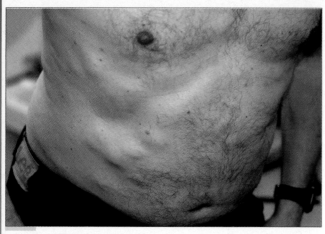

21.31 *Lipomas.* Multiple, rubbery, flesh-colored nodules are palpable on this patient.

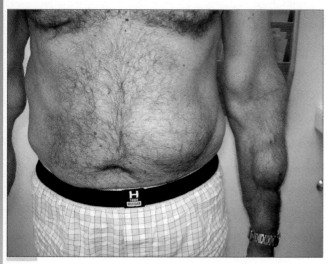

21.32 *Angiolipomas.* This patient has tender, tumor-sized, fatty subcutaneous lesions.

BASICS

- A lipoma is a benign, subcutaneous tumor composed of fat cells.
- **Dercum's disease** is a syndrome of multiple tender lipomas that develop in middle-aged women.
- **Angiolipomas** may be tender or painful.

DESCRIPTION OF LESIONS

- Lipomas are rubbery, generally asymptomatic masses; they range in size from small nodules (Fig. 21.31) to large tumors (Fig. 21.32).
- They are usually irregular in shape and may be greater than 7 cm in length.

DISTRIBUTION OF LESIONS

- Lipomas occur most commonly on the trunk, the back of the neck, the upper arms, and the forearms.

DIAGNOSIS

- The diagnosis is made on clinical grounds.
- A biopsy should be performed if the diagnosis is uncertain.

 DIFFERENTIAL DIAGNOSIS

- As noted earlier, a lipoma may be confused with an epidermoid cyst. However, the latter "feels like an eyeball" and has a regular dome shape.

 MANAGEMENT

- Lesions may be excised or removed using liposuction.

BASICS

- Chondrodermatitis nodularis chronica helicis (CNH) is a relatively common, benign, painful condition of the apex of the helix or on the antihelix of the ear.
- CNH is characterized by one or more spontaneously appearing tender papules.
- CNH occurs most commonly in fair-skinned individuals with severely sun-damaged skin.
- CNH can occur in patients at any age but mostly affects middle-aged to older individuals. It more often occurs in men; 10% to 35% of cases involve women. Age at onset is similar in men and women.
- The onset of CNH may be precipitated by pressure, trauma, or cold. Sleeping on the affected side or holding a telephone instrument to the involved ear can be quite painful.
- Spontaneous resolution is unusual; the condition often continues unless treated.
- The cause of CNH is unknown.
- Neural hyperplasia and a secondary perichondritis probably account for the tenderness associated with this condition.

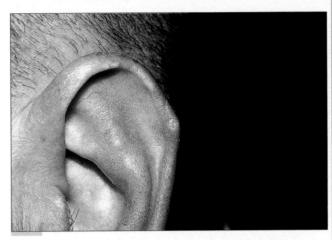

21.33 *Chondrodermatitis nodularis chronica helicis.* This tender papule has a central keratotic punctum. (Note the similarity to Fig. 22.4.)

CLINICAL MANIFESTATIONS

- The nodule—actually papular in size—usually enlarges rapidly to a maximum size, approximately 4 to 8 mm, and remains stable.
- The lesions are firm, tender, well demarcated, and round to oval with a raised, rolled edge and central ulcer or crust (Fig. 21.33).
- The most common location is the apex of the helix. Distribution on the antihelix is more common in women.

 DIFFERENTIAL DIAGNOSIS

See also Chapter 22.

- Actinic keratosis
- Keratoacanthoma
- Squamous cell carcinoma

MANAGEMENT

- Intralesional injections of steroids such as triamcinolone (**Kenalog**; 20 to 40 mg/mL) (Fɪɢ. 21.34) may relieve discomfort and result in resolution. Several visits for these injections may be necessary.
- If the patient sleeps on the affected side, then changing sides or using pressure-relieving pillows or pads may be helpful. A CNH pressure-relieving pillow is available from CNH Pillow, P.O. Box 1247, Abilene, TX 79604; phone (800) 255-7487.
- Biopsy is indicated if the diagnosis is in doubt. The biopsy is necessary to differentiate CNH from actinic keratoses, squamous cell carcinoma, and, less commonly, basal cell carcinoma, because many patients with CNH have chronic solar damage and a history of skin cancer.
- If conservative methods to relieve symptoms are unsuccessful, surgical approaches are almost always needed.
- Wedge excision, curettage, electrocauterization, carbon dioxide laser ablation, and excision of the involved skin and cartilage are often curative.

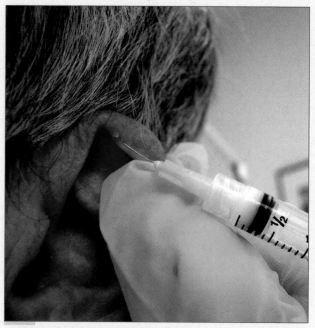

21.34 *Chondrodermatitis nodularis chronica helicis.* Treatment with intralesional triamcinolone is sometimes effective in relieving tenderness and may result in resolution of this lesion.

 HELPFUL HINT

- Most often the patient with CNH seeks medical attention because of the pain associated with the skin lesion(s). In contrast, the cutaneous tumors listed in the differential diagnosis of CNH are usually painless.

Benign Fibrous and Vascular Lesions

Dermatofibromas

BASICS

- Also known as *fibrous histiocytomas* and *sclerosing hemangiomas*, dermatofibromas are common dermal fibrous tumors of unknown cause.
- Dermatofibromas occur most commonly on the legs, trunk, and arms, especially in women older than 20 years of age. The lesions are benign growths that are usually brought to medical attention either to rule out skin cancer or because of cosmetic concerns.

DESCRIPTION OF LESIONS

- A lesion may be a papule or a nodule. It may be elevated with a dome shape, flat, or depressed below the plane of the surrounding skin (FIG. 21.35).
- The color can vary, even in a single lesion, and can be skin-colored, chocolate brown, red, or even purple.
- The surface may be smooth or scaly, depending on whether the lesion has been traumatized (e.g., by shaving).

DIAGNOSIS

- Typically, a dermatofibroma feels like a firm, pea-sized, buttonlike papule that is fixed to the surrounding dermis (accounting for the "dimple" or "collar button" sign) (FIGS. 21.36 A and B).
- It is freely movable over deeper adipose tissue.

DIFFERENTIAL DIAGNOSIS

- **Cysts** and **lipomas** are either compressible or rubbery.
- **MN** (**moles**) are also not as firm as dermatofibromas.
- A **malignant melanoma** is more variable in shape and size than a dermatofibroma.
- **Dermatofibrosarcoma protuberans (DFSP)** is a locally aggressive tumor with a high recurrence rate. DFSP is an uncommon soft tissue neoplasm with intermediate to low-grade malignancy, and metastases rarely occur.

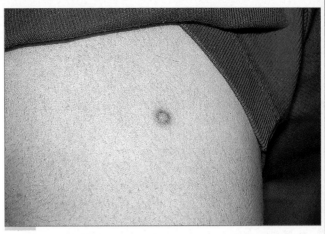

21.35   *Dermatofibroma.* This pigmented, firm papule is a very common finding on the extremities in many patients.

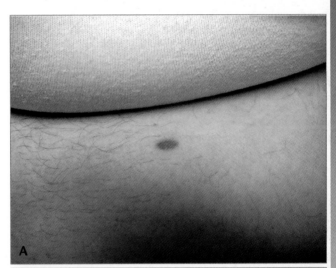

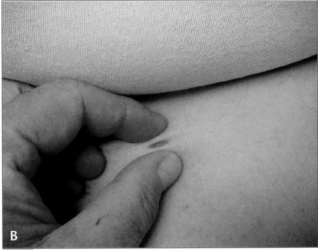

21.36 A and B   *Dermatofibroma.* A: This papule is in a typical location. **B:** Note the "dimple" or "collar button" (retraction) sign that is elicited on compression of the lesion.

POINTS TO REMEMBER

- If there is any doubt about the diagnosis, a biopsy should be performed.
- The patient should be informed that if the lesion is removed, the scar may be more cosmetically objectionable than the original lesion.

 MANAGEMENT

- No treatment is necessary; however, local excision can be performed for biopsy confirmation or cosmetic concerns, or if the lesion is symptomatic.
- Deep shave excision is another alternative; however, the lesion may recur.

Fibrous Papules

BASICS

- Fibrous papules (angiofibromas, fibrous papules of the nose or face; Fig. 21.37) are relatively common benign lesions that may be difficult to distinguish from compound or dermal nevi; furthermore, they often may resemble a basal cell carcinoma (see also Fig. 22.27).
- Histopathology reveals a combined vascular and fibrous proliferation.

DESCRIPTION OF LESIONS

- Generally they are dome-shaped, pale or pink firm papules with a shiny appearance. They usually range from 1 to 5 mm in diameter.
- Lesions appear in adults and usually as a single lesion, but, occasionally, several lesions may be present.
- Most are noted on the nose; less commonly, they are found on the cheeks and chin.

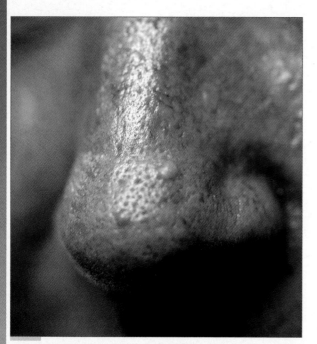

21.37 *Fibrous papules (angiofibromas, fibrous papules of the nose).* These are dome-shaped, pale or pink, firm papules with a shiny appearance and may be difficult to distinguish from compound or dermal nevi. They often may resemble a basal cell carcinoma.

 MANAGEMENT

- No treatment is necessary.
- If necessary, they are biopsied if the diagnosis is in doubt or to rule out a basal cell carcinoma.
- They may also be removed for cosmetic reasons.

BASICS

- A hypertrophic scar is defined as a widened or unsightly scar that does not extend beyond the original boundaries of the original injury. Hypertrophic scars appear within weeks of skin injury.
- A keloid is an overgrowth of dense fibrous tissue, a scar whose size far exceeds that which would be expected from the extent and margins of an injury to the skin. Keloid, derived from the Greek *chele* (crab's claw), describes the lateral growth of tissue into unaffected skin.
- Hypertrophic scars and keloids represent an exaggerated formation of scar tissue in response to skin injuries such as lacerations, insect bites, ear piercing, and surgical wounds.
  - They may also result from healed inflammatory lesions (e.g., acne, chickenpox) (FIGS. 21.38 and 21.39).
  - In recent years, the popularity of skin piercing procedures and tattooing has increased the frequency of these undesirable scars and has expanded the sites on the body where they may occur.
- Exaggerated scars occur less frequently at the extremes of age—the very young and elderly—however, increasing numbers of presternal keloids, as well as hypertrophic scars may be seen in older age groups and result from coronary artery bypass surgery or intravenous Port-A-Caths (peripherally inserted central venous catheters) used to deliver fluids and medications.
- Keloids are more likely to occur in Hispanics, Asians, and particularly individuals of African descent than in Caucasians. There is no racial preponderance noted with hypertrophic scarring.

Pathogenesis

- In susceptible individuals, when there is an overproduction of collagen, the excess collagen becomes piled up in fibrous masses and an exaggerated formation of scar tissue.
- **Hypertrophic scars:** Scanning electron microscopy reveals flattened collagen bundles that are parallel in orientation.
- **Keloid:** Unlike hypertrophic scar formation, the electron microscope reveals a number of distinguishing features, including randomly organized collagen fibers in a dense connective tissue matrix.

DESCRIPTION OF LESIONS

- Hypertrophic scars and keloids are firm, shiny, hairless papules, nodules, or tumors; they may be flesh-colored, tan, or brown.
- If lesions are inflamed or are of recent onset, they may be red (erythematous) or purple (violaceous).

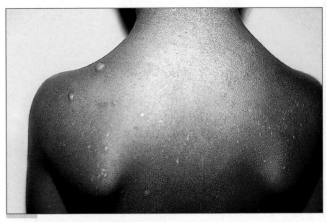

21.38 *Hypertrophic scars.* The scars on this boy's shoulders resulted from healed chickenpox lesions.

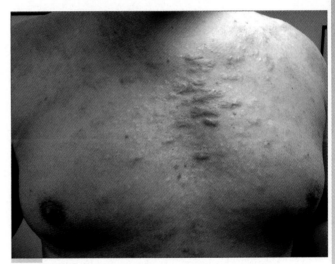

21.39 *Keloid.* These scars appeared in sites of former inflammatory acne lesions.

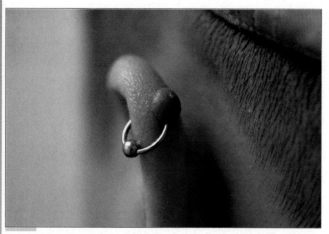

21.40 *Keloid.* The earlobes are a common location. This violaceous lesion is inflamed.

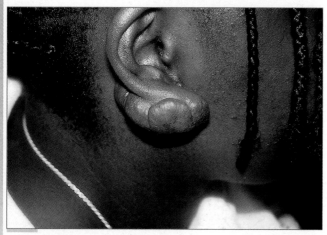

21.41 *Keloid.* This lesion was also caused by earlobe piercing. Large lesions such as this are more likely to occur in African-Americans.

DISTRIBUTION OF LESIONS

- Both hypertrophic scars and keloids most commonly arise in the same anatomic locations: the sternum, the shoulders, the deltoid region of the upper arm, and the upper back.
- The most common sites on the head and neck are the earlobes, mandibular border, and posterior neck. The earlobe is typically affected secondary to earring posts (Figs. 21.40 and 21.41).

CLINICAL MANIFESTATIONS

- Both hypertrophic scars and keloids may be tender, painful, or pruritic; however, keloids, by virtue of their excessive size, are generally more problematic and are of much greater cosmetic concern to patients.
- Unlike keloids, the hypertrophic scar reaches a certain size and subsequently stabilizes or regresses, whereas keloids do not regress without treatment and tend to recur after excision.

DIAGNOSIS

- The diagnosis of hypertrophic scars and keloids is made on the basis of clinical appearance.

 MANAGEMENT

Prevention

- Prevention is essential. Patients who tend to develop hypertrophic scars or keloids should be advised to discontinue or avoid repetitive skin trauma such as tattooing and skin piercing, particularly in areas that are prone to abnormal scarring such as the presternal areas and earlobes.

- Conditions such as inflammatory acne and cutaneous infections should be treated promptly to prevent scarring. Despite preventive measures, keloids may form in simple clean wounds or may occur in the absence of trauma.

Treatment
Hypertrophic Scars
- **Intralesional corticosteroids** with triamcinolone acetate (TAC) in varying concentrations (5 to 40 mg/mL) are

continued on page 387

injected directly into the scar (FIG. 21.42); this has been the mainstay of treatment for hypertrophic scars and keloids. Use of a 25- to 27-gauge needle at 4- to 6-week intervals often helps flatten the lesions. Additionally, these injections are also useful for diminishing itching and tenderness. Side effects from these injections include hypopigmentation, atrophy, and telangiectasias (FIG. 21.43).

- Corticosteroids reduce excessive scarring by reducing fibroblast growth and promoting collagen degradation. Such injections must be administered cautiously to avoid overtreatment, which may result in skin atrophy, telangiectasias, and an overdepressed scar.
- **Topical corticosteroids:** A clear surgical tape that is uniformly impregnated with flurandrenolide, a corticosteroid, has been shown to soften and flatten keloids over time.
- **Pulsed-dye lasers** have been used successfully and safely on some persistent hypertrophic scars.
- If they are in amenable locations, hypertrophic scars can sometimes be removed by simple excision, provided that wound closure can occur without undue tension on the surgical site.

Keloids

- **Intralesional corticosteroid injections**
  - As with hypertrophic scars, intralesional TAC, often in concentrations as high as 40 mg/mL, can help flatten keloids and diminish itching and erythema.
  - Such high concentrations are generally necessary for denser, more recalcitrant lesions. Similarly, complications of repeated corticosteroid injections include atrophy, telangiectasias, and pigmentary alteration.
- **Excision,** in combination with other postoperative modalities, such as TAC injections, compression dressings, radiotherapy, or injected interferon, are sometimes effective.
  - Careful operative technique that closes surgical wounds with minimal tension is important. This is followed by postoperative injection of TAC 2 to 3 weeks postoperatively, followed by repeat injection in 3 to 4 weeks.
  - After excisional treatment alone, keloids frequently recur (more than 50% of the time); however, when excision is combined with injected steroids or other modalities, the recurrence rate is diminished.
  - However, it should be noted that preoperative or intraoperative steroid injection can delay wound healing and increase the possibility of wound dehiscence. A lower steroid dose is preferred because of the potential complications of intralesional steroids, including depigmentation and dermal atrophy.

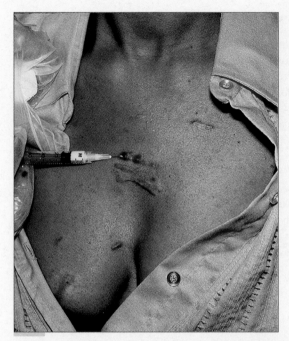

21.42 *Treatment of keloids with intralesional cortisone.* Triamcinolone (Kenalog, Aristocort) is being injected into this patient's presternal lesions.

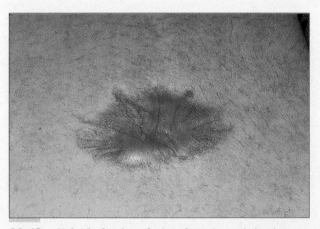

21.43 *Keloid after intralesional cortisone injection.* This shiny scar shows the possible untoward aftereffects of intralesional steroid injections: atrophy, telangiectasias, and perilesional hypopigmentation.

- **Laser therapy.** Lasers have been used as alternatives to cold excision for keloids; however, the use of this equipment is expensive. As with excisional therapy, results are best when laser therapy is combined with postoperative injected steroids.

continued on page 388

- **Combined modality treatment of keloids.** Effective treatment may involve excision followed by:
  - Pressure dressings (compression therapy) during the postoperative period to wounds of patients in whom hypertrophic scars and keloid formation occur. This includes earlobe button compression, pressure earrings, Ace bandages, elastic adhesive bandages, compression wraps, and Lycra bandages. Compression therapy is based on the finding that pressure has long been known to have thinning effects on skin.
  - Occlusive dressings: The application of silicone gel sheeting has not proven to be very effective. Any antikeloidal effects appear to result from a combination of occlusion and hydration, rather than from an effect of the silicone.
- Topical imiquimod (**Aldara**) cream: Postoperative application of imiquimod 5% cream induces local production of interferon alpha, which, in turn, is known to enhance keloidal collagenase activity and reduce the synthesis of collagen. A recent study has demonstrated a lower recurrence rate of keloids when imiquimod is applied postoperatively.
- Other medications: In addition to topical imiquimod, other methods that are sometimes used to treat keloids and hypertrophic scars include intralesional interferon, oral verapamil, intralesional bleomycin, 5-fluorouracil, and botulinum toxin.

Common Angiomas

BASICS

- There are many different types of angiomas, benign growths that consist of small blood vessels. These tumors can be located anywhere on the body. Some of the different types include spider angiomas, cherry angiomas, and angiokeratomas.

Cherry Angiomas

- These lesions, which are also known as Campbell De Morgan spots, ruby spots, and senile angiomas, are extremely common benign vascular neoplasms.
- They are asymptomatic, easily diagnosed, cherry- to plum-colored papules that develop primarily on the trunk (FIG. 21.44).
- The angiomas are found in fair-skinned adults older than 40 years of age.

Venous Lakes

- Venous lakes (venous varices) are another common benign vascular neoplasm. They are generally macules or papules that are dark blue to purple and may be seen on the lower lip (FIG. 21.45), face, ears, and eyelids (see also FIG. 12.18).
- The lesions usually occur in patients older than 60 years of age.

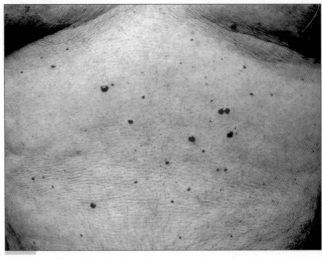

21.44 *Multiple cherry angiomas.* These cherry- and plum-colored papules are common in fair-skinned persons older than 40 years of age.

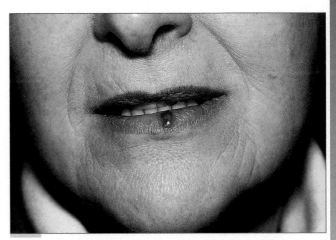

21.45 *Venous lake.* This is a common lesion among seniors. If a patient is concerned about its appearance, the lesion can be removed with electrocautery or laser destruction. They appear on the lower lip and on the external ears.

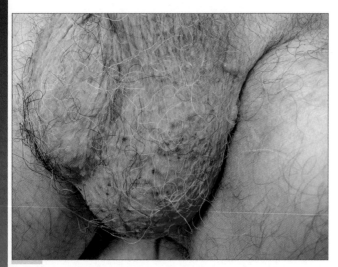

21.46 **Angiokeratomas.** These red-purple papules are most often found on the scrotum; they are usually first noticed when the patient is a young adult.

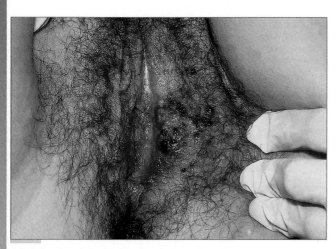

21.47 **Angiokeratomas.** Lesions are seen here on the vulva.

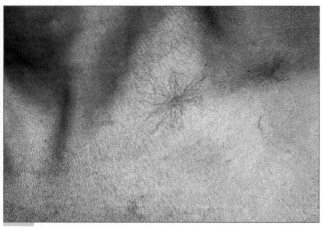

21.48 **Spider angioma.** This lesion is actually a cluster of telangiectasias radiating from a central arteriole. Compression of the central arteriole completely blanches the lesion.

Angiokeratomas (Fordyce Angiokeratomas)

- Angiokeratomas (Fordyce angiokeratomas) are most often found on the scrotum (FIG. 21.46) or vulva (FIG. 21.47), and they consist of multiple red-purple asymptomatic papules ("caviar spots").
- They are usually first noticed in young adulthood.

 DIFFERENTIAL DIAGNOSIS

- The diagnosis of all these lesions is usually made on clinical grounds.

 MANAGEMENT

- Reassure the patient that the lesions are benign.
- If the lesions are a cosmetic concern, they may be treated with electrocautery, cryosurgery with liquid nitrogen, or laser therapy.

Spider Telangiectasias (Spider Angiomas)

- A spider angioma (nevus araneus) is a cluster of telangiectasias, or dilated capillaries, that radiate from a central arteriole (FIG. 21.48).
- It is more commonly seen in women and may be associated with pregnancy or oral contraceptive use. Spider angiomas are also seen in patients with hyperestrogenic conditions, such as chronic liver disease. They may also be seen in healthy children.
- Lesions appear as spokelike capillaries radiating from a slightly raised central arteriole. Compression of the central arteriole completely blanches the lesions.
- Spider angiomas most often occur on the face and trunk. Lesions are asymptomatic and are primarily of cosmetic concern.

 MANAGEMENT

- Light electrocautery or laser destruction of the spider angioma may be performed if the lesion presents a cosmetic problem. Occasionally, lesions regress spontaneously.
- Other types of telangiectasias may serve as a clue to an underlying collagen vascular disease, such as the periungual telangiectasias of systemic lupus erythematosus and dermatomyositis or the telangiectasias seen in scleroderma and the CREST syndrome (*c*alcinosis, *R*aynaud's phenomenon, *e*sophageal motility disorders, *s*clerodactyly, and *t*elangiectasia) (see Chapter 25, "Cutaneous Manifestations of Systemic Disease").

Pyogenic Granuloma

BASICS

- Pyogenic granuloma (PG) is a common vascular hyperplasia of the skin and mucous membranes that occurs most often in children and young adults.
- Lesions can also arise during pregnancy (such a lesion is known as a *granuloma gravidarum*). They are also associated with oral contraceptive use.
- The cause of PGs is unknown, but minor trauma and hormonal factors appear to be factors in their development.

DESCRIPTION OF LESIONS

- PG lesions are benign, rapidly developing, red, purple, or red-brown, dome-shaped papules or nodules. They resemble hemangiomas or granulation tissue ("proud flesh").
- PGs are generally solitary and range in size from a few millimeters to 3 to 4 cm in diameter (FIG. 21.49). The bases of lesions are often surrounded by a collarette of skin. PG papules or nodules may be crusted.
- Lesions are asymptomatic but tend to bleed after minor trauma.

DISTRIBUTION OF LESIONS

- Lesions most frequently occur at sites of minor trauma, such as the fingers and toes, but they also may be seen on the trunk.
- During pregnancy, lesions tend to occur on the lips (FIG. 21.50), gums, and buccal mucosa. Spontaneous resolution often occurs after childbirth.

DIAGNOSIS

- The diagnosis is usually based on the typical clinical appearance and biopsy.

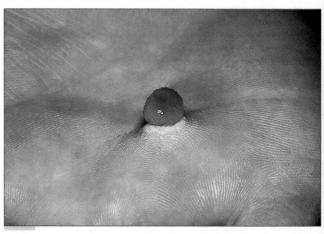

21.49 **Pyogenic granuloma.** This patient has a typical dusky red nodule with a collarette of skin. These lesions tend to bleed when traumatized.

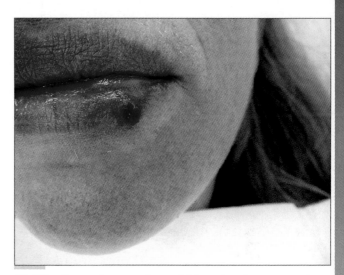

21.50 **Pyogenic granuloma.** This patient is pregnant (see also FIG. 23.5).

 DIFFERENTIAL DIAGNOSIS

In children:

- Hemangioma

In adults:

- Nodular (amelanotic) melanoma
- Skin cancer (e.g., basal cell carcinoma, squamous cell carcinoma)
- Kaposi's sarcoma

 MANAGEMENT

- If there is any doubt about the diagnosis, a biopsy should be performed.
- The lesion is generally destroyed by electrocautery, laser therapy, cryosurgery, or excisional surgery. Recurrences are not uncommon if the lesion is not completely removed.

 POINT TO REMEMBER

- The clinical presentation of a rapidly developing, friable, vascular lesion in a child or pregnant woman suggests a PG.

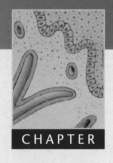

Premalignant and Malignant Skin Neoplasms

- ➤ **SOLAR KERATOSIS**

- ➤ **SQUAMOUS CELL CARCINOMA**

- Bowen's disease (squamous cell carcinoma in situ)
- Squamous cell carcinoma of mucous membranes

- ➤ **KERATOACANTHOMA**

- ➤ **BASAL CELL CARCINOMA**

- Superficial basal cell carcinoma
- Morpheaform basal cell carcinoma

- ➤ **MELANOMA**

- Superficial spreading melanoma
- Nodular melanoma
- Lentigo maligna and lentigo maligna melanoma
- Acral lentiginous melanoma

- ➤ **PAGET'S DISEASE OF THE BREAST AND EXTRAMAM-MARY PAGET'S DISEASE**

OVERVIEW

- This chapter is intended to help health care providers distinguish skin cancers from precancers and benign growths. The ability to make clinical diagnoses, to identify benign versus malignant lesions, especially in their less classic presentations, is an important skill that comes with focused, repetitive visual scrutiny.
- By far, the most important skin lesion for the health care provider to recognize is melanoma.
- The therapy of malignant lesions should be undertaken only by persons experienced in skin cancer therapy.

BASICS

- An aging population that is living longer, in an atmosphere with a declining ozone layer and with more outdoor and leisure time to bask in this ultraviolet environment, has led to a dramatic increase in sun-related skin damage (dermatoheliosis) and precursors to skin cancer such as solar keratoses. It is estimated that 60% of predisposed people older than 40 years have at least one solar keratosis, and many of them have new solar keratoses each year.
- Solar keratosis, also commonly known as *actinic keratosis*, is the most common sun-related skin growth. Whether this lesion is benign (premalignant) or malignant (squamous cell carcinoma in situ) from its onset is controversial. What is accepted, however, is that solar keratoses have the potential to develop into invasive squamous cell carcinomas.
- Solar keratoses are more common in men, particularly those who work, or have worked, in outdoor occupations, such as farmers, sailors, and gardeners, and those who participate in outdoor sports. The incidence of solar keratosis, as with all of the skin cancers described in this chapter, is highest in Australia and in the Sun Belt of the United States.
- It is estimated that 1 in 20 lesions eventually becomes squamous cell carcinoma. It is also accepted that the invasive carcinomas that develop from these actinic keratoses are of a very slow-growing, indolent, unaggressive type, and the prognosis usually is excellent. Distant metastases are extremely rare. Consequently, among dermatologists, there is an ongoing debate regarding the need to be aggressive or *laissez-faire* in the approach to these lesions.

PATHOGENESIS

- The development of solar keratoses, which is directly proportional to sun exposure, is seen in people who are fair-skinned, burn easily, and tan poorly.
- These lesions are rare in dark-skinned persons.

Histopathology
- Cellular atypia is present, and the keratinocytes vary in size and shape. Mitotic figures are common.
- The histologic changes of individual cells are indistinguishable from those seen in squamous cell carcinomas.

DESCRIPTION OF LESIONS

- Lesions usually appear as multiple discrete, flat or elevated, verrucous, scaly lesions. Their texture typically feels rough to the touch (FIG. 22.1).
- They typically have an erythematous base covered by a white, yellowish, or brown scale (hyperkeratosis) (FIG. 22.2).
- Lesions are usually 3 to 10 mm in size and can gradually enlarge, thicken, and become more elevated and thus develop into a **hypertrophic solar keratosis** (FIGS. 22.3 and 22.4) or a **cutaneous horn** (FIGS. 22.5 and 22.6).

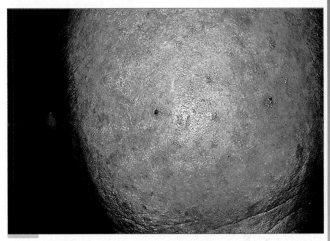

22.1 *Solar keratoses.* Rough, scaly papules are present on the scalp. This is a typical finding in bald, elderly men with fair complexions who have spent much of their lives working outdoors. The lesions in this patient are more easily palpated than visualized.

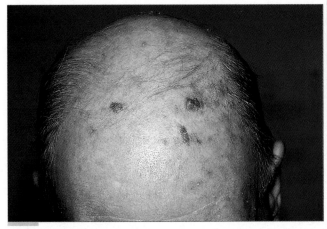

22.2 *Solar keratoses.* Thicker, tan-colored, hyperkeratinized lesions are more obvious in this patient.

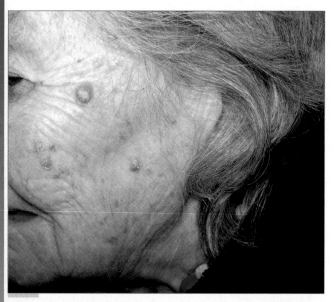

22.3   Solar keratoses, hypertrophic. The solar keratoses occur primarily in areas of sun-exposed skin in this elderly woman.

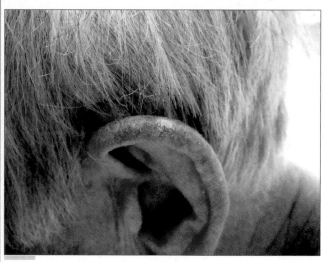

22.4   Solar keratosis. The pinna of the ear is a very common site for these lesions in men. (Note the similarity to Fig. 21.33, an illustration of chondrodermatitis nodularis chronica helicis.)

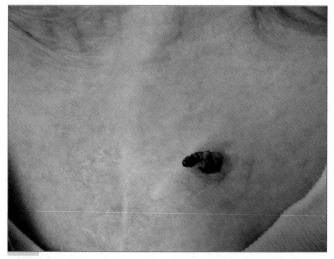

22.5   Solar keratosis. This large cutaneous horn was produced by an underlying hypertrophic solar keratosis.

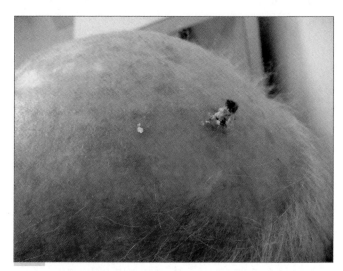

22.6   Solar keratosis. This cutaneous horn was also produced by an underlying solar keratosis. A biopsy was performed to rule out squamous cell carcinoma.

- A cutaneous horn is a hornlike projection of keratin. In addition to solar keratoses, warts and squamous cell carcinomas in situ (**Bowen's disease**) may also produce a cutaneous horn on their surface.
- Sometimes, solar keratoses are tan or dark brown (**pigmented solar keratosis**) (FIG. 22.7) and are often clinically indistinguishable from a solar lentigo (see FIG. 21.4)
- In time, a solar keratosis may develop into a squamous cell carcinoma.

DISTRIBUTION OF LESIONS

- Solar keratoses are most often seen on a background of sun-damaged skin.
- They are found chiefly on sun-exposed areas: the face, especially on the nose, temples, and forehead.
- They are also commonly noted on the bald areas of the scalp and the tops of the ears in men, the dorsa of the forearms (FIG. 22.8) and the dorsa of the hands, the "V" of the neck, and the neck below the occipital hairline and below the ears.
- The vermilion border of the upper lip is another very common site for solar keratoses (FIG. 22.9).

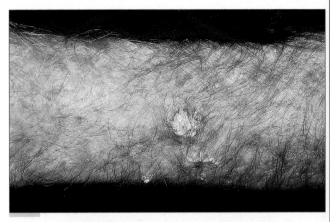

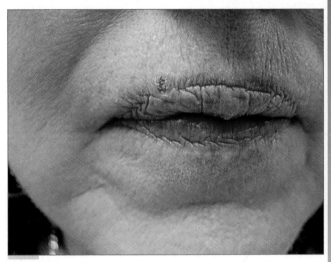

22.8 *Solar keratoses, hypertrophic.* The forearms are a common site of these lesions.

22.9 *Solar keratosis.* The vermilion border of the upper lip is a common site of sun damage.

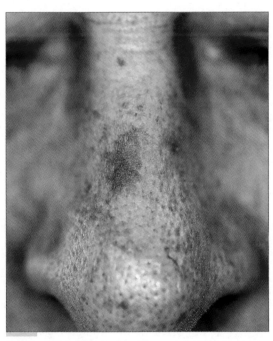

22.7 *Solar keratosis, pigmented.* This lesion is slightly rough to the touch.

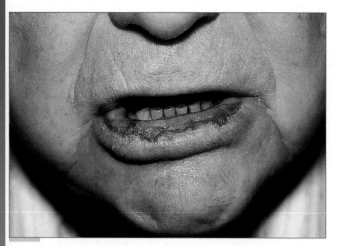

• They may also occur on any area that is chronically or repeatedly exposed to the sun, such as the legs in women.
• Extensive involvement of the mucous membranes of the lower lips (generally the lower lip) is known as *actinic cheilitis* (FIG. 22.10).

CLINICAL MANIFESTATIONS

• Solar keratoses are usually asymptomatic, but they may itch and become tender or irritated. Patients often report one or several "dry" scaly bumps on sun-exposed areas that do not respond to moisturizers.
• They are of cosmetic concern to many patients.
• They may regress spontaneously.

DIAGNOSIS

• Clinically, very small lesions are often better felt than seen. Palpation of these scaly growths reveals a gritty, sandpaper-like texture.
• A shave biopsy is performed if the diagnosis is in doubt.

22.10 *Actinic cheilitis.* This patient is undergoing treatment with topical 5-fluorouracil for multiple solar keratoses of his lower lip.

 DIFFERENTIAL DIAGNOSIS

Squamous Cell Carcinoma
See later discussion.

• Solar keratosis may be indistinguishable from a squamous cell carcinoma.
• Untreated, squamous cell carcinoma becomes indurated, with a tendency to ooze, ulcerate, or bleed.

Basal Cell Carcinoma
See later discussion.

• Classically, this lesion is a pearly, shiny papule with telangiectasias.
• It may be indistinguishable from solar keratosis, particularly when it is small, ulcerated, manipulated, or pigmented.

Verruca Vulgaris (Wart)
• Warts may also be indistinguishable from solar keratoses.

Seborrheic Keratosis
See also Chapter 21, "Benign Skin Neoplasms."

• A seborrheic keratosis may, at times, be indistinguishable from a solar keratosis.
• Seborrheic keratosis has a "stuck-on" appearance and may occur in areas not exposed to the sun.

Chondrodermatitis Nodularis Helicis
See also Chapter 21, "Benign Skin Neoplasms."

• These lesions, when present on the helices or antihelices of the ears, may be easily confused with solar keratoses.

MANAGEMENT

- Prevention begins with educating the patient to limit sun exposure by using sunscreens and wearing protective clothing.
- Treatment is achieved by destruction of solar keratoses (see Chapter 26, "Diagnostic and Therapeutic Procedures").

Destructive Methods

- **Liquid nitrogen** (LN$_2$) is the mainstay of treatment for solar keratoses. LN$_2$ is most useful when lesions are few in number. It is applied to individual lesions for 3 to 5 seconds.
- For thick, hyperkeratotic lesions, **biopsy followed by electrocautery** or **electrocautery alone** is performed.

Chemotherapy

- Topical application of **Efudex**, a 5-fluorouracil (5-FU) cream, is a method that may be used when lesions are too numerous to treat individually. 5-FU interferes with the synthesis of DNA; it destroys dysplastic cells and spares normal cells. Enough medication is applied to cover the entire area with a thin film. This is done twice daily for 2 to 4 weeks for facial lesions. Other body sites require longer treatment (e.g., 6 to 8 weeks for the arms).
- Alternatively, a 0.5% 5-FU cream (**Carac**) may be applied only once daily. This preparation is reportedly less irritating than the stronger 5% 5-FU agents.
- During this treatment, the lesions become increasingly red and crusted, and subclinical lesions become visible. This situation can result in a very red, disfiguring complexion; however, if the patient completes the treatment, the lesions usually heal within 2 weeks of stopping treatment, the skin becomes smooth, and the majority of the solar keratoses are gone (FIGS. 22.11 A and B).

Immunotherapy

- Imiquimod (**Aldara**) 10% cream is a local inducer of interferon. It is applied twice weekly to involved skin for 16 weeks until a response similar to that described with 5-FU agents is elicited.

Other Treatments

- Topical tretinoin (**Retin-A**) has been shown to reverse mild actinic damage to the skin.
- **Photodynamic therapy** can also be used to treat multiple actinic keratoses. In this treatment, topical 5-aminolevulinic acid accumulates preferentially in the dysplastic cells. On exposure to irradiation with light of the appropriate wavelength, oxygen-derived free radicals are generated, and cell death results.

- **Chemical peels** and **dermabrasion** are also used in patients with numerous facial solar keratoses.
- Diclofenac sodium 3% (**Solarase**) gel is a nonsteroidal anti-inflammatory preparation that has been introduced as a topical treatment for solar keratoses. This agent appears to be less irritating than the standard 5-FU products and Aldara; however, its efficacy does not match theirs.

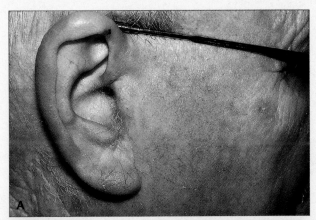

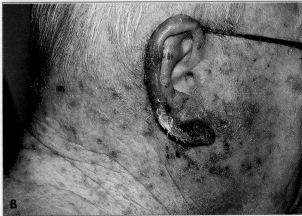

22.11 A and B *Solar keratoses.* **A:** Before treatment, few lesions are clinically visible. **B:** Two weeks after treatment with topical 5-FU, crusting and erythema are evident in areas that had lesions that were not initially apparent.

HELPFUL HINTS

- Because solar keratoses are more often easily felt than seen, the clinician should run ungloved fingers over the patient's skin to detect all lesions.
- The number of solar keratoses is directly related to cumulative sun exposure. Childhood exposure or sun damage is "accumulated like interest on money in the bank"; some of this damage seems to be reversed and prevented by sun avoidance and sun protective measures.
- Sunscreens should also be applied to the lower lip to prevent actinic cheilitis.
- Topical 5-FU treatment can be likened to using a "smart bomb" in which the "bomb" (in this case 5-FU) targets only the "enemy" (the rapidly growing dysplastic cells).
- Imiquimod (**Aldara**) cream may "immunize" patients against their own dysplastic keratinocytes; in fact, some dermatologic surgeons use it prophylactically to prevent recurrence. Aldara is applied two times per week for a full 16 weeks.

POINTS TO REMEMBER

- If a lesion persists or recurs, despite treatment, it should be examined by biopsy.
- The decision to treat solar keratoses can be based on cosmetic reasons, symptom relief, or, most important, the prevention of malignancy.

SEE PATIENT HANDOUTS "Solar Keratosis (Actinic Keratosis)" and "Sun Protection Advice" ON THE SOLUTION SITE

BASICS

- Squamous cell carcinoma (SCC) is a malignant epithelial tumor arising from keratinocytes of the epidermis.
- It is the second most common type of skin cancer. SCC is diagnosed much less frequently than basal cell carcinoma (BCC), but it carries a risk of metastasis. It occurs in an older age group than does BCC.
- Although it is very rare in dark-skinned persons, SCC can be more aggressive in these individuals.
- The majority of SCCs arise in solar keratoses (see earlier discussion). Such SCCs that develop from solar keratoses are slow growing, minimally invasive, and unaggressive, and the prognosis is usually excellent because distant metastases are extremely rare.
- An SCC may appear de novo without a preceding solar keratosis.
- When a metastasis from a cutaneous SCC (non–mucous membrane) does occur, it is more likely to result from lesions that appear on the ears or on the vermilion border of the lips, from lesions that are poorly differentiated, from recurrent lesions, or from tumors larger than 2 cm in diameter.
- Also apt to be more aggressive are SCCs that may occur from causes other than sun exposure. For example, a SCC may arise in long-standing scars or from sites previously exposed to ionizing radiation and long-term exposure to psoralen and ultraviolet A light (PUVA) (see Chapter 3, "Psoriasis"). A SCC may also emerge from pre-existing human papilloma virus infection (**verrucous carcinoma**), in the skin of organ transplant recipients, or chronic inflammatory lesions (e.g., cutaneous lupus erythematosus), as well as cutaneous ulcers (e.g., venous stasis ulcers) or other nonhealing wounds.
- As with solar keratosis and BCCs (see later discussion), SCC is related to sun exposure and is noted more frequently in those with a greater degree of outdoor activity.

Histopathology

- In the in situ type of SCC (**Bowen's disease**), only the full thickness of the epidermis is involved. The basement membrane remains intact. Atypical keratinocytes (squamous cells) show a loss of polarity and an increased mitotic rate.
- An invasive SCC penetrates into the dermis. It has various levels of anaplasia and may manifest relatively few to multiple mitoses and may display varying degrees of differentiation such as keratinization.

Risk of Metastasis

- The risk of metastasis of SCC depends on its degree of differentiation, depth of penetration, and location.
- SCC occurs in several clinical variants that vary in their aggressiveness.
- In situ SCC (Bowen's disease) has a low incidence of metastasis.
- An SCC arising in a solar keratosis also has a low incidence of metastasis.
- Lesions on mucous membranes have the highest risk of metastasis.
- Tumors that are induced by ionizing radiation or those that arise in old burn scars or in inflammatory lesions also are also more likely to metastasize.

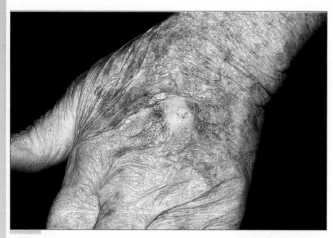

22.12 *Squamous cell carcinoma.* This nodular lesion arose from a solar keratosis.

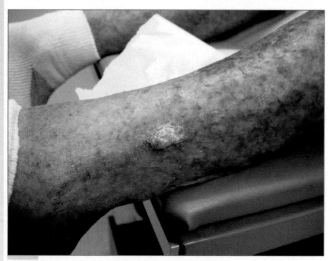

22.13 *Squamous cell carcinoma.* This hyperkeratotic nodule arose in an immunocompromised patient in a site previously exposed to ionizing radiation.

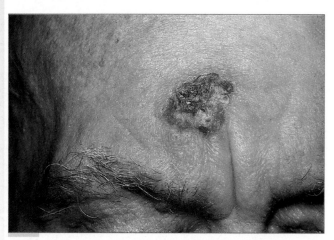

22.14 *Squamous cell carcinoma.* This neglected tumor has ulcerated.

DESCRIPTION OF LESIONS

- Lesions appear as papules, plaques, or nodules (FIG. 22.12) that grow slowly.
- Lesions are scaly or ulcerated.
- Lesions may have a smooth or thick hyperkeratotic surface (FIG. 22.13).
- As with solar keratoses, an SCC may also produce a cutaneous horn on its surface.
- An SCC may appear as a reddish brown nodule. It may, at times, be indistinguishable from a hypertrophic solar keratosis or a BCC.
- Tumors may ulcerate when they are neglected (FIG. 22.14).

DISTRIBUTION OF LESIONS

- Lesions occur in the same locations as do solar keratoses: sun-exposed areas such as the face, the dorsa of the forearms and hands, and the "V" of the neck.
- In men, SCCs tend to arise on the bald areas of the scalp and on the tops of the ears as well as the posterior neck below the occipital hairline.
- In women, lesions tend to occur on the legs as well as other relatively sun-exposed locations.
- In individuals of African origin there is an equal frequency in sun-exposed and unexposed areas.

CLINICAL MANIFESTATIONS

- Most SCCs are asymptomatic, although bleeding, pain, and tenderness may be noted.

- Slow-growing, firm papules with the ability to produce scale (keratinization) tend to be more clearly differentiated and less likely to metastasize.
- Softer, nonkeratinizing lesions are less well differentiated and are more likely to spread (FIG. 22.15).

Clinical Variants

Intraepithelial Squamous Cell Carcinoma
- **Bowen's disease** (SCC in situ) and **erythroplasia of Queyrat** are intraepithelial SCCs that often arise in sites that are not exposed to the sun such as the trunk or extremities. When an SCC in situ lesion occurs on the penis, it is referred to as erythroplasia of Queyrat (FIG. 22.16).
- Bowen's disease (FIG. 22.17) is one of the few skin cancers that should be considered as a diagnosis in African-American, Afro-Caribbean, and African blacks. This non–sun-related skin cancer tends to arise on the extremities de novo (FIG. 22.18).

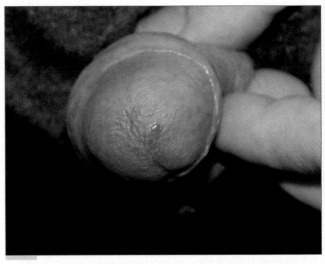

22.16 *Erythroplasia of Queyrat.* This subtle, nonhealing, shiny erosion on the perimeatal area of the glans penis proved to be an SCC in situ. (Courtesy of Joseph S. Eastern, M.D.)

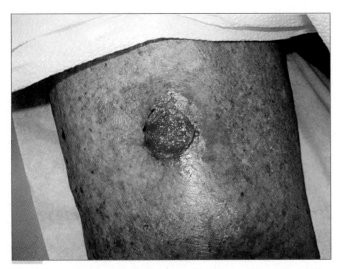

22.15 *Squamous cell carcinoma.* This poorly differentiated nodule has the potential to metastasize.

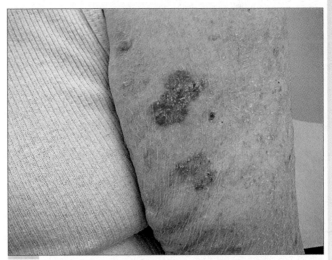

22.17 *Bowen's disease (squamous cell carcinoma in situ).* These lesions closely resemble scaly psoriatic or eczematous plaques.

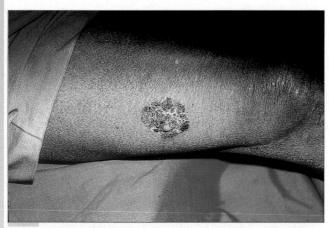

22.18 *Bowen's disease in an African-American woman.*
This plaque arose de novo in a non–sun-exposed location.

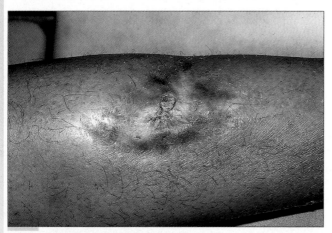

22.19 *Squamous cell carcinoma arising in a burn scar.*
The likelihood of metastasis of this lesion is significant.

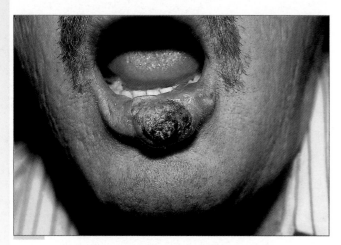

22.20 *Squamous cell carcinoma of the lip.* This lesion
also has a significant metastatic potential.

- If a frank SCC occurs in an old scar (FIG. 22.19) or in a lesion of discoid lupus erythematosus, the lesion should be treated aggressively.

Squamous Cell Carcinoma of Mucous Membranes

- This condition (FIG. 22.20) may present as leukoplakia, nonhealing fissures, or ulcerations. Such lesions have significant metastatic potential.
- Treatment is beyond the scope of this publication.

(text continued on page 405)

DIFFERENTIAL DIAGNOSIS

Solar Keratosis (Actinic Keratosis)
- This lesion is often indistinguishable from SCC (see earlier discussion).

Basal Cell Carcinoma
See later discussion of BCC.

- BCCs are generally pearly and telangiectatic.
- They appear at a younger age than do SCCs.
- BCC may be indistinguishable from SCC, particularly if the lesion is ulcerated.

Keratoacanthoma
See later discussion.

- This lesion also may be clinically and, at times, histopathologically, indistinguishable from a SCC.
- It is fast growing.
- Usually, it has a typical central crater.

Melanoma
See later discussion.

- An amelanotic melanoma (lacking typical pigmentation) or an ulcerated melanoma may also be impossible to distinguish from a SCC.

Psoriasis/Eczema
- Bowen's disease resembles a scaly solitary psoriatic or eczematous plaque (see Chapter 2, "Eczema," and Chapter 3, "Psoriasis").

Seborrheic Keratosis
- This extremely common benign skin growth becomes apparent after 40 years of age (see Chapter 21, "Benign Skin Neoplasms").

Verruca Vulgaris
- A wart may also resemble a SCC (see Chapter 6, "Superficial Viral Infections").

MANAGEMENT

Treatment
- **Electrocautery and curettage** for small lesions (generally smaller than 1 cm). This is done in a fashion similar to that performed for BCC treatment (see subsequent discussion). It is particularly useful on flat surfaces (e.g., forehead, cheek) and SCC in situ (Bowen's disease).
- As with superficial BCCs, selected SCCs may be treated rapidly using **cryosurgery** with LN_2.
- **Total excision**, the preferred method of therapy for SCC, permits histologic diagnosis of the tumor margins.
- **Immunotherapy**
  - Imiquimod (**Aldara**) 5% cream is approved for the treatment of solar keratoses (see previous discussion), for superficial BCCs (see later discussion), and "off-label" for SCC in situ (Bowen's disease).
  - It is applied twice weekly to involved skin for 16 weeks until a significant inflammatory response occurs.
  - **Aldara** may also have some utility in treating selected patients who have highly differentiated SCCs and in some renal transplant patients, who tend to develop numerous SCCs.
- **Micrographic (Mohs')** surgery (see Chapter 26, "Diagnostic and Therapeutic Procedures"; FIGS. 26.26 A–D) is useful for excessively large or invasive carcinomas, for recurrent lesions, for lesions with poorly delineated clinical borders, for SCCs within an orifice (e.g., ear canals or nostrils), and for carcinomas in locations where preservation of normal tissue is extremely important (e.g., tip of the nose, eyelids, nasal alae, ears, lips, and glans penis) (see later discussion). It is also a treatment of choice for a lesion in an area of late radiation change.
- **Radiation therapy** is used for those patients who are physically debilitated or who are unable to, or refuse to, undergo, excisional surgery. It is also suitable for larger, advanced lesions.

Prevention
- Sun avoidance measures
- Sunscreens and hats
- Sunglasses with ultraviolet protection
- Tinted windshields and side windows in cars
- Sun-protective garments
- Avoidance of contact with known carcinogenic compounds

HELPFUL HINTS

- A subungual SCC can easily be mistaken for a verruca.
- High-risk SCCs may require imaging studies
- Lymph node biopsy is indicated for suspected nodal involvement.

SEE PATIENT HANDOUT "Sun Protection Advice" ON THE SOLUTION SITE

SEE PATIENT HANDOUT "Squamous Cell Carcinoma" ON THE SOLUTION SITE

POINTS TO REMEMBER

- An early lesion of SCC is difficult to distinguish from a precursor solar keratosis.
- SCCs that develop from solar keratoses are generally unaggressive.
- An SCC that is histopathologically described as being "poorly differentiated" should be treated more aggressively.
- SCCs arising on a mucous membrane such as the glans penis, lip, or from a chronic ulcer or an SCC arising in an immunocompromised patient should be regarded as potentially metastatic.

BASICS

- A keratoacanthoma (KA) is a unique lesion with a characteristic clinical appearance. There is controversy about the benign versus malignant nature of this lesion. A KA resembles an SCC histologically; some dermatologists and dermatopathologists consider it to be a low-grade variant of an SCC and believe that it should be treated as such. Lesions may be clinically impossible to differentiate from SCCs.
- KAs generally occur in persons older than 65 years of age.
- If ignored, KAs often regress spontaneously. This fact lends support to the theory that this lesion is benign in nature.

DESCRIPTION OF LESIONS

- A KA usually occurs as a single, dome-shaped, erythematous or skin-colored nodule with a central keratin core (central crater) with an overlying crust (FIGS. 22.21 and 22.22). It resembles the appearance of a volcano.
- It generally attains a diameter of 1.0 to 2.5 cm.

DISTRIBUTION OF LESIONS

- As with the nonmelanoma skin cancers such as BCC and SCC, lesions tend to appear on the sun-exposed areas of the face, ears, neck, dorsa of hands, and forearms.

CLINICAL MANIFESTATIONS

- Lesions arise quickly, usually developing in 3 to 4 weeks.
- Spontaneous regression may result in a small depressed scar.

DIAGNOSIS

- An excisional or incisional biopsy is often recommended so that the complete architecture of the lesion can be evaluated histologically. (An insufficient biopsy, such as a shave biopsy, may result in a histology that is indistinguishable from a SCC.)
- When KAs appear in areas in which it is difficult to perform an excisional biopsy, such as the nose and external ears, a deep shave biopsy is often adequate to obtain sufficient tissue.

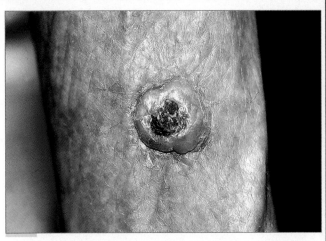

22.21 *Keratoacanthoma.* This "volcanolike" nodule arose over a period of 2 weeks. Note the characteristic crusting in the center.

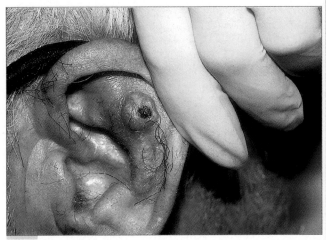

22.22 *Keratoacanthoma.* This nodule arose over a period of 4 weeks in a characteristic location.

POINT TO REMEMBER

- A KA is a lesion that resembles an SCC (FIG. 22.23).

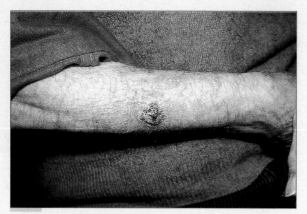

22.23 *Keratoacanthoma.* Clinically this lesion is difficult to distinguish from a hypertrophic solar keratosis or a SCC. (See FIG. 22.8.)

DIFFERENTIAL DIAGNOSIS

- SCC
- Verruca vulgaris

MANAGEMENT

- **Excisional removal** is the treatment of choice; however, a small minority of dermatologists prefer to simply observe these lesions and await spontaneous resolution.
- A **deep shave biopsy with or without electrodesiccation** in selected cases often results in a permanent cure.
- **Intralesional 5-FU** may be used.
- **Micrographic (Mohs') surgery** may be necessary for recurrences.

BASICS

- BCC is the most common skin cancer and the most common cancer overall.
- Although this lesion qualifies as a cancer, its morbidity, if recognized and treated early, is usually inconsequential. A BCC is usually slow growing and very rarely metastasizes, but it can cause significant local invasion and considerable destruction if it is neglected or treated inadequately.

Histopathology

- Cells of nodular BCC typically have large, hyperchromatic, oval nuclei and little cytoplasm. They appear rather uniform, and, if present, mitotic figures are usually scant.
- Nodular tumor aggregates may be of varying sizes, but tumor cells tend to align more densely in a palisade pattern at the periphery of these nests. Cleft formation, known as "retraction artifact," commonly occurs between BCC nests and stroma because of shrinkage of mucin during tissue fixation and staining.

Risk Factors

- Many of the same risk factors that predispose to solar keratoses and SCCs are responsible for the development of BCCs, although BCC tends to occur at a younger age than solar keratosis, SCC, and KA.
- Risk factors for BCC include the following:
  - Age older than 40 years
  - Male sex
  - Positive family history of BCC
  - Light complexion (as in SCCs and solar keratoses, BCCs are rare in blacks and Asians) with poor tanning ability
  - Long-term sun exposure

DESCRIPTION OF LESIONS

- The classic lesion, the nodular BCC, is also the most common type (FIG. 22.24). Nodular BCCs occur most commonly on the head, neck, and upper back and may have some of the following features:
  - A pearly, shiny, semitranslucent, papule or nodule (FIG. 22.25)
  - A rolled (raised) border (FIG. 22.26)
  - Telangiectases over the surface, thus accounting for a history of bleeding with minor trauma
  - Erosion or ulceration ("rodent ulcer") caused by a gnawed appearance (see FIG. 22.24)

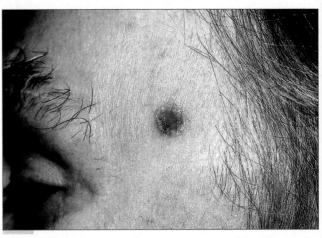

22.24 *Basal cell carcinoma.* A pearly papule with ulceration ("rodent ulcer") and telangiectasias is the "classic" presentation of a nodular BCC.

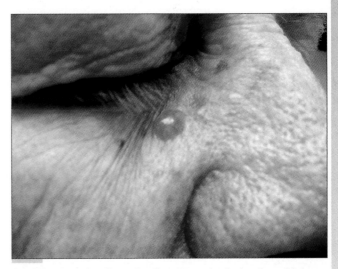

22.25 *Basal cell carcinoma.* Here the lesion is a shiny, pearly, translucent papule.

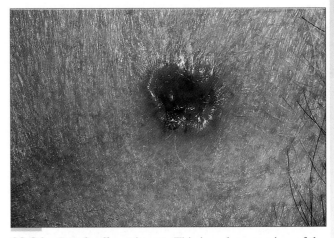

22.26 *Basal cell carcinoma.* This is a close-up view of the lesion shown in FIGURE 22.23, showing rolled borders with telangiectasia.

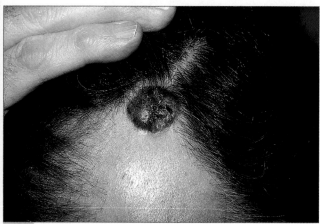

22.27 ***Basal cell carcinoma, pigmented.*** This lesion could easily be mistaken for a melanoma. Note the pearly surface.

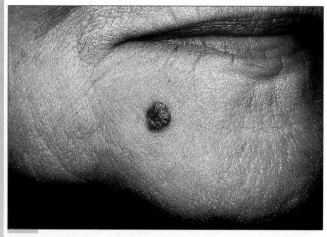

22.28 ***Basal cell carcinoma, pigmented.*** Note the pearly, waxy surface.

- A lesion can sometimes present as a small, nonhealing erosion (FIG. 22.31).
- Brownish to blue-black pigmentation (pigmented BCC) is seen in more darkly pigmented persons (FIGS. 22.27 and 27.28).

DISTRIBUTION OF LESIONS

- Lesions occur on the head and neck in 85% of all affected persons.
- Lesions occur on sun-exposed areas (e.g., the face, especially on the nose, cheeks, forehead, periorbital area, lower face, and the back of the neck) (FIGS. 22.29–22.32).

CLINICAL MANIFESTATIONS

- Lesions are often ignored, asymptomatic, and slow growing.
- Very mild trauma, such as face washing or drying with a towel, may cause bleeding.
- In time, lesions may ulcerate (e.g., "the sore that will not heal").

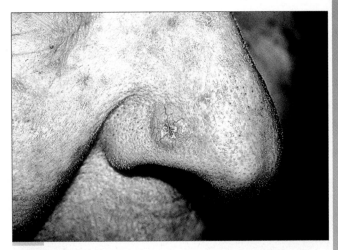

22.30 *Basal cell carcinoma.* The nose is a common site for BCC. Note the central crust, rolled borders, and telangiectasia.

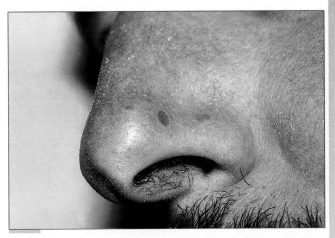

22.31 *Basal cell carcinoma.* This small erosion proved to be a BCC.

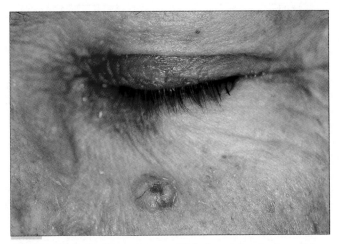

22.29 *Basal cell carcinoma.* This is another lesion with typical features.

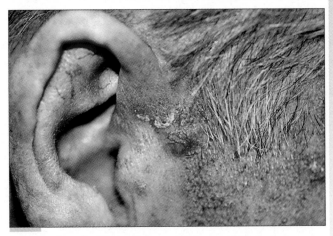

22.32 *Basal cell carcinoma.* The ear, particularly in men, is a frequent site. Note the tortuous telangiectasias.

Clinical Variants

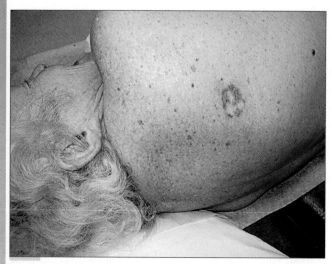

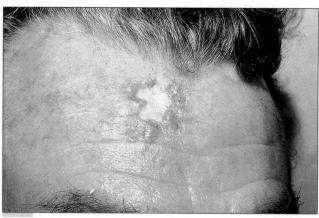

22.33 *Superficial basal cell carcinoma.* The back is a common place to find a superficial BCC. Note the distinct border. Often patients are not aware of these lesions, which resemble psoriatic plaques as well as Bowen's disease.

22.34 *Morpheaform basal cell carcinoma.* A whitish, atrophic, scarlike plaque is present, with surrounding telangiectasias and pearly papules surrounding it.

Superficial Basal Cell Carcinoma

- A superficial BCC occurs as a scaly pink to red-brown patch with a threadlike border (FIG. 22.33).
- The lesions tend to be indolent, asymptomatic, and the least aggressive of BCCs.
- Lesions are sometimes multiple, occurring primarily on the trunk and proximal extremities.
- When solitary, a lesion of superficial BCC may resemble psoriasis, eczema, a seborrheic keratosis, or Bowen's disease (SCC in situ).
- There is no clear association between superficial BCC and sun exposure.

Morpheaform Basal Cell Carcinoma

This is the least common and most aggressive form of BCC.

- Lesions appear as whitish, scarred atrophic plaques with surrounding telangiectasia (FIG. 22.34).
- The margins of these lesions are often difficult to evaluate clinically; as with icebergs, what is seen on the surface is not always what lies under the surface.
- Consequently, morpheaform BCCs are generally more difficult to treat than other BCCs.
- A morpheaform BCC may be mistaken for scar tissue.

DIAGNOSIS

- The diagnosis is generally made by shave or excisional biopsy.
- A shave biopsy suffices for the diagnosis of most BCCs (see Chapter 26, "Diagnostic and Therapeutic Procedures").

 DIFFERENTIAL DIAGNOSIS

- SCC (see earlier discussion)
- Solar keratosis (see earlier discussion)
- Sebaceous hyperplasia (see Chapter 21, "Benign Skin Neoplasms")
- Angiofibroma (fibrous papule of the nose) (see FIG. 21.37) and lesions of sebaceous hyperplasia (see FIG. 21.26), benign neoplasms that are often easily confused with BCC
- Seborrheic keratosis, which may be indistinguishable from a pigmented BCC
- Intradermal nevus (see Chapter 21, "Benign Skin Neoplasms")

MANAGEMENT

Prevention

- Techniques involve sun avoidance, use of sunscreens with a sun protection factor (SPF) of at least 15, and wearing protective clothing.
- People with a history of skin cancer should learn skin self-examination and should have annual skin examinations performed by a physician.

Treatment

See Chapter 26, "Diagnostic and Therapeutic Procedures."

- **Electrodesiccation and curettage.** The overall cure rate exceeds 90% for low-risk BCCs. This method is quick, simple, and less expensive than most other procedures.
- **Cryosurgery** with LN_2. Superficial BCCs may be treated rapidly using this method. However, nodular lesions, particularly selected lesions on the eyelid and ear, are ideally treated with a temperature probe before cryosurgery is performed. Successful treatment is highly dependent on the experience of the operator.
- **Excision,** permitting histologic diagnosis of margins. Cosmetic results compare favorably with those of curettage; however, surgical excision is more time-consuming and costly than curettage.
- **Immunotherapy** with 5% imiquimod cream (**Aldara**), a topical immunomodulator, is approved for the treatment of superficial BCCs. It is applied five times per week for a full 6 weeks.
- **Micrographic (Mohs') surgery** (see Chapter 26, "Diagnostic and Therapeutic Methods"; FIGS. 26.26A–D) for morpheaform, recurrent, or large lesions, as well as for lesions in "danger zones" (e.g., the nasolabial area, around the eyes, behind the ears, in the ear canal, and on the scalp).
  - Mohs' micrographic surgery is a microscopically controlled method of removing skin cancers that allows for controlled excision and maximum preservation of normal tissue. Excisions are repeated in the areas proven to be cancerous until a completely cancer-free plane is reached.
  - Mohs' surgery is time-consuming and expensive, and it may require extensive reconstruction of surgical wounds. However, it provides the most reliable method of determining adequate margins, it has a very high cure rate of 98% to 99% for BCCs, and it preserves the maximum amount of normal tissue around the cancer.
- **Radiation therapy** for elderly debilitated patients or for those who are physically unable to undergo excisional surgery. The disadvantages include the potential for late radiation changes in the skin, as well as the inability to examine skin margins because tissue is not obtained. It is rarely used today.

 HELPFUL HINTS

- Patients should always be undressed for adequate examination of the skin.
- Avoidance of exposure to ultraviolet radiation is encouraged. Preventive measures include carefully planning outdoor activities before 10 a.m. and after 4 p.m., wearing a broad-brimmed hat during outdoor activities, and using sunscreens with an SPF of 15 or greater.

 POINTS TO REMEMBER

- A BCC is, by far, the most common type of skin cancer.
- As with SCC and solar keratoses, BCCs are induced by ultraviolet radiation in susceptible persons.
- Almost 50% of patients with BCC will have another one within 5 years.
- Recurrent BCCs are generally more aggressive than primary lesions.
- Patients with BCC have an increased risk of melanoma.

 SEE PATIENT HANDOUT "Sun Protection Advice" ON THE SOLUTION SITE

 SEE PATIENT HANDOUT "Basal Cell Carcinoma" ON THE SOLUTION SITE

Melanoma

BASICS

- Malignant melanoma, more appropriately referred to (nonredundantly) as melanoma, is a cancer of melanocytes, the cells that produce pigment. Melanoma generally occurs in the skin and, much less commonly, in the eyes, ears, gastrointestinal tract, leptomeninges of the central nervous system, and oral and genital mucous membranes.
- It is the most common cancer in women aged 25 to 29 years and is second only to breast cancer in women aged 30 to 34 years.
- It is also commonly seen in patients with defects of DNA repair such as xeroderma pigmentosum and in patients with familial atypical mole syndrome.
- It is also more often seen in patients who have an abundance of melanocytic nevi.
- Although BCC and SCC (nonmelanoma skin cancers) are associated with long-term exposure to sunlight, melanoma is more likely to occur with infrequent but strong exposures that result in sunburns. Nonmelanoma skin cancers are more likely to be found on chronically sun-exposed areas such as the face; in contrast, melanomas are more likely to occur on areas that are less often exposed and more frequently burned, specifically the backs of men and the legs of women.
- By far, the most important skin lesion for the health care provider to recognize is melanoma. Melanoma is one of the only skin diseases that can be fatal if neglected; consequently, early recognition and prompt removal of a melanoma can save a life.

Risk Factors

Persons at greatest risk for melanoma have the following characteristics:

- Age generally older than 20 years, particularly older than 60 years
- A light complexion, an inability to tan, and a history of sunburns
- Moles that are numerous, changing, or atypical (dysplastic nevi)
- A personal or family history of melanoma (first-degree relatives)
- A personal or family history of BCCs or SCCs

Histopathology

- Superficial spreading melanoma (SSM), lentigo maligna melanoma (LMM), and acral lentiginous melanoma (ALM) have an early in situ (radial growth) phase characterized by increased numbers of intraepithelial melanocytes, which are large and atypical as well as being arranged haphazardly at the dermal-epidermal junction. They show upward (pagetoid) migration and lack the biologic potential to metastasize.

- Invasion into the dermis may confer metastatic potential and is characterized by a distinct population of melanoma cells with mitoses and nuclear pleomorphism within the dermis (papillary, reticular) and, possibly, the subcutaneous fat.

DISTRIBUTION OF LESIONS

- In white women, the most common lesion sites for SSM are the upper back, the lower leg between the knees and ankle, and the arms. Lesions are relatively fewer on covered areas such as under bras and swimsuits.
- In white men, the most common lesion sites for SSM are the upper back, anterior torso, and the upper extremities.
- In both white women and white men, other types of melanoma (e.g., LMM) may occur on the head, neck, and sun-exposed arms. Nodular melanomas are seen on the legs and trunk.
- Malignant melanoma is very rare in dark-skinned persons and Asians. However, when it does occur, it tends to be present on acral, non–sun-exposed areas such as the palms of the hands, soles of the feet, or in the nail bed. It is referred to as acral lentiginous melanoma.

CLINICAL MANIFESTATIONS

Warning Signs

- New, changing (evolving), or unusual moles. A changing mole is the most common sign of melanoma.

- Symptomatic moles (e.g., moles that itch, burn, or are painful). Nevi are generally asymptomatic, unless inflammation or invasion occurs.
- An initial slow horizontal growth phase, if left untreated, is followed in months or years by a vertical growth phase (lesions that extend vertically in the skin), which indicates invasive disease and potential metastasis.
- White coloration may indicate regression or scarring.

Prognosis

- Five-year survival is based on the thickness of the tumor. Once a diagnosis of melanoma is established, further treatment is determined by the scale known as Breslow's measurement (TABLE 22.1). The thickness of the lesion is measured from the top of the granular layer of the skin to the deepest tumor cell. Melanomas that are thicker than 4 mm are associated with a high rate of distant and nodal metastasis.

Table 22.1 BRESLOW'S MEASUREMENT

TUMOR THICKNESS (MM)	5-YEAR SURVIVAL (%)
<0.75	98–99
0.76–1.50	94
1.51–2.25	83
2.26–3.00	72–77
>3.00	<50

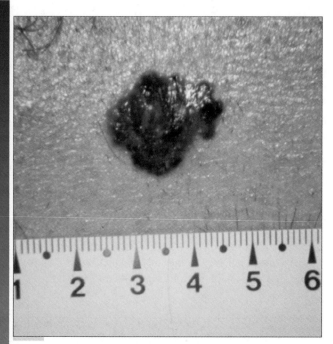

22.35 *Superficial spreading melanoma.* Note the "ABCDE" features: asymmetry, notched border, varied colors, and diameter of more than 6 mm, plus evolution (change in lesion).

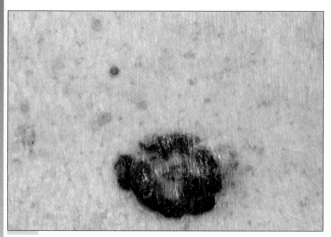

22.36 *Superficial spreading melanoma.* Note the central area (whitish gray) that represents regression.

Table 22.2 CLARK'S LEVELS

GRADE	LOCATION IN DERMIS
I	In situ disease confined to the epidermis
II	Melanoma cells in papillary dermis
III	Melanoma cells filling papillary dermis
IV	Melanoma cells in reticular dermis
V	Melanoma cells in subcutaneous fat

- Prognosis may also be determined by the grade of the melanoma, as determined by its location in the dermis using Clark's levels (TABLE 22.2).
- Sentinel lymph node status is also used for prognostication (see later in this chapter).
- Other important prognostic factors include the sex of the patient (women have a better prognosis than men), age (the prognosis worsens with increasing age), and the presence of ulceration or regional or distant spread.

Superficial Spreading Melanoma

- Of the four major clinicopathologic types of melanoma, SSM is by far the most common (FIGS. 22.35 and 22.36).
- It may arise de novo or in a preexisting nevus.
- The lesions of SSM may conform to some (or all) of the "ABCDE" criteria for melanoma, in which the primary lesion is a macular lesion or an elevated plaque that displays the following:
  A: Asymmetry. If you draw an X and a Y axis through the middle of a lesion and "fold" the lesion on itself, the halves will not match.
  B: Border that is irregular or notched (like a jigsaw puzzle).

C: Color that is varied or has different shades (may have brown, black, pink, blue gray, white, or admixtures of these colors). The blue color results from the Tyndall effect, an optical illusion that occurs when light reflects off brown or black pigment in the deeper layers of the skin. The red color results from an inflammatory response that the immune system is mounting against the tumor. When this response is successful, the tumor regresses, and an ivory-white color results (FIG. 22.36).

D: Diameter greater than 6 mm (the size of a pencil eraser), but a lesion may be smaller when first detected (FIGS. 22.37 and 22.38).

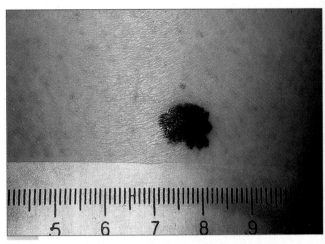

22.37 *Superficial spreading melanoma.* This lesion, which is more brown in color than in the preceding figure, also has color variegation, evidence of regression, and an irregular border. (Note the resemblance to seborrheic keratoses in Chapter 21.)

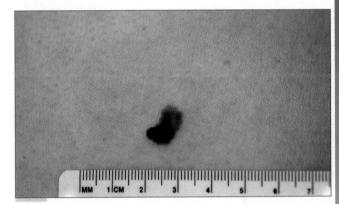

22.38 *Superficial spreading melanoma.* An early melanoma was present on this patient's back. This lesion illustrates two colors. The presence of dark pigmentation and irregular shape prompted biopsy of the lesion.

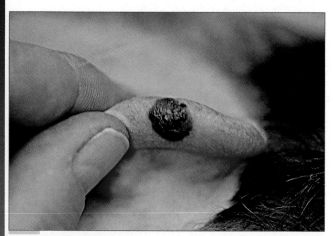

22.39 *Superficial spreading melanoma.* Melanoma of the ear. Note the superficial spreading component (brown color) at the base and the nodule arising from it.

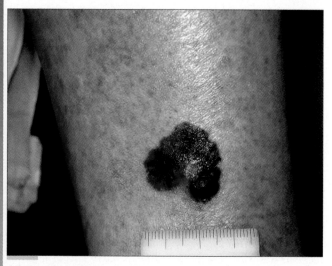

22.40 *Superficial spreading melanoma.* The radial growth phase is represented by the large area; the black, nodular component of this lesion represents the invasive vertical growth phase. The "ABCDE" features are present in this lesion.

E: Evolution, or change in a preexisting lesion, has recently been added to the criteria. Any change—in size, color, elevation—or any new symptom such as bleeding, itching, or crusting (FIGS. 22.39 and 22.41) should prompt suspicion.

DIAGNOSIS

* Clinical diagnosis is based on ABCDE criteria (FIG. 22.40).
* Elliptic excisional biopsy should include all of the visible lesion.

DIFFERENTIAL DIAGNOSIS

See also Chapter 21, "Benign Skin Neoplasms."

Seborrheic Keratosis

- Seborrheic keratosis, particularly if the lesion is variegated in color or jet black (see Chapter 21, "Benign Skin Neoplasms"), should be considered. The "stuck-on" appearing lesions of this condition are most often confused with malignant melanoma by clinicians who are not dermatologists (FIG. 22.42).

Basal Cell Carcinoma

- Pigmented BCC may be clinically indistinguishable from SSM or other types of malignant melanoma (see FIGS. 22.27 and 22.28).

Dysplastic or Atypical Nevus

- A dysplastic nevus or a melanocytic nevus with an atypical appearance may also be clinically indistinguishable from melanoma (see FIG. 21.13).

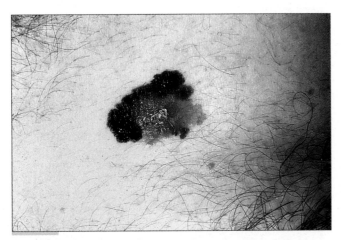

22.41 *Superficial spreading melanoma.* The scaling in the center of this lesion represents ulceration and is a poor prognostic sign.

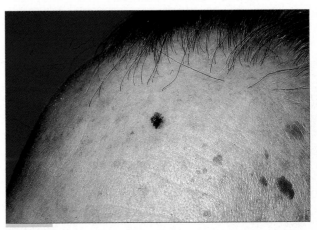

22.42 *In situ melanoma.* Note jet-black coloration of the lesion on this man's forehead in comparison to the surrounding brown seborrheic keratoses. This patient's wife noticed the "ugly duckling" lesion, which was out of character with his usual seborrheic keratoses.

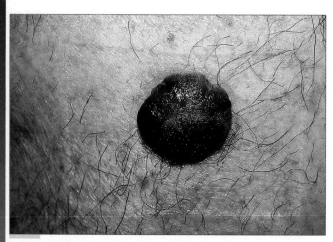

22.43 *Nodular amelanotic melanoma.* This lesion arose de novo; it has a great probability of metastasizing.

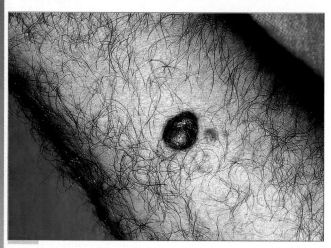

22.44 *Nodular melanoma.* This is a nodule with surrounding satellite lesions that represent local "in transit" metastases.

Clinical Variants

Nodular Melanoma

- The lesion of a nodular melanoma arises de novo as a nodule or plaque (FIGS. 22.43–22.45). It occurs in 10% to 15% of patients. Because of a rapid vertical growth phase, lesions invade early.
- Nodular melanoma lesions have the following characteristics:
  - They are blue, blue black, or nonpigmented (as in amelanotic melanoma); their color is more uniform than that of SSM.
  - They may ulcerate and bleed with minor trauma.
  - They occur most commonly on the legs and trunk.
  - They may be indistinguishable from a pyogenic granuloma (see FIG. 21.49).

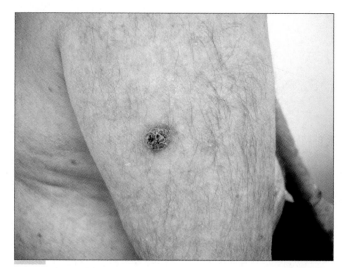

22.45 *Nodular melanoma.* This crusted nodule was initially mistaken for an inflamed seborrheic keratosis. On biopsy the lesion had a Breslow's measurement greater than 4 mm in depth.

Lentigo Maligna and Lentigo Maligna Melanoma

- Lentigo maligna (LM) is a type of lentigo that is found on the face of elderly patients with chronically sun-damaged skin. LM is considered to be a potential precursor to melanoma (FIG. 22.46).
- LM lesions are characterized by:
  - A gradually enlarging tan to brown macule with irregular borders
  - Slow growth over 5 to 20 years
  - An irregular color and border
- When an LM invades the dermis, it is then referred to as an LMM. The prognosis of LMM is similar to that of other subtypes of melanoma and is dependent on the thickness of the tumor (FIGS. 22.47 A and B).

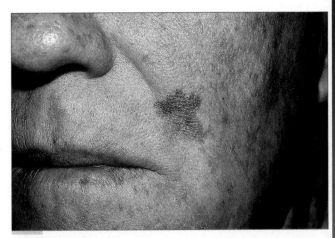

22.46 *Lentigo maligna.* Note in the darker parts of this lesion the irregular border of this malignant melanoma in situ. Note similarity to solar lentigo (see FIG. 21.4).

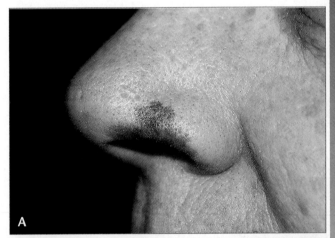

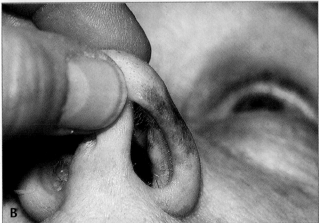

22.47 A and B *Lentigo maligna melanoma.* **A:** Biopsy of this pigmented lesion demonstrated invasion into the dermis. **B:** The same patient; note involvement of the nasal mucosa.

Acral Lentiginous Melanoma

- ALM is the least common subtype of melanoma.
- These malignancies most often appear in blacks and Asians.
- The lesions of ALM tend to occur on areas that do not bear hair, such as the palms, soles, and periungual skin (FIG. 22.49).
- ALM has a tendency toward early metastasis (FIG. 22.49).

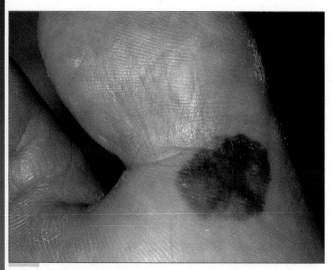

22.48 *Acral lentiginous melanoma.* Note the size and variegated pigmentation of this lesion. (Courtesy of Charles Miller, M.D., San Diego Naval Hospital.)

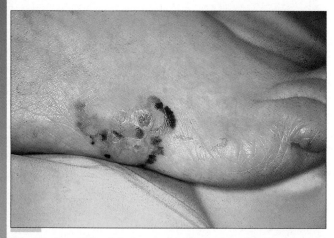

22.49 *Acral lentiginous melanoma.* A podiatrist who was treating the lesion as a wart referred this patient; the lesion did not resolve with destructive therapy. It was, in fact, a level V melanoma (melanoma cells were located in the subcutaneous tissue). (Courtesy of Art Huntley, M.D., University of California at Davis.)

• A subungual ALM presenting as diffuse nail discoloration or a longitudinal pigmented band within the nail plate is potentially confused with subungual hematoma or junctional nevus. Pigment spread to the proximal or lateral nail folds **(Hutchinson's sign)** is a hallmark of ALM (FIGS. 22.50 and 22.51).

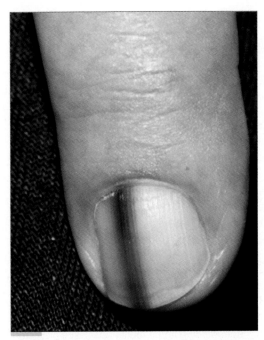

22.50 *Junctional nevus.* This fairly common lesion may present a worrisome quandary (to biopsy or not to biopsy). Note the even, linear bands of pigmentation in this patient's nail bed.

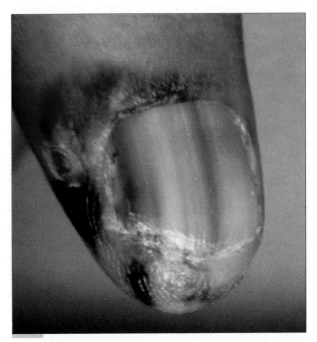

22.51 *Acral lentiginous melanoma.* Hutchinson's sign shows uneven pigmentation spreading beyond the nail into surrounding skin.

MANAGEMENT

Workup for Patients with Melanoma

- The most important aspects of the initial workup for patients with cutaneous melanoma are a careful history, review of systems, and physical examination.
- Recently published data have shown that baseline and surveillance laboratory studies (e.g., lactate dehydrogenase level, liver function tests); chest radiography; and other imaging studies (e.g., computed tomography, positron emission tomography, bone scanning, magnetic resonance imaging) are not typically beneficial for patients without signs or symptoms of metastasis. Such routine tests have not proven to have efficacy in the detection of occult disease in asymptomatic patients with localized melanoma.
- A metastatic workup should be initiated if physical findings or symptoms suggest disease recurrence or if the patient has documented nodal metastasis based on results from a SLNB.

Sentinel Lymph Node Biopsy

- SLNB is a method used to detect the first lymph node draining from the site of a melanoma.
- It is generally indicated for pathologic staging of the regional nodal basin(s) for primary tumors of at least 1 mm depth and when certain high-risk histologic features (e.g., ulceration, extensive regression) are present in thinner melanomas.
- SLNB and lymphatic mapping indicate whether to perform regional lymphadenectomy (in the absence of clinically palpable nodes) in patients with thicker melanomas (1 mm or more in depth).
- The probability of sentinel node positivity increases with increasing tumor thickness, from less than 1% for melanomas measuring 1 mm or smaller to as high as 36% for melanomas measuring 4 mm or larger. The ideal candidate for SLNB is the patient with a melanoma thicker than 1.0 mm without clinical or radiographic evidence of regional lymph node or distant metastases.
- This minimally invasive procedure allows the pathologist to detect micrometastases.
- A negative sentinel node obviates the need for further lymph node dissection.

- Technique
  - A technetium 99–labeled colloid (for the preoperative scanning) and a vital blue dye (for the intraoperative visualization) are injected around the area of the primary melanoma or biopsy scar (at the time of wide local excision/reexcision).
  - The sentinel node is thus identified and excised and examined for the presence of micrometastasis using both routine histology and immunohistochemistry.
  - Sentinel node status (positive or negative) is the most important prognostic factor for recurrence and is the most powerful predictor of survival in melanoma patients.
  - There is conflicting data and controversy about the value of SLNB for melanoma patients. While SLNB enhances metastatic staging for patients with deeper primaries and provides a more accurate determination of the patient's prognosis, its positive therapeutic role has yet to be established.
- If results are positive (i.e., metastatic), an **elective lymph node dissection** (ELND) is usually performed as a separate procedure at a later date. ELND is not recommended for lesions that are less than 1 mm thick unless lymph nodes are palpable. The decision about whether to perform ELND on thicker lesions (1 to 4 mm) is controversial.
- Prophylactic lymph node dissection for primary cutaneous melanoma of intermediate thickness initially was believed to confer a survival advantage on patients with tumors of 1 to 4 mm in depth. Subsequent prospective randomized clinical trials have shown no survival benefit for elective lymphadenectomy for melanomas of varying thicknesses on the extremities and only marginal, if any, benefit for nonextremity melanomas.

Surgical Treatment

- **Elliptic excision** should include the entire visible lesion down to the subcutaneous fat.
- Surgical margins of 5 mm are currently recommended for melanoma in situ.
- For lesions with a thickness of less than 1 mm, a 1-cm margin of normal skin is usually adequate.

continued on page 423

- **Amputation, regional lymph node dissection,** and **regional chemotherapy perfusion** are sometimes necessary for ALMs (FIGS. 22.52 and 22.53).
- In more advanced stages of melanoma, chemotherapy and radiation therapy have not been very effective for achieving remission of metastatic disease.

- **Vaccines, interleukin-2,** and **arterial limb perfusion** are adjuncts to surgery. In fact, an injectable recombinant interferon-alpha 2B (Intron A) has been shown to improve the 5-year survival rate significantly in patients with thick lesions, lymph node involvement, or both.

Long-Term Management
- Patients who have had melanoma should be followed every 3 months for the first 2 years and annually thereafter.
- At each visit, the patient's entire cutaneous surface and lymph nodes should be examined.
- Patients with invasive disease require an annual chest radiograph, complete blood count, and liver function studies.

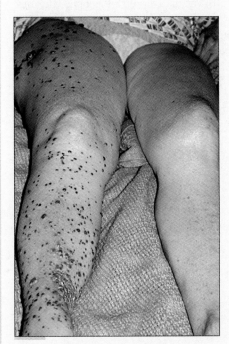

22.52 *Metastatic melanoma.* Note the lymphedema and multiple metastatic nodules on this patient's leg. The skin is the most common organ to which melanoma metastasizes.

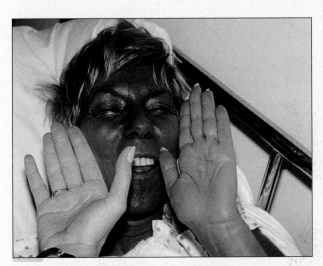

22.53 *Metastatic melanoma.* The unusual brown-blue coloration in this patient is the result of widespread melanin pigmentation in the tissues.

POINTS TO REMEMBER

- Sun protection should be stressed in those with a personal or family history of melanoma. The need to protect children (beginning at an early age) from excessive sun exposure should also be emphasized.
- Anyone who has a history of melanoma needs lifelong skin surveillance, because 3% of these patients will develop a second melanoma within 3 years.
- Patients should be taught self-examination.
- Patients should be advised to have all first-degree relatives undergo a dermatologic examination to check for dysplastic nevi or melanoma.
- Any lesion that looks suspicious must be examined by biopsy.

- An amelanotic melanoma is easily overlooked because of its lack of pigmentation.
- Removal of thin lesions (less than 0.76 mm) is curative in almost all patients.
- Early detection is the key to saving lives, because the treatments for metastatic melanoma are limited. Once a melanoma is metastatic, there is no uniformly effective adjuvant chemotherapy.
- No definite proof of survival benefit has been found for performing SLNB versus a group of people who had similar melanomas but no SLNB.
- Furthermore, there is no evidence to support the necessity of a complete lymph node dissection following a positive sentinel node section.

HELPFUL HINTS

- Trauma from rubbing or irritation does not cause malignant degeneration of moles.
- Total skin examination that includes the legs should be performed when evaluating a female patient for possible skin cancer.
- To identify growing lesions, total body photographs allow for the assessment of existing and new lesions anywhere on the body.
- The use of the "ugly duckling" sign, wherein skin examination is focused on recognition of a lesion that simply looks different from the rest, may assist with detection of lesions that lack the classic ABCDE criteria for melanoma.

SEE PATIENT HANDOUT "Sun Protection Advice" ON THE SOLUTION SITE

BASICS

Paget's disease of the breast (PDB) and extramammary Paget's disease (EMPD) are intraepidermal skin cancers that are often indicative of more severe underlying malignancies. Both diseases—particularly EMPD—can have a subtle, insidious course and tend to be ignored, misdiagnosed, or unrecognized by patients and clinicians alike. A high index of suspicion and prompt identification and treatment of these conditions can be lifesaving.

Paget's Disease of the Breast

- PDB is a relatively uncommon clinical presentation of intraductal carcinoma of the breast. It occurs almost exclusively in postmenopausal women; men are rarely affected. PDB accounts for 1% to 4% of breast cancers. Invariably, the PDB lesion is associated with an intraductal carcinoma of the underlying mammary gland.
- In more than half of the cases, there is no associated palpable breast mass, and mammography results are often normal. Patients with PDB are, on average, 5 to 10 years older than patients with the more common types of breast carcinoma. It is not unusual for PDB patients to remain undiagnosed and untreated for a prolonged period because the PDB lesion is usually insidious and slow growing, and it is often asymptomatic. Furthermore, PDB is often mistakenly diagnosed as a chronic eczematous condition.
- Not infrequently, an elderly patient may be too embarrassed to mention the lesion to her family or clinician, thereby further delaying diagnosis and treatment.

Pathophysiology
- PDB is an underlying intraductal carcinoma of the breast, with retrograde extension into the overlying epidermis through mammary duct epithelium.
- The epidermis becomes infiltrated with characteristic Paget's cells that cause thickening of the nipple and the areolar skin.

CLINICAL MANIFESTATIONS BASICS
- Patients with PDB often present with a chronic **unilateral rash** on the nipple, areola, or surrounding skin; less commonly, the lesion originates and remains on the nipple.
- Typically, the lesion appears as a sharply marginated red plaque with an irregular border and eczemalike appearance (FIG. 22.54).
- When the nipple is involved, it may become scaly, crusted, have a bloody nipple discharge, become deformed, or retracted (FIG. 22.55).

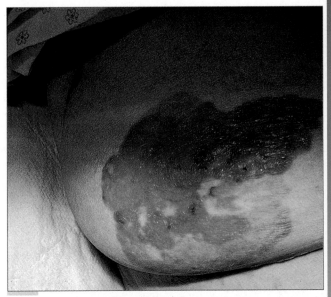

22.54 *Paget's disease of the breast.* This patient had had an eczemalike lesion of the nipple, areola, and surrounding skin for several years. On biopsy, the patient was found to have an infiltrating ductal carcinoma of the underlying breast tissue. (Courtesy of Michael Fisher, M.D., of the Albert Einstein College of Medicine, Bronx, New York.)

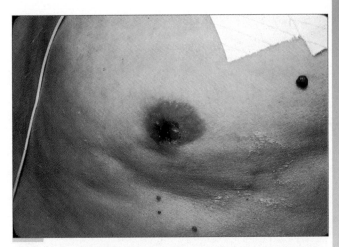

22.55 *Paget's disease of the breast.* Here the nipple and areola are involved. The process began insidiously in one nipple. Note the bloody nipple discharge, which stained the clothing and bras of this patient before she sought treatment. (Courtesy of Michael Fisher, M.D., of the Albert Einstein College of Medicine, Bronx, New York).

DIAGNOSIS

- Punch, wedge, or excisional biopsy of the lesional skin of the nipple-areola complex, including the dermal and subcutaneous tissue for microscopic examination, is performed for the accurate diagnosis of PDB.

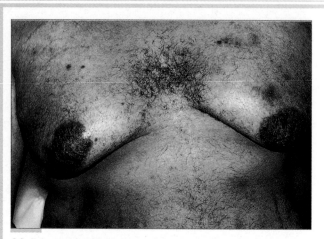

22.56 *Atopic dermatitis on the nipples and areolae (bilateral).* Note the obliteration of the margins of the nipples and areolae, as well as the oozing and fissuring of the left breast. These lesions responded readily to topical corticosteroids.

 DIFFERENTIAL DIAGNOSIS

Atopic Dermatitis

- In addition to various unusual neoplasms, atopic dermatitis of the nipples and areolae should be included in the differential diagnosis.
- Atopic dermatitis often presents bilaterally (FIG. 22.56), but it may present unilaterally.
- Atopic dermatitis occurs in association with a personal or family history of atopy (see Chapter 2, "Eczema"). It should respond rapidly to topical corticosteroid therapy.

Extramammary Paget's Disease

- EMPD is a rare condition that is similar to PDB; the primary difference is the anatomic location. EMPD targets the genital skin, perianal skin, and other cutaneous sites rich in apocrine glands.
- Histologic features of PDB and EMPD disease are similar.
- EMPD is four to five times more likely to occur in women than in men. The condition most commonly appears in patients ages 50 to 60.

Pathophysiology

- EMPD arises as a primary cutaneous adenocarcinoma in most cases. The epidermis becomes infiltrated with characteristic Paget's cells—neoplastic cells that show glandular differentiation.

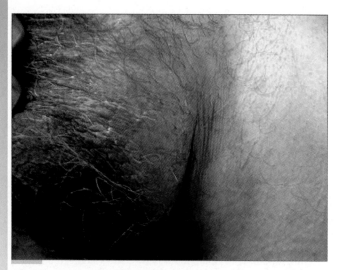

22.57 *Extramammary Paget's disease.* This pruritic eczematous plaque had been present for many years. Biopsy confirmed EMPD. Initially, treatment consisted of both antifungals and topical steroids, with no resolution. Not only is this condition rare, it is especially rare in men.

CLINICAL MANIFESTATIONS

- The initial lesion may present as a unilateral, erythematous, sharply margined, eczema-simulating, slow-growing plaque that may be indistinguishable from PDB (FIG. 22.57).

- Not infrequently, lesions may be ill-defined and resemble eczema, intertrigo, tinea cruris, candidiasis, and other conditions (see "Differential Diagnosis" section).
- EMPD has usually been present for a long time before biopsy is performed to confirm the diagnosis (see FIG. 22.58).
- Some, but not all, cases of EMPD are associated with an underlying adenocarcinoma.

DIAGNOSIS

- The diagnosis of EMPD requires a high degree of clinical suspicion, followed by skin biopsy with pathologic correlation.

 DIFFERENTIAL DIAGNOSIS

- The differential diagnosis of EMPD is more extensive than that of PDB, and EMPD may simulate many neoplastic and inflammatory conditions before the diagnosis is made.

 MANAGEMENT

- It is beyond the scope of this discussion to describe the therapies for breast cancer.
  - However, as in other types of confirmed breast carcinoma, treatment of PDB can include surgery, radiation therapy, chemotherapy, and hormonal treatment as indicated.

- Mastectomy (radical or modified) and lymph node clearance are appropriate for patients with PDB who have a palpable mass and underlying invasive breast carcinoma.
- Because EMPD often extends beyond the visibly involved clinical margins, a wide, controlled surgical excision of all the involved epidermis is the most effective treatment.

 POINTS TO REMEMBER

- PDB is uncommon and unilateral, whereas eczematous dermatitis of the nipples is common and tends to present bilaterally.
- Any unilateral, chronic eczematous lesion of the breast or nipple ("nipple eczema") that is unresponsive to topical corticosteroid therapy should be biopsied.
- EMPD is a rare disorder that is easily overlooked, but it must be considered in the differential diagnosis of patients with chronic genital or perianal dermatitis.
- PDB and EMPD closely resemble eczema. It is important to consider PDB or EMPD among patients in whom supposed eczema of the breast or perineum does not clear with appropriate therapy.

PART TWO

Systemic Conditions and the Skin

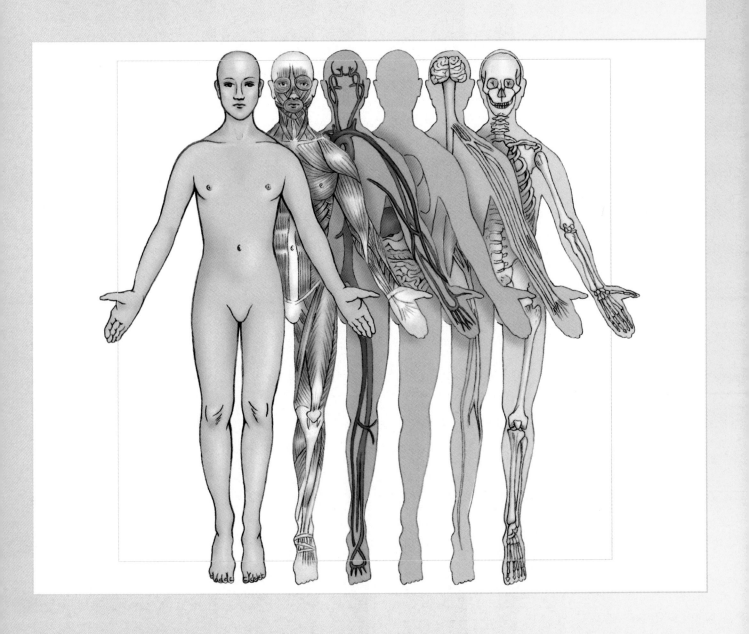

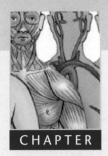

Skin and Hair During Pregnancy

OVERVIEW

During pregnancy, various skin changes occur. Many of these changes are seen so frequently that they are considered normal. Pregnancy can also alter the course of certain preexisting skin conditions or systemic diseases that have cutaneous involvement, for example:

- Systemic lupus erythematosus and scleroderma may flare.
- Acne may improve, or it may worsen.
- Dyshidrotic eczema may appear de novo, or a flare-up of preexisting lesions may occur.
- Condylomata acuminatum may enlarge considerably and may proliferate.

However, it should always be kept in mind that many common skin diseases unrelated to pregnancy should be considered when evaluating a pregnant patient with a skin disorder.

➤ **HYPERPIGMENTATION**

- Linea nigra

➤ **CONNECTIVE TISSUE CHANGES**

- Striae gravidarum
- Keloids

➤ **VASCULAR PHENOMENA**

- Spider telangiectasias
- Palmar erythema

➤ **HAIR CHANGES**

- Telogen effluvium
- Hirsutism

➤ **OTHER FINDINGS**

- Pregnancy gingivitis
- Pyogenic granulomas
- Erythema nodosum

➤ **SPECIFIC DERMATOSES OF PREGNANCY**

- Pruritic urticarial papules and plaques of pregnancy
- Pruritus gravidarum
- Recurrent cholestasis of pregnancy
- Pemphigoid gestationis

➤ **OTHER CONDITIONS**

- Pruritic folliculitis of pregnancy
- Impetigo herpetiformis

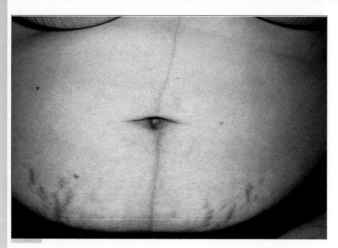

23.1 *Linea nigra and striae gravidarum.* The linea alba darkens during pregnancy, but the normal color usually returns after delivery. In contrast, although the purplish color of striae gravidarum fades over time, the striae themselves are permanent.

 MANAGEMENT

- For patients with melasma caused by pregnancy, it is usually best to keep sun exposure to a minimum and to wait for fading, which often takes place spontaneously. Treatment of persistent nongestational melasma consists of diligent sun avoidance and, frequently, the use of skin bleaching creams (see Chapter 14, "Pigmentary Disorders").
- Darkened freckles, nevi, and linea nigra usually regress postpartum.

Hyperpigmentation

Hyperpigmentation is presumed to be secondary to increased levels of estrogens and melanocyte-stimulating hormone. It frequently manifests as follows:

- Darkening of the linea alba (which becomes the **linea nigra**). There may also be darkening of the nipples and surrounding areolae, as well as darkening of the axillae, thighs, umbilicus, perineum, and external genitalia (FIG. 23.1).

- **Melasma** (for a more complete discussion, see Chapter 14, "Pigmentary Disorders"). The "mask of pregnancy" (formerly known as chloasma) occurs in more than 50% of women. It is worsened by exposure to the sun. Melasma is also seen in women taking oral contraceptives and, on occasion, de novo in women in whom no explanation is obvious.
- Darkening of preexisting freckles and nevi.

 HELPFUL HINT

- Pregnancy does not appear to affect survival adversely in women who have preexisting malignant melanoma.

Connective Tissue Changes

- **Striae gravidarum** (striae cutis distensae related to pregnancy) or "stretch marks." It is thought that these are caused by the combination of increased adrenocortical activity and rapid tissue growth and distension, which result in tearing of the collagen matrix of the dermis and a weakness of elastic fibers. Typically, striae are reddish pink to violaceous, linear, atrophic bands that are located on the abdomen, hips, buttocks, and breasts. The striae are permanent, but the purplish color fades with time.
- Proliferation and enlargement of skin tags, with some persisting after pregnancy.
- Occasional growth of preexisting keloids. For example, this may occur in the scars of an abdominal hysterectomy or a cesarean section (FIG. 23.2). Growth of preexisting keloids is a not-uncommon problem in women of African descent.

 MANAGEMENT

- There is no proven effective treatment for striae.
- If desired, skin tags may be easily removed (see Chapter 21, "Benign Skin Neoplasms").
- Keloids may diminish in size postpartum; if they do not, treatment with intralesional steroids may be helpful (see Chapter 21, "Benign Skin Neoplasms").

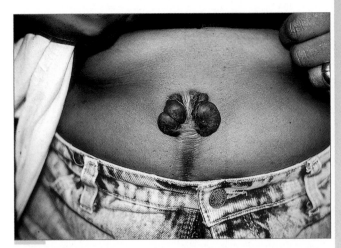

23.2 **_Keloids._** These lesions are growing well beyond the border of the cesarean section scar.

Vascular Phenomena

- Spider telangiectasias. These can result from the high levels of estrogen in pregnancy (FIG. 23.3).
- Scattered petechiae in the lower extremities. These are the result of increased capillary fragility and increased hydrostatic pressure in this region.
- Palmar erythema, flushing, and increased sweating (FIG. 23.4)
- Venous varicosities of the legs and feet
- Hemorrhoids
- Edema of the leg, face, or eyelids

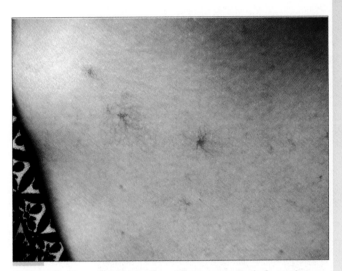

23.3 **_Spider telangiectasias._** These can result from the high levels of estrogens in pregnancy.

 MANAGEMENT

- Most vascular phenomena resolve postpartum. However, varicosities may persist and may worsen with additional pregnancies.

Hair Changes

- Telogen effluvium. Hair loss may occur from 1 to 5 months postpartum and is generally followed by total regrowth. Rarely, the regrowth may not be as thick as prepregnancy hair growth. (See Chapter 10, "Hair and Scalp Disorders Resulting in Hair Loss.")
- Hirsutism. Mild degrees of hirsutism are common. The face is frequently affected, although hair growth may be pronounced on the extremities as well. Hirsutism normally regresses after delivery, but it may recur in subsequent pregnancies. (See Chapter 11, "Hirsutism.")

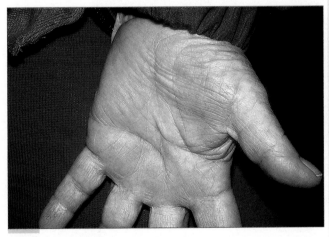

23.4 **_Palmar erythema._** Flushing and increased sweating may also occur during pregnancy.

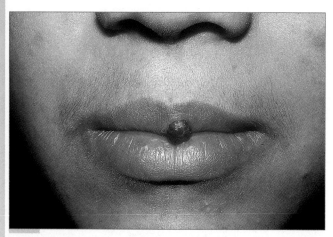

23.5 **Pyogenic granuloma.** Lesions tend to occur on the lips and gums.

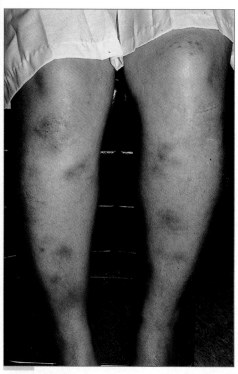

23.6 **Erythema nodosum.** These tender nodules occurred during pregnancy and resolved postpartum.

 MANAGEMENT

- Because both telogen effluvium and hirsutism usually resolve spontaneously, no specific management is needed. However, excessive hirsutism warrants investigation for an endocrinologic abnormality.

Other Findings

Skin conditions during pregnancy can also include the following:

- Increased nail fragility and brittleness and distal separation of the nail plate (onycholysis) may occur.
- Edema and hyperemia of the gums ("pregnancy gingivitis") have been noted.
- Pyogenic granulomas often develop on the lips and gums and usually regress shortly postpartum (FIG. 23.5).
- Erythema nodosum, an apparently autoimmune skin condition, is usually associated with infections, sarcoidosis, malignant diseases, and drugs, but it can also be precipitated by pregnancy alone (FIG. 23.6).
- Erythema multiforme has a variety of causes, including pregnancy.

 MANAGEMENT

Pregnancy Gingivitis
- Good dental hygiene (adequate brushing and flossing) is essential, because the problem is exacerbated by plaque and calculus.

Pyogenic Granulomas
- Treatment may be deferred until after delivery or performed during pregnancy, if necessary. Options include **cryodestruction, electrodesiccation,** and **excisional surgery** (see Chapter 21, "Benign Skin Neoplasms").

Erythema Nodosum
- Erythema nodosum tends to clear postpartum and to recur in subsequent pregnancies. Treatment is with bed rest and mild analgesics.

Erythema Multiforme
- Like erythema nodosum, erythema multiforme resulting from pregnancy tends to clear spontaneously and is managed symptomatically. Underlying causes other than pregnancy (e.g., infection) should be sought and treated.

BASICS

The specific dermatoses of pregnancy are a group of cutaneous eruptions that are unique to pregnancy. Historically, these eruptions have been variously classified, resulting in overlapping and confusing terminology. The following discussion should help to simplify the approach to these entities.

Pruritic Urticarial Papules and Plaques of Pregnancy

- A common dermatosis of late pregnancy, pruritic urticarial papules and plaques of pregnancy (PUPPP), is, as its name suggests, a pruritic eruption consisting of urticarial papules that coalesce into plaques (FIG. 23.7). Initially, the papules are found in the striae cutis distensae (i.e., stretch marks) of the abdomen, and they generally spare the area surrounding the umbilicus. Later, they can be found on the thighs and buttocks, where they coalesce to form plaques. PUPPP tends to spare the face, palms, soles, and mucous membranes.
- The itching, which can become quite intense, generally begins in the last few weeks of the third trimester of pregnancy. It can be sufficiently discomforting to require potent topical—and sometimes oral—corticosteroids.
- The natural history of PUPPP is, in most cases, spontaneous resolution within a few days of delivery. It does not appear to increase infant morbidity. Recurrences in subsequent pregnancies are unlikely, and if they do take place, they tend to be less severe.
- Some dermatologists broaden the clinical description of PUPPP to include the following:
  - A rash resembling that of a drug eruption
  - A targetlike rash that resembles erythema multiforme
  - A vesicular eruption

  These dermatologists thus suggest that PUPPP be renamed "polymorphic eruption of pregnancy."

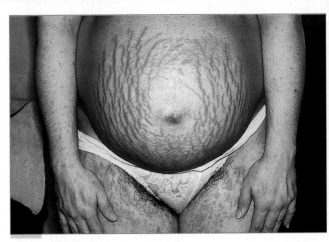

23.7 *Pruritic urticarial papules and plaques of pregnancy.* Lesions are located in the stretch marks. Note the periumbilical sparing.

Pruritus Gravidarum

- This condition, characterized by common, benign, generalized itching, begins in the later stages of pregnancy.
- The patient's complaints often seem to be out of proportion to the visible changes on the skin. There are no primary skin lesions, and the condition clears after delivery.
- Pruritus gravidarum is considered by some investigators to be possibly a variation of PUPPP without lesions.
- Management of pruritus gravidarum is aimed at symptomatic control of pruritus with the use of bland emollients and topical antipruritic agents. Oral antihistamines are sometimes effective.

Recurrent Cholestasis of Pregnancy

- Also known as intrahepatic cholestasis of pregnancy, recurrent cholestasis of pregnancy is a rare form of reversible cholestasis that appears in the second half of pregnancy. It generally occurs during the second or third trimester of pregnancy, although onset in the first trimester has also been reported.
- This condition is caused by hyperbilirubinemia and bile acid accumulation in the skin.
- It initially manifests as severe, generalized pruritus followed by the clinical appearance of jaundice. The degree of itching correlates with levels of serum and skin bile acid. There are no primary skin lesions; however, excoriations may result from the patient's scratching.
- The condition clears after delivery but may recur in future pregnancies. The incidence of premature birth, intrapartal fetal distress, stillbirth, and low birth weight appears to be increased in the children of affected women.
- Ideally, treatment should be directed to decrease maternal bile acid levels; however, traditionally, symptomatic therapy including bland emollients, cholestyramine resins, topical antipruritic agents and, sometimes, oral antihistamines, has been used.
- Recently, oral ursodeoxycholic acid, directed to decrease serum bile acid levels and dosed at 15 mg/kg/day, has been reported to be effective in improving fetal prognosis.

23.8 *Pemphigoid gestationis.* This pregnant woman has multiple pus-filled sterile vesicles and bullae.

Pemphigoid Gestationis

- Pemphigoid gestationis, previously known as herpes gestationis, is a rare, intensely pruritic vesicobullous autoimmune dermatitis that may be clinically confused with PUPPP. The term "herpes" derives from the grouped herpetiform clustering of blisters that sometimes occurs; there is no relation to herpesvirus infection.
- The skin lesions of pemphigoid gestationis are polymorphic, ranging from urticarial papules or plaques to bullae that are small and vesicular or large and tense (FIG. 23.8).
- Lesions tend to appear in the second or third trimester.
- The diagnosis can be confirmed by direct immunofluorescent testing of the skin.
- Treatment generally requires systemic corticosteroids in gradually tapered doses. In mild cases, topical cortico steroids and oral antihistamines may be sufficient.
- Some reports have suggested that women with pemphigoid gestationis may have an increased risk of fetal morbidity and mortality, as well as an increased chance of giving birth prematurely and of having an infant with a lower birth weight; however, the extent, if any, of this increased risk remains controversial. Rarely, a neonate may develop transient blisters.
- Postpartum flares are common. Symptoms may recur with menses or with administration of oral contraceptives; these findings suggest that hormonal factors play a strong role.
- Pemphigoid gestationis often recurs in subsequent pregnancies, with earlier and more florid consequences; however, it has been known to skip an ensuing pregnancy.

Other Conditions

- **Pruritic folliculitis** of pregnancy manifests as a papular, acnelike eruption. Some dermatologists consider this condition a variant of acne.
- **Impetigo herpetiformis,** an extremely rare dermatosis, is considered a form of generalized pustular psoriasis.

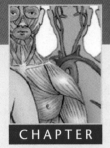

24 Cutaneous Manifestations of HIV Infection

Mary Ruth Buchness

OVERVIEW

- The first organ that may be affected in human immunodeficiency virus (HIV) infection is the skin. Before the advent of highly active antiretroviral therapy (HAART), the inevitable decrease in CD4 cells with disease progression was accompanied by a variety of HIV-associated skin diseases. HIV infection was often suspected initially based on the occurrence of cutaneous diseases, such as Kaposi's sarcoma (KS) or severe molluscum contagiosum, or in a patient with particularly severe or recalcitrant manifestations of a common skin disease, such as psoriasis.

- With the use of HAART, the number and frequency of cutaneous manifestations have plummeted in the United States and other countries. Furthermore, in patients with advanced HIV infection, the cutaneous manifestations often remit spontaneously when HAART is started. Nonetheless, some patients have viral resistance to these drugs or personal or economic reasons for not taking HIV medications, and in this group, the severe cutaneous manifestations of advanced HIV infection may still be seen.

- Acute HIV infection is characterized by a morbilliform rash resembling measles, and fever, lymphadenopathy, sore throat, and malaise may accompany the eruption.

- As the number of CD4 cells decreases to fewer than $200/mm^3$ during the course of infection, signaling the onset of acquired immunodeficiency syndrome (AIDS), skin manifestations become more severe and increase in number.

➤ HIV-ASSOCIATED HERPES SIMPLEX

➤ HIV-ASSOCIATED HERPES ZOSTER

➤ HIV-ASSOCIATED MOLLUSCUM CONTAGIOSUM

➤ HIV-ASSOCIATED CONDYLOMA ACUMINATUM

➤ HIV-ASSOCIATED (EPIDEMIC) KAPOSI'S SARCOMA

➤ HIV-ASSOCIATED BACILLARY ANGIOMATOSIS

➤ HIV-ASSOCIATED SYPHILIS

➤ HIV-ASSOCIATED NORWEGIAN SCABIES

➤ HIV-ASSOCIATED EOSINOPHILIC FOLLICULITIS

➤ HIV-ASSOCIATED ORAL HAIRY LEUKOPLAKIA

➤ HIV-ASSOCIATED ORAL CANDIDIASIS

➤ HIV-ASSOCIATED APHTHOUS ULCERS

➤ HIV-ASSOCIATED DRUG ERUPTIONS

➤ HIV-ASSOCIATED PRURITUS

➤ HIV-ASSOCIATED SEBORRHEIC DERMATITIS

➤ HIV-ASSOCIATED PSORIASIS

➤ HIV-ASSOCIATED LIPOATROPHY

BASICS

- In the immunocompromised host, the clinical manifestations and course of herpes simplex virus (HSV) infection differ in patients with defective cell-mediated immunity, as seen in HIV infection. (See Chapter 6, "Superficial Viral Infections," and Chapter 19, "Sexually Transmitted Diseases," for a full discussion of HSV infections in immunocompetent hosts.)
- Recurrent lesions may affect mucous membranes and possibly become chronic, centrifugally expanding ulcerations. These ulcerations last 1 month or more in an HIV-positive patient and are an AIDS-defining diagnosis.
- Lesions may become resistant to acyclovir, or they may develop into chronic keratotic papules. Because acyclovir resistance is associated with prior treatment of suboptimal doses, it is important not to undertreat HIV-positive patients who also have HSV infections.

DESCRIPTION OF LESIONS

- Initially, there are the typical grouped vesicles on an erythematous base, which evolve into pustules, erosions, and crusts.
- Ultimately, the following lesions may occur:
  - Chronic digital ulcerations (Fig. 24.1)
  - Mucosal erosions or papules (Fig. 24.2)
  - Centrifugally expanding ulcerations with scalloped borders
  - Keratotic or wartlike papules or plaques (Fig. 24.3)

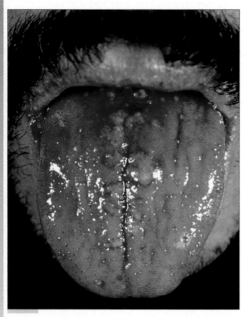

24.1 *Herpes simplex.* Shown here is HIV-associated chronic ulcerated herpes simplex that is resistant to acyclovir. This patient is receiving intravenous foscarnet.

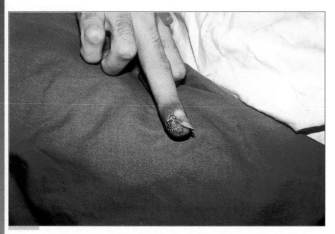

24.2 *Herpes simplex.* Mucosal papules are present in this patient with AIDS.

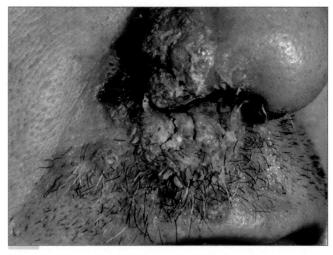

24.3 *Herpes simplex.* Crusted, wartlike papules are noted.

DISTRIBUTION OF LESIONS

- Intraoral areas, including the tongue, buccal mucosa, palate, and gingivae may be involved.
- Chronic ulcerative lesions may appear in perianal areas. These lesions can extend into the intergluteal cleft (FIG. 24.4).
- Keratotic lesions may occur in any location.

CLINICAL MANIFESTATIONS

- Lesions may be more severe and more extensive than in immunocompetent hosts.
- Severe or chronic erosions, ulcerations, or keratotic lesions should alert the clinician to the presence of advanced immunosuppression.

DIAGNOSIS

- See Chapter 6, "Superficial Viral Infections," and Chapter 19, "Sexually Transmitted Diseases," for more detailed discussions.

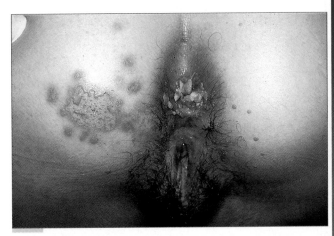

24.4 *Herpes simplex.* Chronic ulcerated lesions and scattered intact vesicles are present in a patient with AIDS.

 DIFFERENTIAL DIAGNOSIS

Herpes Zoster
- Lesions of herpes zoster may involve only part of a dermatome and may be clinically indistinguishable from HSV lesions.
- When in doubt, sufficient doses of antiviral medications are recommended for herpes zoster infection. Underdosing must be avoided.

Decubitus Ulcer
- These lesions affect bony prominences in debilitated patients and do not extend to the intergluteal cleft.

Cutaneous Cytomegalovirus Infection
- In cytomegalovirus infection, perianal ulcers develop as an extension of gastrointestinal involvement. Skin biopsy shows characteristic viral inclusion bodies.

- In the keratotic type of cytomegalovirus infection, disseminated infection is associated with retinal findings, so an ophthalmologic examination is essential.

Disseminated *Mycobacterium avium-intracellulare* Complex
- Patients may have oral ulcerations.
- This infection is associated with severe systemic disease and fever in HIV-infected patients.

Disseminated Histoplasmosis
- Patients may have oral and cutaneous ulcerations.
- Disseminated histoplasmosis is associated with systemic disease.

MANAGEMENT

- If the patient has malabsorption or if lesions do not respond to other treatment, **acyclovir** (5 to 10 mg/kg every 8 hours) is infused over 1 hour. The dosage interval should be increased in patients with renal failure.
- Failure to respond to intravenous acyclovir indicates acyclovir resistance.
- Acyclovir resistance can be prevented by avoiding undertreatment and intermittent treatment.
- **Foscarnet** (40 mg/kg intravenously every 8 hours) is used in acyclovir-resistant patients.
- Strains that recur after treatment with foscarnet are usually acyclovir sensitive.

POINTS TO REMEMBER

- Long-term suppressive therapy with acyclovir has been associated with acyclovir resistance.
- Treatment should continue until clinical lesions resolve completely.
- Clinicians should be careful not to underdose with antiviral agents.

BASICS

- Herpes zoster is most common in elderly patients and in immunocompromised persons, although it may occur in anyone who has a history of chickenpox.
- See Chapter 6, "Superficial Viral Infections," for a more detailed discussion.

DESCRIPTION OF LESIONS

- Grouped vesicles or bullae on an erythematous base affect all or part of a dermatome.
- Lesions evolve into pustules and crusts and may erode. Chronic ulcerations and crusted or verrucous lesions may occur.
- Severe scarring may result (FIG. 24.5).

DISTRIBUTION OF LESIONS

- Any dermatome can be affected.
- Disseminated herpes zoster virus may occur.
  - Occasional dissemination may lead to 25 or more lesions outside of the primary and two contiguous dermatomes (FIG. 24.6).
  - The disease usually begins with typical dermatomal herpes zoster virus that becomes widespread and chronic.
  - The eruption may be indistinguishable from varicella.

CLINICAL MANIFESTATIONS

- Prodromal symptoms of pain and itching may be severe enough to lead to a suspicion of serious illness. For example, the prodromal pain of thoracic zoster has led to critical care unit admission to rule out myocardial infarction.
- Regional adenopathy may occur.
- Varicella pneumonia may develop.
- Cutaneous lesions may become chronic in patients with AIDS.

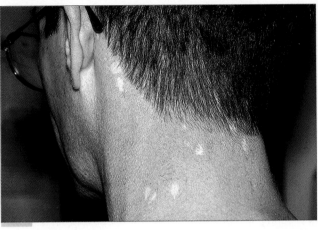

24.5 *Herpes zoster.* This patient developed severe scarring from his infection.

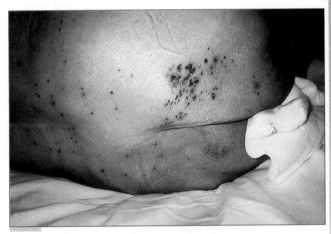

24.6 *Disseminated herpes zoster.* Note the initial dermatomal involvement on the buttock. (Courtesy of Herbert A. Hochman, M.D.)

 MANAGEMENT

- **Intravenous acyclovir** (10 mg/kg every 8 hours) is given for 10 to 14 days.
- Dosage intervals are increased in patients with renal failure.
- If lesions improve but persist beyond 10 to 14 days, treatment is continued until all lesions resolve.
- If lesions fail to resolve, the virus may be resistant to acyclovir.
- Acyclovir-resistant varicella-zoster virus infection responds to **foscarnet** (40 mg/kg every 8 hours until lesions resolve).

 POINTS TO REMEMBER

- Undertreatment may lead to viral resistance.
- Patients with herpes zoster can transmit the virus as chickenpox to nonimmune persons.

HIV-Associated Molluscum Contagiosum

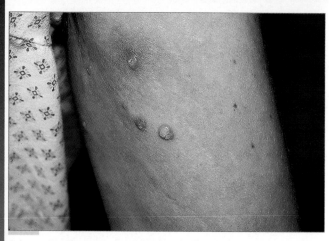

24.7   *Molluscum contagiosum.* This patient has "giant" molluscum lesions on his arm.

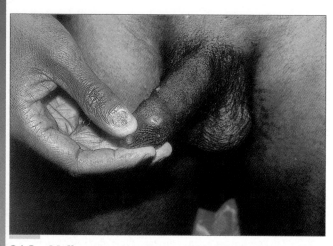

24.8   *Molluscum contagiosum.* This HIV-positive patient has a large molluscum contagiosum lesion on the shaft of his penis as well as other scattered smaller lesions. Also note onychomycosis of his thumbnail, which is another sign of immunodeficiency.

BASICS

- Molluscum contagiosum is caused by a poxvirus; the condition is most commonly seen in immunocompetent children and less commonly in healthy adults.
- Multiple and extensive facial lesions, as well as lesions with atypical morphology, should alert the practitioner to the possibility of HIV infection.
- See Chapter 6, "Superficial Viral Infections," for further discussion.

DESCRIPTION OF LESIONS

- Papules may be dome-shaped or, more commonly, are atypical in appearance.
- Size may be up to, or greater than, 1 cm (giant molluscum contagiosum).
- Lesions may lack central umbilication or may have several umbilications.
- Lesions on hairy areas tend to penetrate hair follicles.
- Lesions may be extensive (hundreds to thousands in number) in patients with advanced AIDS.
- Patients receiving HAART tend to have rare molluscum, with the more typical morphology seen in immunocompetent hosts.
- The appearance of new lesions may follow a downward fluctuation in immunity caused by a concurrent infection, such as influenza.

DISTRIBUTION OF LESIONS

- All areas of the body may be affected (FIG. 24.7), but lesions are most common on the face and genitals (FIG. 24.8).
- In men, possible extensive involvement of the beard area may result from shaving (see FIG. 6.18).

CLINICAL MANIFESTATIONS

- There is occasional tenderness or inflammation.
- Lesions are often a great cosmetic concern to patients.

DIFFERENTIAL DIAGNOSIS

Disseminated Cryptococcosis
- Cutaneous lesions may be clinically identical to those of molluscum contagiosum (FIG. 24.9).
- Affected patients are usually systemically ill, although cutaneous involvement may be the first sign of illness.
- Crush preparation with India ink shows encapsulated yeast.
- When in doubt, biopsy can be used to identify the lesions.
- Patients with cutaneous dissemination have neurologic involvement, and a faster diagnosis can be made by cerebrospinal fluid examination.

Disseminated Histoplasmosis
- This is a less common cause of molluscum contagiosum–like lesions than cryptococcosis.
- Cutaneous histoplasmosis is always indicative of systemic infection.

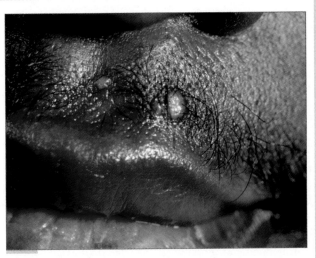

24.9 *Disseminated cryptococcosis.* Note the resemblance of these papules to those of molluscum contagiosum.

MANGEMENT

MANAGEMENT

- Treatment is individualized for each patient. No specific treatment is universally more effective than any other.
- **Topical tretinoin** is a useful adjunctive treatment in cases of molluscum contagiosum of the beard.
- Surgical treatment is with **curettage** or **liquid nitrogen cryosurgery**.
- **Trichloroacetic acid** 25% to 75% may be applied to individual lesions.
- **Podofilox** (Condylox) 5% may be applied to lesions twice per day, 3 days per week.
- Imiquimod 5% (**Aldara**) cream may be effective and should be used daily if possible.
- Treatment is long term and is unlikely to eradicate all lesions unless the patient's immunity improves. Lesions may remit spontaneously after the patient is started on HAART, and knowledge of this fact will sometimes persuade a reluctant patient to begin treatment for HIV infection.

 POINT TO REMEMBER

- Cutaneous lesions of disseminated cryptococcosis and histoplasmosis may look identical to lesions of molluscum contagiosum.

See also Chapter 19, "Sexually Transmitted Diseases."

BASICS

- Ninety percent of HIV-infected men have anal human papillomavirus (HPV) infection.
- Of the many subtypes of HPV, the most common subtype is the oncogenic subtype HPV 16.
- Seventy-three percent of HIV-infected men with HPV have multiple subtypes.
- The increasing rate of anal cancer that has been seen in the United States over the past three decades is a result of the increasing rate of infection with HIV and HPV.
- More than half of HIV-infected men with anal condyloma develop anal intraepithelial neoplasia (AIN). HIV-infected patients with AIN are more likely to develop invasive cancer than nonimmunocompromised patients. Estimated time to progression from AIN to invasive cancer is 10 to 20 years.
- There have been fewer studies of HIV-infected women, but it is known that 49% of HIV-infected women have latent cervical HPV infection, with high oncogenic risk types, persistent infection, and an increased risk of cervical dysplasia and cancer.

DESCRIPTION OF LESIONS

- Four morphologic types of anogenital condyloma acuminata have been described.
- The verrucous type is associated with coinfection with at least four subtypes, including HPV 16. These patients are at high risk for the development of high-grade AIN.
- In the leukoplakic type, a majority of patients have HPV 16, but with fewer numbers of coinfecting subtypes and a lower risk of high-grade AIN.
- The other types are erythroplakic (erythematous, possibly erosive) and bowenoid (flat, tan plaques).

DISTRIBUTION OF LESIONS

- Lesions may occur anywhere on the anogenital skin.
- Lesions may also occur on the vaginal or rectal mucous membranes. Rectal condylomata may be a cause of recurrent anal condyloma, and affected patients should be referred for evaluation by a rectal surgeon.
- In addition, lesions may appear on the skin at the angles of the mouth or on the intraoral membranes.

DIAGNOSIS

- Diagnosis is made on clinical grounds.
- Lesions that appear to be atypical (e.g., with ulcerations), that fail to respond to several treatments, or that grow in spite of treatment should be biopsied to evaluate for malignant degeneration.

 DIFFERENTIAL DIAGNOSIS

Carcinoma (Squamous Cell Carcinoma)
- This is the most important diagnosis to exclude. This can only be done by skin biopsy of atypical lesions or of an atypical area within a lesion.

Inflammatory Conditions
- Atypical, nonverrucous lesions may be confused with an inflammatory dermatosis such as perianal psoriasis, lichen planus, or lichen simplex chronicus.
- For a detailed discussion of the differential diagnosis of condyloma acuminatum, refer to Chapter 19, "Sexually Transmitted Diseases."

 MANAGEMENT

- The treatment of condyloma acuminata in HIV-positive patients is the same as that in HIV-negative patients. However, condyloma acuminata are difficult to eradicate because intact cellular immunity is necessary to clear the skin of viral lesions. See Chapter 19, "Sexually Transmitted Diseases," for treatment information.
- Some experts advocate anal cytology smears in HIV-infected patients with anogenital HPV. This is not currently recommended by the U.S. Centers for Disease Control because the rate of progression of AIN to invasive cancer, the reliability of the screening method, and the safety and effectiveness of treatment for AIN are all unknown.

 POINTS TO REMEMBER

- Condyloma acuminata in HIV-infected patients are often caused by oncogenic subtypes of HPV, and lesions may undergo malignant degeneration.
- Condylomata that appear to be clinically atypical, do not respond to treatment, or enlarge in spite of treatment should be biopsied to evaluate for malignant degeneration.

BASICS

- Epidemic KS is an AIDS-defining diagnosis.
- Because it is found almost exclusively in men who have had homosexual contact, KS is thought to be sexually transmitted.
- KS is exceedingly rare in women, and women with KS are presumed to have had sexual contact with bisexual men.
- KS is associated with infection with human herpesvirus 8 (HHV-8), which has been detected in saliva and in semen of affected patients.
- Lesions may resolve spontaneously as immunity improves. A similar phenomenon has been observed in immunocompromised renal transplant recipients.

DESCRIPTION OF LESIONS

- Violaceous macules, papules, or nodules occur (FIGS. 24.10 and 24.11).
- Limb edema with subtle violaceous discoloration of the skin may be present.

DISTRIBUTION OF LESIONS

- Lesions are most common acrally, on the nose, penis, and extremities.
- Mucous membranes may be affected.
- Lesions may be disseminated in advanced HIV infection.

CLINICAL MANIFESTATIONS

- Most commonly, lesions are asymptomatic.
- Edema occurs with lymphatic involvement, usually in the extremities, but sometimes it affects the face.
- Oral lesions can cause pain, difficulty with eating, and loss of teeth.

 DIFFERENTIAL DIAGNOSIS

- Pyogenic granuloma
- Bacillary angiomatosis
- Disseminated *M. avium-intracellulare* complex (see earlier discussion)

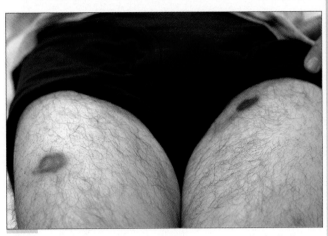

24.10 *Epidemic Kaposi's sarcoma.* Note the resemblance to the lesions of bacillary angiomatosis in FIGURE 24.12.

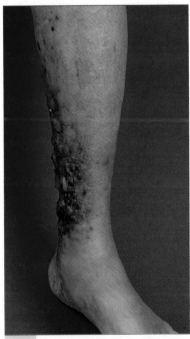

24.11 *Epidemic Kaposi's sarcoma.* Multiple papules and nodules are present on this patient's leg.

MANAGEMENT

- All forms of KS regress spontaneously with successful treatment of immunodeficiency with **HAART**.

Disseminated Cutaneous Kaposi's Sarcoma
- Disseminated involvement that does not regress with HAART requires systemic chemotherapy.

Lymphangitic Kaposi's Sarcoma
- Lymphatic involvement that does not respond to HAART requires systemic chemotherapy.
- Intermittent sequential compression boots can be used to decrease edema and to increase the comfort level of the patient.

Localized Cutaneous or Mucosal Kaposi's Sarcoma
- **Radiation therapy** is used, particularly for facial lesions.
- **Intralesional vinblastine** is given in doses of 0.1 to 0.6 mg/mL.
- **Liquid nitrogen cryosurgery** is used for macular lesions.
- A retinoid gel, alitretinoin (**Panretin**), applied three to four times daily as tolerated, is useful for macular lesions.

POINTS TO REMEMBER
- KS in an HIV-infected patient is an AIDS-defining diagnosis.
- Treatment of individual lesions does not prevent the occurrence of new lesions.
- Lesions may resolve spontaneously in patients receiving effective antiretroviral therapy, so it is beneficial to delay surgical treatment until the patient has been receiving HAART for several months.

BASICS

- Bacillary angiomatosis, which was first reported in 1983, is seen almost exclusively in HIV-positive patients with advanced disease. Cases have been extremely rare in recent years.
- Bacillary angiomatosis is caused by the bacilli *Bartonella henselae* and *B. quintana.*
- Bacillary angiomatosis is a systemic infection, and lesions have been described in nearly every organ of the body.
- Untreated bacillary angiomatosis can be fatal.

DESCRIPTION OF LESIONS

- Lesions may occur as erythematous, dome-shaped papules and nodules (FIG. 24.12); they can also be flatter, violaceous lesions; subcutaneous nodules; or rarely, necrotic tumors.

DISTRIBUTION OF LESIONS

- Bacillary angiomatosis can occur on any location of the skin or internally.

CLINICAL MANIFESTATIONS

- There may be associated fever.
- Untreated lesions can lead to respiratory obstruction, gastrointestinal bleeding, and local or systemic infection.
- Deaths have been reported from laryngeal obstruction and disseminated intravascular coagulopathy.

DIAGNOSIS

- Skin biopsy shows a lesion resembling pyogenic granuloma, with characteristic clusters of bacilli.
- Culture is available only in research centers.

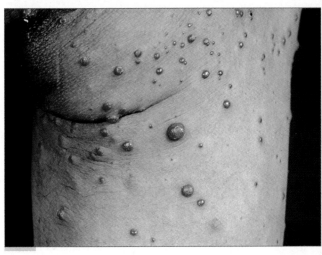

24.12 *Bacillary angiomatosis.* Dome-shaped papules and nodules are present.

DIFFERENTIAL DIAGNOSIS

- Pyogenic granuloma (see FIG. 21.49) may be clinically identical to lesions of bacillary angiomatosis.
- Epidemic KS (HIV-associated) should be considered.

MANAGEMENT

- **Doxycycline** (100 mg twice per day) *or*
- **Erythromycin** (250 to 500 mg four times per day)
- Treat until lesions have resolved (usually 3 to 4 weeks)

BASICS

- An intact cell-mediated immune system is necessary to "cure" the infection.
- Unusual manifestations of syphilis have been reported in patients with coinfection with HIV. These include negative serologic examination for syphilis in the presence of active secondary syphilis, relapse after treatment that should have been adequate, fulminant cutaneous lesions with induration and necrosis (FIG. 24.13), and fulminant neurosyphilis resulting in permanent neurologic deficits.
- See Chapter 19, "Sexually Transmitted Diseases," for a more detailed discussion.

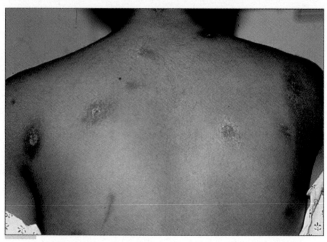

24.13 *Syphilis in a patient with acquired immunodeficiency syndrome.* Note the necrotic lesions.

👉 POINTS TO REMEMBER

- If syphilis is suspected in an HIV-infected patient and the serologic test is negative, then a skin biopsy should be performed.
- The only medication for the treatment of syphilis that adequately penetrates the blood-brain barrier is intravenous **aqueous penicillin,** which should be given at a dosage of 2 to 4 million units every 4 hours for 10 to 14 days in cases of suspected or proven neurosyphilis. Patients who are allergic to penicillin should undergo desensitization.

BASICS

- "Norwegian" scabies is an infestation with *Sarcoptes scabiei* var. *hominis* in an immunocompromised host.
- Immunocompetent hosts are able to limit the number of mites (10 to 12) that remain in the epidermis.
- The rash and itching are the result of a delayed hypersensitivity response to the mite, its eggs, and its fecal products.
- Immunocompromised hosts are not able to contain the population of mites and may be infested with millions of mites. These patients may not itch because of their defective cell-mediated immunity.
- HIV-infected patients with Norwegian scabies infestation pose a significant risk for transmission of scabies to household contacts and medical personnel.
- See Chapter 20, "Bites, Stings, and Infestations," for a more complete description of this condition.

DESCRIPTION OF LESIONS

- Fine, white, linear lesions from female mites may be visualized burrowing into the skin (FIG. 24.14).
- Crusted, keratotic plaques are characteristic in Norwegian scabies.
- Atypical acral lesions may be seen in HIV-infected patients.

DIAGNOSIS

- Mineral oil preparation is done by scraping the epidermal surface of a burrow with a scalpel that has been dipped in mineral oil.
- The scraping is examined with a low-power microscope. Mites, ova, or fecal pellets are seen (FIGS. 24.15 and 24.16).

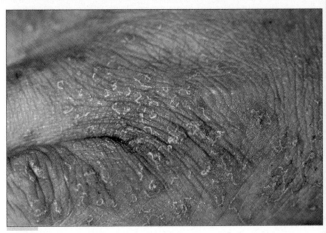

24.14 *Norwegian scabies in a patient with acquired immunodeficiency syndrome.* Note the crusted papules and the white linear burrows.

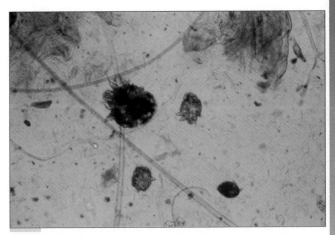

24.15 *Scabies.* Mites, ova, and fecal pellets are shown.

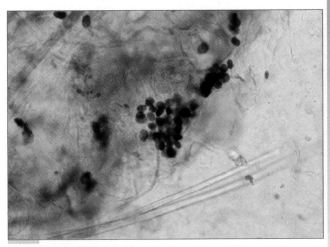

24.16 *Scabies.* Fecal pellets are shown here.

DIFFERENTIAL DIAGNOSIS

Psoriasis

- Psoriatic lesions tend to be located on extensor aspects of the extremities.
- Predominance of scale in the finger webs should lead to suspicion of Norwegian scabies.

Solar Keratoses

- Norwegian scabies on sun-exposed areas in elderly patients can mimic solar keratoses (FIG. 24.17).

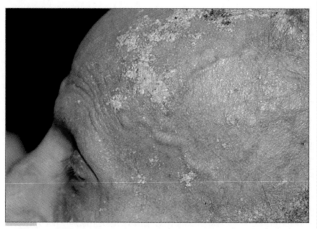

24.17 *Norwegian scabies in a patient with acquired immunodeficiency syndrome.* The lesions resemble solar keratoses.

 MANAGEMENT

Scabicides

- Permethrin 5% (**Elimite**) cream is applied, after a warm bath, to all skin surfaces from head to toe, including the palms, soles, and scalp in small children; it is left on for 8 to 12 hours, usually overnight, and is washed off the next morning; *or*
- Lindane 1% (**Kwell**) lotion is applied from head to toe after bathing. Treatment should be continued once weekly until there is no evidence of residual lesions.

Lindane is not as effective as permethrin and may cause neurologic toxicity, particularly in children and in elderly patients.

- **Ivermectin,** 0.2 mg/kg by mouth, has been shown to be effective in eradicating infection. However, it is not approved by the U.S. Food and Drug Administration for this use.

Keratolytic Agents

- Keratolytic agents, such as 10% to 40% **salicylic acid,** remove crusts and allow penetration of the scabicides.

POINTS TO REMEMBER

- Norwegian scabies is an infestation with millions of scabies mites and is highly contagious. Failure to treat patients promptly has led to epidemics affecting dozens of people.
- Because of the immunodeficiency in patients with Norwegian scabies, prolonged treatment may be necessary.
- Household contacts and medical staff who come into contact with the patient or the patient's bedclothes should undergo treatment as for scabies in an immunocompetent host, regardless of symptoms.

HIV-Associated Eosinophilic Folliculitis

BASICS

- HIV-associated eosinophilic folliculitis, also known as *eosinophilic pustular folliculitis*, is an extremely pruritic rash that is seen in the later stages of HIV infection.
- Eosinophilic folliculitis appears to be a hypersensitivity reaction because of the large numbers of eosinophils that are seen in the skin, but no consistent association with specific allergens has been reported.
- Very few patients with eosinophilic folliculitis respond to antihistamines.
- HIV-infected patients have high circulating levels of interleukins 4 and 5, the cytokines that are chemotactic for eosinophils, so a seemingly allergic manifestation such as eosinophilic folliculitis may be a result of the general immunologic derangement in these patients.
- Eosinophilic folliculitis has become rare now that the use of HAART has decreased the number of cases of advanced HIV infection.

DESCRIPTION OF LESIONS

- Primary lesions are urticarial papules measuring 3 to 5 mm that look like insect bites.
- Pustules may be present, but they are not the predominant lesions.
- In many cases, only excoriations are present because of the intense pruritus.
- Patients with long-standing eosinophilic folliculitis may develop lichenification secondary to repeated scratching.

DISTRIBUTION OF LESIONS

- Lesions may occur anywhere, but they are prominent on the "seborrheic areas" of the skin (e.g., scalp, face, chest, and upper back).

CLINICAL MANIFESTATIONS

- Severe pruritus may interfere with the patient's ability to function.

DIAGNOSIS

- Skin biopsy shows perifollicular and follicular infiltration by eosinophils.
- Occasionally, peripheral eosinophilia may be present.

 DIFFERENTIAL DIAGNOSIS

Bacterial Folliculitis
- See also Chapter 5, "Superficial Bacterial Infections," for a more complete discussion.
- Bacterial folliculitis may be clinically indistinguishable from eosinophilic folliculitis.
- Gram's stain and bacterial culture should be performed.

Pityrosporum Folliculitis
- *Pityrosporum* folliculitis may be clinically indistinguishable from eosinophilic folliculitis.
- Potassium hydroxide preparation of pus shows yeast and hyphae.
- Periodic acid–Schiff stain of skin biopsy specimen shows yeast and hyphae.

Arthropod Bite Reaction
- Arthropod bite reaction may be clinically and histologically indistinguishable from eosinophilic folliculitis.
- Lesions are less likely to be folliculocentric.
- The patient's history should include possible exposure to arthropods (e.g., fleas, lice, scabies, bedbugs, and mosquitoes).

 MANAGEMENT

- **Topical steroids, antihistamines,** and **antibiotics** are usually ineffective.
- **Ultraviolet B phototherapy** is effective. Patients should be referred to a qualified phototherapy center. In the summer, sunlight is effective.
- **Isotretinoin** (40 mg/day) is usually effective. Treatment must be continued for at least 3 months and may need to be continued on a long-term basis. Once the lesions have resolved, an attempt to taper the dosage to the lowest effective dose should be made. Cholesterol and triglyceride levels require monitoring on a monthly basis because of the side effect of hyperlipidemia. Because the protease inhibitors also cause hyperlipidemia, patients may need to be started on a cholesterol-lowering medication concomitantly.
- **Itraconazole** (200 mg twice daily) may be effective.

POINT TO REMEMBER

- Eosinophilic folliculitis, as described herein, is almost always associated with HIV infection.

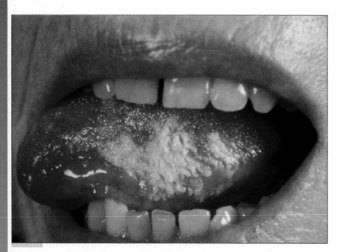

24.18 ***Oral hairy leukoplakia.*** White plaques resembling corrugated cardboard are fixed to the mucosa.

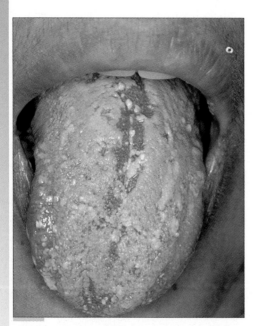

24.19 ***Oral candidiasis.*** These curdlike lesions can be easily removed with gauze.

HIV-Associated Oral Hairy Leukoplakia

BASICS

- Oral hairy leukoplakia is a marker of HIV infection that is thought to be caused by Epstein-Barr virus infection of the oral mucosa. It is rarely seen in patients receiving HAART.
- See Chapter 12, "Disorders of the Mouth, Lips, and Tongue," for a detailed discussion.

DESCRIPTION OF LESIONS

- White plaques resembling "corrugated cardboard" (Fig. 24.18 [see also Fig. 12.12]) are fixed to the mucosa; they are not friable, as in candidiasis (see subsequent discussion).

DISTRIBUTION OF LESIONS

- Lesions most often appear on the lateral aspects of the tongue.

CLINICAL MANIFESTATIONS

- Lesions are usually asymptomatic.
- Patients occasionally complain of a burning sensation of the tongue.

 MANAGEMENT

- Treatment is necessary only in symptomatic cases.
- **Surgical excision** can be performed, but lesions recur at the margins.
- **Acyclovir** (3.2 g/day) is given if lesions recur on cessation of treatment. However, the use of acyclovir for oral hairy leukoplakia may result in the development of acyclovir resistance for concurrent HSV infection.
- **Topical tretinoin** 0.05% solution may be applied for 15 minutes once daily using a gauze sponge.
- **Podophyllin 25% solution** is applied sparingly to one side of the tongue at a time and is allowed to air dry. This is repeated once weekly.

HIV-Associated Oral Candidiasis

- Candidiasis ("thrush") is also seen in immunocompromised patients and in neonates.
- Curdlike or erosive lesions can easily be removed with gauze or a tongue blade (Fig. 24.19).
- Lesions are more common on the dorsal aspect of the tongue, oropharynx, angles of mouth, and buccal mucosa.
- The potassium hydroxide preparation shows yeast.

MANAGEMENT

- In patients with severe immunosuppression, intermittent or prolonged topical or oral antifungal treatment is usually necessary.
- Meticulous dental hygiene and an oral rinse containing 0.12% **chlorhexidine gluconate** may be effective.
- Oral therapy with fluconazole (**Diflucan**) produces remission within approximately 1 week. Fluconazole 100 mg daily is more effective than **nystatin** 500,000 IU four times daily or **clotrimazole** troche 10 mg five times per day.
- Maintenance therapy or intermittent therapy with fluconazole is essential to prevent relapse.

HIV-Associated Aphthous Ulcers

BASICS

- Aphthous ulcers may be severe in HIV-infected patients (Fig. 24.20).
- The pain may interfere with the patient's ability to eat.
- Mucosal pain leads to difficulties with eating and drinking, with resultant weight loss and dehydration.
- See the discussion of mucous membranes in Chapter 12, "Disorders of the Mouth, Lips, and Tongue" (see Figs. 12.1 and 12.2).

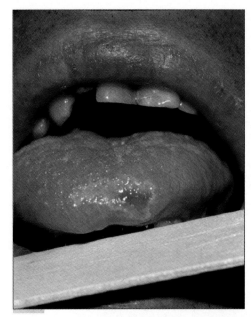

24.20 *Aphthous ulcer in a patient with acquired immunodeficiency syndrome.* These lesions can be quite painful.

MANAGEMENT

- **Topical steroids** may be applied directly to the ulcerations.
- **Stomatitis elixir,** consisting of equal parts of magnesium carbonate or magnesium hydroxide suspension, viscous lidocaine, diphenhydramine elixir 12.5 mg/5 mL, and 1 g tetracycline powder, to be swished and spat out of the mouth as needed, is useful for pain.
- **Thalidomide** (100 mg by mouth twice per day) is effective, with notable toxic effects of sedation, neutropenia, peripheral neuropathy, and teratogenicity.

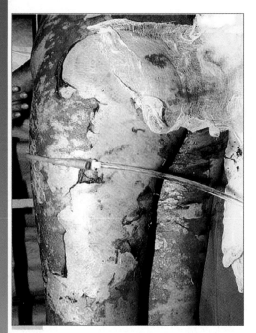

24.21 *Drug eruption.* Toxic epidermal necrolysis has resulted from treatment with nevirapine. (Courtesy of Ashit Marwah, M.D.)

patients with AIDS develop an allergy, followed by the aminopenicillins.

- When the drug allergy causes a typical morbilliform eruption, it is possible to continue the offending medication and treat the patient's symptoms with antihistamines and topical steroids. More serious drug eruptions are characterized by urticaria, mucosal involvement, target lesions, erythroderma, and tenderness of the skin. Any of these signs or symptoms requires prompt discontinuation of the offending medication.
- Mucosal involvement and target lesions are indicative of erythema multiforme or Stevens-Johnson syndrome, whereas erythroderma and skin tenderness are seen in toxic epidermal necrolysis (FIG. 24.21). The nonnucleoside reverse transcriptase inhibitor nevirapine has been associated with severe cases of Stevens-Johnson syndrome. For a complete discussion of drug eruptions, see Chapter 17, "Drug Eruptions."

HIV-Associated Pruritus

BASICS

- Pruritus is a common and troubling symptom in HIV-infected patients. It often has a multifactorial origin.
- Many patients use antibacterial or deodorant soaps with the mistaken belief that these will decrease the risk of infection. In fact, these soaps dry the skin and make the patients itchy and more susceptible to cutaneous infection because of the excoriations that result.
- Patients may become itchy because of subclinical drug eruptions or as a medication-related side effect.
- Patients may be colonized with *Staphylococcus aureus*, which is known to be a cause of pruritus in HIV-infected patients.

HIV-Associated Drug Eruptions

BASICS

- Drug eruptions are common in the HIV-infected population because of the large number of medications taken by these patients. The most commonly implicated medication is sulfamethoxazole/trimethoprim, to which at least 60% of

 MANAGEMENT

- Careful history taking and a physical examination rule out dermatologic disease as the cause.
- Patients should discontinue use of deodorant and antibacterial soaps; superfatted soaps are the least drying.
- Patients should be instructed to limit bathing to once per day.
- **Emollients** should be applied after the patient has bathed and patted dry; ointments are more emollient than creams, which are more emollient than lotions.
- Patients need to try different preparations to find which is most cosmetically acceptable and effective.

- Patients who do not obtain relief with over-the-counter moisturizers often do well with ammonium lactate 12% lotion or cream (**Lac-Hydrin**).
- Anti-itch preparations containing calamine, pramoxine, menthol, camphor, and oatmeal may be soothing.
- Sedating **antihistamines** are useful, especially before bedtime.
- **Topical steroids** should be prescribed for dermatitis, which may result from dry skin.
- **Ultraviolet B phototherapy** is palliative.

   For further discussion of pruritus, see Chapter 15, "Pruritus: The 'Itchy' Patient."

HIV-Associated Seborrheic Dermatitis

BASICS

- Seborrheic dermatitis is a scaly skin condition that affects up to 5% of the human population.
- In immunocompetent patients, it may be associated with an overgrowth of saprophytic *Pityrosporum* yeast on the scalp and face; it is not known whether the same is true in HIV-infected patients.
- The frequency and severity of seborrheic dermatitis are increased in HIV-infected patients, for unknown reasons.
- Seborrheic dermatitis appears commonly in hospitalized patients, probably because of the changes in hygiene (e.g., inability to shampoo the hair) experienced during illness.
- For description and distribution of lesions, as well as management, see Chapter 4, "Inflammatory Eruptions of Unknown Cause."

 POINT TO REMEMBER

- Seborrheic dermatitis is common in HIV-infected patients, and the sudden onset of severe, recalcitrant seborrheic dermatitis should lead to an inquiry regarding risk factors for HIV and HIV testing.

HIV-Associated Psoriasis

BASICS

- Psoriasis is a scaly skin disease that affects 1% to 2% of the general population.
- Psoriasis is not more common in HIV-infected patients, but it may present in a more severe or unusual form and may be recalcitrant to the usual treatments.
- The most severe manifestation is Reiter's disease (see Chapter 25, "Cutaneous Manifestations of Systemic Disease"), which includes psoriatic lesions, arthritis, urethritis, and conjunctivitis. A new onset of severe psoriasis in a patient at risk for HIV should lead to HIV testing.
- Combined treatment with methotrexate and sulfonamides can lead to fatal bone marrow suppression.
- The use of systemic steroids for treatment of psoriasis may result in life-threatening pustular psoriasis.
- See Chapter 3, "Psoriasis," for a more complete discussion.

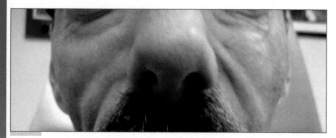

24.22 *Lipodystrophy.* Note the atrophic "nasolabial bands" between the nasolabial lines and the cheeks.

HIV-Associated Lipoatrophy

BASICS

- The complete syndrome of HIV-associated lipodystrophy consists of lipoatrophy of the face and extremities, truncal obesity with the development of a buffalo hump, triglyceridemia, and insulin resistance.
- The cause of the condition is multifactorial. It is associated with treatment with nucleoside reverse transcriptase inhibitors (NRTIs), notably stavudine (Zerit), and with protease inhibitors. In addition, host factors play a role, in that white patients with CD4 counts under 100 cells/mm³ and body mass indices less than 24 kg/m² have a significant risk of developing lipoatrophy independently of HIV medications.
- Facial lipoatrophy is a marker of a person who is infected with HIV. It causes severe psychologic problems and depression in many patients, even after the treatment has lowered the viral load to undetectable levels.

DESCRIPTION OF LESIONS

- There is loss of facial fat to varying degrees.
- In severe cases, there is hollowing of the cheeks and development of a "nasolabial band" between the nasolabial lines and the cheeks (FIG 24.22). Loss of the fat in the temporal, periorbital, and cheek areas gives prominence to the underlying bony structure, producing a skeletal look.

DISTRIBUTION OF LESIONS

- Initially the cheeks are affected.
- Later, the temporal and periorbital fat disappears.

 MANAGEMENT

- Avoidance of NRTIs, especially stavudine.
- Careful selection of protease inhibitors. Atazanavir (Reyataz) does not cause the same lipid abnormalities or body fat changes associated with some of the other protease inhibitors.
- Switching therapy may stop the progression of lipoatrophy.
- Filler substances have been used successfully to treat facial lipoatrophy and to reduce the stigma that is felt by patients with HIV infection. In the United States, poly-L-lactic acid (Sculptra) and calcium hydroxyapatite microspheres (Radiesse) are currently approved for the treatment of HIV-associated lipoatrophy. Many more filler substances are being used in other countries for this indication.

- Treatment of patients with severe lipoatrophy using poly-L-lactic acid requires an average of six treatments over 6 months by a skilled injector to achieve good results; these last an average of 2 years. Results are not immediate but develop 4 to 6 weeks after injection as the skin begins to form new collagen on the poly-L-lactic acid matrix.
- Treatment with calcium hydroxyapatite microspheres results in immediate correction and may require only a single treatment. The microspheres provide a matrix on which new collagen is formed by the skin. Because the reabsorption of the microspheres may occur more rapidly than new collagen formation, a touch-up treatment may be required approximately 3 months after the initial treatment. Results last for a year or more.
- When lipoatrophy is treated by a skilled injector, side effects are rare.

 POINTS TO REMEMBER

- NRTIs and protease inhibitors are the main causes of facial lipoatrophy.
- Patients with HIV are extremely stressed by facial lipoatrophy.
- Facial lipoatrophy can be treated with injections of poly-L-lactic acid or calcium hydroxyapatite microspheres.

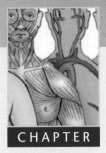

CHAPTER

25

Cutaneous Manifestations of Systemic Disease

Herbert P. Goodheart and Peter G. Burk

OVERVIEW

- The cutaneous surface, nails, hair, and oral cavity often afford clues to many underlying disorders. The skin is sometimes referred to as a "window" to disease. For example, the presence of jaundice, palmar erythema, pruritus, and spider telangiectasias points to liver disease. The appearance of pyoderma gangrenosum, erythema nodosum, or severe aphthous stomatitis may indicate inflammatory bowel disease.
- By appreciating skin signs of systemic diseases, the health care provider can often lead his or her patient to an early diagnosis and expedient and appropriate treatment.
- This chapter reviews some of the cutaneous manifestations of systemic diseases and it highlights recent developments in their management.

➤ **ENDOCRINE DISEASES**

Diabetes-associated lesions
- Necrobiosis lipoidica diabeticorum
- Diabetic bullous disease
- Diabetic neuropathic ulcers
- Acanthosis nigricans
- Eruptive xanthomas
- Diabetic dermopathy
- Perforating folliculitis (Kyrle's disease)
- Disseminated granuloma annulare
- Scleredema of Buschke-Löwenstein

Thyroid Disease
- Pretibial myxedema
- Warm, moist, and velvety skin
- Alopecia with diffuse hair loss
- Nails
- Hair

➤ **LIPID ABNORMALITIES**

- Eruptive xanthomas
- Planar xanthomas
- Xanthelasma
- Tuberous xanthomas
- Tendinous xanthomas

➤ **CONNECTIVE TISSUE DISEASES**

- Systemic lupus erythematosus
- Drug-induced lupus erythematosus
- Subacute cutaneous lupus erythematosus
- Chronic cutaneous lupus erythematosus
- Neonatal lupus erythematosus
- Dermatomyositis
- Scleroderma and morphea
- Crest syndrome and progressive systemic sclerosis

➤ **ERYTHEMA NODOSUM**

➤ **CUTANEOUS SARCOIDOSIS**

➤ **INFLAMMATORY SKIN DISORDERS**

- Reiter's syndrome
- Pyoderma gangrenosum
- Exfoliative dermatitis

➤ **NEUROCUTANEOUS SYNDROMES**

- Neurofibromatosis
- Tuberous sclerosis

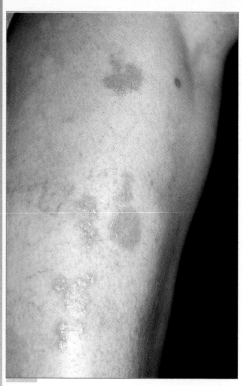

25.1 *Necrobiosis lipoidica diabeticorum.* This diabetic patient has early lesions that consist of yellow-red plaques. Epidermal atrophy and telangiectasias tend to occur later.

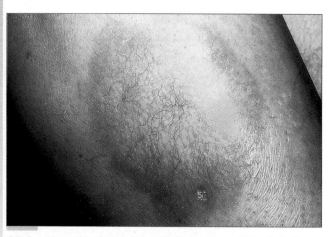

25.2 *Necrobiosis lipoidica diabeticorum.* This diabetic patient has more advanced lesions than those seen in FIGURE 25.1. Epidermal atrophy and telangiectasias are seen here.

BASICS

- Many different skin lesions are seen in conjunction with endocrine diseases. Some cutaneous lesions are directly related to the degree of endocrine dysfunction and may be caused by an excess or lack of a hormone acting on a specific tissue, such as warm and moist skin associated with hyperthyroidism or dry and cool skin associated with hypothyroidism.
- In a disease such as diabetes, it may be difficult to link these skin findings to a specific degree of endocrine dysfunction (e.g., necrobiosis lipoidica diabeticorum with the level of hyperglycemia).

Diabetes Mellitus

- Diabetes mellitus is a disease characterized by a disturbance in the production of insulin or resistance to insulin activity, which results in abnormal glucose metabolism.
- Diabetes causes cellular changes, such as microangiopathy of small blood vessels. This causes organ damage, including retinal disease, renal dysfunction, and possibly cutaneous lesions.
- Diabetes can also affect immune function and can lead to an increase of bacterial, fungal, and yeast infections.

Diabetes-Associated Lesions: Necrobiosis Lipoidica Diabeticorum

- Necrobiosis lipoidica diabeticorum (NLD) is characterized by yellow-red to brown, translucent plaques with epidermal atrophy and telangiectasia (FIG. 25.1). As lesions progress, the center becomes depressed and yellow (FIG. 25.2). Ulceration is not uncommon.
- NLD appears most commonly on the pretibial areas, but it may arise on other sites.
- NLD is more common in women than in men.
- Treatment for NLD is not very satisfactory. The condition is typically chronic with variable progression and scarring.
- NLD is seen more frequently in type 1 than in type 2 diabetes and may occur before the onset of clinical diabetes. Lesions may ulcerate. A minority of patients have no clinical evidence or family history of diabetes; in these patients, the term *necrobiosis lipoidica* is used. Currently, the term *necrobiosis lipoidica* is used to encompass all patients with the same clinical lesions regardless of whether diabetes is present or not.

DIFFERENTIAL DIAGNOSIS

- The lesions of NLD can be similar to those of morphea (see later discussion) and other localized sclerosing lesions.

 MANAGEMENT

- High-potency **topical steroids** or **intralesional steroid injections** are used and can lessen the inflammation of early active lesions and the active borders of enlarging lesions, but these have little beneficial effect on atrophic lesions that are burned out. In fact, with atrophic lesions, steroid use may cause further atrophy.
- Because localized trauma can cause NLD to ulcerate, protection of the legs with **support stockings** may be helpful.
- Antiplatelet aggregation therapy with **aspirin** and **dipyridamole** has produced varied results but overall has shown some beneficial effects.

- Pentoxifylline (**Trental**) is a drug used for the treatment of intermittent claudication. Pentoxifylline is believed to decrease blood viscosity by increasing fibrinolysis and red blood cell deformity. It also inhibits platelet aggregation.
- Topical application of **bovine collagen** is believed to improve granulation tissue by supporting fibroblast activity and promote wound debridement by increasing the number of macrophages and neutrophils at the wound site.
- **Ticlopidine, nicotinamide, clofazimine,** and **perilesional heparin** injections have been used in uncontrolled studies and appeared to benefit some patients with NLD.

Diabetes-Associated Lesions: Diabetic Bullous Disease

- Diabetic bullous disease (bullosis diabeticorum) manifests as large, tense, subepidermal, noninflammatory blisters (FIG. 25.3).
- Lesions most often arise spontaneously on the lower extremities, especially the ankles and feet. The development of multiple lesions at several locations may occur.
- Lesions tend to arise in patients with long-standing diabetes mellitus who have multiple complications of the disease.

 DIFFERENTIAL DIAGNOSIS

- Bullous diabetic lesions can be differentiated from bullous pemphigoid by the characteristic location of lesions and negative direct immunofluorescence of skin biopsies.

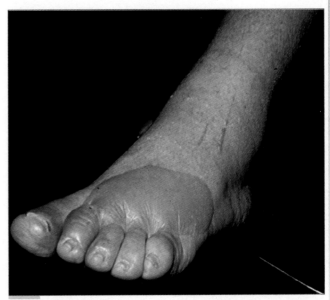

25.3 *Diabetic bullous disease.* This large, tense blister arose spontaneously in a characteristic location.

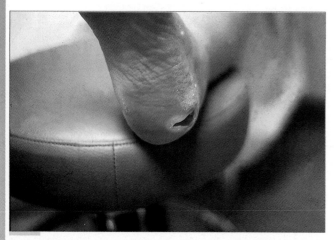

25.4 ***Diabetic ulcer of the heel (mal perforans).*** These lesions are noted at sites of pressure, such as the heel in this patient.

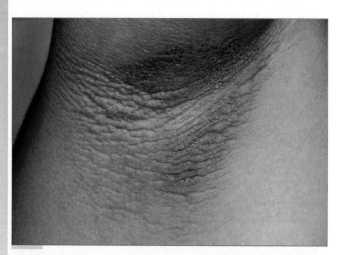

25.5 ***Acanthosis nigricans.*** Note the characteristic hyperpigmentation in a typical location. This patient has insulin-resistant diabetes. (Image courtesy of Bernard Cohen, M.D.)

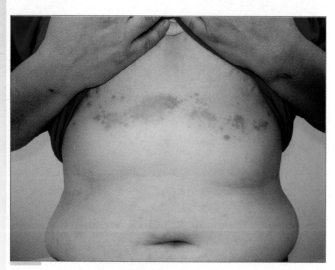

25.6 ***Cutaneous candidiasis.*** These satellite pustules were positive for *Candida albicans*.

 MANAGEMENT

- Blisters generally heal spontaneously within 2 to 6 weeks of onset.
- Topical antibiotics are recommended until the lesions heal.

Diabetes-Associated Lesions: Diabetic Neuropathic Ulcers

- Diabetic neuropathic ulcers (mal perforans) (FIG. 25.4) most often occur at sites of pressure (e.g., the heel), particularly in areas of poor sensory function and poor circulation. They are usually painless as a result of peripheral neuropathy.
- Diabetic foot ulcers occur as a result of the loss of protective sensation.
- Other factors, such as mechanical changes in conformation of the bony architecture of the foot and atherosclerotic peripheral arterial disease, may be contributing causes.

DIAGNOSIS

- Diabetic neuropathic ulcers should be distinguished from infections and other ulcerations and cutaneous neoplasms that may present as ulcerations.

 MANAGEMENT

- It is beyond the scope of this discussion to describe all therapies for diabetic foot ulcers. However, management can include glycemic control, special footwear, topical wound management, daily saline soaks, surgical debridement, and skin grafting when necessary.
- Becaplermin (**Regranex***), a recombinant human platelet-derived growth factor, is available in gel form for topical therapy (in conjunction with good ulcer care) and is reported to promote healing of diabetic neuropathic foot ulcers.
- Hyperbaric oxygen therapy may be useful.

Other Findings in Diabetic Patients

- **Acanthosis nigricans** (FIG. 25.5) sometimes occurs in insulin-resistant diabetes (also see FIGS. 14.19 and 14.20).
- **Cutaneous candidiasis** (FIG. 25.6) may also occur (see also FIGS. 7.31–7.33) (see Chapter 7, "Superficial Fungal Infections").

*There is currently a "black box" warning about an increased risk of cancer from the use of this agent.

- **Eruptive xanthomas** are seen as skin markers for various primary genetic disorders such as certain types of hyperlipidemias or secondary to diabetes (see later discussion).
- **Diabetic dermopathy** is characterized by small brownish, atrophic, scarred, hyperpigmented plaques (Fig. 25.7)
  - Lesions occur primarily on the anterior lower legs in patients with type 1 and type 2 diabetes.
  - It is typically a late manifestation of diabetes and is usually asymptomatic.
  - Diabetic dermopathy must be differentiated from lesions caused by trauma.
- **Perforating folliculitis** (Kyrle's disease) consists of firm, rough, hyperkeratotic papules, which are often hyperpigmented in dark-skinned people.
  - There is a high incidence of perforating folliculitis in patients with long-standing diabetes who are undergoing long-term hemodialysis.
  - Lesions are found most commonly on the extensor surfaces of the extremities. Itching can be intense.
- **Disseminated granuloma annulare** consists of annular dermal papules (see Chapter 4, "Inflammatory Eruptions of Unknown Cause"). It occurs both in patients with clinical diabetes and sometimes in individuals with only abnormal glucose levels.
- **Scleredema of Buschke-Löwenstein** is a rare manifestation of diabetes mellitus. The lesion is a sclerotic, thickened plaque characteristically seen on the upper back.

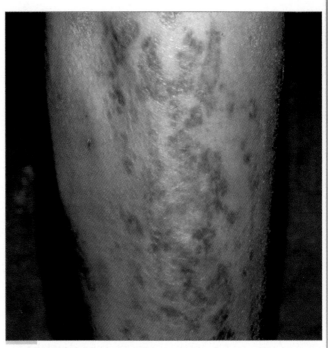

25.7 **_Diabetic dermopathy._** Small, asymptomatic, brownish, atrophic, scarred, hyperpigmented plaques are seen on the shins of this diabetic patient.

DIAGNOSIS

- The diagnoses of many of these entities are generally made on clinical grounds.
- A skin biopsy may be necessary to confirm the diagnosis.

Laboratory Evaluation

- Serum glucose levels and glycosylated hemoglobin A_1 are determined to confirm the diagnosis of diabetes mellitus.
- Skin biopsies of lesions of necrobiosis lipoidica and granuloma annulare demonstrate palisading granulomas with degeneration of collagen.
- Skin biopsy of perforating folliculitis demonstrates basophilic material in the dermis, with transepidermal elimination.
- Skin biopsies of diabetic dermopathy show thickening of blood vessels and mild perivascular infiltrate.
- Diabetic bullous lesions have subepidermal blistering on hematoxylin and eosin staining of skin biopsy tissue; direct immunofluorescence of skin biopsies in these lesions is negative for immunoglobulins.
- Diabetic neuropathic ulcers are rarely examined by biopsy.
- Perforating folliculitis can be differentiated from other keratotic papules by the size and distribution of lesions and by a skin biopsy.

HELPFUL HINT

- Careful consideration should be given before performing a skin biopsy on a patient with diabetes, particularly on areas such as the lower extremities.

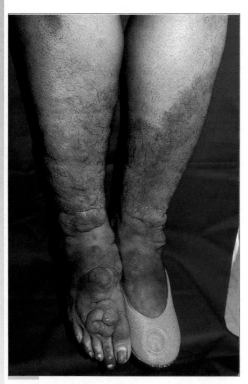

25.8 *Pretibial myxedema, Graves' disease.* Erythematous plaques with early involvement. (Image courtesy of Ashit Marah, M.D.)

25.9 *Pretibial myxedema, Graves' disease.* Note the progressive exuberant hypertrophy with folding of the skin on the shins and tops of the feet.

BASICS

- Thyroid hormones profoundly influence the growth and differentiation of epidermal and dermal tissues.
- Abnormal levels of thyroid hormone produce striking changes in the texture of the skin, hair, and nails.
- Some of the associated skin alterations in thyroid disease are the result of a deficiency or a high toxic level of tissue thyroid hormone. Other skin disorders seen with thyroid disease, such as vitiligo and alopecia areata, are associated clinical findings that are not directly related to thyroid hormone function but are seen on occasion in patients with thyroid disease.
- Findings such as pretibial myxedema are caused by circulating autoimmune γ-globulin, which acts as a thyroid-stimulating hormone.
- Hyperthyroidism may be caused by Graves' disease, subacute thyroiditis, toxic goiter, and thyroid carcinoma.
- Hypothyroidism may be caused by iodine deficiency (cretinism), Hashimoto's thyroiditis, pituitary dysfunction with thyroid-stimulating hormone deficiency, and surgical or radiation ablation of the thyroid.
- Patients with thyroid disease may be hyperthyroid at one point in their clinical course and hypothyroid at another time.

DESCRIPTION OF LESIONS

- Hyperthyroid skin lesions may include the following:
  - Warm, moist, and velvety skin
  - Alopecia with diffuse hair loss
  - Nail changes with onycholysis (Plummer's nails)
  - Hyperpigmentation
  - Pretibial myxedema lesions—flesh-colored, waxy infiltrated translucent plaques (FIGS. 25.8 and 25.9)
- Hyperthyroid findings may include the following:
  - Nervousness and tremor
  - Weight loss
  - Tachycardia with atrial fibrillation
  - Proximal muscle weakness

- Graves' disease
- Exophthalmos (FIG. 25.10)
- Hypothyroid skin lesions may include the following:
  - Myxedema of the skin with generalized thickening and a dry, coarse feel; yellow skin secondary to carotenemia
  - Hair changes—coarse, sparse hair; lateral third of eyebrows lost
- The following conditions may be associated with thyroid disease:
  - Alopecia areata
  - Vitiligo
  - Connective tissue diseases
  - Multiple endocrinopathy syndrome
  - Urticaria

DISTRIBUTION OF LESIONS

- Pretibial myxedema lesions are found most frequently on the lower legs.

CLINICAL MANIFESTATIONS

- Hyperthyroid skin changes that result from the hypermetabolic state (e.g., warm, moist, flushed skin) occur during the active thyrotoxic stage of thyroiditis, during active Graves' disease, and in patients with toxic goiters. These skin changes may gradually resolve when the patient returns to a euthyroid state.
- Graves' disease lesions (pretibial myxedema) occur in up to 4% of patients with this disease. The skin lesions and eye lesions usually do not resolve, even after treatment of the thyroid disease brings a return to a euthyroid state.
- Hypothyroid skin changes (e.g., cool, dry skin) are related to the length and severity of the clinical hypothyroid state. These skin lesions gradually improve some months after the patient returns to a euthyroid state.

DIAGNOSIS

- Diagnosis of both hyperthyroid and hypothyroid disease is made by specific thyroid function tests.
- Graves' disease is diagnosed clinically and with confirmatory thyroid function tests.

Laboratory Evaluation

- Elevated thyroid-stimulating hormone levels are the most sensitive screening test for hypothyroidism.
- Serum thyroid hormone levels can be most accurately measured by obtaining free thyroxine and free triiodothyronine levels.
- Antithyroglobulin antibodies and antithyroid microsomal antibodies are often positive in Graves' disease and Hashimoto's thyroiditis.
- Long-acting thyroid stimulator is elevated in 50% of patients with Graves' disease.
- Skin biopsies in Graves' disease show increased staining of hyaluronic acid with mucin stains in the reticular and papillary dermis.

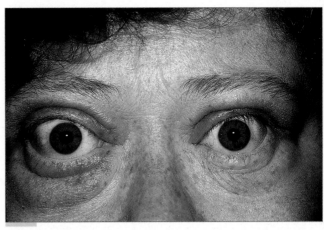

25.10 *Exophthalmos.* This patient has Graves' disease. Note the lid retraction and proptosis.

DIFFERENTIAL DIAGNOSIS

- Pretibial myxedema must be differentiated from other skin diseases with increased mucin production, such as papillary mucinosis and scleredema.

MANAGEMENT

- Functional symptoms (e.g., increase or decrease of sweating, dry skin, hair and nail changes) of hyperthyroidism and hypothyroidism may improve after appropriate treatment of thyroid disease and return to a euthyroid state.
- Treatment of pretibial myxedema lesions can be attempted with **high-potency topical steroids** and **intralesional steroids,** although the response is generally poor.

BASICS

- Abnormalities of lipid metabolism, with high circulating levels of various lipoproteins, can result in deposition of cholesterol and other lipids in the skin, tendons, and other organs.
- Xanthomas result from the deposition of cholesterol and other lipids found in tissue macrophages in the skin and tendons. There is also a high correlation between abnormal lipoproteinemia and the development of atherosclerosis.
- Lipoprotein abnormalities have been classified into primary (genetic) lipoproteinemia and secondary lipoproteinemia resulting from underlying diseases.
- Primary lipoproteinemias are phenotypic expressions of various genetic disorders of lipid metabolism with the following characteristics:
  - Type I, familial lipoprotein lipase deficiency: elevated chylomicrons
  - Type IIA, familial hypercholesterolemia: elevated low-density lipoproteins
  - Type IIB, familial hyperlipidemia: elevated low-density lipoproteins and very-low-density lipoproteins
  - Type III, familial dysbetalipoproteinemia: elevated intermediate-density lipoproteins
  - Type IV, endogenous familial hypertriglyceridemia: elevated triglycerides
  - Type V, familial combined hyperlipidemia: elevated chylomicrons and elevated very-low-density lipoproteins
- Secondary hyperlipoproteinemias result from disturbances in cholesterol and triglyceride metabolism caused by cholestatic liver disease, diabetes mellitus, pancreatitis, multiple myeloma, and nephrotic syndrome. These disorders may mimic any of the genetic lipoprotein abnormalities and may produce similar xanthomatous deposits in tissues.

DESCRIPTION OF LESIONS

- **Eruptive xanthomas** are smooth, yellow, papular lesions (2 to 5 mm) (FIGS. 25.11 A and B). There is sometimes a red halo around the lesions.
- **Planar xanthomas** are flat to slightly palpable yellow lesions.
- **Xanthelasma (xanthoma palpebrarum)** is a form of planar xanthoma (FIG. 25.12).

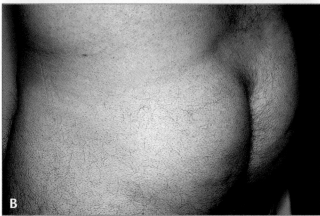

25.11 A and B *Eruptive xanthomas.* **A:** This 28-year-old male patient has a triglyceride level of 31,000 and a cholesterol level of 580 mg/dL. **B:** This is the same patient after 2 months of a low-fat diet and a cholesterol-lowering drug.

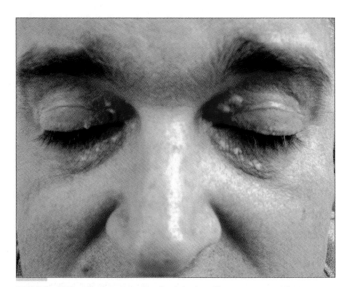

25.12 *Xanthelasma.* Periorbital yellow-orange plaques are present on the upper inner eyelids. This patient was normolipemic when this photograph was taken.

- **Tuberous xanthomas** are small (0.5 cm) to large (3 to 5 cm), firm, yellow papules and nodules (FIG. 25.13).
- **Tendinous xanthomas** are subcutaneous thickenings around tendons and ligaments.

DISTRIBUTION OF LESIONS

- Eruptive xanthomas appear most frequently over the knees, elbows, and buttocks.
- Planar xanthomas are found in the palmar creases but may also be generalized.
- Xanthelasma lesions are usually found on the eyelids and medial canthus.
- Tuberous xanthomas are found on the elbows, knees, and buttocks.
- Tendinous xanthomas affect the Achilles tendon, extensor tendons of the wrists, elbows, and knees.

CLINICAL MANIFESTATIONS

- Eruptive xanthomas tend to appear suddenly over the extensor surfaces and pressure points. These lesions are usually seen in association with very high levels of triglycerides (2,000 to 4,000 mg/dL). Uncontrolled diabetes mellitus and acute pancreatitis are both common underlying causes of their surfacing on the skin.
- Planar xanthomas are usually asymptomatic. Palmar xanthomas are seen with type III lipoproteinemia. Diffuse planar xanthomas are found in patients with multiple myeloma.
- Xanthelasma lesions grow slowly over years. More than 50% of patients with xanthelasma have normal lipoprotein levels.
- Tuberous xanthomas also are slow growing. They are associated with familial hypercholesterolemia but can also occur in patients with high triglyceride levels.
- Tendinous xanthomas occur in patients with hypercholesterolemias.

DIAGNOSIS

- The diagnosis is made by clinical evaluation of skin and subcutaneous lesions.
- Skin biopsy is confirmatory for xanthomas.

Laboratory Evaluation

- Fasting blood levels of triglycerides and cholesterol should be determined.
- Lipoprotein electrophoresis demonstrates specific lipoprotein abnormalities.
- Skin biopsy of xanthomas demonstrates collections of lipids in foamy macrophages in the dermis.
- Serum glucose levels and glycosylated hemoglobin A_1 are determined to rule out diabetes mellitus.
- Serum amylase levels should be examined to rule out pancreatitis.
- Serum protein electrophoresis should be performed to rule out multiple myeloma.

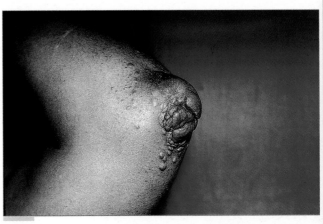

25.13 *Tuberous xanthomas.* These are firm papules and nodules in a patient with hyperlipidemia type II.

 DIFFERENTIAL DIAGNOSIS

- Eruptive xanthomas must be differentiated from cutaneous sarcoid papules and cutaneous histiocytosis.
- Tuberous xanthomas can be confused with rheumatoid nodules and subcutaneous granuloma annulare.

 MANAGEMENT

- Patients with lipid disorders and xanthomas must be appropriately evaluated for primary and secondary lipoprotein abnormalities. Treatment of the underlying cause may reverse both eruptive and tuberous xanthomas over time.
- **Dietary restrictions** and **cholesterol-lowering drugs** may reverse some changes associated with hypercholesterolemia.
- Xanthelasmas of the eyelids can be removed by application of 25% to 50% **trichloroacetic acid,** by local **electrodesiccation, laser therapy,** and **excision;** however, lesions can recur.

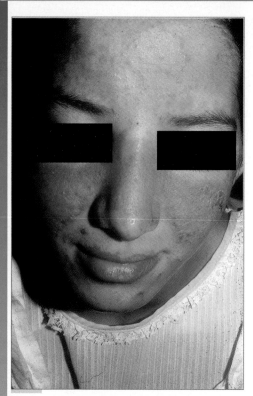

25.14 *Systemic lupus erythematosus.* A "butterfly rash" is evident. Note the sparing of the nasolabial areas that are often involved with seborrheic dermatitis.

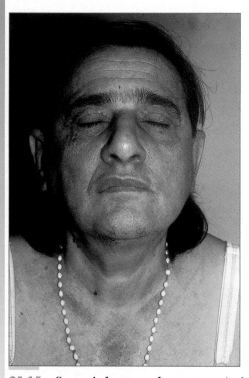

25.15 *Systemic lupus erythematosus.* A photodistribution on the face and the "V" of the neck are evident in this patient. Note the violaceous color suggestive of connective tissue disease. Similar findings are noted in dermatomyositis.

Systemic Lupus Erythematosus

BASICS

- Systemic lupus erythematosus (SLE) is a chronic, idiopathic, multisystemic, autoimmune disease associated with polyclonal B-cell activation. Fibrinoid degeneration of connective tissue and the walls of blood vessels associated with an inflammatory infiltrate involving various organs may result in arthralgia or arthritis, kidney disease, liver disease, central nervous system disease, gastrointestinal disease, pericarditis, pneumonitis, myopathy, and splenomegaly, as well as skin disease.
- The cutaneous manifestations of SLE result from the production of multiple autoantibodies that deposit immune complexes at the dermal–epidermal junction.
- Current investigators have reclassified lupus skin lesions into three distinct groups:
  - **Acute cutaneous lupus erythematosus (ACLE)** lesions are strongly associated with active SLE; however, ACLE lesions may occasionally be seen in **subacute cutaneous lupus erythematosus (SCLE)**.
  - SCLE comprises the second category.
  - **Chronic cutaneous lupus erythematosus (CCLE)** traditionally had been referred to as discoid lupus erythematosus (DLE). DLE lesions may be seen in both SLE and CCLE.
- SLE is seen in a 9:1 female-to-male ratio; it is more common in blacks and Hispanics.
- Approximately 10% of patients with SLE have a first-degree relative with the disease. An association of lupus and human leukocyte antigens (HLA) -DR2 and -DR4 has been seen.
- The following 4 of the 11 American Rheumatologic Association criteria for lupus are related to the skin and are considered lupus-specific lesions:
  - The classic malar or **"butterfly" rash** (FIG. 25.14) is a persistent erythema over the cheeks that tends to spare the nasolabial creases. Sometimes, this is the initial symptom of lupus, and it often occurs after sun exposure.
  - **Photosensitivity** (FIG. 25.15) occurs as an exaggerated or unusual reaction to sunlight. The reaction may resemble a drug eruption.

- **Discoid lesions (discoid lupus erythematosus)** are erythematous lesions that evolve into scaly, atrophic scarring plaques (FIG. 25.16). Such discoid lesions affect 10% to 15% of patients with SLE.
- **Oral ulcerations** may develop, often on the hard palate or nasopharynx.
- Nonspecific lesions of lupus that may be seen in SLE and other connective tissue diseases include the following:
  - The **"spider" type of telangiectasia** is usually seen in SLE, scleroderma, and dermatomyositis. Macular (mat-like) telangiectasias usually occur in scleroderma.
  - **Periungual telangiectasias** are seen in SLE, as well as in dermatomyositis and scleroderma.
  - Palmar telangiectasias are usually seen in SLE.
  - **Vasculitis,** palpable purpura, and vasculitic ulcers usually occur in SLE and scleroderma.
  - **Raynaud's phenomenon** is associated with SLE and scleroderma.
  - **Livedo reticulitis,** panniculitis, thrombophlebitis, urticaria, urticarial vasculitis, frontal alopecia ("lupus hair") and diffuse nonscarring alopecia, palmar erythema, and bullae are associated primarily with SLE.

DISTRIBUTION OF LESIONS

- The lesions of ACLE tend to occur in sun-exposed areas such as the face, dorsa of the forearms, the hands, and the "V" of the neck.
- The lesions of DLE may occur on the face, scalp, ears, neck, or oral mucosa, or they may be widespread (see later discussion).
- On the lower extremities, livedo reticularis (FIG. 25.17) and vasculitic ulcers (FIG. 25.18) may be seen.

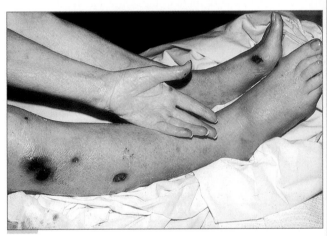

25.17 *Systemic lupus erythematosus.* Livedo reticularis is present.

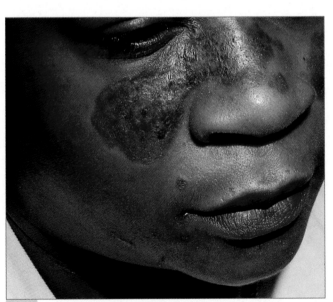

25.16 *Systemic lupus erythematosus (discoid lupus erythematosus).* Lesions of DLE, consisting of erythematous, scaly, disc-shaped scarring plaques, are present in this patient, who has SLE.

25.18 *Systemic lupus erythematosus.* Vasculitic ulcers are seen on this patient's legs.

- On the dorsal hands, violaceous plaques that spare the skin overlying the joints are characteristic of SLE. Conversely, in dermatomyositis, the joints are affected (Gottron's papules). Ulcerated vasculitic lesions on the fingertips may also develop (FIG. 25.19).

CLINICAL MANIFESTATIONS

- Fatigue, fever, and malaise may be the presenting nonspecific symptoms.
- Signs or symptoms are related to the specific organ or area involved (e.g., arthralgia).
- Flare of lupus is common during pregnancy.
- The following hematologic abnormalities may be associated with SLE: idiopathic thrombocytopenic purpura, hemolytic anemia, leukopenia, and clotting abnormalities, which may be related to the anticardiolipin syndrome. Other associated conditions and symptoms include rheumatoid arthritis, Sjögren's syndrome, seizures, and the occurrence of multiple spontaneous abortions.

DIAGNOSIS

According to the American Rheumatologic Association, a person has SLE if four or more of the following criteria are present:
1. "Butterfly" rash
2. Lesions of CCLE or DLE
3. Photosensitivity
4. Oral ulcers
5. Arthritis in two or more joints
6. Serositis
7. Renal disorder
8. Neurologic disorder
9. Hematologic disorder
10. Immunologic disorder: anti-DNA, anti-Smith (anti-Sm) antibody, or a false–biologic-positive syphilis serologic result
11. Antinuclear antibodies (ANAs)

Laboratory Evaluation

- Antinuclear antibody (ANA) titers are positive in 95% of patients with SLE. The peripheral rim pattern is associated most strongly with lupus erythematosus, although other patterns commonly are present.
- Anti-dsDNA (antibody to native double-stranded DNA) is present in 60% to 80% of patients and is more specific for SLE.
- Anti-Sm antibody has a strong specificity for SLE. This is particularly relevant in patients in whom anti-dsDNA results are negative and may help exclude underlying systemic involvement.
- Antiphospholipid antibodies are present in 25% of patients.
- The erythrocyte sedimentation rate is usually elevated.

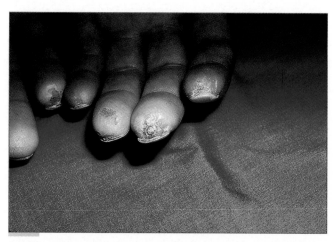

25.19 *Systemic lupus erythematosus.* Necrotic, painful, vasculitic ulcers are present on the fingertips.

- Hypocomplementemia occurs in 70% of patients and is noted especially when there is renal involvement in active SLE.
- The lupus band test involves the direct immunofluorescence of uninvolved, non–sun-exposed skin. When positive, it is suggestive of the presence of renal disease. This test has been largely supplanted by the aforementioned serologic tests.

 DIFFERENTIAL DIAGNOSIS

Facial Lesions

Rosacea
See Chapter 1, "Acne and Related Disorders."
- Presence of acnelike papules and pustules in addition to malar erythema
- Absence of systemic complaints
- Negative ANA titers

Seborrheic Dermatitis
See Chapter 2, "Eczema."
- Patients respond readily to topical steroids
- Lack of systemic complaints
- Negative ANA titers

Other Conditions
- Other connective tissue diseases, such as scleroderma and dermatomyositis (see later discussion)
- Other photosensitivity conditions, such as polymorphous light eruption
- Other causes of renal, hematologic, and central nervous system (CNS) disease

Drug-Induced Lupus Erythematosus

BASICS

- The clinical and serologic picture of drug-induced lupus erythematosus is often indistinguishable from that of SLE.
- A syndrome resembling SLE can be induced by certain drugs: hydralazine, procainamide, phenytoin, isoniazid, quinidine, beta-blockers, sulfasalazine, and lithium; however, patients with drug-induced lupus syndromes develop cutaneous lesions much less commonly than is typically seen in SLE.

- Arthralgia or arthritis, generally affecting the small joints, is often the only clinical symptom. Myalgia, pleuritis, pericarditis, fever, and hepatosplenomegaly may occur.
- The classic SLE-type lesions of butterfly rash and mucosal ulcerations, for example, are usually absent in drug-induced lupus erythematosus. CNS manifestations and renal involvement are also rare.
- In 90% of patients, ANAs are present in a homogenous or speckled pattern.
- Withdrawal of the offending drug, followed by a regression of symptoms, helps confirm the diagnosis.

MANAGEMENT

Sun-Related Symptoms

- Excessive sun exposure should be avoided; the patient should be counseled in the use of broad-spectrum sunscreens.

Cutaneous DLE

- See the later discussion of the management of CCLE.

Severely Ill Patients

- The mainstays of therapy for systemic disease are systemic steroids (prednisone), given in a dosage of 0.5 to 1 mg/kg/day.
- Administration of oral antimalarials such as hydroxychloroquine (**Plaquenil**) and chloroquine (**Aralen**) are sometimes used as first-line therapy. They both may be very effective in the treatment of skin lesions.
- Other therapeutic agents include:
  - **Dapsone, gold, oral retinoids** such as isotretinoin (**Accutane**), and immunosuppressive drugs such as azathioprine (**Imuran**) and cyclophosphamide (**Cytoxan**) and **methotrexate** may be helpful.
  - Mycophenolate (**CellCept**) as well as interferon alpha-2a and alpha-2b (**Roferon and Intron A**) may also be used.
- Immunosuppressive and antimalarial agents are used as adjuvant therapy to treat systemic disease because of their steroid-sparing effects.
- Thalidomide and intravenous γ-globulin are used to control recalcitrant cases.

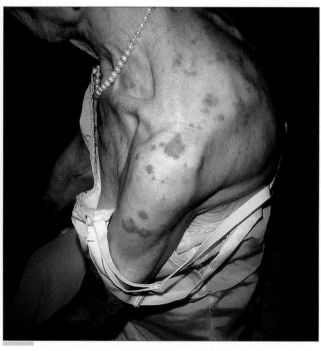

25.20 *Subacute cutaneous lupus erythematosus.* This patient has scaly, papulosquamous lesions. (Image courtesy of Herbert A. Hochman, M.D.)

Subacute Cutaneous Lupus Erythematosus

BASICS

- SCLE tends to be less severe than SLE and rarely progresses to renal or CNS involvement.
- SCLE is characterized by photodistributed erythematous lesions that are nonscarring.
- SCLE occurs most commonly in young and middle-aged white women.
- Patients may have some of the American Rheumatologic Association criteria for SLE, but serious disease with renal involvement is uncommon.

DESCRIPTION OF LESIONS

- Lesions are papulosquamous and closely resemble psoriasis or pityriasis rosea (FIG. 25.20).

- Lesions are often annular and heal without scarring (Fig. 25.21).

DISTRIBUTION OF LESIONS

- Lesions occur on the upper trunk, the "V" of the neck, and the extensor surfaces of the arms and hands.
- The face is often spared.

DIAGNOSIS

- Sjögrens anti-SS-A (anti-Ro) and anti-SS-B (anti-La) antibodies are often found, although the absence of these antibodies does not exclude the diagnosis.
- Low titers of ANA may be present.

CLINICAL MANIFESTATIONS

- Fatigue, malaise, and arthralgias may be noted.
- Sjögren's syndrome, idiopathic thrombocytopenic purpura, urticarial vasculitis, and morphea also have been reported in association with SCLE.

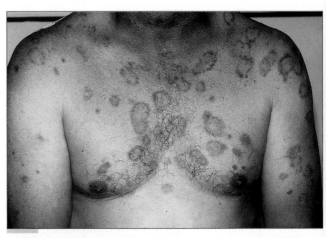

25.21 *Subacute cutaneous lupus erythematosus.* Note the annular plaques.

 DIFFERENTIAL DIAGNOSIS

- Psoriasis
- Pityriasis rosea

 MANAGEMENT

- Treatment of SCLE is much like that of CCLE and SLE.
- It focuses mainly on the avoidance of excessive sun exposure and the use of **broad-spectrum sunscreens** and **topical steroids**, **oral antimalarials, dapsone, gold,** **oral retinoids, thalidomide,** and **immunosuppressive drugs**.
- Because patients with SCLE have a better prognosis than patients with SLE, the clinician must weigh the potential toxicities of these agents against their benefits before initiating therapy.

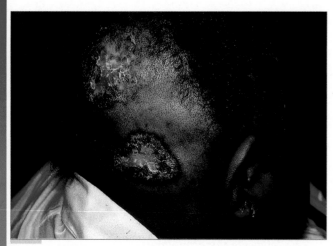

25.22 ***Chronic cutaneous lupus erythematosus.*** Lesions of DLE have caused scarring alopecia in this patient who has no evidence of SLE.

Chronic Cutaneous Lupus Erythematosus

BASICS

- CCLE consists of scarring plaques.
- DLE is, by far, the most common form of CCLE.
- Other CCLE variants include hypertrophic lupus erythematosus, lupus erythematosus panniculitis, and lupus profundus.
- DLE is a chronic, scarring, photosensitive dermatosis. DLE may occur in patients (approximately 25%) with SLE.
- If the initial workup of patients who present solely with localized lesions of DLE shows no evidence of SLE, then those patients are considered to be at low risk (less than 5%) for SLE to develop.

DESCRIPTION OF LESIONS

- Lesions begin as well-defined, erythematous plaques that evolve into atrophic, disc-shaped plaques, characterized by scale, accentuated hair follicles, follicular plugging, and a combination of hypopigmentation and hyperpigmentation.
- DLE often involves the scalp and produces scarring alopecia (FIG. 25.22), which can be quite extensive (FIG. 25.23).

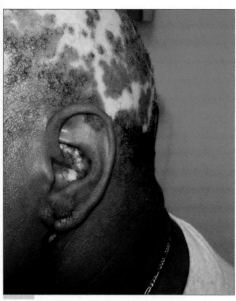

25.23 ***Chronic cutaneous lupus erythematosus.*** Extensive, progressive scarring alopecia and external ear involvement are evident in this patient, who has neither serologic nor clinical evidence of systemic disease.

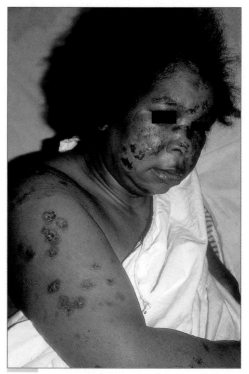

25.24 ***Chronic cutaneous lupus erythematosus.*** Widespread lesions of DLE are noted. Note the postinflammatory hyperpigmentation.

DISTRIBUTION OF LESIONS

- Patients with DLE often are divided into two groups: those with localized disease and those with widespread disease. Localized DLE occurs when only the head, neck, and external ears (see Fig. 25.23) are affected, whereas widespread DLE occurs when other areas are involved (Fig. 25.24).
- SLE is more likely to develop in patients with widespread involvement of DLE.

CLINICAL MANIFESTATIONS

- Lesions of DLE are relatively asymptomatic, but they may itch or be tender.
- Rarely, squamous cell carcinoma develops in hypertrophic chronic lesions.

DIAGNOSIS

- The clinical appearance is confirmed by a punch biopsy of the skin.

 DIFFERENTIAL DIAGNOSIS

- Sarcoidosis should be considered.
- Lichen planus is another possible diagnosis.
- CCLE variants include the following:
  - Hypertrophic lupus erythematosus is a warty-appearing form of CCLE.
  - Lupus erythematosus panniculitis is an inflammation of subcutaneous tissue.
  - When lupus panniculitis occurs with a lesion of CCLE overlying it, it is referred to as lupus profundus.

 MANAGEMENT

- Excessive sun exposure should be avoided.
- **Broad-spectrum sunscreens** that block both ultraviolet A (UVA) and ultraviolet B (UVB) are used.
- **Potent topical steroids** are generally effective for treating isolated lesions. Facial lesions should be treated with low- to medium-potency agents. If necessary, high-potency or superpotent agents may be used for short periods.
- **Intralesional steroid injections** are helpful in CCLE lesions that are refractory to topical therapy.
- Systemic agents may be indicated when lesions are widespread or unresponsive to topical or intralesional therapy. Agents such as the antimalarials hydroxychloroquine (**Plaquenil**) and chloroquine (**Aralen**) comprise the first line of systemic therapy.
- **Systemic steroids, dapsone, oral retinoids, gold, clofazimine, methotrexate, thalidomide, tetracycline** or **erythromycin combined with niacinamide,** and **mycophenolate mofetil (CellCept)** have proved to be helpful in selective cases.

 POINTS TO REMEMBER

- Patients with widespread involvement are more likely to develop SLE.
- Most patients with CCLE do not have and will not develop SLE. Even so, many patients who are given the diagnosis of CCLE describe themselves as having "lupus" and are convinced that they have the more serious disease.

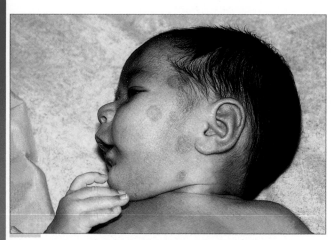

25.25 *Neonatal lupus erythematosus.* These annular erythematous plaques that look like "ringworm" appeared shortly after birth in this 3-month-old infant of an Ro-positive mother.

 MANAGEMENT

Cutaneous Manifestations
- **Low-potency,** nonfluorinated **topical steroids** are given.
- Sun exposure should be avoided.

Heart Block
- Experimental therapy using **dexamethasone,** which crosses the placental barrier, has been used to treat heart block in utero with minimal success.
- **Pacemaker implantation** is frequently required.

Neonatal Lupus Erythematosus

BASICS

- Neonatal lupus erythematosus (NLE) is a rare autoimmune syndrome that affects 1% to 2% of infants born of mothers who are anti-Ro (SS-A) antibody positive.
- Mothers may or may not show any of the signs or symptoms of connective tissue disease at the time of birth of the affected infant; however, some features of Sjögren's syndrome or lupus erythematosus (e.g., dry mouth, dry eyes, or arthralgias) do ultimately develop in most of these women. This situation may occur many years after the birth of the child; however, in most of these women, SLE does not develop.

DESCRIPTION OF LESIONS

- The rash of NLE is a benign, self-limited eruption that appears at birth and tends to disappear by approximately 6 months of age.
- The rash is characterized by annular (ringlike) erythematous plaques or smaller erythematous patches that generally are apparent at birth or several days thereafter (FIG. 25.25).

CLINICAL MANIFESTATIONS

- NLE is characterized by either benign skin disease or congenital heart block, or both, in about 10% of cases.
- Involvement of joints, kidneys, and CNS is rare.
- Congenital heart block presents a 20% mortality risk and often requires the insertion of a pacemaker. The onset of heart block generally occurs a few weeks before term and is seen at birth.
- Unlike the skin lesions, the cardiac problems associated with NLE are permanent.

Dermatomyositis

BASICS

- Dermatomyositis is an inflammatory skin and muscle disease that is related to polymyositis; in fact, both conditions are considered to be the same disease except for the presence or absence of the rash. Cutaneous manifestations without detectable muscle disease are known as *amyopathic dermatomyositis*.
- The female-to-male ratio is 2:1.
- An autoimmune origin, which may be initiated by a virus in genetically susceptible people, has been proposed as a possible cause of dermatomyositis. As a result, antibodies that attack the skin and muscle are produced.
- An overlap syndrome with scleroderma or lupus (**mixed connective tissue disease**) is characterized by the presence of antiribonucleoprotein (anti-RNP) antibodies.
- Adults with dermatomyositis appear to have an increased risk of malignant diseases. The skin disease often follows the clinical course of exacerbations and remissions of the cancer. Most malignant diseases are the common cancers (e.g., colon and breast cancer) that occur in a general aging population.

DESCRIPTION AND DISTRIBUTION OF LESIONS

- The **heliotrope rash** consists of red or violaceous coloration around the eyes and is associated with periorbital edema (FIG. 25.26). (The change in color may be a subtle clinical finding, particularly in dark-skinned patients.)
- **Gottron's papules** consist of erythematous or violaceous, flat-topped papules on the dorsa of the hands (FIG. 25.27). Lesions are located on the joints of the fingers; they begin as papules and later become atrophic and hypopigmented.
- **Poikiloderma** is a characteristic rash of dermatomyositis, consisting of telangiectasia, atrophy, hyperpigmentation, and hypopigmentation. Poikiloderma occurs on the extensor aspects of the body, upper back (shawl sign), forearms, and "V" of the neck (see also FIG. 25.15). Atrophic lesions occur particularly on the knees and elbows.
- **Periungual telangiectasias** and nail dystrophy occur. Nail fold changes consist of periungual telangiectases and/or a characteristic hypertrophy of the cuticle (FIG. 25.28).

CLINICAL MANIFESTATIONS

- Progressive, bilateral, symmetric, proximal muscle weakness develops, as suggested by difficulty with brushing or combing hair and standing from a seated position.
- Muscle tenderness or pain is usually not a complaint.
- Photosensitivity is evidenced in areas of poikiloderma.
- Arthralgias occur in one third of patients.
- There may be features of an overlap syndrome.

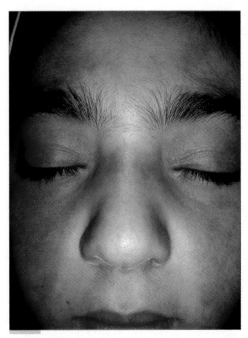

25.26 *Dermatomyositis.* This child has the characteristic heliotrope (pink-purple) erythema of the upper eyelids, as well as lesions on the cheeks, nose, and "butterfly" area, that are suggestive of SLE.

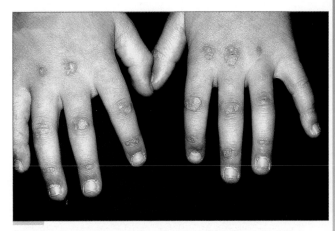

25.27 *Dermatomyositis.* Gottron's papules are violaceous, flat-topped papules located on the *knuckles* of the fingers in this child with juvenile dermatomyositis.

- Pulmonary fibrosis affects 10% of patients, particularly in the presence of anti-Jo 1 (histidine) or anti-PL 12 (alanine) antibodies.
- Evidence of vasculitis (e.g., palpable purpura or ulcers) may be present.
- Calcinosis cutis is seen in the juvenile form of dermatomyositis.
- Myocardial disease may be an associated finding.
- Dysphagia may occur.

DIAGNOSIS

- The findings on skin biopsy are often nonspecific but are generally suggestive of a connective tissue disease.
- Elevation of creatine phosphokinase levels is often a reliable indicator of muscle involvement.
- Aldolase levels may be increased.
- Electromyography may aid in the diagnosis.
- Muscle biopsy may aid in the diagnosis as well.
- The presence of autoantibodies, such as anti-DNA, anti-RNP, and anti-Ro, may be found. Anti-M-1 antibody is highly specific for dermatomyositis, but it is present in only 25% of patients.

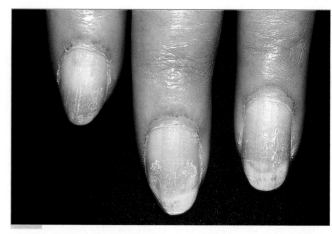

25.28 *Dermatomyositis.* Periungual telangiectasias are present. Note the thickening of the cuticles and the nail dystrophy in this patient.

 DIFFERENTIAL DIAGNOSIS

- SLE should be considered.
- Mixed connective tissue disease or overlap syndrome is another possibility.
- When only the muscle is involved, other myopathies should be considered.

 MANAGEMENT

Skin
- Avoidance of excessive sun exposure
- Use of broad-spectrum sunscreens
- Antimalarial drugs: hydroxychloroquine (**Plaquenil**), 5 mg/kg/day for 4 to 6 weeks; then titrate according to clinical response
- Low-dose oral **methotrexate**

Systemic Symptoms
- Physical therapy
- **Systemic steroids** (when used for systemic symptoms, may also improve skin conditions)

- Immunosuppressive therapy, including **low-dose oral methotrexate**
- **Cyclosporine**
- **Cyclophosphamide**
- **Azathioprine**
- **Plasmapheresis**
- **Interferons**
- **Intravenous high-dose γ-globulin**

 POINT TO REMEMBER

- The adult form of dermatomyositis may be associated with internal malignant diseases; patients older than age 50 years should be evaluated with this possibility in mind.

Scleroderma and Morphea

BASICS

- Scleroderma is an autoimmune connective tissue disease in which excess collagen results from an increase in number and activity of fibroblasts. Induration and thickening of the skin and subcutaneous tissues result. This process is triggered by vascular inflammation and infiltration of activated T4 cells.
- The origin of scleroderma is unknown. As in lupus, scleroderma may be seen either in a systemic or localized cutaneous form.

Classification

- Morphea, or localized scleroderma, is limited to the skin and has rarely been reported to progress to systemic scleroderma. The female-to-male ratio is 3:1.
- Systemic scleroderma may be divided as follows:
  - CREST syndrome (defined subsequently), which accounts for 90% of the cases of systemic sclerosis, is a relatively benign variant with a delayed appearance of visceral involvement.
  - Progressive systemic sclerosis is a chronic multisystem disease that affects the skin and internal organs and has a very poor prognosis.
  - In systemic sclerosis, the female-to-male ratio is 4:1.

DESCRIPTION OF LESIONS

Morphea

- A localized, indurated, hairless plaque has a characteristic "lilac" border (FIG. 25.29).
- Patients may have a single plaque or multiple plaques.
- White, ivory, or hyperpigmented permanent scars result when lesions heal.

CREST Syndrome and Progressive Systemic Sclerosis

- **Acrosclerosis** refers to ill-defined, indurated fibrotic skin, which occurs peripherally and gradually involves the forearms.
- **Sclerodactyly** consists of thickened, sausage-shaped digits in which the skin becomes tight and bound down. Gradually, the skin becomes shiny, stiff, waxy, and atrophic (FIG. 25.30).

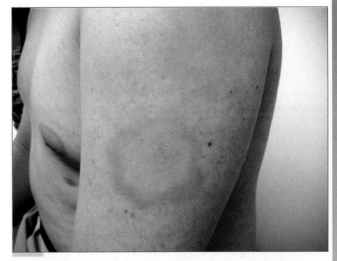

25.29 *Morphea.* This ivory-colored plaque has the characteristic "lilac" border. This boy has multiple plaques.

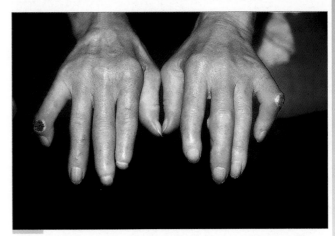

25.30 *Scleroderma with acrosclerosis and sclerodactyly.* The patient has tapered, shiny, stiff, waxy fingers. Note the painful vasculitic lesions on the fingertips.

DISTRIBUTION OF LESIONS

- In morphea, lesions are commonly found on the trunk; they may become widespread (generalized morphea) or linear (linear morphea), which may have the characteristic frontoparietal distribution (*coup de sabre*) (Fig. 25.31).
- In CREST syndrome, the cutaneous involvement is usually limited to acral areas (hands, feet, face, and forearms).
- Patients with progressive systemic sclerosis often have widespread, progressive disease.

CLINICAL MANIFESTATIONS

- Morphea (localized scleroderma) is generally asymptomatic, usually "burns out" spontaneously, and leaves a scar.
- CREST syndrome consists of the following:
  - *C*alcinosis cutis, most commonly occurring on the palms, fingertips, and bony prominences
  - *R*aynaud's phenomenon
  - *E*sophageal dysfunction
  - *S*clerodactyly ("claw deformity")
  - *T*elangiectasia (macular lesions) on the face, lips, palms, back of hands, and trunk
- Manifestations of progressive systemic sclerosis include the following:
  - Raynaud's phenomenon, often an early symptom, which consists of pain and a characteristic sequence of color changes of the distal fingers from white to purple to red in response to cold exposure
  - Diffuse involvement and symptoms secondary to the tightening of the skin, with difficulty in opening the mouth and loss of manual dexterity; later, contractures of the hands, painful fingertip ulcers resulting from vasculitis, and shortening of fingers resulting from distal bone resorption (Fig. 25.32)
  - Esophageal dysfunction, dysphagia, bloating, and diarrhea
  - Systemic symptoms including shortness of breath, difficulty in swallowing, and arthralgia
  - Masklike facies
  - Possibly, rapid progression of kidney disease, reduced breathing capacity, cardiac disease, and renal failure

DIAGNOSIS

Morphea
- The diagnosis is generally made on clinical grounds and skin biopsy.
- The serologic examination is generally negative.

CREST Syndrome
- The diagnosis is generally made on clinical grounds.
- Positive anticentromere antibody is seen in 70% of patients.

Progressive Systemic Sclerosis
- The diagnosis is generally made on clinical grounds.
- The Scl-70 antibody is present in approximately 30% of patients.

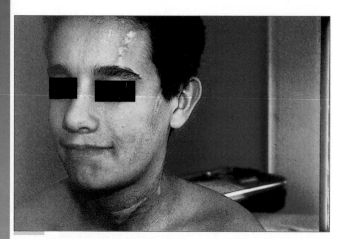

25.31 ***Linear morphea.*** Coup de sabre lesions are present.

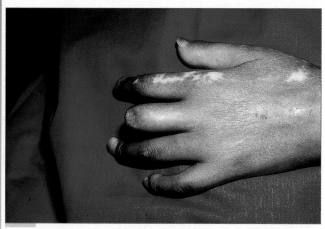

25.32 ***Scleroderma.*** Note the shortened finger resulting from distal bone resorption.

DIFFERENTIAL DIAGNOSIS

- Other connective tissue diseases
- Mixed connective tissue disease
- Overlap syndromes
- Lichen sclerosis

MANAGEMENT

Localized Scleroderma
- **Topical**, **intralesional**, and **systemic steroids** may be helpful in the early inflammatory stage.
- Vitamin D analogues (**calcitriol, calcipotriene**), **UVB, UVA,** and **methotrexate** may also be of some benefit.

CREST Syndrome and Progressive Systemic Sclerosis
These conditions are difficult to treat and remain a great challenge. The following agents and approaches have been used with minimal success:
- The following drugs are currently under investigation for this indication: **nifedipine, angiotensin-converting enzyme inhibitors, prostaglandins, immunosuppressive agents, D-penicillamine, colchicine, γ-interferon,** and **relaxin.**
- **Systemic steroids, minocycline,** psoralen and UVA light, **lung transplantation, autologous stem cell transplantation, etanercept,** and thalidomide have also been used.

POINT TO REMEMBER

- CREST syndrome has a more favorable prognosis than progressive systemic sclerosis, although visceral involvement may occur late in the course of the disease.

HELPFUL HINTS

- Therapy of systemic scleroderma should include full range-of-motion exercises.
- Some evidence suggests that some European cases of morphea may result from *Borrelia burgdorferi* infection. This connection has not been demonstrated in the United States.

Erythema Nodosum

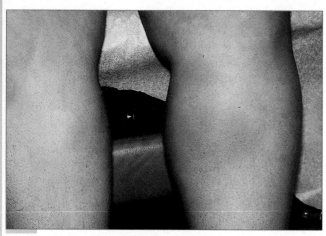

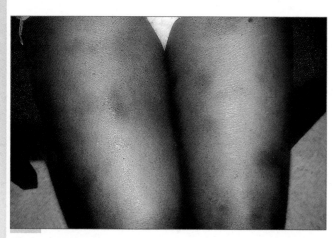

25.33 *Erythema nodosum.* Acute red, tender nodules appeared in this patient after she began taking oral contraceptives.

25.34 *Erythema nodosum.* These are healing "contusiform" lesions.

 MANAGEMENT

- Treatment is symptomatic, consisting of **bed rest, leg elevation**, **nonsteroidal anti-inflammatory drugs** (NSAIDs), or **iodides**.
- **Systemic corticosteroids,** which often bring dramatic improvement, can be used if an infectious cause is excluded.
- Treatment or avoidance of the underlying cause, if discovered, should be attempted.

BASICS

- Erythema nodosum (EN) is an acute inflammatory reaction of the subcutaneous fat. It is considered a delayed hypersensitivity reaction to various antigenic stimuli.
- EN is three times more common in females than in males and has a peak incidence between 20 and 30 years of age.
- Sarcoidosis, streptococcal infections, pregnancy, and the use of oral contraceptives are the most common causes of EN in the United States.
- In children, streptococcal pharyngitis is the most likely underlying cause.
- Approximately 40% of cases are idiopathic.
- In addition to sarcoidosis and pregnancy, EN is associated with a variety of conditions: deep fungal infections (in endemic areas), including coccidioidomycosis, histoplasmosis, and blastomycosis; tuberculosis; *Yersinia enterocolitica* infection; inflammatory bowel disease, including ulcerative colitis and Crohn's disease; malignant disease, including lymphoma and leukemia; radiation therapy; and Behçet's syndrome. Drugs such as sulfonamides, penicillin, gold, amiodarone, and opiates also have been implicated as causes of EN.

DESCRIPTION OF LESIONS

- Lesions begin as bright red, deep, extremely tender nodules (FIG. 25.33).
- During resolution, lesions become dark brown, violaceous, or bruiselike macules ("contusiform") (FIG. 25.34).

DISTRIBUTION OF LESIONS

- EN tends to occur in a bilateral distribution on the anterior shins, thighs, knees, and arms.

CLINICAL MANIFESTATIONS

- Malaise, fever, arthralgias, and periarticular swelling of the knees and ankles may accompany the panniculitis.
- Other symptoms may also be present, depending on the cause of EN.
- Spontaneous resolution of lesions occurs in 3 to 6 weeks, regardless of the underlying cause.
- Generally, EN indicates a better prognosis in patients who have sarcoidosis.

DIAGNOSIS

- The diagnosis of EN is usually made on clinical grounds, but a biopsy may be helpful for confirmation.

Laboratory Evaluation

- Usually, a complete blood count, erythrocyte sedimentation rate, throat culture, antistreptolysin titer, purified protein derivative skin test, and chest film are all that are necessary.
- A excisional skin biopsy will show panniculitis with infiltration of lymphocytes in the septa of the fat.
- Additional tests, such as gastrointestinal tract evaluation and serum angiotensin-converting enzyme determination, can be performed if suggested by the review of systems and physical examination.

BASICS

- Sarcoidosis is an example of a systemic disease in which cellular granulomatous infiltrates produce dermal skin lesions.
- Sarcoidosis is a chronic multisystemic disease of unknown origin. Most often, it presents with bilateral hilar adenopathy, pulmonary infiltration, eye lesions, and arthralgias; less commonly, there is involvement of the spleen and salivary and lacrimal glands, as well as gastrointestinal and cardiac manifestations.
- Sarcoidosis is seen most commonly in young adults, particularly in blacks in the United States and South Africa. It is also more common in Scandinavians.
- Of patients with sarcoidosis, 20% to 35% have cutaneous involvement. It usually accompanies systemic involvement but may be the only site of involvement.
- African-Americans have a greater risk of developing more serious problems such as cystic bone lesions, chronic uveitis, and chronic progressive disease.

DESCRIPTION OF LESIONS

- Specific lesions of cutaneous sarcoid include the following:
  - Dermal papules, nodules, or plaques that are brown or violaceous (FIG. 25.35).
  - Lesions that may be annular, serpiginous, or atrophic.
  - Lesions that can also appear on dorsa of hands, fingers, toes, and forehead.
  - **Lupus pernio,** a distinct variant, which consists of reddish purple plaques around the nose, ears, lips, and face (FIG. 25.36). Lupus pernio also occurs with a higher frequency in African-Americans and Puerto Ricans than in whites.
  - Subcutaneous nodules (**Darier-Roussy nodules**). These usually nontender, firm, oval, flesh-colored or violaceous 0.5- to 2-cm nodules are found on the extremities or trunk.
- Nonspecific cutaneous lesions associated with sarcoid include the following:
  - EN may occur in acute sarcoidosis (see the earlier discussion of EN). It more commonly affects Scandinavian populations.
  - Ichthyosis may be noted.

DISTRIBUTION OF LESIONS

- Lesions tend to be located periorifically (e.g., around the eyelids, nasal ala, tip of nose, earlobes, and lips).
- Lesions may occur in old scars anywhere on the body. Scars from previous traumas, surgery, venipuncture, or tattoos may become infiltrated and may be red or purple.
- Scalp lesions may produce scarring alopecia.
- Ichthyosiform and lesions of EN tend to occur on the pretibial area.

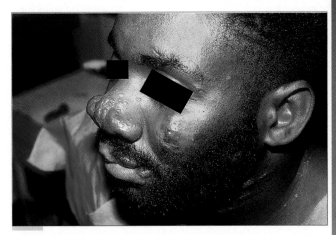

25.35 *Cutaneous sarcoidosis.* Dermal nodules are seen in a periorificial distribution (i.e., around the mouth, eyes, and nares). Note the sarcoidal lesions arising in the scars of this patient's neck.

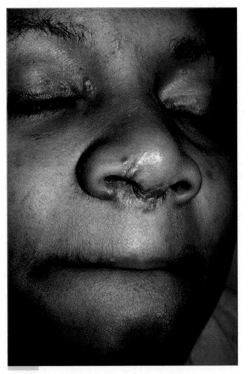

25.36 *Cutaneous sarcoidosis (lupus pernio).* These reddish purple and "apple jelly" beaded papules are located periorifically.

CLINICAL MANIFESTATIONS

- Skin lesions are generally asymptomatic; however, they are often of great cosmetic concern because they occur commonly on the face.
- EN associated with sarcoidosis generally resolves spontaneously and suggests a better prognosis.
- **Löfgren's syndrome** (EN and arthritis) is a clinical variant of sarcoidosis.

DIAGNOSIS

- "Apple jelly" nodules are seen on blanching lesions with a glass slide (diascopy). These nodules represent the gross appearance of granulomas.
- Skin biopsy demonstrates noncaseating granulomas (sarcoidal granulomas).
- A chest radiograph may demonstrate bilateral hilar adenopathy and other characteristic changes.
- Abnormal laboratory evaluations may include the following:
  - Elevated angiotensin-converting enzyme levels
  - Hypergammaglobulinemia
  - Hypercalcemia

HELPFUL HINTS

- Systemic steroids should not be used routinely to treat cutaneous lesions; rather, potent topical steroids, intralesional steroids, or oral antimalarials should be tried first. If possible, systemic steroids are best reserved for more serious systemic involvement.
- Oral antimalarials can lead to irreversible retinopathy and blindness. Eye examination is necessary before and during antimalarial therapy.
- Granulomatous acne rosacea may mimic sarcoidosis clinically and histopathologically. It is referred to as *lupus miliaris disseminatus faciei.*

DIFFERENTIAL DIAGNOSIS

Granuloma Annulare
- This condition is discussed in Chapter 4, "Inflammatory Eruptions of Unknown Cause."

Cutaneous Tuberculosis
- This is also known as lupus vulgaris.

MANAGEMENT

- **Potent topical steroids** are applied under occlusion, if necessary.
- **Intralesional steroid injections** can help flatten lesions.
- Oral **antimalarial agents** such as hydroxychloroquine (**Plaquenil**) and chloroquine are administered for therapeutically unresponsive or widespread disease.
- **Oral corticosteroids** should be used only on a short-term basis.
- If corticosteroids are not effective, **immunosuppressants** such as **methotrexate** and **azathioprine** may be effective. Other agents that have been used to treat cutaneous sarcoidosis include **cyclosporine, oral isotretinoin, allopurinol,** and **thalidomide. Chlorambucil** also has been reported to be effective, but the risk of malignant disease is great with this medication.

Reiter's Syndrome

BASICS

- Reiter's syndrome (RS), also referred to as reactive arthritis, is an idiopathic inflammatory process affecting the skin, joints, and mucous membranes. The classic triad of **urethritis, conjunctivitis,** and **arthritis** is found in only 40% of cases at the time of the initial clinical presentation.
- RS is seen most commonly in young white men of European origin.
- Initial symptoms often occur after nongonococcal urethritis (e.g., chlamydial infection) or infection with an enteric pathogen (e.g., *Shigella* and *Yersinia*).
- HLA-B27 is frequently positive in patients with RS and portends a poorer prognosis.

DESCRIPTION OF LESIONS

Skin lesions are often indistinguishable from psoriasis; however, RS often manifests certain characteristic findings such as the following:

- **Keratoderma blennorrhagicum** (FIG. 25.37) consists of scaly, red, inflammatory, psoriasislike lesions on the palms and soles. The lesions may have a thick scale and may be pustular.
- Scaling red plaques or erosions may be found on the glans penis (**circinate balanitis**) (FIG. 25.38).
- Nail changes may include findings such as those seen in psoriasis (e.g., onycholysis and subungual hyperkeratosis); furthermore, subungual pustules with resultant shedding of nails may occur.
- Oral lesions are usually painless, irregularly shaped, white plaques on the tongue that resemble geographic tongue.

DISTRIBUTION OF LESIONS

- Keratoderma blennorrhagicum is most often noted on the palms and soles.
- Psoriasislike plaques may be seen on the scalp, elbows, knees, buttocks, shaft of the penis, and scrotum.

CLINICAL MANIFESTATIONS

- RS is a multisystemic disease that may present with fever, malaise, dysuria, arthralgias, and red irritated eyes with accompanying cutaneous lesions.
- Frequently, RS has a self-limited course, but it may become a chronic, relapsing condition.
- RS is common in patients with human immunodeficiency virus (HIV) disease. (See Chapter 24, "Cutaneous Manifestations of HIV Infection.")
- The arthritis of RS is an asymmetric oligoarthritis that commonly involves large joints (elbows, knees); it may also

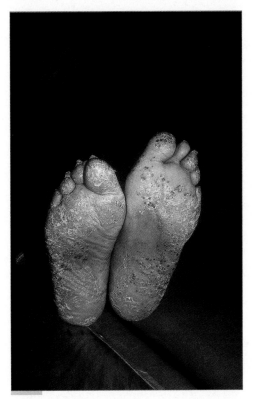

25.37 *Reiter's syndrome.* Keratoderma blennorrhagicum. Scaly, red-brown, inflammatory, pustular, psoriasislike lesions are present on the soles.

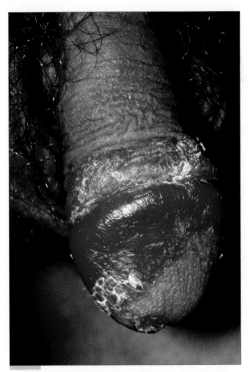

25.38 *Reiter's syndrome.* In circinate balanitis, psoriasiform lesions occur on the glans penis and the scrotum.

involve smaller joints. Sacroiliitis and ankylosing spondylitis may occur.

- Ocular disease may include conjunctivitis with intense red conjunctival injection and, less commonly, iritis and keratitis.
- Urethritis is a nonspecific urethral inflammation with a purulent exudate and dysuria.

DIAGNOSIS

- The diagnosis is generally made on clinical grounds.

Laboratory Evaluation

- HLA-B27 is positive in 75% of patients.
- ANA and rheumatoid factor are usually negative.
- The histopathologic features of skin lesions in RS are indistinguishable from those of psoriasis.
- HIV testing should be performed.

 DIFFERENTIAL DIAGNOSIS

Psoriasis with Arthritis
See Chapter 3, "Psoriasis."
- Psoriasiform skin lesions
- Arthritis similar to that seen in RS
- No ocular symptoms
- No urethritis

Behçet's Syndrome
- Painful oral ulcers
- Arthritis
- Iritis
- Vasculitic skin lesions

Candidal Balanitis
- Positive potassium hydroxide examination or fungal culture

 MANAGEMENT

Mild Cases
- RS may be treated with **topical steroids** for the skin lesions.
- **NSAIDs** are prescribed for pain.

Severe Cases
- Oral **methotrexate** is sometimes used on a weekly basis for severe cases.

- **Oral steroids** may be necessary; however, tapering of steroids can produce an extreme flare of the pustular lesions.
- Oral retinoids such as 13-*cis*-retinoic acid (**Accutane**) and acitretin (**Soriatane**) have also been used to treat skin lesions.
- **Methotrexate, cyclosporine, UVB/UVA,** and infliximab (**Remicade**) have also been used to treat the cutaneous manifestations.

 POINT TO REMEMBER

- During initial or recurrent episodes, most patients with RS do not manifest the complete triad of urethritis, conjunctivitis, and arthritis.

Pyoderma Gangrenosum

BASICS

- Pyoderma gangrenosum (PG) is an uncommon condition of uncertain origin.
- It is a unique, painful, inflammatory, ulcerative process of the skin.
- It is often seen in association with certain systemic diseases including ulcerative colitis, regional enteritis, rheumatoid arthritis, and leukemia; however, some investigators believe it to be a distinct disease.

DESCRIPTION OF LESIONS

- Skin ulcers are 2 to 10 cm in diameter.
- They are deep ulcerations with an erythematous to violaceous border. The border is often undermined (a probe can be placed under the overhanging edge of the lesion).
- Lesions may be multiple.
- Lesions heal with scarring (FIG. 25.39).

DISTRIBUTION OF LESIONS

- Skin ulcers are most commonly found on the lower extremities (shins and ankles).

CLINICAL MANIFESTATIONS

- Lesions can appear as a rapidly expanding, painful, skin ulcer (FIG. 25.40).
- It is usually self-limited, and spontaneous healing may occur.
- Patients often have associated oligoarticular arthritis.
- Ulcerations of PG occur after trauma or injury to the skin in some patients; this process is termed *pathergy.*
- Diseases associated with PG include the following:
  - Ulcerative colitis
  - Regional enteritis (Crohn's disease)
  - Rheumatoid arthritis
  - Myelogenous leukemia
- In 50% of patients, no underlying systemic disease is present.

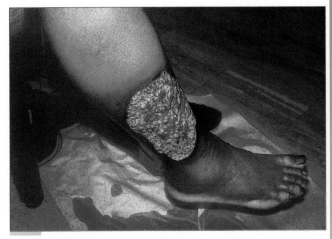

25.39 *Pyoderma gangrenosum.* This large ulceration is beginning to heal with a craterlike (cribriform) scar.

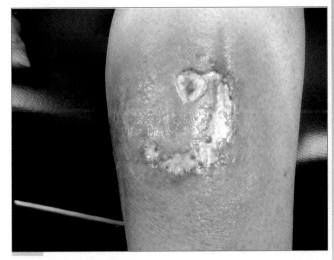

25.40 *Pyoderma gangrenosum.* This acute ulceration was initially considered to be a necrotic reaction to a spider bite. The patient was found to have regional enteritis (Crohn's disease).

DIAGNOSIS

- The diagnosis of PG is generally made on a clinical basis. This is often done by excluding other causes of similar-appearing cutaneous ulcerations including infection, stasis ulcers, malignant disease, vasculitis, collagen vascular diseases, diabetes, and trauma, as described subsequently.

Laboratory Evaluation

- Skin biopsy of the edge of the ulcer may be performed to rule out other causes of skin ulcers, such as infections or malignant disease; however, the pathologic findings for PG are nonspecific.
- Bacterial, fungal, and viral cultures of the ulcer are performed if clinically indicated.
- Workup for systemic disease should include complete blood count with differential, erythrocyte sedimentation rate, sequential multichannel autoanalyzer 20, ANA, Venereal Disease Research Laboratory test, rheumatoid factor, and a chest radiograph.
- Serum or urine protein electrophoresis, peripheral smear, and bone marrow aspirate are performed, if indicated, to evaluate for hematologic malignant diseases.
- A gastrointestinal series for inflammatory bowel disease should be done if clinically indicated.

 DIFFERENTIAL DIAGNOSIS

Cutaneous Malignant Diseases
- Basal cell carcinoma
- Squamous cell carcinoma

Infectious Processes
- Bacterial infections
- Deep fungal infections
- Herpes simplex virus infections

Inflammatory Processes
- Collagen vascular diseases
- Polyarteritis nodosa
- Behçet's disease
- Wegener's granulomatosis
- Antiphospholipid antibody syndrome

MANAGEMENT

- The treatment of underlying associated diseases does not necessarily promote the healing of PG.

Topical and Intralesional Therapy
- Local compresses, antiseptic washes, and topical antibiotics may be useful.
- **Superpotent topical corticosteroids, cromolyn sodium 2% solution, nitrogen mustard,** and **5-aminosalicyclic acid** may be tried.
- **Intralesional steroid injections** (triamcinolone acetonide, 10 mg/mL) are administered into the edge of the ulcer.

Systemic Therapy
- **Oral steroids** for several weeks to months (starting at 60 to 80 mg prednisone daily and tapering the steroid slowly). Systemic steroids may be given alone or in combination with **dapsone, azathioprine,** or **chlorambucil.**

In patients with steroid-resistant PG, **oral cyclosporine** has been shown to be effective.
- The following drugs have also met with some success: **mycophenolate mofetil (CellCept), tacrolimus, cyclophosphamide, thalidomide,** and **nicotine** chewing gum.
- Intravenous therapy can be administered using **pulsed methylprednisolone, pulsed cyclophosphamide,** or **human immunoglobulin.**
- **Surgical grafting** and **microvascular free flaps** are best reserved for after the disease has become inactive.

Other Therapies
- Hyperbaric oxygen has been used.
- Biologics such as etanercept (**Enbrel**), adalimumab (**Humira**), and infliximab (**Remicade**) may prove useful. See Chapter 3, "Psoriasis," for a discussion of the biologics.

 POINT TO REMEMBER

- Surgical débridement of the lesions of PG should be avoided, if possible, because of the pathergy that may occur with surgical manipulation or grafting. This can result in further wound enlargement.

Exfoliative Dermatitis

BASICS

- Exfoliative dermatitis (ED), known as *erythroderma* in the United Kingdom and *l'homme rouge* in France, refers to a total, or almost total, redness or scaling of the skin.
- It is an uncommon disorder seen more often in male patients; 50 years is the average age of occurrence.
- In children, ED most often is secondary to severe atopic dermatitis.
- In adults, psoriasis is the most frequently associated skin disease (see Chapter 3, "Psoriasis").
- ED may appear suddenly or gradually, occasionally accompanied by fever, chills, and lymphadenopathy.
- ED may be a stage in the natural history of severe eczematous dermatitis or psoriasis.
- Less commonly, ED has been reported as a finding in the following skin disorders:
  - Allergic contact dermatitis
  - Stasis dermatitis with secondary autoeczematization

- Papulosquamous dermatitis of acquired immunodeficiency syndrome
- Graft-versus-host disease
- Seborrheic dermatitis (Leiner's disease) in infants
- Pemphigus foliaceus
- Pityriasis rubra pilaris (a rare disorder of keratinization)
- ED may occur as a reaction to the following drugs: sulfonamides; penicillins; antimalarials; lithium; phenothiazines; barbiturates; gold; allopurinol; NSAIDs, including aspirin; captopril; codeine; and phenytoin.
- It may be a complication or presenting symptom of the following malignant diseases:
  - Mycosis fungoides (cutaneous T-cell lymphoma)
  - Sézary syndrome (leukemic variant of mycosis fungoides)
  - Hodgkin's disease
  - Non-Hodgkin's lymphoma and leukemia
- It is an idiopathic phenomenon in 20% to 30% of cases without any preceding dermatosis or systemic disease.

DESCRIPTION OF LESIONS

- Marked **generalized erythema** is followed by scaling (FIGS. 25.41 and 25.42).
- Pruritus may be severe.
- There is edema and increased warmth of the skin.
- Lymphadenopathy, usually a reactive type (**dermatopathic lymphadenopathy**), is often present.
- Unlike toxic epidermal necrolysis, ED spares the mucous membranes.

DISTRIBUTION OF LESIONS

- ED usually begins in a limited area; however, it may rapidly become generalized.

CLINICAL MANIFESTATIONS

- Unless patients have a known preexisting skin condition or concurrent physical evidence of a skin disease such as psoriasis, the clinical appearance and symptoms of most cases of ED tend to be similar, consisting of the following:
  - Erythema is followed by scaling.
  - Pruritus may develop.
  - Edema and increased warmth of skin are usually present.
  - Lymphadenopathy, usually a reactive type (dermatopathic lymphadenopathy) and secondary to the marked inflammatory changes in the skin, may be seen; however, lymphoma should be considered, particularly if the lymph nodes are large or unilateral.
  - Thermoregulatory disturbances are manifested by fever or, more frequently, by hypothermia. If widespread inflammation occurs, the barrier efficiency of the skin may be impaired secondary to extensive vasodilatation.
  - Protein loss secondary to a massive shedding of scale may occur, with resultant hypoalbuminemia.

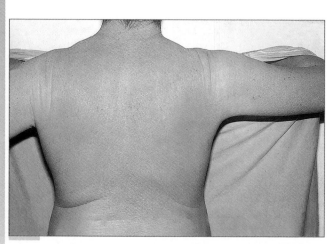

25.41 *Exfoliative erythroderma* (**exfoliative dermatitis**). This patient has generalized erythema (l'homme rouge, "red man syndrome"). The etiology of his erythroderma was never determined.

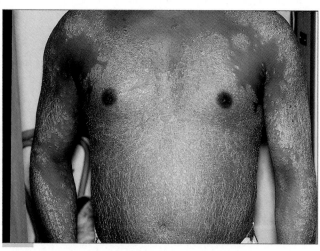

25.42 *Exfoliative erythroderma.* This patient has severe, widespread psoriasis. Note the marked scaling.

- Rarely, high-output cardiac failure may develop, particularly in patients with a history of cardiac disease.
- The following chronic changes may also be seen:
  - Scaling of palms and soles (keratoderma)
  - Thickening and lichenification of the skin
  - Scalp involvement, occasionally producing nonscarring alopecia
  - Nail dystrophy, onycholysis (separation of the nail plate from the nail bed), or nail shedding
  - Pigmentary changes (postinflammatory hypopigmentation or hyperpigmentation)
  - Persistent generalized erythema
  - Conjunctivitis, keratitis, or ectropion

DIAGNOSIS

- The diagnosis of ED is made on a clinical basis. The diagnosis of the underlying cause is often elusive. Clinical findings, such as the characteristic lichenification and crusting of atopic dermatitis or nail pitting that suggests psoriasis, may be found.
- Eliciting a history of drug ingestion or a preexisting dermatosis may be valuable.
- Laboratory testing can provide serologic evidence of Sézary's syndrome or leukemia.
- Patch testing during a period of remission may uncover a contact allergen.

Histopathology

- Histologic findings of the various causes are similar and are generally nondiagnostic; however, a diligent search for lymphoma, particularly mycosis fungoides, must be pursued with repeated skin biopsies.

Laboratory Evaluation

The following are possible positive laboratory findings:

- Anemia (usually the anemia of chronic disease)
- Decreased serum levels of protein and albumin
- Leukocytosis
- Eosinophilia
- Elevated sedimentation rate
- Elevated immunoglobulin E level (possibly supporting the diagnosis of atopic dermatitis)
- Leukemia (found by peripheral blood smear)
- Imaging studies with computed tomography or magnetic resonance imaging if lymphoma or Hodgkin's disease is suspected

DIFFERENTIAL DIAGNOSIS

- Toxic epidermal necrolysis is a potentially fatal condition that involves the skin and mucous membranes. Marked erythema is quickly followed by sloughing of the skin. This condition is often the result of a severe drug reaction.

MANAGEMENT

- Treatment is directed toward the underlying cause, if it is known. For example, suspected etiologic drugs or contactants should be eliminated.
- **Bed rest, cool compresses**, lubrication with emollients, antipruritic therapy with **oral antihistamines,** and **low- to intermediate-strength topical steroids** are used.
- Systemic antibiotics can be administered if signs of secondary infection are observed
- In severe cases, patients frequently require hospitalization, where measures such as fluid replacement, temperature control, expert topical skin care, and systemic corticosteroids may be used.
- Isotretinoin (**Accutane**) has been used when pityriasis rubra pilaris is the underlying cause

Exfoliative Dermatitis Secondary to Psoriasis

- Possible precipitating factors (e.g., ultraviolet exposure) or drugs that are suspected to provoke ED (e.g., antimalarials) should be avoided.
- **Systemic and topical steroids** are helpful, except that they may worsen psoriasis and have been known to precipitate ED or an acute fulminant form of pustular psoriasis, known as pustular psoriasis of Von Zumbusch. This worsening of psoriasis tends to occur after steroid withdrawal.

- If conservative therapy fails, **methotrexate, cyclosporine,** and **retinoids** (e.g., acitretin) are additional therapeutic options.
- Phototherapy, photopheresis, and photochemotherapy, as well as monoclonal antibodies such as infliximab (**Remicade**) and Adalimumab (**Humira**), may be effective.
- For a further discussion of psoriasis, see Chapter 3, "Psoriasis."

Prognosis

- The course of ED depends on its underlying origin. ED resulting from a drug eruption may clear in days to weeks, whereas in some cases, the disease may persist for many years, with exacerbations and remissions and no diagnosis.
- The prognosis of ED depends largely on the underlying etiology.
- In patients with an identified underlying cause, the course and prognosis generally parallel the primary disease.
- ED caused by a drug eruption usually clears when the drug is stopped.
- Acute, severe episodes, particularly in elderly persons or in persons with preexisting heart disease, have a more guarded prognosis.
- In patients with idiopathic ED, the prognosis is poor, and recurrences are not uncommon.

POINTS TO REMEMBER

- In its more severe manifestations, ED is a medical and dermatologic emergency. Consultation and ongoing management, using the expertise of both disciplines, are often necessary.
- In many cases, the underlying cause is never established.

Neurocutaneous Syndromes

Neurocutaneous diseases are genetically determined disorders that show both cutaneous and neurologic involvement.

Neurofibromatosis

BASICS

- Neurofibromatosis (NF), or **von Recklinghausen's disease,** is an autosomally inherited disease in which macular pigmented skin lesions (café au lait spots) and skin tumors (neurofibromas) occur in patients in whom a wide range of CNS or spinal cord lesions may ultimately develop.
- The incidence of NF is 4 per 10,000 births. Fifty percent of cases are thought to be inherited in an autosomal dominant fashion; the remaining cases are the result of spontaneous new mutations.
- There are two genetic types of NF:
  - NF1 is caused by a mutation in a gene on chromosome 17q11.2. This gene has been isolated and encodes neurofibromin. This protein may act as a tumor-suppressor gene by binding to Ras protein.
  - NF2, which is localized to chromosome 22q11, is characterized by bilateral acoustic neuromas and fewer skin manifestations. The protein for this gene has not been isolated, but it may also act as a tumor-suppressor gene.

DESCRIPTION OF LESIONS

- **Café au lait spots** are multiple, light brown macules that are greater than 1 cm in diameter (Fig. 25.43).
- **Cutaneous neurofibromas** are soft, rubbery, skin-colored or tan papules and nodules (Fig. 25.44).
- **Plexiform neuromas** manifest as large, drooping tumors, which on palpation feel like a "bag of worms" (Fig. 25.45).
- Axillary or inguinal freckling **(Crowe's sign)** consists of small pigmented macules in some patients and is considered to be pathognomonic for NF1 (Fig. 25.46).

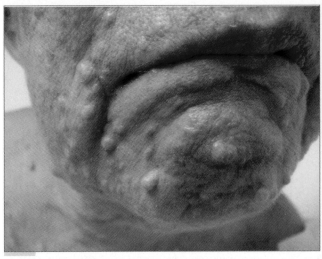

25.44 *Neurofibromatosis 1.* Soft, rubbery, flesh-colored papules and nodules are seen on this patient's face.

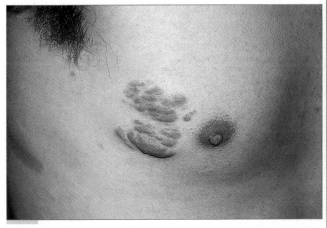

25.45 *Neurofibromatosis 1.* This plexiform neuroma feels like a "bag of worms."

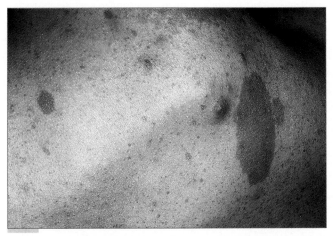

25.43 *Neurofibromatosis 1.* The multiple light brown macules are café au lait spots.

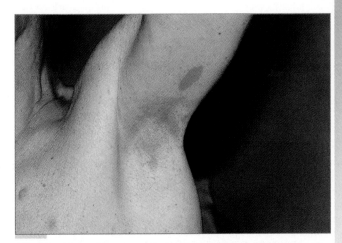

25.46 *Neurofibromatosis 1.* Crowe's sign (axillary "freckles") is considered pathognomonic for the disease.

DISTRIBUTION OF LESIONS

- Café au lait spots most often appear on the trunk and extremities.
- Neurofibromas may appear on the face, trunk, and extremities.

CLINICAL MANIFESTATIONS

- Café au lait spots are usually present at birth or shortly thereafter.
- Cutaneous neurofibromas may first develop in adolescence, and new lesions may continue to emerge during the patient's lifetime. Up to 5% of skin tumors may develop into neurofibrosarcomas.
- Ocular lesions (Lisch nodules) are asymptomatic, pigmented iris hamartomas seen in 80% of patients with NF.
- CNS tumors, optic gliomas, and spinal cord tumors may develop at any age.
- CNS involvement usually consists of benign lesions such as optic gliomas, acoustic neuromas, and meningiomas. CNS lesions may become astrocytomas.
- CNS involvement may occur in up to 10% of patients with NF.
- Spinal cord tumors may produce spinal cord damage and paraplegia.
- Many patients with NF have seizure disorders and mental retardation.
- Macrocephaly may be present in up to 16% of patients.
- Musculoskeletal disorders are uncommon, but pseudoarthrosis of the tibiae and kyphoscoliosis may be diagnostic in some patients with NF.
- Gastrointestinal symptoms may occur in some patients in whom intussusception and obstruction of the small intestine develop from intraabdominal neurofibromas.
- Endocrine disorders occur; 3% to 5% of affected children have sexual precocity associated with short stature.
- Pheochromocytomas characterized by life-threatening severe hypertension occur in less than 1% of patients with NF.

DIAGNOSIS

Neurofibromatosis 1

- Café au lait spots are seen in 10% to 20% of the general population; however, six or more café au lait spots that are greater than 0.5 cm in diameter in infants or greater than 1 cm in diameter in adults are supportive of the diagnosis of NF1.
- A first-degree relative with NF1 supports the diagnosis.
- Other findings supportive of the diagnosis include the following:
  - Crowe's sign
  - Lisch nodules
  - Distinctive osseous lesions such as sphenoid dysplasia or thinning of long bone cortex

Neurofibromatosis 2

- Bilateral masses of the eighth cranial nerve (acoustic neuromas) are suggestive.
- A first-degree relative with NF2 supports the diagnosis.

Laboratory Evaluation

- Skin biopsies of café au lait macules may show macromelanosomes on electron microscopy, but these findings are not diagnostic.
- Biopsies of neurofibromas show characteristic Schwann cells and neuronal cells.
- Magnetic resonance imaging studies of the brain and cervical spine may be helpful in NF1 patients with symptoms of CNS disease and in patients with suspected NF2 disease.

DIFFERENTIAL DIAGNOSIS

Segmental Neurofibromatosis

- Café au lait macules localized to one area of the body
- Cutaneous localized neurofibromas
- Absence of CNS tumors
- Lack of inheritance (somatic mutation)

McCune-Albright Syndrome

- Pigmented macular lesions
- Polyostotic fibrous dysplasia
- Precocious puberty

MANAGEMENT

- Surgical removal of symptomatic or disfiguring neurofibromas
- Follow-up for the development of neurofibrosarcomas, optic gliomas, acoustic neuromas, and pheochromocytomas
- Genetic counseling for patients and their families

Tuberous Sclerosis

BASICS

- Tuberous sclerosis (TS; **Bourneville's disease**) is a disease in which cutaneous lesions may be seen in association with hamartomatous tumors of the CNS and other organs. The classic triad of TS includes the following:
  - **Adenoma sebaceum**
  - **Epilepsy**
  - **Mental retardation,** although at least 50% of affected persons show no evidence of mental retardation
- TS, which is inherited in an autosomal dominant fashion, is found in fewer than 1 per 10,000 births.
  - Two genetic loci have been identified. The first gene (*TSC1*) is on chromosome q34 and produces tuberin. The second gene (*TSC2*) is on chromosome 16p13 and produces a second protein, hamartin.
  - Tuberin and hamartin are thought to act together to regulate cell differentiation and proliferation. Defects in these gene products may result in the growth of multiple hamartomas in TS.

DESCRIPTION OF LESIONS

- **Ash-leaf macules** are hypopigmented, characteristically oval, and sometimes linear or "confetti-shaped" macular lesions.
- So-called **adenoma sebaceum** (actually angiofibromas) are pink to reddish-brown, dome-shaped papules (FIG. 25.47).
- Periungual fibromas (**Koenen's tumors**) are smooth, firm, skin-colored papules.
- A pebbly, skin-colored "*peau d'orange*" or "pigskinlike" dermal plaque ("**shagreen patch**") has fine hypopigmentation resembling confetti.

DISTRIBUTION OF LESIONS

- Ash-leaf spots are more common on the trunk and proximal extremities.
- Adenoma sebaceum papules are symmetric in distribution and are most commonly located on the nose, nasolabial folds, and cheeks. More widespread distribution involves the forehead, ears, and scalp.
- Periungual fibromas occur around and under the nails on the periungual areas of the fingers and toes (FIG. 25.48).
- "Shagreen patches" appear on the trunk, most often in the lumbosacral region.

CLINICAL MANIFESTATIONS

- Ash-leaf macules and "shagreen patches" are usually present at birth.
- Adenoma sebaceum may begin to develop in late childhood and adolescence.

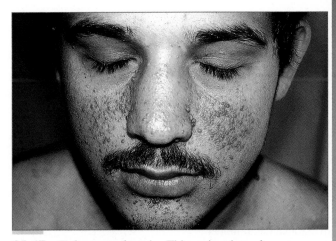

25.47 *Tuberous sclerosis.* This patient has adenoma sebaceum (angiofibromas). Note the similarity to acne lesions.

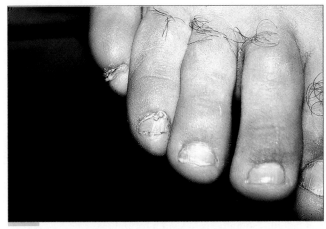

25.48 *Tuberous sclerosis.* Periungual fibromas (Koenen's tumors) are noted.

Central Nervous System Lesions

- Gliomatous brain tumors (tubers), which may calcify in 50% of patients
- Seizure disorders in 60% to 70% of patients, with fewer than 50% showing evidence of mental retardation
- Retinal and optic nerve gliomas

Other Findings

- In 50% to 60% of patients, cardiac rhabdomyomas of the atrium, which rarely cause cardiac obstructive disease
- Renal hamartomas
- In about 15% of patients, renal tumors (angiomyolipomas) and polycystic kidneys, which must be differentiated from renal carcinoma
- Gastrointestinal tumors with microhamartomatous polyps of the rectum
- Possible bone cyst formation and periosteal new bone growth and sclerosis

DIAGNOSIS

Two major or one major and two minor criteria are necessary for a definite diagnosis of TS.

Major Diagnostic Criteria

1. Adenoma sebaceum
2. Hypopigmented ash-leaf macules (three or more)
3. Shagreen patch
4. Periungual fibroma
5. Cortical tuber
6. Cardiac rhabdomyosarcoma
7. Subependymal nodule
8. Subependymal giant cell astrocytoma
9. Lymphangiomatosis
10. Renal angiolipoma

Minor Diagnostic Criteria

1. Multiple dental enamel pits
2. Hamartomatous rectal polyp
3. Bone cyst
4. Gingival fibroma
5. Nonrenal hamartoma
6. Retinal achromic patch
7. Confetti skin lesions: fine, hypopigmented macules (2 to 4 mm) that look as though they are "sprinkled" on the lower legs
8. Multiple renal cysts

Laboratory Evaluation

- Cranial magnetic resonance imaging
- Posteroanterior and lateral skull films (for adults) to demonstrate calcifications of gliomas of the brain
- Echocardiography for rhabdomyomas
- Renal ultrasonograms to search for tumors
- Skin biopsy of cutaneous lesions

DIFFERENTIAL DIAGNOSIS OF ADENOMA SEBACEUM

Acneiform Papules

- They often resemble adenoma sebaceum.
- Acne has a waxing and waning course.
- A skin biopsy is necessary only if the diagnosis is in doubt.

MANAGEMENT

- Follow-up of infants with ash-leaf spots to monitor the development of seizure disorder or mental retardation
- Follow-up of patients with TS to monitor the development of cardiac or renal lesions
- Removal of cosmetically objectionable or disfiguring adenoma sebaceum by **excision, electrocautery, dermabrasion**, or **laser resurfacing**
- Surgical removal of painful periungual fibromas
- **Genetic counseling** of patients with TS and their families after computed tomographic scanning is performed on the parents and siblings of the affected patient (these studies have demonstrated CNS lesions in asymptomatic parents of TS patients)

PART THREE

Dermatologic Procedures

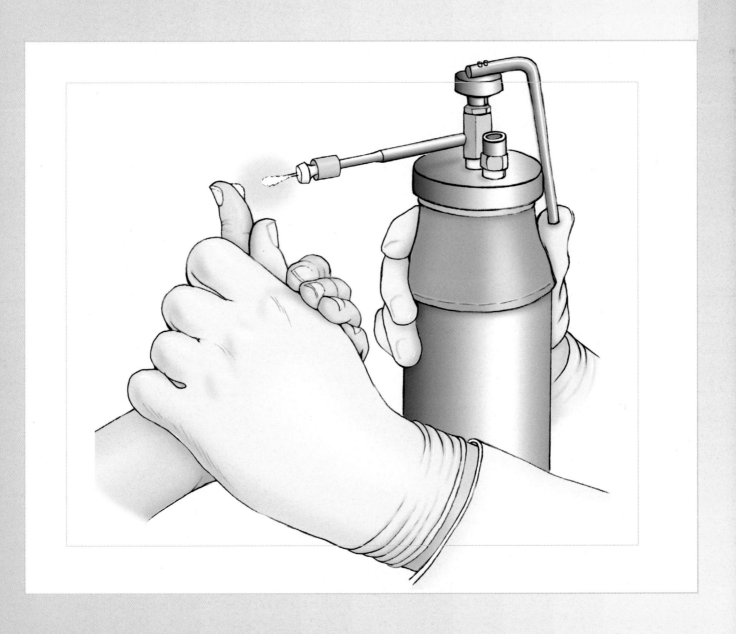

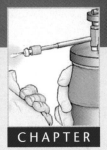

Diagnostic and Therapeutic Procedures

OVERVIEW

- Because of the ready availability of the skin to examination, a number of diagnostic measures—many of which are non-invasive—can lead to a specific diagnosis.
- Examples include potassium hydroxide (KOH) examination and fungal culture (see later discussions), Tzanck preparation (see FIG. 6.26), scabies preparation (see FIG. 20.18), Wood's light examination (see FIG. 14.4), and patch testing (see FIG. 2.33).
- Skin biopsies using punch, shave, snip, or excisional methods are relatively free of complications.
- Therapeutic modalities such as cryosurgery (see later discussion), phototherapy (discussed in Chapter 3, "Psoriasis") and advanced surgical procedures such as Mohs' micrographic surgery (see later discussion) are but a few of the many available treatments for skin disorders.

➤ **FUNGAL TESTS**

- Potassium hydroxide test
- Fungal culture

➤ **SKIN BIOPSY**

- Local anesthesia
- Shave biopsy and shave removal
- Scissor (snip) biopsy and snip excision
- Punch biopsy

➤ **SIMPLE ELLIPTICAL EXCISION**

- Undermining technique
- Wound closure
- Suture material
- Suturing

➤ **COMEDO EXTRACTION**
   SIMPLE PUNCH BIOPSY METHOD TO REMOVE CYSTS
   ELECTRODESICCATION AND CURETTAGE

- Curettage
- Electrodesiccation

➤ **CRYOSURGERY**

- Cotton tip applicator technique
- Cryospray technique
- Postoperative course and wound care

➤ **MOHS' MICROGRAPHIC SURGERY**
   DRESSINGS AND WOUND MANAGEMENT

Potassium Hydroxide Test

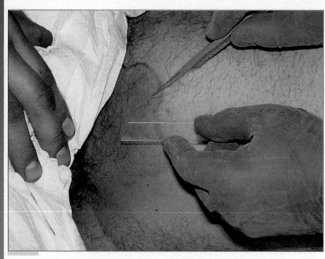

26.1 *Potassium hydroxide examination.* Collection of scale from the "active" border of a lesion.

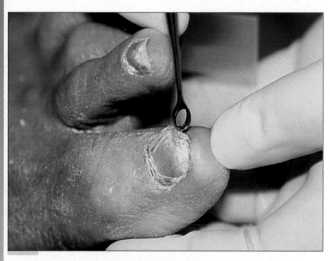

26.2 *Potassium hydroxide examination.* Collection of scale from under the nail after trimming.

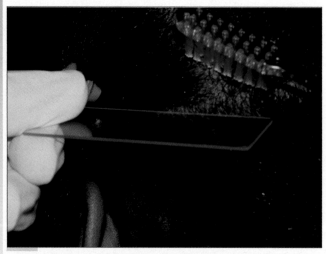

26.3 *Potassium hydroxide examination.* Collection of scale from the scalp of a child using a toothbrush.

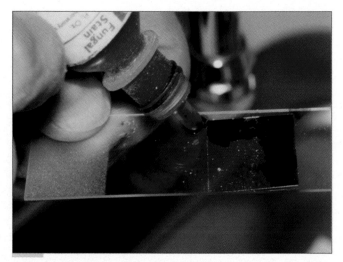

26.4 *Potassium hydroxide examination.* A single drop of a KOH solution is placed at the edge of the coverslip.

BASICS

- The KOH examination has the advantage of providing an immediate diagnosis of a superficial fungal infection, rather than having to wait weeks for the results of a fungal culture.
- It is a simple, rapid method to detect fungal elements in skin, nails, and hair.

TECHNIQUE

Collection of Specimen

- Collection is optimal when no surface artifacts (e.g., topical medications) are present.

Skin

- Gently scrape scale from the "active border" with a no. 15 scalpel blade (FIG. 26.1).

Nails

- Trim the nail.
- Use a no. 15 scalpel blade or a 1- to 2-mm curette (FIG. 26.2) under the nail surface to obtain scale.

Hair

- Pluck broken hairs with forceps or use a toothbrush to obtain scale and hairs (FIG. 26.3).

Preparation

- Use a KOH solution such as Swartz-Lamkins fungal stain or a KOH solution with dimethyl sulfoxide.
- Gather a thin layer of scale or scale plus hair on a slide and cover it with a coverslip.
- With an eyedropper, place a single drop of a KOH solution at the edge of the coverslip and allow it to spread under the coverslip by capillary action (FIG. 26.4).

- Heat the undersurface of the slide gently with a lighter or a match until bubbling begins.
- Blot excess KOH solution with tissue paper held at the edge of the coverslip.

Observation
- Examine under low light intensity (condenser down).
- Begin with a low-power scan to identify scale and possibly hyphae.
- Become aware of artifacts that are easily confused with hyphae and spores, such as hairs, clothing fibers, keratinocyte cell borders, and air bubbles (FIG. 26.5).
- Use high power to confirm the presence of hyphae or spores (FIGS. 26.6–26.11).

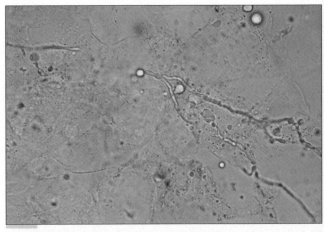

26.6 *Potassium hydroxide examination.* Dermatophyte. Note the wavy, branched hyphae with uniform widths coursing over cell borders.

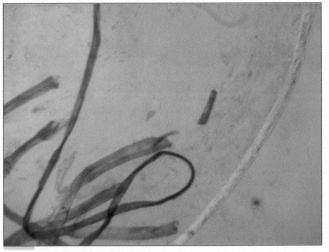

26.5 *Potassium hydroxide examination.* Artifacts. Note the clothing fibers on the left and the single hair shaft on the right.

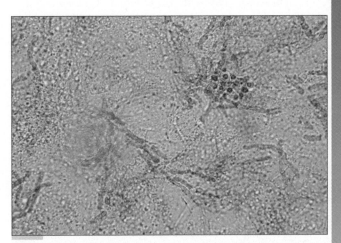

26.7 *Potassium hydroxide examination.* Tinea versicolor. Note the short, stubby hyphae ("spaghetti") and the clusters of spores ("meatballs").

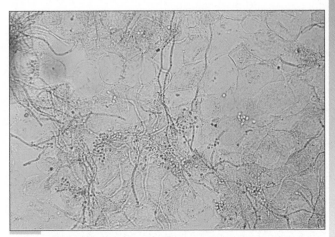

26.8 *Potassium hydroxide examination.* *Candida.* Spores and pseudohyphae (spores lack septae).

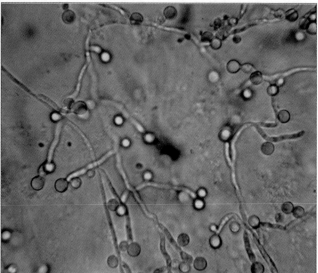

26.9   *Potassium hydroxide examination.* *Candida.*
Pseudohyphae with budding spores (higher magnification).

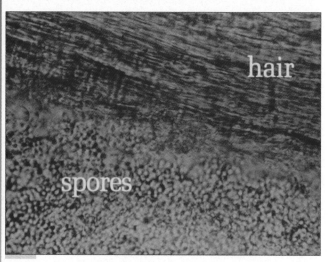

hair

spores

26.10   *Potassium hydroxide examination.* Ectothrix. Note the spores outside the hair shaft.

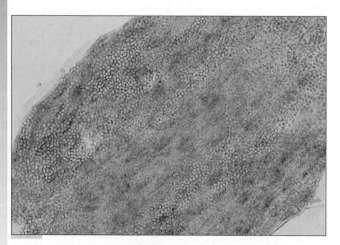

26.11   *Potassium hydroxide examination.* Endothrix.
Note spores inside the hair shaft ("sack of marbles").

Culture

- Place fungal cultures on Sabouraud's agar or on Dermatophyte test medium and incubate for 1 to 4 weeks (FIG. 26.12).
- Clinical Laboratory Improvement Act guidelines may require the practitioner to use outside laboratory facilities for performing fungal cultures.

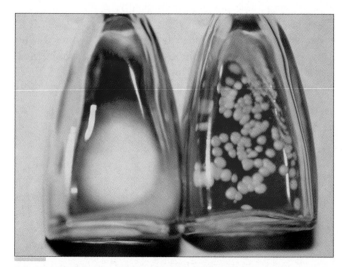

26.12   *Fungal culture using the Dermatophyte test medium.* Note the positive result on the left indicated by the color change from yellow to red and the monomorphic colony growth. On the right are discrete mucoid growths of a yeast contaminant that confirm that the color change to red is a false-positive result.

- Various skin biopsy techniques are available to the practitioner: shave biopsy, scissor or snip biopsy, punch biopsy, and excisional biopsy. The surgical tools and approaches vary according to size, shape, depth, and location of a lesion.
- Obtaining the appropriate amount of tissue to provide adequate information about the disease is the most important factor to keep in mind when deciding on the proper biopsy technique.
- Do not choose the biopsy specimen site indiscriminately.
  - Evaluate the site according to the clinical impression, the lesion's location, the estimated depth of the pathologic process, the planned tissue studies, and the ensuing cosmetic result.
  - The choice of biopsy technique requires some knowledge of where the pathologic process is likely to be located.

Local Anesthesia

Methods to decrease pain caused by injections include the following.

- Use a small, 30-gauge needle.
- Add a buffer (sodium bicarbonate) to the lidocaine.
- Inject very slowly.
- Distract the patient by talking continuously.
- Minimize the number of injection sites by reinjecting into areas that are already numb.

Shave Biopsy and Shave Removal

BASICS

- This is used for the diagnosis and therapeutic removal of superficial (epidermal and upper dermal) skin lesions, such as melanocytic nevi, warts, seborrheic and solar keratoses, pyogenic granulomas, and skin tags, as well as other benign and malignant skin tumors.
- It is used to obtain biopsy specimens to confirm skin disease before a more definitive surgical procedure (e.g., basal or squamous cell carcinoma).
- It is very useful for flattening and diagnosing nevi, particularly in the facial area.

Advantages

- It is fast and economical.
- The technique is easy to learn.
- Wound care is simple.
- Cosmetic results are generally excellent.
- It does not use sutures.
- It is useful for difficult-to-reach sites (e.g., ear canal, orbit of the eye).
- It is useful in areas of poor healing (e.g., the lower leg in elderly or diabetic patients).

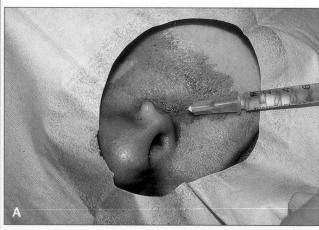

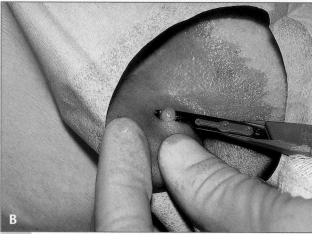

26.13 A and B *Shave biopsy.* **A:** Local anesthesia creates a wheal that elevates the lesion above the surrounding skin. **B:** The lesion is stabilized with the free hand; the blade, which is parallel to the skin surface, is drawn through the lesion.

Disadvantages

- It is not indicated for lesions that extend into the subcutaneous layer.
- It is not indicated when a full-thickness biopsy is necessary (e.g., inflammatory dermatoses).
- It should not be performed on lesions suspected of being melanoma because of the difficulty in clinically determining the maximum thickness or extent of a lesion.

TECHNIQUE

- Anesthetize the area adjacent to the lesion with an injection into the superficial dermis with 1% plain lidocaine using a 30-gauge needle. If necessary, use epinephrine in a 1:100,000 or 1:200,000 dilution. Use lidocaine without epinephrine in finger and toe areas to avoid vascular compromise.
- Administer local anesthesia with lidocaine to create a wheal and elevate the lesion above the surrounding skin (FIG. 26.13A).
- Apply traction with the thumb and index finger of the free hand on either side of the lesion to stabilize it.
- Place a no. 15 scalpel blade flat on the skin; use in a slight sawing motion with smooth strokes parallel to the skin surface and draw the middle of the blade through the lesion (FIG. 26.13B).
- Release traction when the lesion becomes sufficiently free; use small forceps with teeth to hold and elevate the lesion to complete the "shave" and then to deliver it to a bottle of formalin.
- Use electrocautery or further shaving to "feather" jagged edges.
- Apply Monsel's solution (ferric subsulfate) or aluminum chloride 35% with a cotton pledget (Q-Tip) to rapidly achieve hemostasis. Hemostasis is possible only if the field is wiped dry of blood.
- Send all pigmented lesions to a pathologist; nonpigmented skin tags do not need to be sent for pathologic evaluation.

Scissor (Snip) Biopsy and Snip Excision

BASICS

- Various lesions can be removed from the skin in a short period of time.
- Certain elevated or pedunculated lesions, such as warts, nevi, seborrheic keratoses, and skin tags, are ideally suited for removal with scissors. Many can be precisely removed level to the skin.

Advantages

- It is fast; many lesions can be removed in one visit.
- It is economical.
- Frequently, it can be performed without anesthesia.

Disadvantages

- None exist, except for the possibility of obtaining an inadequate amount of tissue if a specimen is to be sent for histopathologic examination.

TECHNIQUE

- It may be possible to snip off thin, small lesions without any anesthesia; larger lesions require the administration of local anesthesia. Anesthetize the area of larger lesions in the same manner as for scalpel shave excisions.
- Gently hold the lesion with small forceps without teeth and pull it to cause slight tenting of the epidermis and upper dermis (Fig. 26.14).
- Use straight or curved sharp iris scissors with fine points to snip off the lesion.
- Use light electrodesiccation at the base of the lesion, or apply a styptic (e.g., Monsel's solution) or aluminum chloride 35% to cause hemostasis (stinging or burning may result if the lesion has not been anesthetized). Local pressure also is effective in preventing blood flow.
- Trim away any slight elevation or irregularity of the margin with scissors.

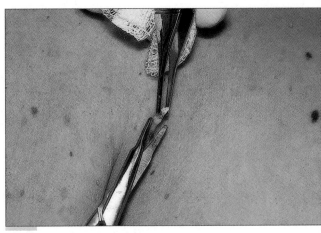

26.14 *Snip excision.* This filiform wart is snipped off after having been anesthetized with lidocaine.

Punch Biopsy

BASICS

- Performance of a punch biopsy involves the use of a 3- to 5-mm cylindric cutting instrument ("punch") to remove all or part of a lesion.
- This method is most useful for biopsy of relatively flat, inflammatory lesions such as seen in psoriasis, lichen planus, and vasculitis.

Advantages

- The specimen obtained is uniform.
- This is an effective method to evaluate inflammatory skin diseases.
- It is an efficient biopsy method for full-thickness skin.
- The operative site heals rapidly.
- Skin closure establishes a barrier to infection almost immediately after the procedure.

Disadvantages

- The sample may not adequately show the entire lesion; a second technique (i.e., an elliptic biopsy) may be necessary for adequate demonstration of tumor architecture.
- It is not suited for lesions primarily located in the subcutaneous tissue.
- Areas to be avoided are the digits, around the facial nerve, or in any region where the operator is unfamiliar with the underlying anatomy.

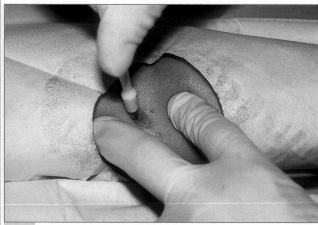

26.15 *Punch biopsy.* Traction of surrounding skin is provided by the fingers while the punch is rotated.

TECHNIQUE

- In contrast to shave biopsy, a more thorough approach to sterile technique is necessary.
- Cleanse the lesion and surrounding skin with 70% isopropyl alcohol, povidone-iodine (**Betadine**), or chlorhexidine (**Hibiclens**).
- Anesthetize the area with an injection into the deep dermis of 1% plain lidocaine using a 30-gauge needle. If necessary, use epinephrine in a 1:100,000 or 1:200,000 dilution (Fig. 26.15).
- With the fingers of the nondominant hand, stretch the skin at a 90-degree angle to the natural wrinkle lines.
- Hold the punch between the thumb and forefinger.
- Gently push the punch downward into the dermis while advancing it slowly and twirling it back and forth until it "gives." Caution should be used over thin tissue or over vital structures.
- It is important to push the punch deep enough to obtain underlying fat tissue for an adequate sample.
- Withdraw the punch along with the tissue sample. If the sample does not come out with the punch, cut it at the base while depressing the surrounding skin.
- Remove the tissue specimen with forceps with teeth and then cut the specimen, if necessary, with iris scissors. Take care to avoid crushing the specimen and distorting the tissue sample.
- Place firm pressure on the circular skin wound to curtail bleeding.
- A single suture for closure is all that is usually necessary.

BASICS

- Excisions are useful for obtaining tissue samples for biopsy specimens and for the removal of many benign and cancerous lesions.
- **Excisional biopsies** may be performed on discrete lesions, such as cysts, basal or squamous cell carcinomas, malignant melanomas, or other solitary tumors and nevi.
- An **incisional biopsy** is the incomplete or partial removal of a lesion that may be too big or poorly located to perform a complete excision (e.g., a suspected melanoma that is too large to remove).

Advantages

- It provides a more extensive tissue sample of a lesion that is too large for a shave or a punch biopsy.
- The margins of submitted tissue can be examined for possible involvement (e.g., basal cell carcinoma, squamous cell carcinoma and melanoma).
- It often affords a definitive cure for many benign and malignant lesions.

Disadvantages

- It is time-consuming.
- It is less economical than shaves or snips.
- It usually requires a return visit for suture removal.

TECHNIQUE

- The operator should be familiar with the underlying and surrounding anatomy.
- A thorough approach to sterile technique is necessary: sterile gloves and sterile drapes should be used.
- To achieve the best cosmetic results, place the lines of incision in or parallel to the relaxed skin tension lines. This placement is demonstrated by observing wrinkle lines and the effect of pinching the skin.
- Once a direction for the long axis of the ellipse has been chosen, draw an ellipse around the lesion before administering a local anesthetic. This approach minimizes tissue distortion, which may cause difficulty in subsequent planning of the ellipse. Use gentian violet or a surgical skin marker to mark the skin.
- Make sure that the excision has a length-to-width ratio of at least 3:1 and that the apices are at a 30-degree angle.
- Anesthetize the area by local infiltration with lidocaine and epinephrine 1:100,000.
- Use a No. 15 scalpel blade to make the incision. Use the dominant hand with the index finger and thumb of the other hand placed on either side of the incision. This pushes the skin under tension downward and away from the scalpel (FIG. 26.16 A).
- Start the incision using the point of the scalpel held in a vertical position at the apex of the ellipse (FIG. 26.16 B). Use the belly of the scalpel along the side of the ellipse to elongate the incision.

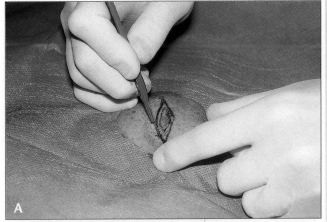

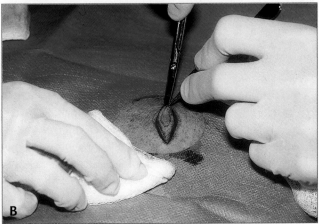

26.16 A and B *Excision.* **A:** The incision is started using the point of the scalpel, held in a vertical position, at the apex of the lesion. Traction is accomplished with the nondominant hand. **B:** The tissue is dissected free of the underlying fat. Forceps are used to hold the apex of the skin being removed.

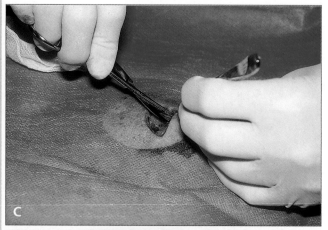

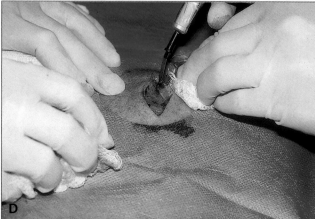

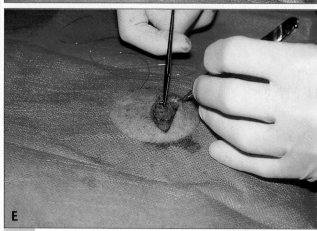

26.16 C, D and E *Excision.* **C:** Undermining is performed using blunt-tipped scissors while the skin edge is elevated by forceps. **D:** Hemostasis is achieved with an electrocautery device. **E:** Deeper, nonabsorbable sutures are used to approximate the wound edges.

- Obtain an optimal tissue sample for histologic examination. The scalpel should cut through the full thickness of the skin, including the upper subcutaneous fat.
- Dissect the tissue free of the underlying fat after making incisions on both sides of the ellipse. Use forceps with teeth to hold the apex of the skin being removed.
- If the defect is large, dissect (undermine) the ellipse using curved, blunt-tipped scissors (e.g., **Steven's tenectomy** or **Gradle scissors**), making certain that the plane of the dissection is at the same level throughout. Undermining allows for the mobilization of tissue so that it can be advanced to close the defect; it also allows skin edges to come together with less tension and allows eversion of the wound edges with suturing.

Undermining Technique

- To perform undermining, use blunt-tipped scissors while elevating the skin edge by forceps with teeth or a skin hook (Fig. 26.16 C).
- Advance scissors to the desired degree and open them to stretch the underlying skin. If necessary, repeat this procedure several times to achieve the desired skin mobility for wound closure.
- Remove any remaining tissue septa using the open blades of the scissors.
- Undermining is most effective when performed at the level of superficial fat tissue. This reduces the possibility of injury to nerves and blood vessels in the facial and neck areas.
- Wound repair is facilitated if an adequate ellipse has formed, the edges are perpendicular to the skin, and skin lines are followed.
- Meticulous hemostasis must occur after undermining. Apply direct pressure or perform electrocoagulation (Fig. 26.16 D).
- Place subcutaneous sutures after undermining; this will allow approximation of the edges of the wound to close the wound (Fig. 26.16 E).

Wound Closure

- Wounds should be closed in layers.
- The closure of dead space is necessary when large, subcutaneous vacuities have been created, such as after removal of subcutaneous cysts.
- Dermal, buried sutures are important on areas of the body that overlie large muscle groups, such as the upper trunk.

Suture Material

- Obtain hemostasis (a "dry field") before initiating wound closure.
- Choice of suture material depends on the size and degree of tension on the wound and the area of placement.
- For facial or limb areas, **Vicryl** or **Dexon** sutures are suitable for the deeper layers as they are absorbable. 5-0 or 6-0 synthetic (**Prolene** or **Ethilon**) sutures are recommended for epidermal closure on the face.
- On the upper trunk, greater skin support is required for proper wound closure. Therefore, **Maxon** or polydioxanone sutures are recommended; 3-0 or 4-0 are preferred.
- An absorbable suture, Monocryl, is very easy to handle, causes little tissue reaction, excellent tensile strength, and lasts up to 3 months in tissue.

Suturing

- Simple, interrupted skin sutures are most commonly used in this procedure.
- The method of "halving" is the most effective technique for wound closure. "Halving" allows for equal distribution of wound tension (FIG. 26.16 F).
- Place the first suture in the center of the ellipse.
- Place the second and third sutures in the centers of the remaining wound lengths.
- Repeat this procedure until the wound is completely closed.
- Apply an occlusive dressing (a perforated plastic film or sheet with an absorbable pad) or pressure dressing, if necessary, to prevent postoperative bleeding (FIG. 26.16 G).
- Suture removal depends on wound tension, area of location, and depth of placement.
- Generally, removal of facial sutures may be necessary in 5 days; removal of sutures in the trunk and extremities may be required in 1 to 2 weeks.

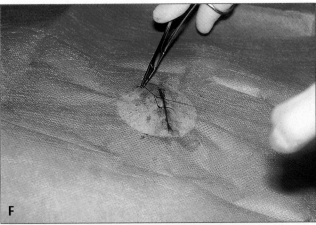

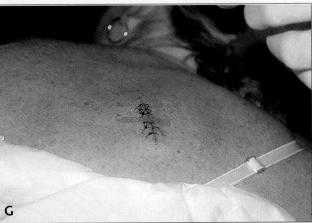

26.16 F and G *Excision.* **F:** Closure. Interrupted skin sutures are placed using the method of "halving." The first suture was placed in the center of the ellipse. **G:** Dressing. A transparent dressing overlying Steri-Strips allows for visualization of the wound as it heals.

Comedo Extraction

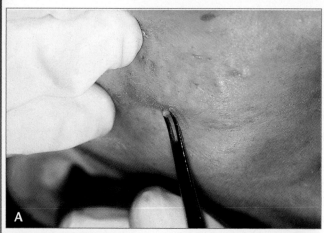

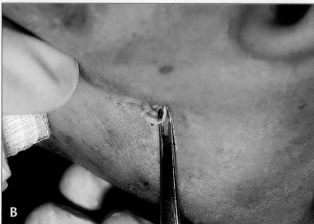

26.17 *Comedo extraction.* **A:** Gentle pressure is exerted along the rim of this closed comedo. **B:** The contents are extruded.

- Removal of comedones involves a comedo extractor, an instrument that minimizes skin injury. Use a round loop extractor to apply uniform, smooth pressure to dislodge comedonal contents (FIGS. 26.17 A and B).
- To loosen lesions that offer resistance, insert a pointed instrument, needle, or a no. 11 blade to carefully incise and expose the contents.
- Extraction can be a useful adjunct to topical therapy when blackheads and whiteheads are somewhat resistant to topical retinoids.
- Pretreatment with a topical retinoid for 4 to 6 weeks often facilitates the procedure. Performance of comedo extraction is now less common since the use of topical retinoids.

Simple Punch Biopsy Method to Remove Cysts

- A large lesion such as an epidermoid or pilar cyst can be removed through a small hole and heals with excellent aesthetic results.
- If the results of this procedure are not completely satisfactory, a standard excision can be performed at a future date.

TECHNIQUE

- Superficially administer local anesthesia over the cyst (FIG. 26.18 A).
- Punch the center of the cyst (the "pore") with a 4-, 6-, or 8-mm disposable punch (FIG. 26.18 B).
- Dissect the cyst wall using forceps, iris scissors, and manual pressure around the cyst (FIGS. 26.18 C and D).
- Close the defect with a 4-0 nylon stitch.

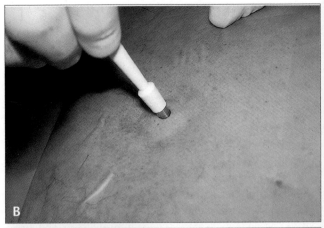

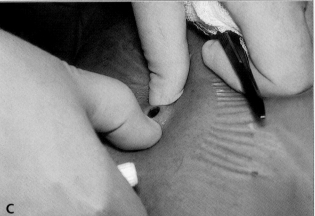

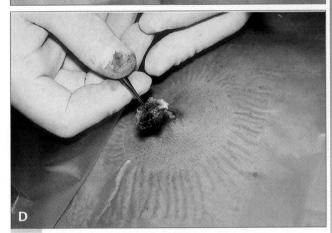

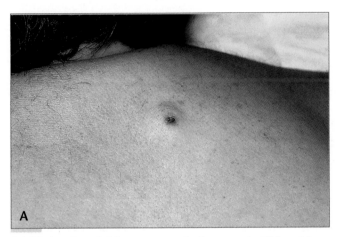

26.18 A   *Punch biopsy removal of a cyst.* **A:** This epidermoid cyst has a central "pore."

26.18 B, C and D   *Punch biopsy removal of a cyst.* **B:** A 6-mm disposable punch creates an opening. **C:** After dissection with iris scissors, pressure is exerted with the operator's thumbs. **D:** The cyst wall is extracted.

BASICS

- The technique of electrodesiccation and curettage is a means to remove or destroy many types of benign superficial skin lesions such as warts, seborrheic keratoses, solar keratoses, pyogenic granulomas, and skin tags.
- In experienced hands, it is often used as a method to treat skin cancers such as small basal cell and squamous cell carcinomas.
- Electrodesiccation uses monopolar high-frequency electric currents to destroy lesions; curettage is a scraping or scooping technique performed with a dermal curette, which has a round or oval sharp ring.
- Electrodesiccation without curettage (as an alternative to shave procedures) is often used to eliminate warts, skin tags, and spider angiomas and to flatten lesions (e.g., melanocytic nevi). Conversely, curettage without electrodesiccation may also be used to remove many of these epidermal lesions.
- Curettage is a "blind technique" in which the specimen cannot be examined for margin control.

Advantages

- It is fast and economical.
- It is useful for difficult-to-reach sites, e.g., ear canal, orbit of the eye.
- It is useful in areas of poor healing, e.g., the lower leg in elderly or diabetic patients.
- Secondary infection is uncommon.

Disadvantages

- The procedure is "blind"; margins of lesions can only be guessed.
- Cosmetic results are unpredictable; hypopigmentation and scarring may result.
- Healing is by secondary intention and takes 2 to 3 weeks, which is longer than healing after an excisional procedure.
- Obtaining biopsy specimens from curettage is discouraged.

Curettage

TECHNIQUE

- Anesthetize the area to be biopsied in a similar manner to that described in the sections "Skin Biopsy" and "Shave Biopsy and Shave Removal." The local anesthetic creates a wheal and elevates the lesion above the surrounding skin.
- Apply traction with the thumb and index finger of the free hand on either side of the lesion; this stabilizes it and keeps it taut.
- Hold a sharp curette like a pencil and draw it through the tissue with strokes pushed away with the thumb until an adequate amount of tissue is removed (usually when the dermis is reached) (FIG. 26.19).
- Obtain hemostasis with **Monsel's solution** (ferric subsulfate) or aluminum chloride 35% after wiping the field dry of blood.

Electrodesiccation

- Electrodesiccation may be used before or after curettage or used alone.
- It causes superficial destruction with a charring of the skin.

TECHNIQUE

- Perform this procedure after administering local anesthesia.
- Use the lowest possible setting to prevent unnecessary tissue destruction.

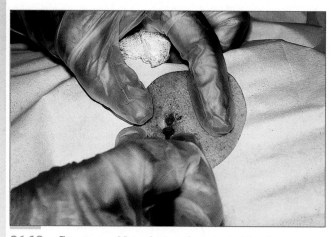

26.19 *Curettage.* Note the traction exerted by the operator's fingers.

BASICS

- Cryosurgery entails the destruction of tissue by freezing in a controlled manner to produce sharply circumscribed necrosis. Tissue destruction results from intercellular and extracellular ice formation, denaturing of liquid protein complexes, and cell dehydration. Second or subsequent freeze–thaw cycles result in more cellular damage than a single cycle.
- Liquid nitrogen (LN_2) at $-195.8°C$ is the standard agent that is used. It is applied with a cotton swab, a cryospray gun, or a cryoprobe, and it is stored in a special vacuum container.
- Cryosurgery should be used only when a confident clinical diagnosis has been made.
- It is most commonly used on warts and solar keratoses.

Advantages

- Cryosurgery is an inexpensive, rapid, and simple technique that does not require complicated apparatus.
- Anesthesia is usually not necessary.
- Postoperative pain is minimal.
- Bleeding is not a problem during or after treatment.
- Sutures are not necessary, and scarring is generally minimal or absent.
- It is a relatively risk-free treatment for the cryosurgeon who treats some skin conditions in patients who are infected with human immunodeficiency virus. These include patients with molluscum contagiosum, condylomata acuminatum, Kaposi's sarcoma, and warts.

Disadvantages

- Young children do not tolerate cryosurgery well.
- Scarring may occur, particularly if lesions are overzealously frozen or if the patient tends to heal with hypertrophic scars or keloids.
- Postinflammatory pigmentary alterations may occur; more often, hypopigmentation results because of the destruction of melanocytes.

TECHNIQUE

Standardization of freeze times is difficult to categorize for the treatment of benign and premalignant lesions. The goal is to produce, with either the swab or spray technique, a solid ice ball that extends 2 mm onto normal skin.

Cotton Tip Applicator Technique

- Place LN_2 in a Styrofoam cup.
- Dip a cotton swab into the cup.
- Touch the lesion with the saturated cotton-tipped applicator, with a minimal amount of pressure, and create a 2- to 3-mm zone of freeze around the lesion for a total of 4 to 5 seconds (FIG. 26.20).
- The skin turns white. Care must be taken to avoid dripping onto surrounding normal skin.

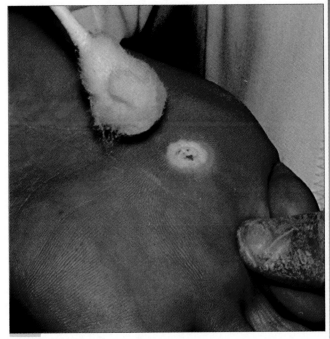

26.20 Cryosurgery. Liquid nitrogen is applied with a cotton pledget.

Cryospray Technique

- A handheld **Cryogun,** which operates under a working pressure of approximately 6 psi, is the standard instrument. Nozzle attachments with apertures of varying diameter for spray application are available (the "A" nozzle applies the greatest amount of spray; the "D" applies the least amount for delicate work) (FIGS. 26.21 and 26.22).
- Generally, no local anesthesia is necessary.
- For smaller lesions, this procedure involves treating the center of the lesion and allowing the freeze to spread laterally.
- The time of application varies, depending on the thickness of the lesion.

Postoperative Course and Wound Care

- Mild to moderate swelling may occur at the lesion site.
- A blister or blood blister may form within 24 hours and resolves in 2 to 7 days (FIG. 26.23).
- The lesion site may be cleansed with soap and water during the exudative stage.
- The lesion site starts to dry at the end of the exudative stage and then sloughs.
- A crust, which loosens spontaneously, commonly occurs.

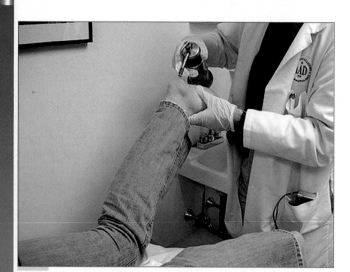

26.21   *Cryosurgery.* A prone position is helpful in examining and treating plantar lesions.

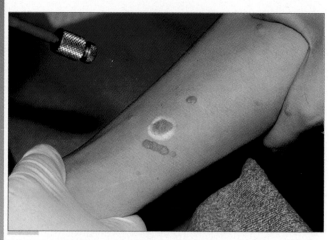

26.22   *Cryosurgery.* Here liquid nitrogen is delivered with a cryospray gun. Note the 2- to 3-mm zone of freeze around the lesion.

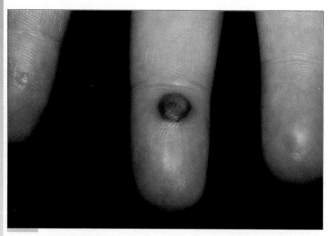

26.23   *Cryosurgery.* Note the wart on the surface of a hemorrhagic blister that appeared 24 hours after treatment.

HELPFUL HINTS

- It is best to underfreeze lesions; they can be retreated at a later date.
- For anxious children, a topical anesthetic such as **EMLA cream** (eutectic mixture of local anesthetics) can be applied under occlusion 1 hour before cryosurgery to decrease the discomfort associated with the procedure.
- Alternative delivery methods that can help minimize pain are shown in Figures 26.24 and 26.25. (See also FIGS. 21.24 and 21.25.)

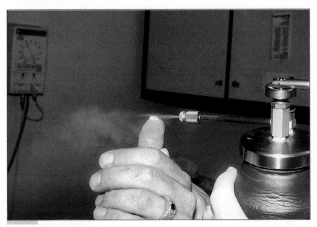

26.24 *Cryosurgery.* Application with a Cryogun apparatus. Freezing the lesion at a right angle may lessen the pain.

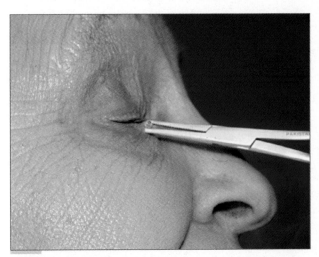

26.25 *Cryosurgery.* Treatment of a cutaneous horn with a hemostat that has been immersed for 30 seconds in liquid nitrogen. This simple, relatively painless procedure causes very little collateral damage to the surrounding skin.

Mohs' Micrographic Surgery

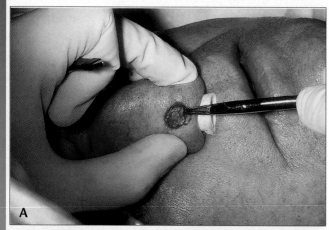

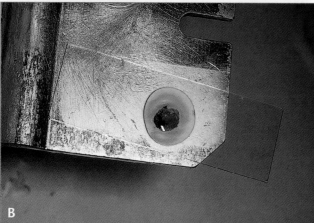

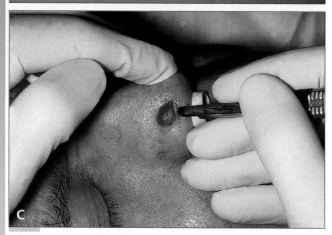

26.26 A, B and C *Mohs' micrographic surgery.* **A:** First stage of excision of lesion (image courtesy of Michael J. Mulvaney, M.D.). **B:** The excised tissue is color-coded and then evacuated by frozen section. (Image courtesy of Michael J. Mulvaney, M.D.) **C:** A second stage of excision is performed, because the first section had positive margins. (Image courtesy of Michael J. Mulvaney, M.D.)

BASICS

- Mohs' micrographic surgery is a microscopically controlled method of removing skin cancers that allows for controlled excision and maximum preservation of normal tissue.

Advantages
- Most reliable method in determining adequate margins
- Cure rate of 98% to 99% for basal cell carcinomas
- Preserves the maximum amount of normal tissue around the cancer

Disadvantages
- Time-consuming
- Expensive
- May require extensive reconstruction of surgical wounds

Indications
Mohs' surgery is best suited for:

- Recurrent basal and squamous cell carcinomas, particularly those on the face
- Excessively large (more than 2 cm) or invasive carcinomas
- Carcinomas within an orifice (e.g., ear canals or nostrils)
- Carcinomas in locations where preservation of normal tissue is extremely important (e.g., tip of the nose, ala nasi, eyelids, ears, lips, glans penis)
- Carcinomas in locations known to have a high rate of recurrence (e.g., ala nasi, nasal labial folds, medial canthi, pinnae of the ears, postauricular sulcus)
- Morpheaform or sclerotic (desmoplastic) basal cell carcinoma
- Lesions of the finger or penis

TECHNIQUE

- Tissue is excised in a circular pie-shaped fashion (FIG. 26.26 A); then it is systematically mapped and examined by means of frozen sections.
- While the patient waits in the examining room, tissue is submitted to a histotechnician for the surgeon to review (FIG. 26.26 B).
- Excisions are repeated in the areas proven to be cancerous until a complete cancer-free plane is reached (FIG. 26.26 C). Several stages may be necessary.

- Surgical wounds may be left to heal by secondary intention or corrected by plastic reconstructive procedures (FIG. 26.26 D).

Wound Care and Healing

- Infections after simple skin surgery are unusual.
- Administration of systemic antibiotics is generally unnecessary.
- Meticulous hemostasis during surgery is essential.
- Small amounts of necrosis normally occur in wound healing.
- Hemostasis induced by electrosurgery, suture ligature, or cautery always produces tissue necrosis.
- Wound healing is delayed when necrosis is extensive.
- Hemostasis can be achieved with a pressure dressing, which is applied for 24 hours.
- When wounds are closed with a considerable amount of tension or if the patient has been taking steroids, the wound should be closed with sutures that are nonabsorbable and buried (nylon or **Prolene**) or have prolonged tensile strength (**polydioxanone, Dexon, Vicryl**). Under the former conditions, skin sutures may be left in place for longer periods of time.
- External splinting using tape provides additional support until the tensile strength of the wound increases after suture removal.
- Exercise that stretches the skin should be avoided to minimize spreading of the scar.

Dressings and Wound Management

- For small ellipses, dry, sterile gauze covered with paper tape may be all that is necessary.
- An occlusive dressing or pressure dressing should be applied, if necessary, to prevent postoperative bleeding.
- After 24 hours, the patient can remove the dressing and compress the wound with tap water or hydrogen peroxide. The hydrogen peroxide mechanically softens the wound and removes any debris.
- A topical antibiotic such as bacitracin is applied to the surface of the wound before applying a clean, occlusive dressing.
- Patients repeat this procedure daily at home until the wound is covered with fresh epidermis.
- Patients are advised to return for follow-up if there is any pain, swelling, tenderness, purulent drainage, discharge, or bleeding of the wound.
- Postoperative pain usually is negligible, and patients are advised to call the surgeon should any pain occur.

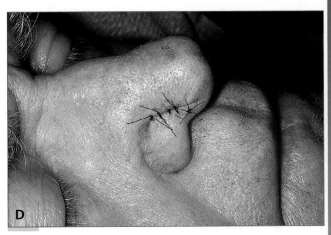

26.26 D *Mohs' micrographic surgery.* Primary closure after the second tissue excision was found to be free of malignancy. (Image courtesy of Michael J. Mulvaney, M.D.)

PART FOUR

Dermatologic Disorders in Special Populations

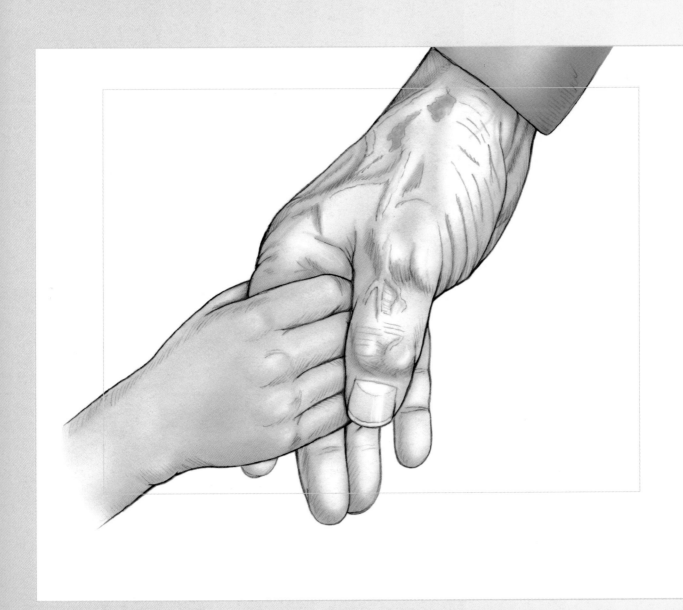

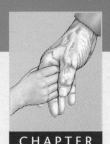

Special Considerations in the Skin of Pediatric and Elderly Patients

OVERVIEW

An individual's age, as well as gender and ethnic background, often influences the presence and severity of various skin disorders. This chapter provides a thumbnail description of dermatologic concerns in pediatric and elderly patients that are not discussed in previous chapters. It is intended to complement the earlier descriptions of common skin disorders and to present some less common conditions and rare skin diseases that may affect a patient seeking medical attention from any health care provider.

TO SEE LARGER IMAGES, GO TO THE WEB SITE AT www.goodheartsskindisorders.com.

Pediatric Skin Disorders

BASICS

- The overwhelming majority of pediatric skin disorders that present to pediatricians, family practitioners, and dermatologists consist of acne, atopic dermatitis, diaper rash, congenital lesions, warts, molluscum contagiosum, as well as a multitude of viral, bacterial, and idiopathic rashes.
- Common as well as various rare dermatoses and congenital lesions are briefly summarized in TABLE 27.1.

Table 27.1 DERMATOSES AND CONGENITAL LESIONS IN PEDIATRIC POPULATIONS

CONDITION	DESCRIPTION	MANAGEMENT	IMAGE
Superficial hemangioma (formerly called "strawberry" or capillary hemangioma)	Benign proliferation of endothelial cells that starts as macule and grows into dome-shaped papule or nodule Most often followed by spontaneous involution ("graying")	Observation or treatment with intralesional or systemic steroids, or laser ablation, especially if lesions compromise function	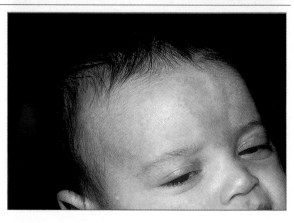
Deep hemangioma (formerly called "cavernous" hemangioma)	Deep dermal and subcutaneous red to violaceous nodule; regression often incomplete	Observation or treatment with intralesional, systemic steroids, or laser ablation, especially if lesions compromise function	
Macular stains ("angel's kisses," "salmon patches")	Red macules located on forehead, eyelids, nose, or upper lip Most often regress by 2 years of age	None indicated	

continued on page 521

Table 27.1 DERMATOSES AND CONGENITAL LESIONS IN PEDIATRIC POPULATIONS *(Continued)*

CONDITION	DESCRIPTION	MANAGEMENT	IMAGE
Stork bites	Red macules on back of neck Persist in 25% of adults	None indicated	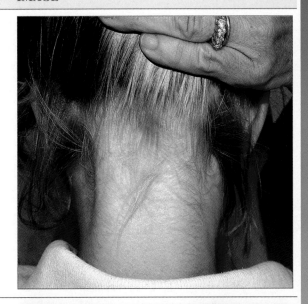
Nevus flammeus (port-wine stain)	Congenital malformation of blood vessels Usually appears at birth	Laser therapy	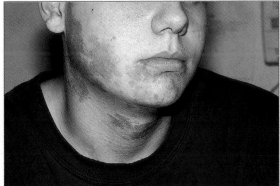
Nevus spilus (speckled lentiginous nevus)	Tan patches characterized by numerous darker macules or papules	Surgical excision for cosmetic reasons only	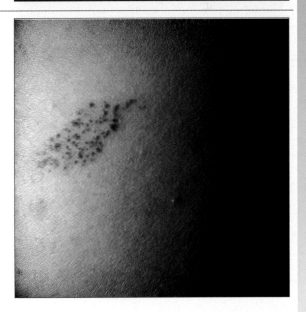

continued on page 522

CONDITION	DESCRIPTION	MANAGEMENT	IMAGE
Becker's nevus (pigmented hairy nevus)	Pigmented hairy nevus that is located over chest, shoulder, or back Often appears at puberty	None; surgical excision or laser ablation for cosmetic reasons only	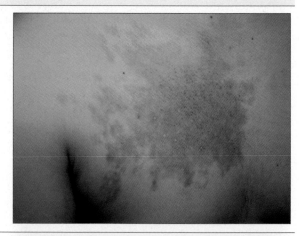
Nevus sebaceous	Congenital hamartoma, with plaques on head or neck Thickens at puberty Small risk of malignant degeneration, mainly to basal cell carcinoma	Excision	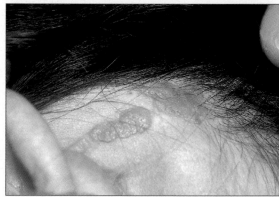
Nevus lipomatosis	Solitary or grouped proliferation of fatty tissue Lesions are asymptomatic, soft, skin-colored to yellow papules, nodules, or plaques, with predilection for upper thighs, pelvic, lumbar, and buttock areas	Surgical excision for cosmetic reasons only	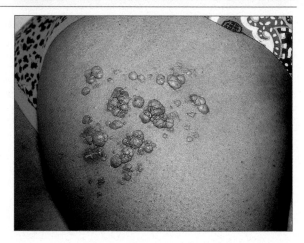

continued on page 523

Table 27.1 DERMATOSES AND CONGENITAL LESIONS IN PEDIATRIC POPULATIONS *(Continued)*

CONDITION	DESCRIPTION	MANAGEMENT	IMAGE
Epidermal nevi	Congenital hamartomas with various presentations: verrucous, inflammatory, linear, multiple, or comedonal	Excision, observation, or cryotherapy, with topical steroids for inflammatory type, topical retinoids for comedonal type	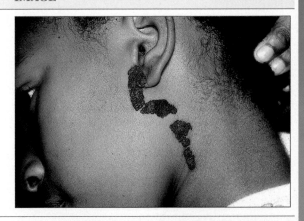
Mongolian spots	Macular, flat, blue or blue-gray skin markings that appear at birth or shortly thereafter on the sacral area and back Most prevalent among Asians and African Americans Often fade spontaneously	None	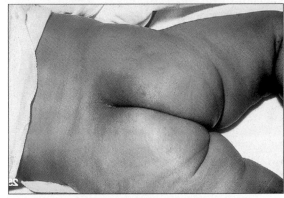
Nevus of Ota	Gray-blue melanin pigmentation of sclera of the eye Seen in Japanese, as well as in Africans, African Americans, and East Indians	Laser therapy	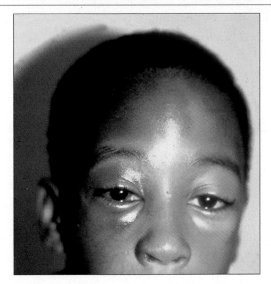

continued on page 524

Table 27.1 DERMATOSES AND CONGENITAL LESIONS IN PEDIATRIC POPULATIONS *(Continued)*

CONDITION	DESCRIPTION	MANAGEMENT	IMAGE
Acropustulosis of infancy	Recurrent crops of small pruritic vesicles that evolve into pustules Involves the palms and soles, most often in black newborns and infants Remits spontaneously	Topical steroids	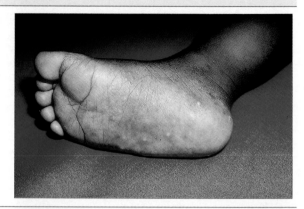
Gianotti-Crosti syndrome (acrodermatitis papulosa)	Self-limited, sometimes pruritic exanthem associated with many viral agents and immunizations Pale, pink to flesh-colored papules (sometimes flat-topped) in symmetric distribution on extremities	None	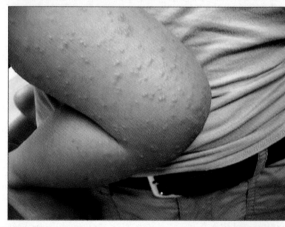
Urticaria pigmentosum	Multiple red-brown macules, usually on the trunk	Antihistamines and/or topical steroids, if symptomatic	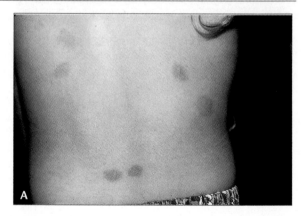

continued on page 525

CONDITION	DESCRIPTION	MANAGEMENT	IMAGE
Solitary mastocytoma (the **mastocytosis syndrome** can involve multiple organs and become chronic; it is not discussed here)	Lesions become a wheal (urticate) when rubbed or stroked; this change is referred to as **Darier's sign,** which is explainable on the basis of mast cell degranulation induced by physical stimulation Most cases resolve spontaneously Usually yellow-brown rubbery plaque that urticates or blisters (bullous urticaria pigmentosum) after rubbing Resolves spontaneously	No treatment necessary	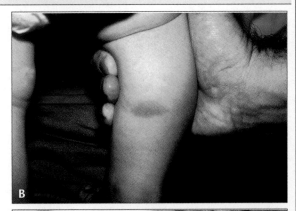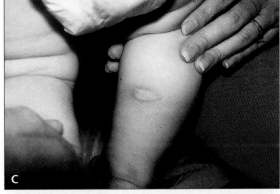
Tinea amiantacea	Thick, adherent scale on scalp and in hair	Keratolytics, followed by topical steroids when scale is cleared	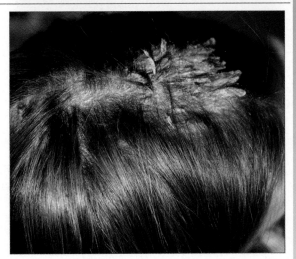

continued on page 526

CONDITION	DESCRIPTION	MANAGEMENT	IMAGE
Talon noir (tennis heel)	Self-limited, multiple, black petechiae of heel after minor trauma	Paring, protective heel pad	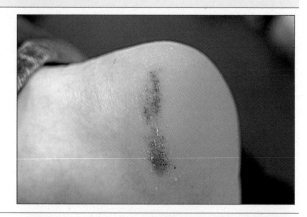
Pitted keratolysis	Pits in stratum corneum of soles; caused by prolonged occlusion, hyperhidrosis, and bacterial proteinase proliferation Malodorous	Topical erythromycin, clindamycin, or oral erythromycin Wearing cotton socks to prevent moisture buildup	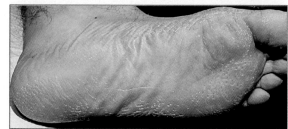
Lichen striatus	Idiopathic linear inflammatory eruption Consists of papules that coalesce into linear, unilateral plaques that appear most often on extremities Resolves spontaneously	Topical steroids	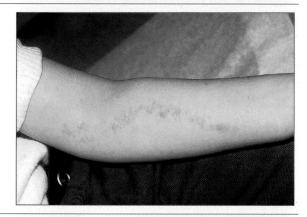
Perianal streptococcal dermatitis (perianal cellulitis)	Affects children 3 to 4 years of age Caused by group A beta-hemolytic streptococci Bright pink to red erythema that extends 2 to 3 cm from anus; infrequently accompanied by itching, fissuring, pain, and mucoid discharge May become more of a cellulitis, with possible pain on defecation	Penicillin V combined with topical Bactroban (mupirocin) ointment or cream twice a day	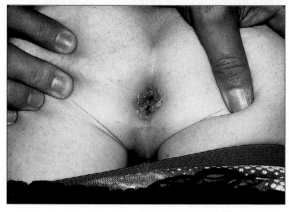

continued on page 527

CONDITION	DESCRIPTION	MANAGEMENT	IMAGE
Juvenile xanthogranuloma	Occurs in infancy and early childhood Lesions composed of histiocytic cells; benign, smooth, firm, red-brown papules and nodules that change to yellow Resolves spontaneously	None necessary	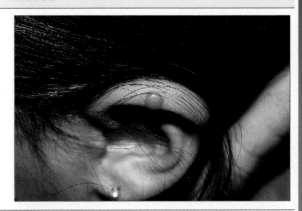
Lichen nitidus	Occurs on thighs, arms, trunk, and genitalia Idiopathic, asymptomatic, small (1 to 2 mm), flat-topped, shiny, skin-colored papules	Topical steroids, if necessary	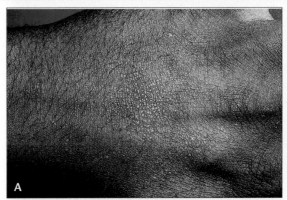 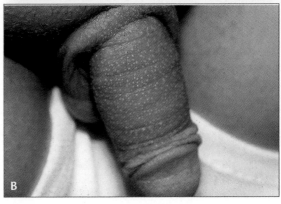

continued on page 528

CONDITION	DESCRIPTION	MANAGEMENT	IMAGE
Hyperhidrosis	Usually starts in early teen years Excessive sweating, particularly axillae, palms, and soles	**Topical:** Aluminum and zirconium antiperspirants Topical 20% aluminum chloride hexahydrate in absolute alcohol, anticholinergics, aldehydes, and tannic acid Iontophoresis **Systemic:** Oral anticholinergic medications Injection: botulinum toxin **Surgical:** Liposuction Sympathectomy	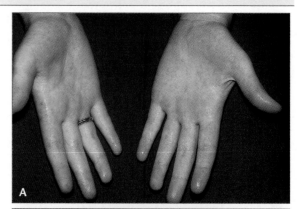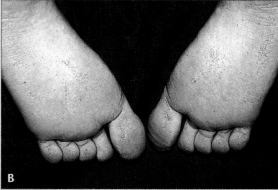
Subcutaneous fat necrosis of newborn	Firm, erythematous nodules and plaques on trunk, arms, buttocks, thighs, and cheeks in otherwise healthy infants Self-limited	None necessary	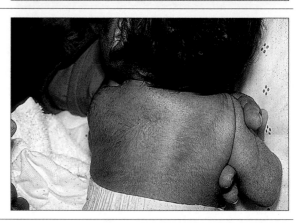
Lymphangioma circumscriptum	Congenital hamartoma of lymphatics Consists of small clusters of vesicles ("frog spawn")	Surgical excision, laser ablation, cryosurgery, electrocautery, or sclerotherapy	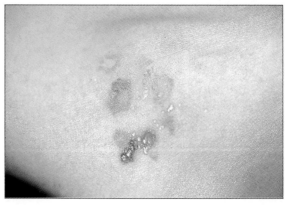

continued on page 529

CONDITION	DESCRIPTION	MANAGEMENT	IMAGE
Acute hemorrhagic edema of infancy (Finkelstein's disease)	Large, urticarial or annular, targetoid, purpuric plaques found primarily on face, ears, and extremities; presumably immune complex–mediated Self-limited	None necessary	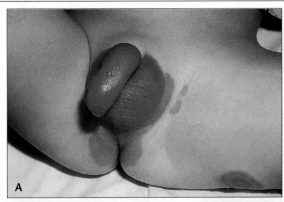 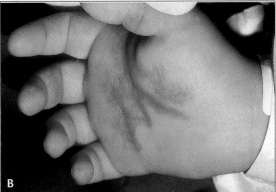 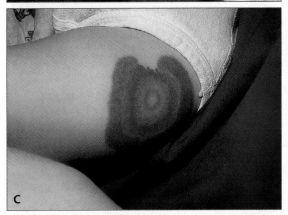 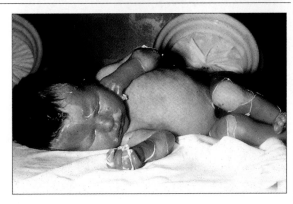
Staphylococcal scalded skin syndrome (SSSS)	Occurs mostly in neonates in neonatal or day care nurseries Toxin-mediated type of exfoliative dermatitis caused by toxigenic strains of *Staphylococcus aureus* Lesions range from localized bullous impetigo to extensive blistering and exfoliation	Dicloxacillin	

See TABLE 27.2.

BASICS

- The consequences of aging are most obvious on the skin.
- Genetics and sun exposure are the most important factors in determining the rate of aging and seem to influence susceptibility to certain types of disorders, including benign as well as precancerous and cancerous skin lesions.

Table 27.2 SKIN DISORDERS IN OLDER PATIENTS

CONDITION	DESCRIPTION	MANAGEMENT	IMAGE
Solar elastosis (dermatoheliosis, cutis rhomboidalis nuchae)	Caused by chronic sun exposure; results from breakage and clumping of elastic fibers in skin and thickening of epidermis Skin looks older than chronologic age Skin becomes wrinkled, furrowed, and unevenly pigmented, and it may have yellow hue	Sun protection measures, tretinoin, chemical peels, and/or laser resurfacing	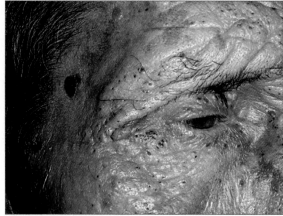
Favre-Racouchot syndrome	Chronic sun exposure results in multiple, bilaterally symmetric, open and closed comedones in periorbital and temporal areas	Comedone extraction or topical tretinoin	

continued on page 531

Table 27.2 SKIN DISORDERS IN OLDER PATIENTS *(Continued)*

CONDITION	DESCRIPTION	MANAGEMENT	IMAGE
Giant comedones	Commonly seen in elderly, particularly on the back Lesion is large dilated pore of epidermal inclusion cyst	Comedone extraction Excision	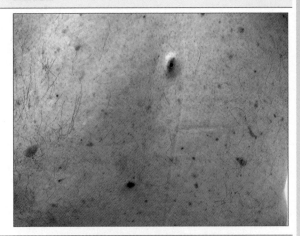
Nonspecific balanitis	Erythema, pruritus Erosions are seen primarily in uncircumcised males	Low-potency topical steroids, pimecrolimus, or tacrolimus Consider circumcision in recalcitrant cases	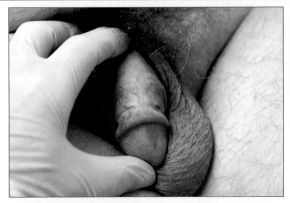
Genital lichen sclerosis (lichen sclerosis et atrophicus) in women	Chronic, idiopathic inflammatory dermatosis that results in white vulvar plaques with epidermal atrophy	Class 1 topical steroids Oral retinoids	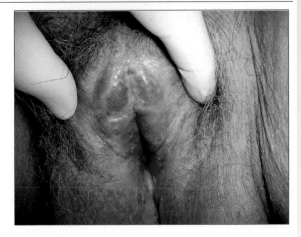

continued on page 532

Table 27.2 SKIN DISORDERS IN OLDER PATIENTS *(Continued)*

CONDITION	DESCRIPTION	MANAGEMENT	IMAGE
Genital lichen sclerosis (balanitis xerotica obliterans) in men	Chronic, idiopathic, sclerosing, inflammatory dermatosis of penis and prepuce	Class 1 topical steroids or topical testosterone Oral retinoids Circumcision or laser vaporization	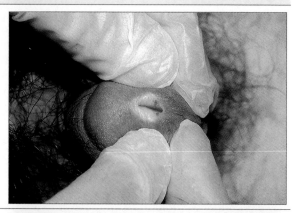
Grover's disease (transient acantholytic dermatosis)	Most often seen in elderly men Multiple pruritic, red, scaly, or eroded papules on trunk	High-dose vitamin A or high-potency topical steroids	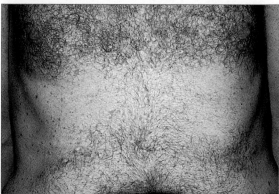
Bullous pemphigoid	Autoimmune blistering disease characterized by numerous tense vesicles and bullae May begin with nonspecific pruritic eruption; caused by autoantibodies	**Mild:** class 1 topical steroids, combination of tetracycline and niacinamide **Severe:** prednisone, azathioprine, cyclophosphamide, mycophenolate mofetil, dapsone, or methotrexate	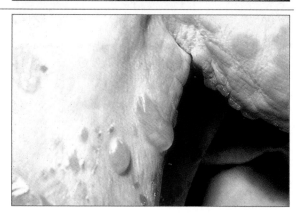

continued on page 533

Table 27.2 SKIN DISORDERS IN OLDER PATIENTS *(Continued)*

CONDITION	DESCRIPTION	MANAGEMENT	IMAGE
Pemphigus vulgaris	Autoimmune blistering disease characterized by numerous superficial (flaccid) vesicles and bullae of skin and mucous membranes Caused by autoantibodies	Prednisone, class 1 topical steroids, and intralesional steroids Steroid-sparing agents: azathioprine, cyclophosphamide, mycophenolate mofetil, dapsone, cyclosporine, and intravenous immune globulin	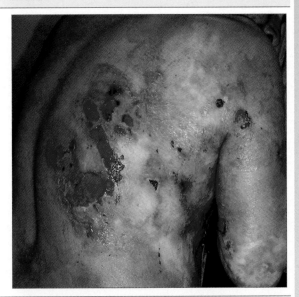
Onychogryphosis	Nail plate enlargement with increased thickening and marked curvature	Ongoing podiatric care and appropriate footwear	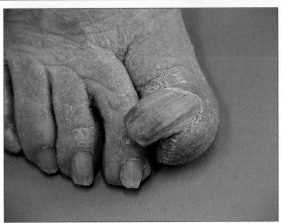
Fissured heels	Linear parallel epidermal fissures Painful when lesions involve dermis	Keratolytics, emollients, and occlusive dressings	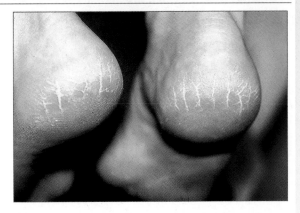

continued on page 534

Table 27.2 SKIN DISORDERS IN OLDER PATIENTS *(Continued)*

CONDITION	DESCRIPTION	MANAGEMENT	IMAGE
Nonepidemic Kaposi's sarcoma	Affects older men of Mediterranean or eastern European origin Violaceous patches, plaques, and nodules, most often on lower extremities	None indicated for indolent lesions Radiation therapy, cryotherapy, or surgical excision or laser ablation, when indicated	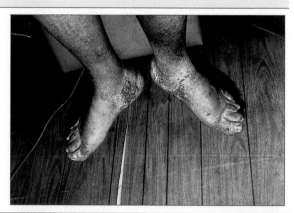
Lupus vulgaris (cutaneous tuberculosis)	Solitary, slowly evolving, red-brown papules or plaques of head and neck	Isoniazid, rifampin, pyrazinamide, ethambutol, or streptomycin	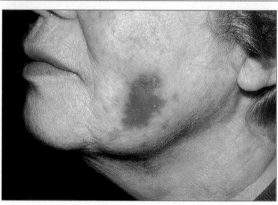

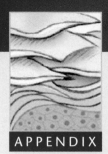

Brand Names of Dermatologic Medications in Various Countries

GENERIC NAME	UNITED STATES	FRANCE	GERMANY	UNITED KINGDOM	INDIA	CANADA
For acne and rosacea: Oral						
Minocycline	Minocin	Mestacine Mynocine	Skid, Lederderm	Minocin	Cynomycin	Minocin
Doxycycline hyclate	Vibramycin	Vibromycine	Vibramycin	Vibramycin	Doxt	Nu-doxycycline
Erythromycin	E-Mycin	Érythrocyne	Monomycin, Erythrocin	Erymax	Eltocin	Eryc
13-cis retinoic acid	Sotret Claravis Amnesteen	Roaccutane	Roaccutan	Roaccutane	Sotret Isotroin	Accutane, Clarus
For acne and rosacea: Topical						
Azelaic acid	Azelex	Skinoren	Skinoren	Skinoren	Aziderm	NA
Metronidazole	Noritate, MetroGel, MetroCream	Rosiced Rozagel	Metrogel	Rozex	Metrogyl	Metrocream, Metrolotion, Metrogel, Noritate
Clindamycin	Cleocin-T	Dalacine T	Basocin	Dalacin T	ClindacA	Dalacin-T, Clindets, Clinda-T
Erythromycin	Emgel	Éryacné	Aknemycin, Stiemycine	Stiemycin	NA	Erysol
Tretinoin	Retin-A	Aberel Effederm	Eudyna, Airol	Retin-A	Retino-A	Retin-A micro, Retin-A, Stieva-A, Vitamin A Acoid
Adapalene	Differin	Différine	Differin	Differin	Adaferin	Differin, Differin-XP
Tazarotene	Tazorac	Zorac	Zorac	Zorac	Tacroz	Tazorac
Benzoyl peroxide	Oxy-5, Oxy-10	Panoxyl Éclaran	Benzaknen, PanOxyl	PanOxyl	Benzac AC	Benoxyl, Benzac, Panoxyl, Solugel

continued on page 536

GENERIC NAME	UNITED STATES	FRANCE	GERMANY	UNITED KINGDOM	INDIA	CANADA
For psoriasis: Topical						
Salicylic acid	Keralyt gel	Cold cream salycilé	Squamasol, Psórimed	NA	Sa6, Sa12	NA
Calcipotriene	Dovonex	Daivonex	Psorcutan, Daivonex	Dovonex	Daivonex	Dovonex
Calcipotriene/ betamethasone dipropionate	Taclonex	Daivobet	Daivobet	Dovobet	Daivobet	Dovobet
Antifungals: Topical						
Terbinafine	Lamisil	Lamisil	Lamisil	Lamisil	Lamisil, Zimig	Lamisil
Ketoconazole	Nizoral	Nizoral	Terzolin, Nizoral	Nizoral	Nizral	Nizoral
Tolnaftate	Tinactin	Sporilline	Tonaftal	Tinaderm	Tinaderm	NA
Econazole	Spectazole	Dermazol	Epi-Pevaryl	Ecostatin	NA	NA
Ciclopirox	Loprox	Mycoster	Batrafen	NA	NA	Loprox, Stieprox
Antifungals: Oral						
Griseofulvin	Fulvacin-PG	Fulcine	Likuden, Fulcin	Grisovin	GrisOD	NA
Terbinafine	Lamisil	Lamisil	Lamisil	Lamisil	Lamisil, Zimig	Lamisil
Itraconazole	Sporanox	Sporanox	Sempera	Sporanox	Sporanox	Sporonox
Fluconazole	Diflucan	Triflucan	Diflucan	Diflucan	Zocon, Fusys	Diflucan
Antihistamines						
Hydroxyzine	Atarax	Atarax	Atarax, AH3	Atarax	Atarax	Atarax
Cyproheptadine	Periactin	Périactine	Peritol	Periactin	Practin	NA
Loratadine	Claritin	Clarytine	Lisino, Lorano	Clarityn	Lorfast	Claritin
Cetririzine	Zyrtec	Zyrtec	Zyrtec	Zirtek	Zyrtec	Reactine
Doxepin	Sinquan	Quitaxon, Sinquan	Aponal, Sinquan	Sinquan	Spectra	Sinequan
Alopecia						
Minoxidil (topical)	Rogaine	Regaine	Regaine	Regaine	Mintop	Rogaine
Finasteride	Propecia	Propécia	Propecia	Propecia	Finpecia	Propecia
Antimitotic: Topical						
5-Fluorouracil	Efudex Carac	Efudix	Efudix	Efudix	Flonida	Efudex
Scabacides: Topical						
Permethrin	Elimite Acticin	Nix Charlieu anti-poux	Infectopedicul	Lyclear	Permite	Nix, Kwellada-P
Lindane	Kwell	Aphtiria	Jacutin	Quellada		
Scabacides: Oral						
Ivermectin	Stromectol	NA	NA	Mectizan	Ivermectol	NA

The brand name of this product is either unavailable or was not obtained at the time of publication.

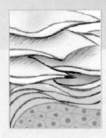

Index

Note: Page numbers followed by "f" indicate figure, and "t" indicate table.

Ivermectin (Stromectol)
   for lice, 357
   for Norwegian scabies, HIV-associated,
      450
   for scabies, 353, 353t
Ixodes tick, 344, 348, 348f

J

Jellyfish sting, 358–359, 358f
Jock itch, 176–177, 176f, 177f
Junctional melanocytic nevi, 364–365,
      364f, 365f, 419f–421f, 421
   vs. freckles, 365, 365f
   vs. solar lentigenes, 365, 365f, 419f,
      420f
Junctional nevus, of nail, 272, 272f
Juvenile xanthogranuloma, 527t

K

Kaposi's sarcoma
   HIV-associated, 445–446, 445f
   nonepidemic, in elderly, 534t
Kaposi's varicelliform eruption, 159,
      159f, 329
Kawasaki's syndrome, 211–213, 212f, 213f
Keloid, 3, 3f, 385–388, 385f–387f
   basics of, 385, 385f
   clinical manifestations and diagnosis
      of, 386
   lesion distribution in, 386, 386f
   lesions in, 385
   management of, 386–388, 387f
   pathogenesis of, 385
   in pregnancy, 433, 433f
Keratoacanthoma, 405–406, 405f, 406f
Keratolytic agents, 95t. *See also* Salicylic
      acid, topical
   for cradle cap, 81
   for seborrheic dermatitis, 81
Keratosis pilaris, 56, 56f
   vs. adolescent acne, 29, 29f
Ketoconazole (Nizoral), 170t
   for cutaneous candidiasis, 189
   for paronychia, 268
   for perlèche, 248
   for psoriasis, scalp, 105
   for seborrheic dermatitis, 81, 82, 82t
   for tinea capitis, 180
   for tinea pedis, interdigital, 170, 170t
   for tinea versicolor, 192, 192t
Köbner reaction, 122f
   in psoriasis, 90, 90f, 104
   in sunburn, 90, 90f
Koenen's tumors, 493
KOH test, 498–500, 498f–500f
Koilonychia, 271, 271f
Kojic acid, for melasma, 283
Kyrle's disease, 461

L

Labial melanotic macule, 252, 252f
Lactic acid cream, for brittle nails, 260

Lactic-salicylic acid (Duofilm, Occlusal-HP),
      for flat warts, 148
Lanugo, 214
Laser therapy
   for adolescent acne, 35–36
   for rosacea, 44
   for warts, 147
Lemon oil, phytophotodermatitis from, 285
Lentigo maligna, 419, 419f
Lentigo maligna melanoma, 419, 419f
Leser-Trélat, sign of, 374
Lesions, 2–8. *See also specific types and
      disorders*
   configuration of, 12, 12f
   follicular, 12, 12f
   grouped, 12, 12f
   linear, 11, 11f
   primary, 2–5, 2f–5f (*See also specific
      lesions*)
   secondary, 6–8, 6f–8f (*See also specific
      lesions*)
   shape of, 11, 11f
Leukocytoclastic vasculitis, 298, 300,
      316–317
Leukoderma, chemical, *vs.* vitiligo
      vulgaris, 277, 277f
Leukonychia striata, 270, 270f
Leukoplakia
   oral, 250, 250f
   oral hairy, 251, 251f
Leukotrichia, 275
L'homme rouge, 487–490, 488f
Lice infestations, 355–357, 355f
Lichenification
   atopic dermatitis with, 9, 9f
   in eczema, 50, 50f, 53f
Lichen nitidus, 527t
Lichenoid eruptions, drug-induced, 301
Lichen planopilaris, 228–229, 228f
Lichen planus, 122–125, 250, 250f
   basics of, 122
   clinical manifestations of, 123
   clinical variants of, 124, 124f
   diagnosis of, 124
   differential diagnosis of, 124–125, 124f
   hyperpigmentation from, 284, 284f
   lesion distribution in, 124, 124f
   lesions in, 122, 122f, 123f
   management of, 125
   oral, 250, 250f
   other clinical findings with, 123
   pathophysiology of, 122
   point to remember on, 125
Lichen sclerosis, genital
   in men, 532t
   in women, 531t
Lichen sclerosis et atrophicus, 531t
Lichen simplex chronicus, 55f, 73–74, 73f
   vs. lichen planus, 124, 124f
   vs. psoriasis, 93, 93f
   vs. tinea cruris (jock itch), 175, 175f

Lichen striatus, 526t
Lidocaine, topical (Xylocaine)
   for aphthous stomatitis, 245
   for herpes simplex genitalis, 331
Lidocaine patches, for postherpetic
      neuralgia, 166
Light-induced urticaria, 307, 308, 308f
Light therapy. *See also* UVA (ultraviolet
      light A); UVB (ultraviolet light B)
   for adolescent acne, 35–36
   for rosacea, 44
Lindane (Kwell, Scabene)
   for lice, 357
   for Norwegian scabies, HIV-associated,
      450
   for scabies, 353
Linea nigra, 432, 432f
Linear lesions, 11, 11f
Linezolid, for MRSA impetigo, 129
Lip disorders. *See* Oral disorders; *specific
      disorders*
Lipid abnormalities, 464–465, 464f, 465f
Lipoatrophy (lipodystrophy), HIV-
      associated, 455, 455f
Lipodermatosclerosis, 84, 84f
Lipodermosclerosis, with stasis dermatitis,
      84, 84f
Lipoma, 380, 380f
   multiple, 10, 10f
Liquid nitrogen (cryosurgery). *See*
      Cryosurgery (liquid nitrogen)
Lithium, on acne, 48
Livedoid vasculopathy, *vs.* purpura, 318,
      318f
Livedo reticulitis, 467, 467f
Liver spot. *See* Solar lentigenes
Löfgren's syndrome, 482
Longitudinal ridging of nails, 260, 260f
Loratadine (Claritin)
   for drug eruptions, 302
   for urticaria and angioedema, 309
Lotions, 13, 15. *See also specific types*
Lupus, drug-induced, 469–470
Lupus erythematosus
   acute cutaneous, 466
   chronic cutaneous, 466, 472–473, 472f
      hair loss from, 227–228, 228f
   neonatal, 474, 474f
   subacute cutaneous, 466, 470–471,
      470f, 471f
   systemic, 466–469, 466f–468f
Lupuslike drug eruption, drug-induced, 301
Lupus pernio, 481–482, 481f
Lupus vulgaris, 534t
Lyme borreliosis. *See* Lyme disease
Lyme disease, 344–349
   basics of, 344
   clinical manifestations of, 345
   diagnosis of, 346
   differential diagnosis of, 347, 347f
   erythema migrans rash of